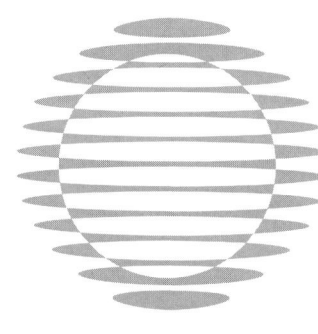

Medical Management of AIDS in Children

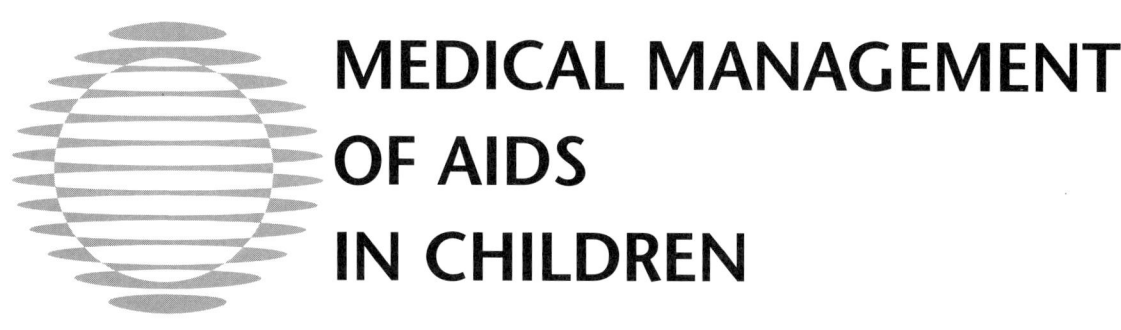

MEDICAL MANAGEMENT OF AIDS IN CHILDREN

William T. Shearer, MD, PhD
Professor of Pediatrics and Immunology
Baylor College of Medicine
Chief, Allergy and Immunology Service
Texas Children's Hospital
Houston, Texas

I. Celine Hanson, MD
Bureau Chief
Bureau of HIV/STD Prevention
Texas Department of Health
Austin, Texas

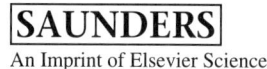

An Imprint of Elsevier Science

SAUNDERS
An Imprint of Elsevier Science

The Curtis Center
Independence Square West
Philadelphia, PA 19106

MEDICAL MANAGEMENT OF AIDS IN CHILDREN   ISBN 0-7216-8284-7
Copyright © 2003, Elsevier Science (USA). All rights reserved.

No part of this publication may be reproduced or transmitted in any form or by any means, electronic or mechanical, including photocopy, recording, or any information storage and retrieval system, without permission in writing from the publisher.

Library of Congress Cataloging-in-Publication Data

Medical management of aids in children/William T. Shearer [editor].
    p. cm.
  ISBN 0-7216-8284-7
    1. AIDS (Disease) in children. 2. AIDS (Disease) in children—Treatment. 3. AIDS (Disease) in children—Patients—Family relationships. I. Shearer, William T.
  RJ387.A25 M43 2003
618.92′9792—dc21   2002030245

Acquisitions Editor: Judith Fletcher
Publishing Services Manager: Frank Polizzano

Printed in the United States of America
Last digit is the print number: 9 8 7 6 5 4 3 2 1

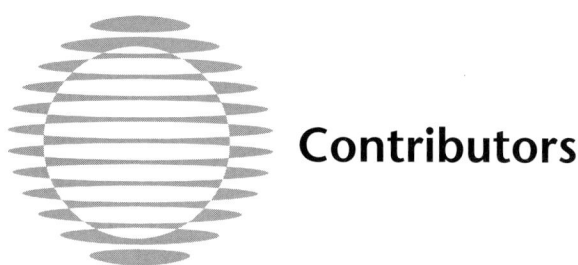
Contributors

Donna T. Beck, MD
Centers for Disease Control and Prevention, Division of HIV/AIDS Prevention, Atlanta, Georgia
Depression of Blood Cells in HIV-infected Children and Adolescents

Jeanne M. Bertolli, MPH, PhD
Senior Epidemiologist, Prevention Support Office, Office of the Director, National Center for HIV, STD and TB Prevention, Centers for Disease Control and Prevention, Atlanta, Georgia
Infectious Complications of Pediatric HIV Infection

Pim Y. Brouwers, PhD
Professor of Pediatrics and Neuroscience, Baylor College of Medicine; Director, Clinical Neurosciences, Texas Children's Cancer and Sickle Cell Centers, Texas Children's Hospital, Houston, Texas
HIV-Induced CNS/Developmental Abnormalities in Childhood

Yvonne J. Bryson, MD
Professor and Chief, Pediatric Infectious Diseases, David Geffen UCLA School of Medicine, Los Angeles, California
Vertical Transmission of HIV-1: Timing of Transmission and Risk Factors

Traci C. Burgess, MD
Department of Obstetrics and Gynecology, The Perinatal Center, Maimonides University and Medical Center, Brooklyn, New York
Identification and Treatment of the HIV-Infected Pregnant Woman

Javier Chinen, MD, PhD
Staff Clinician, National Human Genome Research Institute, National Institute of Health, Bethesda, Maryland
Immune-Based Therapies for HIV Infection

Ellen R. Cooper, MD
Associate Professor of Pediatrics, Division of Infectious Diseases, Boston University School of Medicine, Clinical Director of Adolescent and Pediatric HIV Programs, Boston Medical Center, Boston, MA
Infection Control in Hospital, School and Community: Distinguishing Real Risk from Perceived Danger

Margaret R. Coyne, RN, MSN, CPNP
Instructor, Baylor College of Medicine; Pediatric Nurse Practitioner, Texas Children's Hospital, Houston, Texas
Primary Care of the HIV-Infected Infant and Child

Timothy Dilon Daniel, MD, PhD
Internal Medicine Resident, Baylor College of Medicine, Internal Medicine Department, Houston, Texas
Cutaneous Manifestations in Pediatric HIV Infection

Wayne M. Dankner, MD
Adjunct Associate Professor of Pediatrics, Duke University School of Medicine; Senior Medical Director, Parexel International, Durham, North Carolina
Infectious Complications of Pediatric HIV Infection

Jaime G. Deville, MD
Assistant Clinical Professor, Department of Pediatrics, Division of Pediatric Infectious Diseases, UCLA School of Medicine; Attending Physician, Mattel Children's Hospital at UCLA, UCLA Medical Center, Los Angeles, California
Vertical Transmission of HIV-1: Timing of Transmission and Risk Factors

Joanna Dobroszycki, MD
Centers for Disease Control and Prevention, Division of HIV/AIDS Prevention, Atlanta, Georgia
Depression of Blood Cells in HIV infected Children and Adolescents

Dawn M. D'Orlando, MSN, MPH
New Jersey Department of Health and Senior Services, Division of AIDS Prevention and Control, Trenton, New Jersey
Managed Care for Children with HIV Infection

Kim D. Evans, RN, MSN, CPNP, ACRN
Instructor in Pediatrics, Baylor College of Medicine, Pediatric Nurse Practitioner, Allergy and Immunology Department, Texas Children's Hospital, Houston, Texas
Primary Care of the HIV-Infected Infant and Child

Stacey D. Fisher, MD
University of Rochester Medical Center and Golisano Children's Hospital at Strong, Rochester, New York
Abnormal Cardiovascular Function in HIV-Infected Infants and Children

Catherine M. Flaitz, DDS, MS
Professor, Department of Diagnostic Sciences and Director, Surgical Oral and Maxillofacial Pathology, The University of Texas Dental Branch; Courtesy Staff, Texas Children's Hospital, Active Teaching Staff, Memorial Hermann Hospital, Houston, Texas
Oral Manifestations in Pediatric HIV Infection

Toni Frederick, PhD, MSPH
County of Los Angeles, Department of Health, Pediatrics-Spectrum of Diseases, Los Angeles, California
Infectious Complications of Pediatric HIV Infection

Samuel Grubman, MD
Associate Professor of Clinical Pediatrics, New York Medical College, Valhalla; Vice Chairman, Department of Pediatrics, and Chief, Allergy and Immunology, St. Vincent's Catholic Medical Centers, St. Vincent's Hospital-Manhattan, New York, New York
Palliative Care for Children Infected with HIV

Colleen M. Hadigan, MD, MPH
Assistant Professor in Pediatrics, Harvard Medical School; Massachusetts General Hospital, Department of Pediatric Gastroenterology and Nutrition, Boston, Massachusetts
Gastrointestinal Illness and Wasting in Pediatric Patients with HIV Infection

I. Celine Hanson, MD
Adjunct Professor of Pediatrics, Baylor College of Medicine, Houston; Bureau Chief, Texas Department of Health, Bureau of HIV and STD Prevention, Austin, Texas
Primary Care of the HIV-Infected Infant and Child

Jennifer F. Havens, MD
Associate Clinical Professor of Psychiatry, Columbia University College of Physicians and Surgeons; Director, Child and Adolescent Psychiatry, Children's Hospital of New York-Presbyterian Hospital, New York, New York
Psychosocial Challenges in Pediatric HIV Infection

M. John Hicks, MD, DDS, MS, PhD
Associate Professor of Pathology, Baylor College of Medicine; Director of Surgical and Ultrastructural Pathology, Department of Pathology, Texas Children's Hospital, Houston, Texas
Oral Manifestations in Pediatric HIV Infection

Victor S. B. Jorden, MD, MPH
Associate Medical Director, Anesthesia and Sedation, Abbott Laboratories, Inc., Abbott Park, Illinois
Managed Care for Children with HIV Infection

Meyer Kattan, MD
Professor of Pediatrics, Mount Sinai School of Medicine; Chief, Pediatric Pulmonary and Critical Care Division, Mount Sinai Medical Center, New York, New York
Respiratory Compromise in Children Infected by HIV

Marcie J. Keesler, BA
Clinical Research Coordinator, University of Rochester, Rochester, New York
Abnormal Cardiovascular Function in HIV-Infected Infants and Children

Paul R. Langevin, Jr., BS, MS
President, Health Care Association of New Jersey, Hamilton, New Jersey
Managed Care for Children with HIV Infection

Moise L. Levy, MD
Professor, Dermatology and Pediatrics, Baylor College of Medicine; Chief, Dermatology Service, Texas Children's Hospital, Houston, Texas
Cutaneous Manifestations in Pediatric HIV Infection

Steven E. Lipshultz, MD
Professor of Pediatrics and Oncology; Associate Chairman of Pediatrics, University of Rochester School of Medicine and Dentistry; Chief of Pediatric Cardiology and Director of the Children's Heart Center at Strong, University of Rochester Medical Center and Golisano Children's Hospital at Strong, Rochester, New York
Abnormal Cardiovascular Function in HIV-Infected Infants and Children

Kenneth L. McClain, MD, PhD
Professor of Pediatrics, Baylor College of Medicine, and Texas Children's Cancer Center, Houston, Texas
Childhood Malignancies in AIDS

Ross E. McKinney, Jr., MD
Vice Dean for Research and Chief, Pediatric Infectious Diseases, Duke University Medical Center, Durham, North Carolina
Prophylactic Antiretroviral Treatment of HIV Infection in Neonates

Howard L. Minkoff, MD
Distinguished Professor of Obstetrics/Gynecology, State University of New York Downstate; Chairman, Obstetrics/Gynecology Department, Maimonides Medical Center, Brooklyn, New York
Identification and Treatment of the HIV-Infected Pregnant Woman

Lynne M. Mofenson, MD
Branch Chief, Pediatric Adolescent, and Maternal AIDS Branch, Center for Research for Mothers and Children, National Institute of Child Health and Human Development, National Institutes of Health, Rockville, Maryland
Pediatric HIV Infection in Developed and Developing Countries: Epidemiology and Natural History

Warren Yiu Kee Ng, MD
Assistant Clinical Professor, Department of Psychiatry, Columbia University College of Physicians and Surgeons; Director, Special Needs Clinic-Columbia Presbyterian, New York Presbyterian Hospital-Columbia Site, New York, New York
Psychosocial Challenges in Pediatric HIV Infection

James M. Oleske, MD, MPH
François-Xavier Bagnoud, Professor of Pediatrics, New Jersey Medical School, Newark, New Jersey
Palliative Care for Children Infected with HIV

Paul Palumbo, MD
Professor of Pediatrics and Professor of Biochemistry and Molecular Biology, University of Medicine and Dentistry of New Jersey, New Jersey Medical School, Newark, New Jersey
Diagnostic Methods for Infants Born to HIV-Infected Women

Sindy M. Paul, MD, MPH
Assistant Clinical Professor, University of Medicine and Dentistry of New Jersey, Piscataway; Medical Director, Division of AIDS Prevention and Control, New Jersey Department of Health and Senior Services, Trenton, New Jersey
Managed Care for Children with HIV Infection

Michael Rosenberg, MD, PhD
Centers for Disease Control and Prevention, Division of HIV/AIDS Prevention, Atlanta, Georgia
Depression of Blood Cells in HIV-infected Children and Adolescents

William T. Shearer, MD, PhD
Professor of Pediatrics and Immunology, Baylor College of Medicine; Chief, Allergy and Immunology Service, Texas Children's Hospital, Allergy and Immunology Department, Houston, Texas
Immune-Based Therapies for HIV Infection

Jill Simone, MD
New Jersey Department of Health and Senior Services, Division of AIDS Prevention and Control, Trenton, New Jersey
Managed Care for Children with HIV Infection

Stephen A. Spector
Professor of Pediatrics and Chief, Division of Infectious Diseases; Director, Mother, Child, and Adolescent HIV Program; Member, Center for Molecular Genetics and Center for AIDS Research, University of California, San Diego, La Jolla, California
Treatment and Virologic Monitoring of Primary HIV-Infection in Children

Stuart E. Starr, MD
Emeritus Professor of Pediatrics, University of Pennsylvania School of Medicine, Philadelphia, Pennsylvania
Immunopathogenesis of Pediatric HIV Infection

Patrick S. Sullivan, DVM, PhD
Associate Director for Scientific Support, HIV Vaccine Trials Network, Fred Hutchinson Cancer Research Center, Seattle, Washington
Depression of Blood Cells in HIV-infected Children and Adolescents

Ruth E. Tuomala, MD
Assistant Professor of Obstetrics and Gynecology, Harvard Medical School, Director of Obstetrics and Gynecologic Infectious Diseases, Brigham and Women's Hospital, Boston, Massachusetts
Perinatal HIV Infection: Obstetrical Issues

Carol A. Vincent, MSN, CRNP
Project Manager, Pediatric AIDS Clinical Trials Unit and CRNP, Special Immunology, The

Children's Hospital of Philadelphia, Philadelphia, Pennsylvania
Nursing Care in Pediatric HIV Infection

Lori S. Wiener, PhD, DCSW
Coordinator, Pediatric HIV Psychosocial Support and Research Program, HIV and AIDS Malignancy Branch, National Cancer Institute, National Institutes of Health, Bethesda, Maryland
Psychosocial Challenges in Pediatric HIV Infection

Harland S. Winter, MD
Associate Professor of Pediatrics, Harvard Medical School; Director, Pediatric IBD Center, and Pediatrician, Massachusetts General Hospital for Children, Boston, Massachusetts
Gastrointestinal Illness and Wasting in Pediatric Patients with HIV Infection

Pamela L. Wolters, PhD
Principal Investigator, Neuropsychology Group, National Cancer Institute and Medical Illness Counseling Center, Bethesda, Maryland
HIV-Induced CNS/Developmental Abnormalities in Childhood

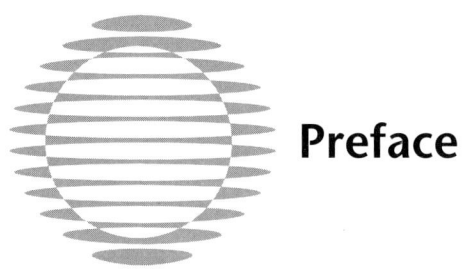

Preface

Medical Management of AIDS in Children is designed to be a reference for physicians, nurses, and other health care workers who diagnose, treat, and care for HIV-infected children. This book, although rooted in the immunopathogenesis and antiretroviral therapy of pediatric HIV infection, is intended for the translational clinical care of patients that basic and clinical science research have made possible. The book is intended to be the definitive reference for the day-by-day maintenance of pediatric patients infected by HIV. The sections of the book have been carefully chosen to quickly inform readers of the essentials of host: viral interaction (Section 1), prevention and treatment issues (Section 2), control of HIV-induced complications (Section 3), and special features of pediatric HIV infection and AIDS (Section 4). Chapter topics have been chosen for their timeliness of present knowledge and their relevance to clinicians seeking rapid updates on important issues.

Throughout the text, authors have stressed the unique features of pediatric HIV infection that clearly mandate different approaches to patients and their infected parent(s), as compared with those methods used with adult HIV patients. Some of these unique aspects are: the intimate nine-month exposure to an HIV-infected mother, a more precise timing of infection, HIV attack of developing immune system, prolonged levels of HIV in the blood of infants, obstetrical risk factors, acquisition of infection by breastfeeding, alternate diagnostic methods, antiretroviral prevention of HIV infection, potential for thymic immunoreconstitution, neurodevelopment abnormalities and loss of childhood milestones, early cardiovascular compromise, pain management, primary care of HIV-infected children, quality of life and psychosocial issues, and managed care issues for HIV-afflicted families.

All of the chapter authors have been carefully selected for their total involvement, vast experience, and preeminent reputations as leaders in the field of pediatric AIDS. All of these authors share the same daily management experiences as the readers of the book, and their chapters will be an extension of their own long-term experience.

The book will appeal not only to pediatricians but also to obstetricians, family practice physicians, nurses, social workers, community workers, and family members affected by HIV infection. There will be a need for short intervals between revised versions of this book, due to the constantly changing database of pathophysiology, treatment regimen, and patient management issues.

WILLIAM T. SHEARER, MD
I. CELINE HANSON, MD

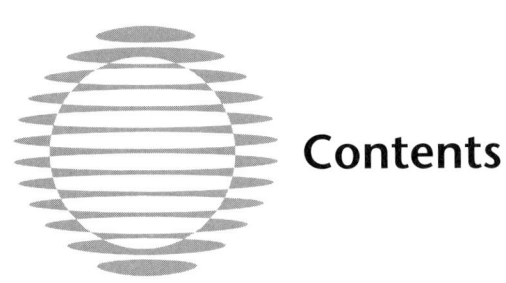

Contents

1 Pediatric HIV Infection in Developed and Developing Countries: Epidemiology and Natural History 1
Lynne M. Mofenson

2 Vertical Transmission of HIV-1: Timing of Transmission and Risk Factors 29
Jaime G. Deville and Yvonne J. Bryson

3 Immunopathogenesis of Pediatric HIV Infection 53
Stuart E. Starr

4 Identification and Treatment of the HIV-Infected Pregnant Woman 69
Howard L. Minkoff and Traci C. Burgess

5 Perinatal HIV Infection: Obstetric Issues 87
Ruth E. Tuomala

6 Diagnostic Methods for Infants Born to HIV-Infected Women 107
Paul Palumbo

7 Prophylactic Antiretroviral Treatment of HIV Infection in Neonates 117
Ross E. McKinney, Jr.

8 Treatment of Virologic Monitoring of Primary HIV-1 Infection in Children 127
Stephen A. Spector

9 Immune-Based Therapies for HIV Infection 139
Javier Chinen and William T. Shearer

10 Infectious Complications of Pediatric HIV Infection 155
Wayne M. Dankner, Toni Frederick, and Jeanne M. Bertolli

11 Respiratory Compromise in Children Infected with HIV 193
Meyer Kattan

12 Infection Control in Hospital, School and Community: Distinguishing Real Risk from Perceived Danger 205
Ellen R. Cooper

13 HIV-Induced Central Nervous System and Developmental Abnormalities in Childhood 227
Pim Y. Brouwers and Pamela L. Wolters

14 Oral Manifestations in Pediatric HIV Infection 249
Catherine M. Flaitz and M. John Hicks

15 Cutaneous Manifestations in Pediatric HIV Infection 271
Timothy Dilon Daniel and Moise L. Levy

16 Gastrointestinal Illness and Wasting in Pediatric Patients with HIV Infection 291
Colleen M. Hadigan and Harland S. Winter

17 Abnormal Cardiovascular Function in HIV-Infected Infants and Children 303
Marcie J. Keesler, Stacey D. Fisher, and Steven E. Lipshultz

18 **Depression of Blood Cells in HIV-Infected Children and Adolescents** 321
Patrick S. Sullivan, Donna T. Beck, Michael Rosenberg, and Joanna Dobroszycki

19 **Childhood Malignancies in AIDS** 337
Kenneth L. McClain

20 **Palliative Care for Children Infected with HIV** 349
Samuel Grubman and James M. Oleske

21 **Primary Care of the HIV-Infected Infant and Child** 361
Margaret R. Coyne, Kim D. Evans, and I. Celine Hanson

22 **Psychosocial Challenges in Pediatric HIV Infection** 373
Lori S. Wiener, Jennifer F. Havens, and Warren Yiu Kee Ng

23 **Nursing Care in Pediatric HIV Infection** 395
Carol A. Vincent

24 **Managed Care for Children with HIV Infection** 419
Sindy M. Paul, Paul Langevin, Dawn M. D'Orlando, Victor S. B. Jorden, and Jill Simone

Index 435

Pediatric HIV Infection in Developed and Developing Countries: Epidemiology and Natural History

Lynne M. Mofenson

By the end of 2001, the Joint United Nations Programme on HIV/AIDS (UNAIDS) estimated that 3 million children were living with HIV infection, 90% residing in developing countries.[1] In the United States, an estimated 6000 infants are born to HIV-infected women annually.[2] Prior to 1994, approximately 25% of these infants became infected with HIV. However, the pediatric HIV epidemic in the United States and other developed countries changed dramatically after February 1994, when the results of Pediatric AIDS Clinical Trials Group (PACTG) protocol 076 became available.[3] This study showed that a regimen of zidovudine (ZDV) given during pregnancy after the first trimester, during labor, and to the neonate for 6 weeks could reduce the risk of perinatal transmission by nearly 70%. A significant decline in perinatal transmission has been observed with incorporation of this regimen into clinical practice. Transmission rates of 3% to 6% have been reported with ZDV prophylaxis in various cohort studies, and 2% or less when ZDV is combined with elective cesarean delivery or when women are treated with highly active antiretroviral regimens that reduce maternal viral load to unquantifiable levels.[4–9]

This success is in stark contrast to the continuing perinatal HIV epidemic in developing countries, where intervention strategies that are affordable, implementable, and effective in breastfeeding women have not been available. Several short antiretroviral regimens have been shown to decrease perinatal transmission, with reduced but persistent efficacy through at least age 6 months in breastfeeding infants.[10–15] However, many developing countries are having difficulty in implementing these regimens; barriers to implementation include inadequacies in maternal-child health care infrastructure, lack of antenatal HIV counseling and testing programs, and the economic reality of severely limited resources.

Similar dichotomies exist in the treatment of HIV-infected children. In the developed world, the use of highly active antiretroviral therapy and prophylaxis against opportunistic infections has significantly modified the natural history of HIV disease. However, these treatments are generally not available in developing countries, where an estimated 580,000 children die annually of HIV infection. In Southern Africa, the HIV epidemic threatens to eliminate gains in infant and child survival achieved with childhood immunization and oral rehydration programs.

This chapter reviews the current epidemiology and natural history of pediatric HIV infection, emphasizing differences between developed and developing countries.

EPIDEMIOLOGY

The UNAIDS estimates that 40 million people were living with HIV infection at the end of 2001, including 18.5 million women and 3 million children; an additional 14 million children had one or both parents die of HIV/AIDS.[1] Almost 12 million of these infected individuals are youths between 15 and 24 years of age, and about half of all new adult

All material in this chapter is in the public domain with the exception of any borrowed figures or tables.

infections are occurring among adolescents. During 2001 alone, an estimated 2 million women and 800,000 children became infected with HIV.

The global distribution of HIV infection is shown in Figure 1–1. Almost 4 million infected people reside in India alone.[16] Two countries, South Africa and Nigeria, each have more than 3.5 million infected people, and an additional three countries, Ethiopia, Kenya, and Zimbabwe, each have over 2 million infected individuals. The United States has an infected population nearing 1 million, and China, Russia, Brazil, and Thailand each have 500,000 individuals currently infected with HIV. Although most HIV-infected persons reside in sub-Saharan Africa, substantial growth in HIV prevalence has occurred in Asia and the former Soviet Union.

Perinatal transmission accounts for virtually all new cases of HIV infection in children. Prior to the use of antiretroviral prophylaxis, perinatal transmission rates ranged between 15% and 25% in the United States and other developed countries where HIV-infected women are advised not to breastfeed and between 25% and 40% in Africa and Haiti, where most women breastfeed.[17] Although the most obvious reason for differences in transmission between developed and developing countries is the frequency of breastfeeding, other factors that can vary geographically may also play a role, including coinfections, maternal nutritional status, genetic factors, mode of delivery, and viral subtype, phenotype, or genotype. In studies from both developed and developing countries, peripheral blood and cervicovaginal viral load has been identified as a critical risk factor for transmission.[18–21]

HIV-1 is divided into 2 groups, M (major) and O (outlier).[22] Within the M group, multiple subtypes have been identified, designated as subtypes A through J. Viruses in the highly divergent group O, which have limited distribution at this time, have not been able to be subtyped in a similar fashion. In the United States, subtype B is the primary subtype found in infected individuals, while in the developing world, other subtypes predominate (Table 1–1). The greatest subtype diversity is in Africa, with subtype A most common in West and Central Africa, A and D in East Africa, and C in North and South Africa. Recombinant subtypes (mosaics) have also been described; the A/E subtype is common in Thailand and other parts of Asia and Central Africa. The relationship between biologic phenotype, chemokine receptor utilization, and envelope tropism of HIV has been less studied for non-B subtypes, and it is possible that some differences between transmission rates in the developed versus developing world are related to differences in transmissibility between subtypes.[22–24]

HIV Infection in Women

Because most pediatric infection is perinatally acquired, an understanding of HIV epidemiologic trends among women of childbearing age is critical to understand the HIV epidemic in children.

United States

Women of childbearing age (15–44 years) represent the most rapidly growing group of persons with AIDS in the United States. In 1985, women

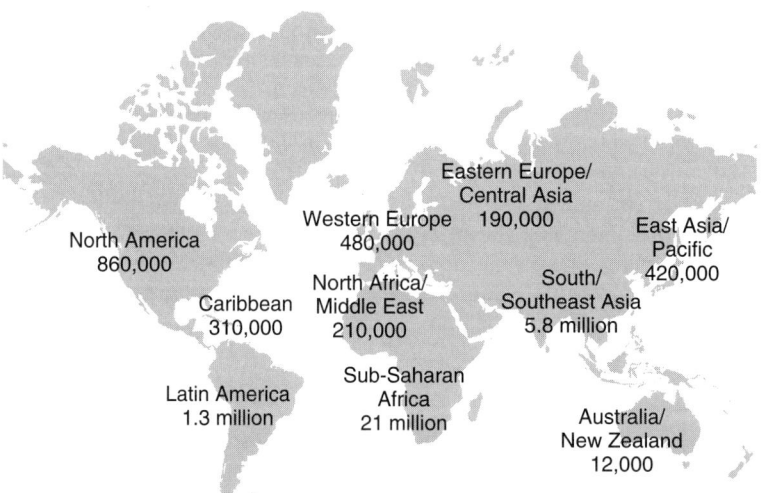

Figure 1–1. Estimated global distribution of HIV infection in adults and children in 2001 (40 million estimated total number infected) from the Joint United Nations Programme on HIV/AIDS and World Health Organization.

Table 1-1
Global Distribution of HIV Subtypes

HIV SUBTYPE	PRIMARY COUNTRY OR REGION
HIV-1	
A	West, Central, and East Africa
B	North and South America, Europe, Caribbean, Thailand, Japan
C	Central and South Africa, India
D	Central and East Asia
E	Southeast Asia, Japan, India
F	Central Africa, South America, Eastern Europe
G	West Africa
H	West and Central Africa, Taiwan
I	Cyprus, Zaire (identified in only a small number of individuals)
J	Central Africa
O	Cameroon, West and Central Africa
HIV-1 Mosaic Subtypes	
A/E	Asia, Central Africa
G/A	West and Central Africa, Eastern Europe
A/G	East and West Africa
Other mosaics	Africa, Asia, South America
HIV-2	
A	West Africa, India
B	West Africa

accounted for only 7% of reported AIDS cases in adults, whereas in 2000, 25% of all reported cases were in women.[25] Nearly 10,500 women were newly diagnosed with AIDS in 2000, giving an incidence rate of 8.7 per 100,000 women. HIV infection was the third leading cause of death among all women aged 24 to 44 years and the leading cause of death among black women in this age group.

Seventy-eight percent of women with AIDS are of minority race/ethnicity, compared with 52% of men. In 2000, the incidence of AIDS was 21 times higher among black women and six times higher among Hispanic women than among white women (45.9 and 13.8, respectively, versus 2.2 per 100,000). Heterosexual contact is currently the predominant mode of exposure for women with AIDS. In 1989, 31% of AIDS cases in women overall were acquired through heterosexual contact; by June 2001, this had risen to 41%. While AIDS in women continues to be concentrated in the Northeast and large metropolitan areas, the epidemic now affects all regions, particularly the South, as well as rural areas.[26] Regions with the highest AIDS rates in women correspond to regions in which HIV seroprevalence is highest among male injecting drug users, reflecting heterosexual spread from these men to their sexual partners.

AIDS surveillance does not accurately reflect the incidence and prevalence of HIV infection among women. The Centers for Disease Control and Prevention (CDC) estimated in 1994 that only 15% of more than 100,000 women aged 15 to 44 years living with HIV infection had developed AIDS. Data from HIV-reporting states indicate that women accounted for 31% of HIV-infected adults reported between July 2000 and June 2001, compared with 25% of AIDS cases reported during the same time period and 45% of newly acquired HIV infections in adolescents and young adults aged 13 to 24 years old.[25]

In some inner cities, the incidence of heterosexually acquired HIV infection is similar to that reported in some developing countries. In a study of 449 HIV-negative women followed prospectively in an inner city clinic in Brooklyn, the cumulative incidence of seroconversion after 24 months of follow-up was 1.2%, comparable to the 2-year seroconversion rate of 1.2% in a population with improved treatment services for sexually transmitted diseases in Tanzania.[27, 28] The mode of acquisition in all seroconverters was heterosexual, and the rate of pregnancy among seroconverters (55.5 pregnancies per 100 person-years) was five times higher than among non-seroconverters.

Data on HIV infection among women giving birth are more directly relevant to HIV infection in children. Data on HIV seroprevalence among childbearing women are available from the Survey of

Childbearing Women, which was conducted in 45 sites between 1989 and 1995.[2] During this time, an estimated 6000 to 7000 HIV-infected women gave birth annually. HIV seroprevalence among childbearing women remained stable nationwide, ranging from 1.5 to 1.7 per 1000 women, although there were differing regional trends.[29] In the Northeast, seroprevalence declined between 1989 and 1995 (from 4.1 to 3.2 per 1000), whereas seroprevalence significantly increased in the South through 1991 and then stabilized (from 1.6 to 2.0 per 1000). However, seroprevalence among black women in some southern states continued to significantly increase through 1995. Rates in the Midwest and West remained stable at approximately 0.6 per 1000. The highest seroprevalence rates were observed in urban areas, particularly on the East Coast, but high rates were also observed in some rural areas, particularly in the South. Rates among black women were 3 to 35 times higher than among white women, regardless of geographic area of residence.

Europe

HIV/AIDS epidemiology in Europe differs substantially between countries. Most reported AIDS cases have been in Western Europe, predominantly in France, Italy, and Spain. Central and Eastern Europe have been less affected, although recent increases in HIV seroprevalence among injecting drug users in some countries, such as the Ukraine and Russia, have been reported; a rapid evolution of the HIV epidemic from drug users to women via heterosexual spread has been observed in countries such as Thailand. A marked increase in the incidence of sexually transmitted diseases in countries of the former Soviet Union and Eastern Europe presages the potential for future widespread HIV transmission to women in these countries.[30]

Substantial increases in cases of AIDS among women in Europe have been reported. Between 1991 and 1995, women older than 13 years of age accounted for 18% of AIDS cases in Europe overall and 20% of cases in Southern Europe.[31] The incidence of AIDS among women between 1991 and 1995 increased by 100% in Southern Europe, 60% in Central Europe, 113% in Northern Europe, and 367% in Eastern Europe. The predominant mode of HIV acquisition varies by region; for example, in Southern Europe, 54% of AIDS cases among women were acquired via injecting drug use, while in Northern Europe, 71% of cases were attributed to heterosexual contact.

In population-based estimates of HIV infection in 2001 in Europe from UNAIDS, women between 15 and 49 years of age accounted for 33% of all infected persons in Italy, 27% in France, and 20% in Spain and Germany.

HIV seroprevalence among childbearing women also varies significantly between countries (Table 1–2). In a study of trends in 14 European countries, estimated HIV prevalence among pregnant women having live births showed statistically significant increases through 1993 in Portugal, Spain, and the United Kingdom and, to a smaller magnitude, in France and Italy.[32] The prevalence of infection in childbearing women in Europe is generally similar to that observed in the United States.

Latin America and the Caribbean

The HIV epidemic in Latin America, as in the United States, began with the primary affected populations being homosexual men and injecting drug users. By the late 1980s, however, heterosexual transmission began to increase. In Brazil, heterosexual transmission accounted for only 7.5% of AIDS cases in 1987 but increased to 26% by 1994, while the male-female ratio of AIDS cases decreased from 16:1 to 3:1 in 1996.[33] HIV seroprevalence among injecting drug users is as high as 60% in some areas of Brazil and Argentina, foreshadowing potential for further spread heterosexually and then from women to children. In 2001, women of childbearing age accounted for 36% of all HIV-infected persons in Brazil.[1]

In the Caribbean, heterosexual transmission has been the predominant mode of transmission since early in the epidemic. In Haiti, up to 10% of urban and 5% of rural adults are infected, predominantly through heterosexual acquisition. A seroprevalence study in the Commonwealth of the Bahamas showed that 2.9% of pregnant women were HIV-infected; the highest incidence was in women aged 25 to 34 years and in women with multiple pregnancies.[34] HIV seroprevalence rates among pregnant women have reached 4% in the Bahamas, Haiti, and Trinidad/Tobago[1] (see Table 1–2).

Sub-Saharan Africa and Asia

Ninety percent of HIV-infected adults live in developing countries, with sub-Saharan Africa most affected. On a global basis, approximately 46% of HIV-infected adults are women, and this proportion is growing. Heterosexual transmission is responsible for more than 75% of HIV infections worldwide.[33]

Seroprevalence rates of HIV among pregnant women in Africa vary between and also within countries (see Table 1–2). Seroprevalence has generally, although not universally, been higher in urban than

Table 1–2
HIV-1 Seroprevalence Among Pregnant Women in Selected Countries*

	HIV PREVALENCE IN WOMEN IN ANTENATAL CARE			
	MAJOR URBAN AREAS		OUTSIDE OF URBAN AREAS	
COUNTRY	YEAR	MEDIAN %	YEAR	MEDIAN %
North America				
United States	1994	0.15	—	—
Canada	1993	0.20	—	—
Caribbean				
Bahamas	1995	3.6	1993	3.6
Dominican Republic	1999	1.2	1999	2.1
Haiti	2000	3.8	2001	3.4
Latin America				
Argentina	1998	0.9	1998	0.2
Brazil	2000	1.6	2000	0.4
Honduras	1998	2.9	1998	3.0
Western Europe				
France	1994	0.42	—	—
Germany	1997	0.10	1997	0.0
Italy	1992	0.15	1993	0.10
Spain	1997	0.10	1996	0.15
United Kingdom	1997	0.20	1997	0.0
Eastern Europe & Central Asia				
Bulgaria	—	—	1997	0.01
Czech Republic	—	—	1996	0.01
Ukraine	1996	0.2	1996	0.05
Africa				
North Africa				
Sudan	1998	0.5	1998	3.8
East Africa				
Kenya	2000	15.3	2000	14.0
Rwanda	2000	23.0	1999	7.0
Uganda	2000	11.3	2000	6.0
Central Africa				
Cameroon	2000	9.0	2000	10.7
Congo	2000	10.0	1993	4.0
West Africa				
Burkina Faso	2000	6.3	2000	6.6
Cote d'Ivoire	2000	9.0	2000	8.8
Nigeria	2001	4.2	2001	5.3
Southern Africa				
Botswana	2001	44.9	2001	34.8
Malawi	2001	20.1	2001	16.1
South Africa	2000	24.3	2000	22.9
Zambia	2001	30.7	1998	13.0
Zimbabwe	2000	31.1	2000	33.2
South & Southeast Asia				
Cambodia	2000	2.7	2000	1.7
India	1999	2.0	2000	2.0
Thailand	2000	1.6	2000	1.5
East Asia & Pacific				
China	2000	0.0	2000	0.5
Japan	1999	0.0	1999	0.0

Data from Joint United Nations Programme on HIV/AIDS: Report on the Global HIV/AIDS Epidemic, 2002. Geneva, World Health Organization/UNAIDS, 2002.

rural areas. In a rural health district in South Africa, serial seroprevalence surveys among pregnant women at an antenatal clinic indicate an explosive rise in infection, from less than 5% in 1990 to 41.2% in 1999.[35] Seroprevalence in pregnant women in Malawi rose by 16-fold between 1985 and 1996.[36] In Botswana, HIV seroprevalence among pregnant women in urban areas was 38.5% in 1997 and increased further to 44.9% in 2001[1] (Table 1–2). In other countries, such as Kenya and Zambia, seroprevalence among pregnant women has appeared to stabilize at high levels.[37,38] In contrast, in Kampala, Uganda, where effective HIV/AIDS prevention programs are in place, seroprevalence in pregnant women has dropped from a high of 29.5% in 1992 to 11.3% in 2001.[1]

The HIV epidemic was introduced later into Asia but is escalating rapidly. Although initially introduced into this region in injecting drug users, the epidemic has become increasingly heterosexually spread. While prevalence levels have not reached those observed in sub-Saharan Africa, HIV is well established across the continent. It is estimated that 6.6 million persons are infected in Asia, with more than 50% being in India.[1,16] HIV prevalence was examined in women attending a sexually transmitted disease clinic in Pune, India, between 1993 and 1996, and was found to be 50% in female sex workers and 14% in women who were not sex workers.[39] Most of the non–sex workers were married, and the primary risk factor for infection was sexual contact with a single partner (generally her spouse) who had been diagnosed with a sexually transmitted disease, implying that it is likely that these women were infected by their spouses.

Southeast Asian countries, particularly Thailand, Cambodia, Vietnam, and Myanmar, have had an increasing prevalence of HIV infection in their populations; prevalence in China has been low, although an increasing number of cases are being reported.[1] In Bangkok, Thailand, the prevalence of HIV among pregnant women has increased steadily from 1.2% in 1991 to 2.3% 1996.[40] Similar to the report from India, sex with a current partner was the only identified risk for 52% of infected women. Seroprevalence rates of more than 8% in pregnant women have been reported in northern Thailand.[33] More recently, implementation of large-scale prevention programs by the Thai government has been associated with a decline in seroprevalence in pregnant women to 1.6% in 2001.[1] Based on national surveillance data, it is estimated that about 23,000 HIV-infected women give birth annually in Thailand.

HIV Infection in Children

United States and Other Developed/Mid-Developed Countries

In the United States, as in other countries, most children have become infected via perinatal transmission. As of June 2001, 8994 cases of AIDS have been reported in children in the United States; 91% were acquired perinatally and 7% through receipt of infected blood, blood products, or tissue or through contaminated blood products for hemophilia treatment.[25] AIDS in children reflects the HIV epidemic in women, with children of minority race/ethnicity disproportionately affected: 59% of children with AIDS are black; 23% Hispanic; 17% white; and 1% Native American or Asian/Pacific Islander. Children with AIDS have been reported from all states and from Puerto Rico, the Virgin Islands, and the District of Columbia. New York, California, Florida, Texas, and New Jersey have the highest proportion of pediatric AIDS cases, reflecting HIV prevalence among childbearing women. Eighty-five percent of children with AIDS have been reported from metropolitan areas with 500,000 or more population.

HIV antibody screening of donors of blood, blood products, and tissue and heat treatment of clotting factors has virtually eliminated transmission of HIV via blood or tissue. The number of cases of AIDS secondary to blood products peaked in the 1980s and has steadily decreased since 1990. Newly reported AIDS cases in children secondary to blood products are almost exclusively in children who were infected prior to screening of blood for HIV.

While transmission of HIV by blood products is unusual in the United States and Europe, transmission of HIV to children in Romania is unique. More than 4000 cases of pediatric AIDS have been reported in Romania. More than 95% of the children acquired HIV infection through blood transfusions or injection with unsterilized needles and syringes.[41] Microtransfusions of blood were administered repeatedly to malnourished children in orphanages, for an alleged "nutritional" effect. HIV seroprevalence among children in Romanian orphanages ranges between 5% and 20%. A similar outbreak occurred in Russia, where reuse of unsterilized injecting equipment resulted in the infection of approximately 100 children.[42]

Remarkable changes in the epidemiology of perinatal AIDS have been observed in the United States following the results of PACTG 076, showing that ZDV prophylaxis could reduce the risk of mother-to-child transmission.[3] Epidemiologic studies demonstrated decreases in perinatal transmission in the United States as early as 1995, temporally associated with increased prenatal HIV testing and use of ZDV prophylaxis.[4,43,44] In a study from 18 states with HIV reporting, the percentage of HIV-exposed infants whose mothers were tested for HIV prior to giving birth increased from 70% to 94% between 1993 and 1997, and the percentage of women receiving ZDV increased from 7% to 91% during this same time period.[43] Similar to the United States, the use of ZDV prophylaxis has had a significant impact on perinatal transmission in Europe, Latin America, and the Caribbean.[6,45,46]

The widespread incorporation of ZDV prophylaxis into clinical practice has already been reflected in a substantial decrease in reported perinatal AIDS cases in the United States. The number of perinatal AIDS cases peaked in 1992 and then declined by nearly 80% from 1992 through 2000.[25,43] This decline has been most dramatic in the youngest age groups. AIDS cases declined by over 85% for infants younger than 1 year of age and 70% for those aged 1 to 5 years, while little decline was observed in children older than 5 years, who would have been born prior to 1994. Perinatal AIDS cases have declined in all regions of the country and among all racial and ethnic groups.

An important barrier to elimination of perinatal HIV infection in the United States is the continued rise in HIV infection among women of childbearing age, particularly among adolescent women of minority race/ethnicity.[47,48] These same women are also at high risk of becoming pregnant, often unintentionally. Inadequate prenatal care constitutes another significant barrier to prevention of transmission. In one study from four states, 14% of HIV-infected women received no prenatal care, and 23% started care only in the third trimester.[49] Lack of prenatal care was most common among infected women who used illicit drugs and those who were not diagnosed as infected until after the birth of their infant (35% and 50% lacked prenatal care, respectively). Identification of HIV-infected women before or during pregnancy is critical, to enable initiation of appropriate treatment for their infection and provide prophylaxis to prevent perinatal transmission.[50] However, there is significant geographic variation in prenatal HIV testing in the United States, despite Public Health Service recommendations for universal counseling and testing.[51] The Institute of Medicine recommended in 1999 that HIV testing be integrated into the standard prenatal test battery and that a national policy of universal prenatal testing, with patient notification and right of refusal, be instituted.[52]

Strategies to enable detection of any potential short- or long-term adverse consequences of in utero and neonatal antiretroviral drug exposure on the infant are critical, particularly now that the vast majority of infants will not be infected. ZDV prophylaxis appears safe in the short-term for women and infants followed for as long as 5.6 years[53–55]; however, long-term data are not yet available. Some nucleoside analogue drugs are carcinogenic in rodent studies and can induce mitochondrial dysfunction.[56,57] Additionally, an increasing number of pregnant women are receiving antiretroviral therapy with multiple drugs for treatment of their HIV disease, but there is minimal information regarding the safety of these drugs in pregnancy or to the child. Thus, follow-up into adulthood is recommended for all children with in utero or neonatal exposure to antiretroviral drugs.[50]

Sub-Saharan Africa and Other Developing Countries

In developed countries, children account for only about 2% of all AIDS cases; however, in the developing world, where a greater proportion of women of childbearing age are infected, pediatric AIDS accounts for 10% to 15% of cases. By the end of 2001, 6 million children will have been infected with HIV, 3 million of whom have died; and over 2000 newly infected infants continue to be born daily.[1] Most of these infected children live in sub-Saharan Africa.

Mother-to-child transmission accounts for at least 90% of pediatric infection worldwide. Transmission rates in developing countries are higher than in developed countries, in large part due to HIV transmission by breastmilk.[58] In many developing countries, a safe alternative to breastfeeding is unavailable because of lack of clear water and affordable formula, and feeding with breastmilk substitutes would pose a significant risk of malnutrition, infections, and death to the infant. Additionally, more than 9 of 10 HIV-infected women in developing countries do not know they are infected, and therefore they are unable to make informed choices about infant feeding.

Epidemiologic data indicate that breastfeeding is associated with approximately a doubling of HIV transmission risk. A meta-analysis indicated that the attributable risk for HIV transmission through breastmilk was 14% (95% CI, 7–22%) for women with established HIV infection at delivery, and 29% (95% CI, 16–42%) for those who seroconverted postpartum.[59] However, the proportion of transmission occurring during early and late breastfeeding is not well defined. Colostrum and early milk have high cellular content and could be more infectious than later milk, and the neonate could have enhanced susceptibility to early transmission due to an immature immune system and increased gut permeability. However, the volume of later milk ingested by the infant is considerably larger, and at least one study suggests that the prevalence of HIV RNA is higher in mature than early milk.[60] Additionally, specific and nonspecific immune substances in breastmilk decrease over time, and intercurrent gastrointestinal infections, possibly related to introduction of supplemental foods and liquids, could compromise gastrointestinal mucosal integrity, facilitating HIV transmission. If a significant proportion of transmission occurs late, then early weaning might be able to maximize early nutrition of the infant and minimize the risk of HIV transmission. On the other hand, if the majority of transmission occurs during the first few weeks of breastfeeding, early weaning may not provide much benefit, but provision of an antiretroviral drug for a short critical high-risk period might provide an effective intervention.

The risk of late postnatal transmission (after age 4 months) was 3.2% per year of breastfeeding (95% CI, 3.1–3.8%) in a pooled analysis of eight cohorts, with an overall risk of 9.2% after 36 months of breastfeeding.[61] The risk of early breastmilk transmission is not easy to quantify, because it is difficult to distinguish intrapartum from early postnatal transmission through breastmilk. A study in Malawi found that there was a relatively high risk of HIV transmission during the early breastfeeding period (0.7% and 0.6% per month for months 1–5 and 6–11, respectively), with a lower but continuous risk afterward (0.3% and 0.2% per month for months 12–17 and 18–23, respectively).[62] The cumulative risk of postnatal transmission was 3.5%, 7.0%, 8.9%, and 20.3% after 5, 11, 17, and 23 months of breastfeeding, respectively. Other factors may also play a role, including the presence of mastitis, nipple pathologic conditions, and variation in feeding practices.[63–65] Two studies have suggested that mixed infant feeding (breastmilk and other liquid such as cows' milk, water, tea, or juice) is associated with a higher risk of transmission than exclusive breastfeeding.[64,65] Theoretically, mixed feeding could introduce contaminated fluids that could predispose to gastrointestinal infections and inflammation.

A number of clinical trials in breastfeeding women have identified several antiretroviral regimens that are effective in reducing transmission. These include oral ZDV given for 2 to 4 weeks antenatally and intrapartum; ZDV and 3TC, given either orally antenatally for 4 weeks, intrapartum, and to the mother and infant for 1 week postpartum, or, with somewhat lower efficacy, only intrapartum and postnatally; and oral nevirapine given as a single dose at the onset of labor and to the infant at the age of 48 hours.[10,12–14] Efficacy of these regimens is maintained during continued breastfeeding for at least 4 to 6 months, and possibly as long as 15 to 24 months for the ZDV regimens and single dose nevirapone regimen, although there is diminution of efficacy with continued breastfeeding.[15] These regimens offer the potential to significantly decrease perinatal transmission in the developing world.

While perinatal transmission accounts for the majority of pediatric infection, transmission via blood products or contaminated needles accounts for a significant minority (about 10%) of pediatric infection in developing countries. Many countries in the developing world do not routinely screen blood donations for HIV. In Africa, more than half of all transfusions are given to children, primarily for anemia caused by malaria.[66] In a study of children aged 2 to 14 years admitted to the hospital in Zaire in 1984–85, 11% of 368 children were found to be HIV seropositive; seropositivity was associated with prior hospitalizations, receipt of a blood transfusion prior to the current hospitalization, and receipt of medical injections during the past year.[67] Other practices with the potential for parenteral exposures to contaminated blood, such as scarification with unsterilized needles, have also been implicated.

NATURAL HISTORY OF HIV INFECTION IN CHILDREN

In contrast to HIV infection in adults, infection in perinatally infected children occurs in the context of an immature and developing immune system. As a consequence, there are differences in the manifestations of HIV disease between children and adults. Primary HIV infection in adults is characterized by an initial burst of viremia, with HIV RNA levels as high as 10^5 to 10^6 log copies per milliliter, followed by a 100- to 1000-fold decline over the subsequent 2 to 3 months to reach a steady-state plateau that may persist for years.[68] In contrast, in perinatally infected children, HIV RNA levels peak at 10^6 log copies/mL or higher within a month of birth, and remain high (mean, 10^5 log copies/mL) for several years.[69,70] Progression to symptomatic disease occurs more rapidly in children, in part due to their inability to control HIV replication. In infected adults, the onset of HIV-related symptoms occurs at a mean 4.4 years post infection, and progression to AIDS occurs after 9.8 to 15 years.[71] In contrast, the onset of HIV-related symptoms occurs in perinatally infected children at a mean age of 4 to 5 months and progression to AIDS at 4 to 6 years.[72,73] As HIV-induced immunologic dysfunction progresses, opportunistic infections with pathogens associated with defects in cell-mediated immunity are seen in infected children and adults. In adults, these generally reflect reactivation of latent infection acquired earlier in life, with some preexisting immunity at the time of reactivation. In young children, however, infections with opportunistic organisms generally reflect primary infection in an individual without any prior immunity, and more fulminant disease may result.

In both developed and developing countries, HIV disease manifestations in children predominantly reflect the consequences of perinatal HIV acquisition. Early symptoms are similar in developed and developing countries and generally nonspecific, distinguished primarily by their persistence, recurrence, and severity. However, progression to HIV disease appears more rapid in developing countries. Additionally, because the opportunistic infections children develop depend on the organisms they are exposed to in their environment, differences may be seen between developed and developing countries in the types of opportunistic infections that develop. Other chapters in this book will discuss evolution of the virologic and immunologic consequences and organ system manifestations of HIV infection in children. This chapter gives a general review of HIV disease in children, emphasizing differences between developed and developing countries.

United States and Other Developed Countries

Pregnancy Outcome

Data are conflicting regarding the effect of HIV on pregnancy outcome. Early studies from the United States and Europe reported no increase in adverse pregnancy outcomes in infected and uninfected pregnant women from similar demographic groups.[74–77] Some (although not all) recent studies have suggested that infected women may be more likely to have preterm and low birth weight infants than uninfected women.[78–80] A higher prevalence of chorioamnionitis and placental inflammatory cytokine expression in placentas of infected women has been described, which could predispose to these adverse outcomes.[81,82] A significant decrease in preterm and low birth weight infants was associated with maternal use of ZDV monotherapy, compared with infants born to infected women receiving no treatment in the European Collaborative Study.[83] However, a small Swiss study in 30 women reported that combination antiretroviral therapy was associated with an increase in preterm delivery when compared with women receiving no therapy or ZDV monotherapy.[84] These results were not corroborated in a retrospective evaluation of prenatal records from more than 400 infected pregnant women delivering between 1998 and 1999 at 32 clinical trial sites in the United States.[85] However, as the use of combination antiretroviral therapy and new agents in pregnant women increases, continued surveillance for potential effects on pregnancy outcomes is important.

Mortality

Initial reports on the natural history of perinatal HIV infection described rapid disease progression and short survival. In a report on 172 infected children from Miami, perinatally infected children presented with symptomatic disease at a median age of 8 months and only 21% were free of symptoms at 2 years of age.[86] The median survival was 38 months from the time of diagnosis and the highest mortality rate, 17%, was during the first year of life. Early age at diagnosis and presentation with *Pneumocystis carinii* pneumonia (PCP) or encephalopathy was associated with high mortality rate. Similar data were reported from a cohort of 111 children in New York City; the median survival of perinatally infected children was 1.9 years, and 25% of children died within a year of developing an HIV-associated illness.[87] However, these early reports were based on children whose HIV infection had been ascertained because of symptomatic disease and therefore were biased toward including those children with most rapidly progressive disease.

Later reports of children prospectively followed from birth described a longer time to development of AIDS and death than in these initial reports. Prospective cohorts have also shown bimodal disease progression, with 20% to 30% of children having onset of HIV disease and/or death before 2 or 3 years of age and a larger group of 70% to 80% of children with more slowly progressive HIV disease and longer survival.[72, 88–91] Data from cohorts in the United States and Europe indicate that only 6% to 16% of infected children die during the first year of life, and only 25% to 29% by the age of 5 years (Table 1–3).[72, 90, 92] In the Italian Register for HIV in Children, after the first year of life, the mortality rate decreased to 3.5% per year through age 7 years, and increased again to 8% to 12% per year at age 8 to 9 years.[91] The median survival in these studies has ranged from 7.1 to 8.0 years.

The risk of rapid disease progression has been associated with severity of maternal HIV disease, low birth weight, a positive virologic test result during the first week of life, early onset of symptoms and low CD4+ count, high viral load after the first week of life, viral phenotype, and possibly host genotype (e.g., chemokine receptor genotype).[69,70,90,91,93–98] Development of PCP or encephalopathy was associated with particularly short survival and development of lymphoid interstitial pneumonitis (LIP) with longer survival in a number of studies.[86,87,91]

Long-term survival in a subset of perinatally infected children was described even before current potent antiretroviral drugs were available, with reports of small cohorts of perinatally infected children who did not have their HIV infection recognized until preadolescence or adolescence.[99–102] However, true long-term survival with the absence of clinical symptoms or immunosuppression is unusual. In a study from New Jersey of 42 children with perinatal infection older than 9 years of age, only 24% were asymptomatic; 19% had HIV-related symptoms, 57% had AIDS, and 79% had moderate or severe immunodeficiency.[100] In two studies involving 253 perinatally infected children over the age of 5 years in Texas and Italy, only 5% to 15% had no symptoms.[93, 101] Similarly, in a report from five clinical sites in California, Florida, and New Jersey, only 20% of 143 perinatally infected and 54 neonatal transfusion-infected children over the age of 8 years were without HIV-related symptoms.[102] In all studies, the most common AIDS-defining conditions in long-term survivors was LIP and recurrent bacterial infections.

The primary cause of death in 58 infected children who died between 1990 and 1996 in New York City was infectious (70%), with PCP and *Mycobacterium avium-intracellulare* (MAI) the most common causes.[103] The lung was most frequently affected in children who died (78%), with PCP and LIP being the most common findings at autopsy. The central nervous system was involved in 61% of deaths, with the primary diagnosis of encephalopathy prior to death. Gastrointestinal involvement, primarily manifest as diarrhea, was present in 44% of those who died, cardiac disease in 41%, and nephropathy in 20%.

Morbidity

In studies in the United States and Europe, conducted prior to widespread use of potent antiretroviral therapy, approximately 20% to 36% of infected children developed AIDS by the age of 1 to 2 years and 36% to 50% by the age of 5 or 6 years (Table 1–4).[72, 89, 90, 92] Although most infected children do not have rapidly progressive disease, studies from the United States and Europe have shown that 69% to 96% of infected children develop some HIV-related symptoms by 1 year of age and only 6% to 15% have no symptoms at 5 years of age.[72,93,94, 104,105] The median age at development of HIV-related symptoms in perinatally infected infants was 5 months in studies from Italy and the United States.[92, 94] Early symptoms tend to be nonspecific, such as lymphadenopathy and hepatosplenomegaly, but in comparison to uninfected children, the incidence of these symptoms is higher (Table 1–5).

A clinical classification system for pediatric HIV infection was developed by the CDC that divided the natural history of pediatric disease into stages: stage N, no signs or symptoms; stage B, moderate signs or symptoms; and stage C, severe signs or symptoms[106] (Table 1–6). In a Markov model based on data from 2148 perinatally infected children born between 1982 and 1993 in the Pediatric Spectrum of Disease Project, the mean estimated time in each stage was as follows: N, 10 months; A, 4 months; B, 65 months (5.4 years); and C, 34 months (2.8 years) (Table 1–7).[72] The estimated mean and median time from birth to stage C disease was 6.6 and 5.0 years, respectively, and the mean and median survival was 9.4 and 8.0 years. Markov modeling from other U.S. and European cohorts has had similar results.[92,107]

Since the early 1990s, there has been remarkable progress in the ability to diagnose and treat HIV infection and its complications in children. These changes have resulted in change in the clinical spectrum of HIV disease and survival in children as well as adults.

A decline in opportunistic infections was first observed after prophylaxis guidelines were published, and a further decline after the availability of highly active antiretroviral therapy. Opportunistic infection with *P. carinii* is the most common

Table 1-3
Mortality in Children with Perinatal HIV Infection in Developed and Developing Countries

LOCATION	Infected Children, n	Years Enrolled	PROBABILITY OF DEATH BY AGE, %						MEAN/MEDIAN SURVIVAL FROM BIRTH
			1 Year	2 Years	3 Years	4 Years	5 Years	6 Years	
Developed Countries									
United States: Pediatric Spectrum of Disease Project[72]	2148	1982–93	—	—	—	16	25	—	8.0/9.4 years (median/mean)
Connecticut[105]	75	1985–93	16	—	31	—	—	—	7.1 years (median)
New York City[104]	116	1986–95	16	27	—	—	—	—	—
Europe[89]	392	1986–94	—	—	—	21%	—	26%	—
United States: Women and Infants Transmission Study[92]	128	1989–95	6	11	—	—	—	—	—
Italy[91,93]	141	to 1992	14	—	—	—	29	32	8.0 years (median)
Developing Countries									
Zaire[128]	92	1986–87	26	41	44	—	—	—	—
Haiti[136]	22	1985–94	—	64	—	—	—	—	—
Rwanda[139]	54	1988–89	26	45	—	—	62	—	12.4 months (median)
South Africa[138]	48	1990–93	29	35	—	—	—	—	34.2 months (mean)
Malawi[127]	155	1994–95	—	30	45	—	—	—	—

Table 1-4
Progression to HIV-Related Symptoms and AIDS in Children with Perinatal HIV Infection in Developing and Developed Countries

LOCATION	INFECTED CHILDREN, n	YEARS ENROLLED	% WITH ANY SYMPTOMS BY AGE		% DEVELOPING AIDS BY AGE				MEAN/MEDIAN AGE AT AIDS DIAGNOSIS	MEAN/MEDIAN SURVIVAL AFTER AIDS DIAGNOSIS
			1 Year	2 Years	1 Year	2 Years	5 Years	6 Years		
Developed Countries										
United States: Pediatric Spectrum of Disease Project[72]	2148	1982–93	69	—	—	—	50	—	6.6 years (median)	2.8 years (mean)
Connecticut[105]	75	1985–93	79	—	12	—	—	—	—	—
New York City[104]	116	1986–95	83	92	36	—	—	—	—	1.8 years (median)
Europe[89]	392	1986–94	88	—	20	25	—	36	—	1.9 years (median)
United States: Women and Infants Transmission Study[92]	128	1989–95	74	84	21	34	—	—	4 years (median)	—
Italy (91)	573	to 1991	96	—	—	—	—	—	—	—
Developing Countries										
Haiti[136]	51	1984–92	—	96	33	—	84	—	19 months (median)	—
Rwanda[138]	54	1988–89	—	100	17	28	35	—	14 months (median)	9 months (median)

Table 1-5
Early HIV-Related Clinical Conditions in 116 Children with HIV Infection Compared to 396 Uninfected Children in New York City

CLINICAL FINDING	FREQUENCY OF SYMPTOM, %		MEDIAN AGE OF ONSET, MO		RATIO OF INCIDENCE RATES (Infected/Uninfected)
	Infected	Uninfected	Infected	Uninfected	
Lymphadenopathy	85	17	3.7	5.5	18.6
Hepatomegaly	83	22	3.6	2.6	12.6
Splenomegaly	79	9	4.2	3.1	27.9
Failure to thrive	47	16	6.2	11.3	3.9
Dermatitis	40	25	5.6	6.0	1.8
Persistent oral candida	35	2	7.0	1.9	29.0
Fever for 30 days or more	22	2	10.9	11.1	21.7
Parotid enlargement	22	1	19.6	7.1	23.0
Hepatitis	14	3	6.1	0.4	4.1
Weight loss	12	0.3	18.6	36.0	46.0
Recurrent diarrhea	12	0.3	27.6	3.4	47.0
Chronic diarrhea	10	0.8	26.7	26.3	13.3
Respiratory infection (persistent or recurrent)	9	0	14.7	—	—
Zoster	6	1	42.7	15.8	5.7
Disseminated varicella	3	0	69.2	—	—
Nephropathy	2	0	16.0	—	—
Herpes simplex	2	0	32.6	—	—
Cytomegalovirus	0.9	0.3	4.0	58.7	3.0

Data from Bamji M, Thea DM, Weedon J, et al: Prospective study of human immunodeficiency virus 1-related disease among 512 infants born to infected women in New York City. Pediatr Infect Dis J 1996;15:891–898.

AIDS-defining condition in cases of pediatric HIV infection and a leading cause of death. Most cases occur between 3 to 6 months of life and are fatal in approximately one third of infants.[108] The first guidelines for prevention of PCP in children were published in 1992 and were based on age-related CD4+ cell count. These guidelines were expanded in 1995 to recommend initiation of prophylaxis in all children born to HIV-infected women at age 4 to 6 weeks, continuing until infection is ruled out or age 12 months, when prophylaxis is continued in infected children based on age-related CD4+ cell count.[109] Early use of primary PCP prophylaxis by infected infants was shown to be highly effective in decreasing the frequency of PCP and early death.[110,111] Among infected children followed from birth in New York City between 1986 and 1993 who did not receive prophylaxis, the incidence of PCP in the first year of life was 25% and it caused 31% of deaths, while for children receiving early PCP prophylaxis, PCP incidence was reduced two- to sixfold and mortality by 4.4-fold.[110] The number of children newly diagnosed with AIDS has decreased by more than twofold at 10 medical centers in New York City between the period of 1991 through 1994 and the period of 1995 through 1998, and change in types of AIDS diagnoses have been observed; the finding of PCP has declined from 17% to 11% of new AIDS diagnoses (Table 1–8).[112]

In 1993, the first guidelines for use of antiretroviral drugs in children were issued, recommending ZDV treatment for children with low CD4+ cell count or clinical symptoms.[113] New, more aggressive treatment guidelines were issued in 1998, as new antiretroviral drugs such as protease inhibitors became available for children; these guidelines recommend treatment with highly active combination antiretroviral therapy for all HIV-infected children younger than 12 months of age regardless of symptoms.[114] Dramatic changes in the natural history of HIV disease have been observed in adults following widespread use of highly active antiretroviral therapy.[115,116] Data in children are more limited but suggest that similar changes are occurring. Significant decreases in hospital admissions, duration of

Table 1-6
Centers for Disease Control and Prevention Pediatric HIV Disease Classification: Clinical Categories

Category N: Not Symptomatic
Children who have no signs or symptoms considered to be the result of HIV infection or who have only one of the conditions in Category A.

Category A: Mildly Symptomatic
Children with two or more of the following conditions in the absence of Category B or C conditions:
  Lymphadenopathy
  Hepatomegaly
  Splenomegaly
  Dermatitis
  Parotitis
  Recurrent or persistent upper respiratory infection, sinusitis, or otitis media

Category B: Moderately Symptomatic
Children with signs or symptoms related to HIV infection, examples of which include but are not limited to:
  Anemia (<8 g/dL), neutropenia (<1000/mm^3), or thrombocytopenia (<1,000,000/mm^3) persisting more than 30 days
  Bacterial meningitis, pneumonia or sepsis (single episode)
  Oropharyngeal candidiasis, persisting for >2 months in a child aged >6 months
  Cardiomyopathy
  CMV infection, with onset before 1 month of age
  Diarrhea, recurrent or chronic
  Hepatitis
  HSV stomatitis, recurrent (> two episodes within 1 year)
  HSV bronchitis, pneumonitis, or esophagitis with onset before age 1 month
  Herpes zoster involving at least two episodes or more than one dermatome
  Leiomyosarcoma
  Lymphoid interstitial pneumonitis or pulmonary lymphoid hyperplasia complex (note: this condition meets 1987 surveillance case definition of AIDS)
  Nephropathy
  Nocardiosis
  Persistent fever lasting >1 month
  Toxoplasmosis with onset before 1 month of age
  Varicella, disseminated

Category C: Severely Symptomatic
Children with any condition listed in the 1987 surveillance case definition for AIDS except for lymphoid interstitial pneumonitis (which is a Category B condition):
  Multiple or recurrent serious bacterial infections (sepsis, pneumonia, meningitis, bone or joint infection, or abscess of internal organ)
  Candidiasis, esophageal or pulmonary
  Coccidioidomycosis, disseminated
  Cryptococcosis, extrapulmonary
  Cryptosporidiosis or isosporiasis with diarrhea persisting >1 month
  CMV disease with onset of symptoms at >1 month of age
  CMV retinitis (with loss of vision)
  Encephalopathy in the absence of a concurrent illness other than HIV infection that could explain the findings
  HSV infection causing a mucocutaneous ulcer persisting for >1 month, or pneumonitis, bronchitis, or esophagitis with onset after 1 month of age
  Histoplasmosis, disseminated
  Kaposi sarcoma
  Primary central nervous system lymphoma
  Lymphoma, Burkitts, large cell, or immunoblastic
  Mycobacterium tuberculosis infection, disseminated or extrapulmonary
  Mycobacterium infections other than tuberculosis, disseminated
  Pneumocystis carinii pneumonia
  Progressive multifocal leukoencephalopathy
  Toxoplasmosis of the brain with onset at >1 month of age
  Wasting syndrome in the absence of concurrent illness other than HIV infection

CMV, cytomegalovirus; HSV, herpes simplex virus.

Table 1-7
Progression in Pediatric HIV Disease Clinical Category in Children with Perinatal HIV Infection in the Pediatric Spectrum of Disease Project, United States 1982-1993

CLINICAL CATEGORY	MEAN TIME SPENT IN CATEGORY, MO(Y)	MEAN TIME TO DEVELOP CATEGORY C DISEASE, Y	% DEVELOPING CATEGORY C DISEASE WITHIN 5 YEARS (RANGE)	% SURVIVING AT LEAST FIVE YEARS (RANGE)	MEDIAN SURVIVAL, Y
N	10 (0.9)	6.6	50 (40-60)	75 (68-82)	8.0
A	4 (0.3)	5.7	58 (47-69)	67 (61-74)	7.1
B	65 (5.4)	5.4	60 (49-71)	65 (56-73)	6.8
C	34 (2.8)	—	—	17 (10-24)	1.9

Data from Barnhart HX, Caldwell MB, Thomas P, et al: Natural history of human immunodeficiency virus disease in perinatally infected children: An analysis from the Pediatric Spectrum of Disease Project. Pediatrics 1996;97:710–716.

Table 1-8
Trends in AIDS Diagnosis and Death in HIV-Infected Children Followed in 10 Medical Centers in New York City Between the Periods of 1991-1994 and 1995-1998

PARAMETER	PERIOD	
	1991–1994	1995–1998
Children newly diagnosed with AIDS, n	404	184
New AIDS conditions diagnosed (children can have more than one), n	751	371
Lymphoid interstitial pneumonitis, %	20	12
Pneumocystis carinii pneumonia, %	17	11
Mycobacterium avium-intracellulare, %	11	18
Wasting, %	10	12
Candida esophagitis, %	5	8
HIV encephalopathy, %	15	16
Recurrent bacterial infections, %	6	5
Mortality, %	11	6

Data from Peters V, Bornschlegel K, Brooks A, et al: Evidence for improved outcome in HIV-infected New York City children. The Second Global Conference for the Prevention of HIV Transmission from Mothers to Infants. Montreal, Canada, September 1–6, 1999 (abstract 205).

hospitalization, and use of antibiotics was seen in Italian infected children receiving protease inhibitor–containing therapy.[117] Data from 1500 infected children enrolled between 1995 and 1998 in a prospective long-term observational study, PACTG 219, indicate that the use of protease inhibitor–containing antiretroviral therapy increased from 0% prior to 1996 to 73% by 1999.[118] Coincident with the increase in the use of potent antiretroviral therapy, the mortality rate has declined from 5.3% in 1996 to 2.1% in 1997, 0.9% in 1998, and 0.7% in 1999; this has occurred in all age groups. Similarly, in New York City, overall mortality in infected children decreased from 11% in 1991–94 to 6% in 1995–98.[112]

Data comparing children who died in 1996 with those who died in 1990, prior to advances in HIV treatment, indicate that those who died in 1996 were older (9.2 versus 2.1 years, respectively), more immunosuppressed, had more organ system involvement, and were more likely to have received antiretroviral therapy (70% versus 33%) and prophylaxis against PCP (100% versus 27%) and MAI (100% versus 0%).[103] PCP was the primary cause of death in 53% of children who died in 1990 but none of those who died in 1996, when the primary causes of death were MAI and infection with *Pseudomonas aeruginosa*. Thus, as survival has increased over time and HIV infection has become more chronic, management of HIV disease has become more complex, with multisystem organ involvement.

However, as children live longer due to potent antiretroviral therapy, concerns about possible drug toxicity increase. Abnormal body fat distribution, lipodystrophy, hyperlipidemia, and insulin resistance have been reported in HIV-infected adults receiving protease inhibitors, along with diabetes mellitus, coronary artery disease, and possible accelerated atherosclerosis.[119] The implications of such toxicities are especially significant for infected children, who are beginning possible life-long therapy during early childhood. Data on the incidence of such toxicity in children are very limited, however. In a survey of 16 pediatric clinical trials units, 61% of children were receiving treatment with a protease inhibitor.[120] Abnormal body fat distribution was reported in 0.4% of children not receiving non-protease inhibitor therapy, compared with 1.5% of those receiving such therapy. Abnormalities in lipid profiles of children receiving protease inhibitor regimens have also begun to be described.[121,122]

Use of ZDV prophylaxis has significantly reduced the number of newly infected infants in the United States, although some children become infected despite maternal antiretroviral therapy. Few data exist on the natural history of HIV disease in children who have become infected despite ZDV prophylaxis. The Italian Register for HIV Infection in Children compared HIV disease progression in 38 children who became infected despite ZDV prophylaxis to that of 178 infected children of untreated women.[123] ZDV-exposed infected infants had a 1.8-fold increase in the risk of rapid clinical progression, a 2.4-fold increase of developing severe immune suppression, and a 1.9-fold increase in the risk of death in the 3 years following birth. No virologic data were available. In contrast, data from PACTG 076 found no difference in timing of HIV transmission, progression of clinical or immunologic disease, or levels of plasma HIV-1 RNA through age 18 months in infected infants in the ZDV group compared with the placebo group.[124] Additionally, no genotypic ZDV resistance developed in infected infants during the 6-week neonatal ZDV prophylaxis treatment period in infants with sequential viral isolates available. Further data are needed to better assess whether the course of HIV disease is favorably or negatively affected by antiretroviral prophylaxis of the mother and infant.

Developing Countries

Data on the natural history of HIV infection in developing countries are relatively sparse.

High maternal, infant, and child mortality rates existed in these countries prior to the HIV epidemic. Although significant improvements in infant and child survival in developing nations have been realized through safe motherhood initiatives, promotion of breastfeeding, childhood immunization, and oral rehydration programs, these gains are in danger of being reversed by HIV infection in women and children. Advances in the treatment of HIV disease and its complications taken for granted in the United States and other developed countries are generally not available in the developing world. As a result, progression of HIV disease in children in developing countries is more rapid than in developed countries.

Pregnancy Outcome

In contrast to the data from developed countries, most studies from developing countries have reported higher rates of adverse outcomes among HIV-infected compared with uninfected women. In a meta-analysis of 31 studies, 21 from developing countries, increased rates of spontaneous abortion or stillbirth, intrauterine growth retardation, low birth weight, and preterm delivery were observed among HIV-infected pregnant women, but these were primarily confined to studies from developing countries.[125] A higher incidence of confounding factors such as sexually transmitted diseases or vitamin deficiency in infected women from developing countries could account for higher rates of adverse outcomes. However, in a study of HIV-infected and uninfected women followed in an antenatal clinic in Rwanda, where screening and treatment for malaria and sexually transmitted diseases was performed monthly, premature birth was observed in 23% of infected versus 14% of uninfected women and low birth weight in 26% of infected versus 15% of uninfected women.[126] Thus, HIV infection itself appears to contribute to some adverse pregnancy outcomes in developing countries.

Mortality

Significantly higher perinatal and infant mortality rates in infants born to HIV-infected than in those born to uninfected women have been described in many studies from Africa.[127–131] In the previously mentioned meta-analysis, infants born to infected women had a 1.8-fold higher risk of perinatal death and a 3.7-fold higher risk of infant death than infants of uninfected women.[125] Preterm delivery and low birth weight induced by HIV disease or other factors may account for these early deaths. For example, increased infant mortality among HIV-infected women correlated with the degree of maternal vitamin A deficiency in a study in Malawi[132]; multivitamin supplementation of HIV-1–infected women during pregnancy has been shown to significantly decrease the risk of low birth weight, preterm delivery, and small for gestational age infants.[133,134] In another study in Malawi, infants born to women coinfected with HIV and malaria were 4.5 times more likely to die than infants born to women with malaria but not coinfected with HIV.[135] These factors could increase the risk of mortality regardless of the HIV infection status of the infant.

Rapidly progressive HIV infection may also be playing a significant role in early as well as late infant mortality, however. Early in the HIV epidemic, before the availability of HIV DNA polymerase chain reaction or RNA assays, discerning the contribution of infant HIV infection to these early infant deaths was difficult because diagnosis of infection was not possible. A more recent prospective study of the natural history of HIV infection in Haitian infants found that significantly more infected than uninfected infants died during the first 6 months of life.[136]

In contrast to developed countries, in developing countries the reported mortality rate has been as high as 29% during the first year of life and more than 60% by age 5 years (see Table 1–3). A bimodal risk of death has been described in infected children in developing as well as developed countries.[137] However, the proportion of children with rapid progression in developing countries and the mortality rate among the "slower progressors" appears higher than in developed countries. For example, the mean survival time for infected children in the United States in the Pediatric Spectrum of Disease Study was 9.4 years,[72] compared with 34.2 months in infected children in South Africa[138] and 12.4 months in Rwanda.[139]

In a study of 181 infants born to HIV-infected women in Durban, South Africa, the overall mortality rate was 35% among infected children, with 83% of deaths occurring prior to the age of 10 months and only 3 after the age of 12 months.[138] The mean age at symptom onset was younger in those who died compared with those who did not (3 vs 5 months), but both groups had early evidence of symptoms. Most children who died had low birth weight, failure to thrive, or marasmus at the time of death, and half had neurologic signs or developmental delay.

Mortality in children who were short-term survivors (alive at 1 year) was evaluated in 702 children born to HIV-infected women and uninfected women in Malawi; 83 died during follow-up.[140] HIV-infected children were nine times more likely to die than uninfected children. The mortality rate was 339 per 1000 person-years for infected children but similar in the uninfected children born to infected or uninfected women (46 versus 36 per 1000 person-years, respectively). Thirty percent of infected children died by the age of 24 months, and 45% by 36 months. All children with severe immunosuppression (CD4+ <15%) died by the age of 32 months.

Description of the specific causes of mortality in the developing world is incomplete because of infrequent autopsies and limited resources. The leading causes of death in HIV-infected children in these countries are similar to those in uninfected children and include diarrheal disease, failure to thrive or malnutrition, respiratory disease or pneumonia, and systemic infections (meningitis, sepsis). In Durban, South Africa, 71% of deaths in HIV-infected children were related to either diarrheal disease or respiratory infection or both, and the main presenting symptoms just before death were cough, diarrhea, and fever.[138] Similarly, in Malawi, diarrheal disease, respiratory infections, and failure to thrive were the most common causes of death.[140]

In an autopsy study of 78 HIV-infected and 77 HIV-uninfected children who died in Abidjan, Côte d'Ivoire, respiratory diseases were the predominant causes of death in HIV-infected children, and the causes were heterogeneous.[141,142] Interestingly, the prevalence of PCP was 31% in infected children under 15 months of age, similar to the frequency of PCP in infected children in developed countries. Compared with uninfected children, there was an increased prevalence of pulmonary disease associated with measles in infected children 15 months or older. Tuberculosis was found in only 1% of infected children.

Morbidity

The diagnosis of AIDS in children in developing countries is complicated by poor access to technologies needed to diagnose opportunistic infections, malignancies, and neurologic HIV disease, rendering the AIDS definition used in the United States of limited utility. The World Health Organization (WHO) developed a simpler clinical case definition based on clinical signs and symptoms for countries with limited laboratory facilities (Table 1–9). However, diseases that could be indicative of severe HIV infection are frequent in uninfected as well as infected children. In a study of children in Abidjan, Côte d'Ivoire, the specificity of the WHO AIDS definition was 98%, but the sensitivity was only 19% and the positive predictive value was 45%.[143]

The long-term natural history of HIV infection during the first 5 years of life was evaluated in a prospective study of children born to HIV-infected and uninfected women in Kigali, Rwanda.[139] All infected children presented with at least one nonspecific HIV-related condition during the first 13 months of life, and while most symptoms of HIV were nonspecific, they occurred earlier, occurred

Table 1–9
Modified World Health Organization Clinical Case Definition for Pediatric AIDS

Pediatric AIDS is suspected in a child presenting with at least two major signs associated with at least two minor signs in the absence of any known cause for immunosuppression:
Major signs
Weight loss or failure to thrive
Chronic diarrhea persisting for >1 month
Prolonged fever persisting for >1 month
Minor signs
Generalized lymphadenopathy
Oropharyngeal candidiasis
Repeated common infections
Generalized pruritic dermatitis
Confirmed maternal HIV infection

more frequently, and were more severe among infected infants. The most frequent clinical signs were chronic cough, failure to thrive, and generalized lymphadenopathy, which occurred in more than 90% of all infected children (Table 1–10). Clinical findings that were most specific for HIV infection were recurrent oral candidiasis and chronic parotitis. The cumulative probabilities for WHO-defined clinical AIDS at 1, 2, and 5 years of age were 17%, 28%, and 35%. Development of AIDS was more frequent in children who presented with failure to thrive or persistent generalized lymphadenopathy, and a higher mortality rate was associated with symptom onset before 6 months of age. The uninfected children of HIV-infected women did not differ from children born to uninfected women in morbidity, mortality, or use of health care services. Disease progression was more rapid in infected children from Haiti, where AIDS developed in 33% of 51 infected children by the age of 12 months and 84% by the age of 5 years (see Table 1–4).[144]

In a study of HIV-related disease in 4480 hospitalized children in Abidjan, Côte d'Ivoire, HIV seroprevalence was 8.2%.[143] As in the Rwandan study, the clinical presentations of HIV disease in these children resembled that of other common illnesses in African children. More than 80% of children, irrespective of age or HIV status, were diagnosed with six clinical syndromes—acute respiratory infection, malaria, malnutrition, meningitis, anemia, or diarrheal disease. The dominant diagnoses in hospitalized HIV-positive children were respiratory infection (26%) and malnutrition (26%), whereas the most common diagnoses for HIV-negative children were malaria (30%) and respiratory infection (19%). Overall mortality was 2.4-fold higher in hospitalized HIV-positive than HIV-negative children: 20.8% compared with 8.7%, respectively.

In the developing world, malnutrition and growth abnormalities are common in children in general, but these problems are compounded by HIV infection. In prospective studies in the Congo, Rwanda, and Malawi, early, severe, and sustained impairment in weight, height, and head circumference growth were observed among infected compared with uninfected children.[145-147] Low weight for age and low height for weight (stunting) were more common than low weight for height (wasting); development of wasting was associated with a history of severe and/or persistent infections. In multivariate analyses that included maternal clinical, immunologic, and sociodemographic factors, only infant HIV infection status and HIV symptoms were independently associated with growth retardation. Infants born to infected women had lower birth weight and height than infants born to uninfected women, but seroreverting children had rapid "catch up" growth and within several months

Table 1–10
Clinical Findings in 54 Children with Perinatal HIV Infection Compared with 347 Uninfected Children in Kigali, Rwanda

	FREQUENCY, %		MEDIAN AGE AT ONSET, MO		HAZARD RATIO
	Infected	Uninfected	Infected	Uninfected	(Infected/Uninfected)
Chronic cough	100	100	9.0	6.2	0.9
Failure to thrive	90	60	9.5	11.9	2.8
Lymphadenopathy	90	70	9.7	20.7	3.5
Hepatomegaly	80	20	11.9	15.0	6.6
Dermatitis	70	20	12.4	18.1	6.5
Chronic diarrhea	70	20	18.0	19.5	5.4
Severe pneumonia	70	30	14.9	17.7	3.0
Lymphoid interstitial pneumonitis	70	20	20.9	20.9	4.9
Splenomegaly	60	20	6.1	14.9	4.3
Oral candidiasis	50	5	11.8	9.0	12.7
Chronic fever	40	10	20.8	23.5	5.9
Parotitis	40	3	24.0	47.9	11.1

Data from Spira R, Lepage P, Msellati P, et al: Natural history of human immunodeficiency virus type 1 infection in children: A five-year prospective study in Rwanda. Pediatrics 1999;104:e56 (URL: *http://www.pediatrics.org/cgi/content/full/104/5/e56*).

had anthropomorphic characteristics similar to those of infants born to uninfected women.

Similar to studies in developed countries, frequent central nervous system involvement has been reported in infected African children. HIV-infected infants in Uganda and Rwanda demonstrated greater deficits in motor development and neurologic status and more frequent and earlier onset of motor and neurologic abnormalities compared with seroreverters and infants born to uninfected women.[148,149] At 6 months of age, 62% of Ugandan infants had an abnormal neurologic examination finding, 30% had motor abnormalities, and 26% had cognitive impairments, whereas seroreverters had similar neurodevelopmental findings to infants of uninfected women.[148]

Opportunistic Infections

The specific types of opportunistic infections seen in infected children may differ geographically depending on the prevalence of various infectious organisms in that region in general. For example, *Penicillium marneffei* is a dimorphic fungus that is an endemic pathogen in Southeast Asia, found in various species of bamboo rats as well as the soil. In northern Thailand, disseminated infection with *P. marneffei* is a common opportunistic infection in HIV-infected children and adults.[150] PCP, tuberculosis, malaria, measles, and diarrheal disease in developing countries are discussed in the following sections.

Pneumocystis carinii Pneumonia

Respiratory infections are a leading cause of death for infected children in developing countries, but assays to permit accurate diagnosis are not easily available. It had been thought that PCP was an infrequent cause of disease in Africa. However, more recent studies suggest that PCP may be common in children and adults in developing as well as developed countries.[142,143,151–153] In South Africa, postmortem lung biopsies were examined on 36 HIV-infected and 36 uninfected children who died of severe pneumonia.[152] *P. carinii* and cytomegalovirus were the most frequently detected organisms in HIV-infected children, found in 16 children each; in comparison, none of the uninfected children had *P. carinii* and only 4 had cytomegalovirus. In an autopsy study in Abidjan, Côte d'Ivoire, *P. carinii* was diagnosed in 31% of HIV-infected children younger than 15 months of age, compared with only 3% of infected adults.[142,143] In another necropsy study in Zimbabwe, *P. carinii* was found in 16% of all infected children and cytomegalovirus in 7%, with the vast majority of cases found in children younger than 6 months of age; many of these patients had bacterial coinfection.[154]

Pneumocystis carinii pneumonia has also been reported in children in Asia. In a study of 279 hospitalized HIV-infected children in Bangkok, Thailand, pneumonia accounted for 46% of all hospitalizations.[155] Twenty percent of children with pneumonia had severe disease, and 35% of those with severe pneumonia were diagnosed with PCP; a bacterial cause was seen in the other cases and bacterial coinfection was seen in 33% of children with PCP. Children with PCP were significantly younger than those with non-PCP pneumonia; 44% were younger than 6 months of age. Following change in PCP prophylaxis guidelines in June 1996, from use only in symptomatic infected children to prophylaxis in all HIV-exposed infants from 1 to 6 months of age, the number of PCP cases decreased from 9 in 1996 to 0 in 1997.[155] Additionally, the rate of severe pneumonia decreased from 16% to 7%, suggesting a potential benefit of PCP prophylaxis against bacterial pneumonia. A recent study of trimethoprim-sulfamethoxazole prophylaxis of infected adults in Abidjan showed a significant decrease in clinically severe infections, primarily bacterial infections, with prophylaxis.[156] These data indicate that PCP may be a common cause of serious respiratory disease in young HIV-infected infants in developing countries, and that prophylaxis might be explored as an inexpensive and effective strategy to decrease morbidity and mortality of HIV disease in children in these countries.

Tuberculosis

In many areas of the developing world where the HIV epidemic is flourishing, infection with *Mycobacterium tuberculosis* (TB) is endemic. The impact of these overlapping epidemics in resource-poor countries is a major public health concern. TB has become a frequent opportunistic infection among infected adults in these communities and is increasing among HIV-infected children. A major impediment to defining the problem of HIV-TB coinfection in children in the developing world has been problems with TB diagnosis in young children due to their inability to produce adequate sputum samples and the absence of sensitive tests to provide an alternative to culture. Additionally, HIV-infected children are often anergic, making tuberculin skin testing less useful for diagnosis.[157–159] As a consequence, in many pediatric studies, TB diagnosis is based on epidemiologic, clinical, and radiologic findings without mycobacteriologic confirmation.

Most pediatric studies have evaluated the prevalence of HIV infection among children already diagnosed with TB. In the Dominican Republic, HIV prevalence was 5.8% among children with TB.[160] In Lusaka, Zambia, HIV seroprevalence in children hospitalized with newly diagnosed TB increased from 24% in 1989 to 37% in 1990, 57% in 1991, and 69% in 1992, while HIV seroprevalence among children hospitalized with other diagnoses was stable at 10% to 11% between 1990 and 1992.[161, 162] HIV prevalence was highest among the youngest children with TB, ranging from 79% to 81% in children younger than 18 months, 50% to 64% in children 19 months to 9 years, and 19% in children 10 to 14 years old.[162] The clinical presentation of TB was similar in infected and uninfected children, with the predominant clinical site of disease being pulmonary in both groups. However, HIV-infected children were slightly more likely to have miliary or lymphadenopathic disease than uninfected children. The mortality rate was 24% among HIV-TB coinfected children, compared with no deaths in children with TB without HIV infection. In a similar study in Abidjan, Côte d'Ivoire, HIV-1 seroprevalence among children with TB rose from 11% in 1989–90 to 19% in 1994–95, and the mortality rate in HIV-TB coinfected children was 23%, 3.6 fold higher than in children without HIV.[159, 163]

Adverse drug reactions to anti-TB therapy were more common among infected than uninfected children.[159,160,162,164] Dermatologic reactions were most common and included several fatal cases of Stevens-Johnson syndrome.[161,162,164] HIV-infected children were more likely to fail standard TB treatment than uninfected children in most studies.

These data do not address the prevalence and incidence of TB in HIV-infected children. Although the prevalence of HIV in children with already diagnosed TB in Abidjan was 19%, among hospitalized HIV-infected children, the prevalence of TB was 1.9% overall, with an age-specific prevalence of 0.7% at less than 15 months of age, 1.7% at 15 to 59 months, and 5.6% in children 5 years of age or older.[143] The comparatively low prevalence of TB among infected children is consistent with an autopsy study in Abidjan, where TB was found in only 1% of HIV-infected children who died.[141,142] Similarly, in an autopsy study in Zimbabwe, TB was present at death in 4% of 184 HIV-infected children examined. In contrast, in cohorts of infected children in Haiti, Zambia, and South Africa, 10% to 25% of HIV-infected children developed TB during follow-up.[144,164,165] These differences could reflect differences in the prevalence of TB in the populations in the countries or under-recognition of TB due to diagnostic difficulties in pediatric patients.

Malaria

Similar to TB, malaria is endemic in many developing nations. However, prospective studies have not reported a significant increase in malarial episodes among HIV-infected compared with uninfected infants.[166–168] In a large study of children born to HIV-infected and uninfected women in Zaire, no significant differences were found in the incidence, severity, and response to therapy between HIV-infected children and seronegative control subjects.[168] Similar data were reported from Malawi.[167] In a study in Uganda, the incidence of malaria among infected children (3.5 episodes per 100 child-months) was actually lower than in uninfected children (5.0 per 100 child-months in seroreverters and 5.5 in children of uninfected women).[166] While the level of parasitemia did not differ between infected and uninfected children, infected children in Uganda had more severe malaria, as evidenced by more frequent hospitalizations and blood transfusions than uninfected children; these findings suggest that while episodes were not more frequent, HIV-infected children may have had difficulty in clearing the parasitemia, leading to more complications.[167]

Measles

Measles is a significant cause of death of children in the developing world. In an autopsy study in Côte d'Ivoire, measles giant cell pneumonia was found in 19% of HIV-infected children older than 15 months of age compared with 4% of uninfected children.[141] A study in Nairobi found that the risk of acquiring measles prior to vaccination at the age of 9 months was 3.8 times higher in infants born to HIV-infected women than in those born to uninfected women.[169] The morbidity and mortality rates of early measles were considerable in these children, regardless of HIV infection status. Low levels of anti-measles antibody were found in cord blood of three of seven HIV-exposed infants who developed measles, suggesting that their HIV-infected mothers may have had reduced levels of circulating antibodies or a defect in placental transfer of IgG. Consistent with this, a study in Brazil found that neonatal antibody titers to measles, tetanus toxoid, and *Streptococcus pneumoniae* were significantly lower in infants born to HIV-infected than in those born to uninfected women.[170] These findings suggest that infants born to infected women may be more susceptible to measles regardless of the infants' HIV infection status, and that an earlier schedule of measles immunization may be needed for these children in developing countries.

Diarrheal Disease

Chronic diarrhea is a common problem in developing countries in children, regardless of HIV infection status, but appears to be more frequent in infected children and is a significant contributor to mortality. In studies in Tanzania and Zambia, 25% to 40% of children admitted to the hospital for diarrhea were found to be HIV-infected.[171, 172] Diarrhea-causing parasites were detected in approximately 40% to 50% of infected children with chronic diarrhea, while in the remainder of children the cause remained unidentified. In Zaire, the incidence of acute diarrhea was 170 per 100 child-years in infected infants compared with 100 per 100 child-years in uninfected infants, and the incidence of persistent diarrhea was 19 per 100 child-years in infected infants compared with 4 per 100 child-years in uninfected infants.[173] Diarrhea was the leading cause of death for all infants, accounting for 36% of deaths, and HIV-infected infants had an 11-fold increased risk of death from diarrhea compared with uninfected children. Interestingly, the incidence of persistent diarrhea in uninfected infants of seropositive mothers was nearly double that of uninfected infants of seronegative mothers (4.9 vs 2.7 episodes per 100 child-years). This risk increased if the mother was symptomatic or died, suggesting that it was related to her ability to care for her infant and maintain infant hygiene and nutrition.

SUMMARY

Marked changes in the epidemiology of pediatric HIV/AIDS have been seen in the last 5 years in the United States and other developed countries with increasing use of ZDV prophylaxis. However, these benefits have not yet been extended to developing countries. With the availability of simple and less expensive interventions that could reduce perinatal transmission in developing countries, the next decade offers the opportunity to significantly affect perinatal transmission in these countries as well. New potent antiretroviral therapies and the use of prophylaxis against opportunistic infections has dramatically modified the natural history of pediatric HIV disease in developed countries. Although the use of expensive and complex antiretroviral regimens may not be immediately possible in developing countries with limited resources, implementation of more inexpensive interventions, including nutritional supplementation,[174] immunization, and prophylaxis against common opportunistic infections, such as PCP and bacterial infections, could improve the quality and duration of life for infected children in these countries.[175]

REFERENCES

1. Joint United Nations Programme on HIV/AIDS: AIDS epidemic update: 2002. Geneva, World Health Organization, 2002.
2. Davis SF, Rosen DH, Steinberg S, et al: Trends in HIV prevalence among childbearing women in the United States, 1989–1994. JAIDS 1998; 19:158–164.
3. Connor EM, Sperling RS, Gelber R, et al: Reduction of maternal-infant transmission of human immunodeficiency virus type 1 with zidovudine treatment. N Engl J Med 1994; 331:1173–1180.
4. Fiscus SA, Adimora A, Schoenbach VJ, et al: Trends in human immunodeficiency virus (HIV) counseling, testing and antiretroviral treatment of HIV-infected women and perinatal transmission in North Carolina. J Infect Dis 1999; 180:99–105.
5. Wade NA, Birkhead GS, Warren BL, et al: Abbreviated regimens of zidovudine prophylaxis and perinatal transmission of the human immunodeficiency virus. N Engl J Med 1998; 339:1409–1414.
6. Mayaux M-J, Teglas J-P, Mandelbrot L, et al: Acceptability and impact of zidovudine for prevention of mother-to-child human immunodeficiency virus transmission in France. J Pediatr 1997; 131:857–862.
7. The European Mode of Delivery Collaboration: Elective cesarean-section versus vaginal delivery in prevention of vertical HIV-1 transmission: A randomised clinical trial. Lancet 1999; 353:1035–1039.
8. The International Perinatal HIV Group: The mode of delivery and the risk of vertical transmission of human immunodeficiency virus type 1: A meta-analysis of 15 prospective cohort studies. N Engl J Med 1999; 340:977–987.
9. Cooper E, Charuvat M, Mofenson L, et al: Effectiveness of potent antiretroviral therapies on reducing perinatal transmission of HIV-1. JAIDS 2002; 29:484–494.
10. Guay LA, Musoke P, Fleming T, et al: Intrapartum and neonatal single-dose nevirapine compared with zidovudine for prevention of mother-to-child transmission of HIV-1 in Kampala, Uganda: HIVNET 012 randomised trial. Lancet 1999; 354:795–802.
11. Shaffer N, Chuachoowong R, Mock PA, et al: Short-course zidovudine for perinatal HIV-1 transmission in Bangkok, Thailand: A randomised controlled trial. Lancet 1999; 353:773–780.
12. Wiktor SZ, Ekpini E, Karon JM, et al: Short-course oral zidovudine for prevention of mother-to-child

12. transmission of HIV-1 in Abidjan, Cote d'Ivoire: A randomised trial. Lancet 1999; 353:781–785.
13. Dabis F, Msellati P, Meda N, et al: 6-month efficacy, tolerance, and acceptability of a short regimen of oral zidovudine to reduce vertical transmission of HIV in breastfed children in Cote d'Ivoire and Burkina Faso: A double-blind placebo-controlled multicentre trial. Lancet 1999; 353:786–792.
14. The Petra Study Team: Efficacy of three short-course regimens of zidovudine and lamivudine in preventing early and late transmission of HIV-1 from mother to child in Tanzania, South Africa, and Uganda (Petra Study): a randomized, double-blind placebo-controlled trial. Lancet 2002; 359:1178–1186.
15. Leroy V, Kavon JM, Alioum A, et al: Twenty-four month efficacy of a national short-course zidovudine regimen to prevent mother-to-child transmission of HIV-1 in West Africa. AIDS 2002;16:631–641.
16. Schwartlander B, Stanecki KA, Brown T, et al: Country-specific estimates and models of HIV and AIDS: Methods and limitations. AIDS 1999; 13:2445–2448.
17. Mofenson LM: Mother-child HIV-1 transmission. Obstet Gynecol Clin North Am 1997; 24:759–784.
18. Mofenson LM, Lambert JS, Stiehm ER, et al: Risk factors for perinatal transmission of human immunodeficiency virus type 1 in women treated with zidovudine. N Engl J Med 1999; 341:385–393.
19. Shaffer N, Roonpisuthipong A, Siriwasin W, et al: Maternal virus load and perinatal human immunodeficiency virus type 1 subtype E transmission, Thailand. J Infect Dis 1999; 179:590–599.
20. Katzenstein DA, Mbizvo M, Zijenah L, et al: Serum level of maternal human immunodeficiency virus (HIV) RNA, infant mortality, and vertical transmission of HIV in Zimbabwe. J Infect Dis 1999; 179:1382–1387.
21. Chuachoowong R, Shaffer N, Siriwasin W, et al: Short-course antenatal zidovudine reduces both cervicovaginal human immunodeficiency virus type 1 RNA levels and risk of perinatal transmission. J Infect Dis 2000; 181:99–106.
22. Expert Group of the Joint United Nations Programme on HIV/AIDS: Implications of HIV variability for transmission: Scientific and policy issues. AIDS 1997; 11:1–15.
23. Tscherning C, Alaeus A, Fredriksson R, et al: Differences in chemokine usage between genetic subtypes of HIV-1. Virol 1998; 241:181–188.
24. Hu DJ, Buve A, Baggs J, et al: What role does HIV-1 subtype play in transmission and pathogenesis? An epidemiological perspective. AIDS 1999;13:873–881.
25. Centers for Disease Control and Prevention: U.S. HIV and AIDS cases reported through December 2000. HIV/AIDS Surveillance Report 2001; 12:1–47.
26. Wortley PM, Fleming PL: AIDS in women in the United States: Recent trends. JAMA 1997; 278:911–916.
27. Chirgwin KD, Feldman J, Dehovitz JA, et al: Incidence and risk factors for heterosexually acquired HIV in an inner city cohort of women: Temporal association with pregnancy. JAIDS 1999; 20:295–299.
28. Gilson L, Mkanje R, Grosskurth H, et al: Cost-effectiveness of improved treatment services for sexually transmitted diseases in preventing HIV-1 infection in Mwanza Region, Tanzania. Lancet 1997; 350:1805–1809.
29. Wasser SC, Gwinn M, Fleming P: Urban-nonurban distribution of HIV infection in childbearing women in the United States. JAIDS 1993;6:1035–1042.
30. UNAIDS: Report on the global HIV/AIDS epidemic June 1998. Geneva, World Health Organization, 1999.
31. Franceschi S, Dal Maso L, Serraino D, et al: Increasing incidence of AIDS among women. JAMA 1998; 279:354–355.
32. Law MG, Downs AM, Brunet J-B, Kaldor JM: Time trends for HIV infection among pregnant women in Europe. AIDS 1998; 12:211–216.
33. Quinn TC: Global burden of the HIV pandemic. Lancet 1996; 348:99–106.
34. Gomez MP, Bain RM, Major C, et al: Characteristics of HIV-infected pregnant women in the Bahamas. JAIDS 1996; 12:400–405.
35. Wilkinson D, Connolly C, Rotchfor K: Continued explosive rise in HIV prevalence among pregnant women in rural Southern Africa. AIDS 1999; 13:740.
36. Taha TE, Dallabetta GA, Hoover DR, et al: Trends of HIV-1 and sexually transmitted diseases among pregnant and postpartum women in urban Malawi. AIDS 1998; 12:197–203.
37. Fylkesnes K, Musonda RM, Kasumba K, et al: The HIV epidemic in Zambia: Socio-demographic prevalence patterns and indications of trends among childbearing women. AIDS 1997; 11:339–345.
38. Jackson DJ, Ngugi EN, Plummer FA, et al: Stable antenatal HIV-1 seroprevalence with high population mobility and marked seroprevalence variation among sentinel sites within Nairobi, Kenya. AIDS 1999; 13:583–589.
39. Gangakhedkar RR, Bentley ME, Divekar AD, et al: Spread of HIV infection in married monogamous women in India. JAMA 1997; 278:2090–2092.
40. Siriwasin W, Shaffer N, Roonpisuthipong A, et al: HIV prevalence, risk and partner serodiscordance among pregnant women in Bangkok. JAMA 1998; 280:49–54.
41. Patrascu IV, Dumitrescu O: The epidemic of human immunodeficiency virus infection in Romanian children. AIDS Res Human Retroviruses 1993; 9:99–104.
42. Mintz M, Boland M, O'Hara M-J, et al: Pediatric HIV infection in Elista, Russia: Interventional strategies. Am J Public Health 1995; 85:586–588.

43. Lindegren ML, Byers RH, Thomas P, et al: Trends in perinatal transmission of HIV/AIDS in the United States. JAMA 1999; 282:531–538.
44. Cooper ER, Nugent RP, Diaz C, et al: After AIDS Clinical Trials Group 076: The changing patterns of zidovudine use during pregnancy, and the subsequent reduction in the vertical transmission of human immunodeficiency virus. J Infect Dis 1996; 174:1207–1211.
45. Pinto J, Chaves M, Carvalho I, et al: Impact of zidovudine use on the perinatal tranmission rates of HIV in Belo Horizonte, Brazil. Paper presented at the Second Conference on Global Strategies for the Prevention of HIV Transmission from Mothers to Infants, Sept 1–6, 1999, Montreal, Canada (abstract 369).
46. Read SE, Gomez MP, Bain RM, et al: Prevention of HIV transmission from mothers to babies in the Bahamas: Lessons learned from application of a strategy based on ACTG 076. Paper presented at the Second Conference on Global Strategies for the Prevention of HIV Transmission from Mothers to Infants, Sept 1–6, 1999, Montreal, Canada (abstract 372).
47. Valleroy LA, MacKellar DA, Karon JM, et al: HIV infection in disadvantaged out-of-school youth: Prevalence for U.S. Job Corps entrants, 1990 through 1996. JAIDS 1998; 19:67–73.
48. Mofenson LM: Can perinatal HIV infection be eliminated in the United States? JAMA 1999; 282:577–579.
49. Centers for Disease Control and Prevention: Success in implementing Public Health Service guidelines to reduce perinatal tranmission of HIV: Louisiana, Michigan, New Jersey and South Carolina, 1993, 1995 and 1996. MMWR 1998; 47:688–691.
50. Centers for Disease Control and Prevention: Public Health Service Task Force recommendations for use of antiretroviral drugs in pregnant women infected with HIV-1 for maternal health and for reducing perinatal HIV-1 transmission in the United States. MMWR 1998; 47:1–30.
51. Centers for Disease Control and Prevention: U.S. Public Health Service recommendations for human immunodeficiency virus counseling and voluntary testing for pregnant women. MMWR 1995; 44:1–15.
52. Institute of Medicine, National Research Council: Reducing the Odds: Preventing Perinatal Transmission of HIV in the United States. Washington D.C., National Academy Press, 1999.
53. Sperling RS, Shapiro DE, McSherry GD, et al: Safety of the maternal-infant zidovudine regimen utilized in the Pediatric AIDS Clinical Trials Group 076 Study. AIDS 1998; 12:1805–1813.
54. Culnane M, Fowler MG, Lee SS, et al: Lack of long-term effects of in utero exposure to zidovudine among uninfected children born to HIV-infected women. JAMA 1999; 281:151–157.
55. Hanson IC, Antonelli TA, Sperling RS, et al: Lack of tumors in infants with perinatal HIV type 1 exposure and fetal/neonatal exposure to zidovudine. JAIDS 1999; 20:463–467.
56. Olivero OA, Anderson LM, Diwan BA, et al: Transplacental effect of 3'-azido-2',3'-dideoxythymidine (AZT): Tumorigenicity in mice and genotoxicity in mice and monkeys. J Natl Cancer Inst 1997; 89:1602–1608.
57. Blanche S, Tardieu M, Rustin P, et al: Persistent mitochondrial dysfunction and perinatal exposure to antiretroviral nucleoside analogues. Lancet 1999; 354:1084–1089.
58. The Working Group on Mother-to-Child Transmission of HIV-1 in Africa, America, and Europe: Results from 13 perinatal studies. JAIDS 1995; 8:506–510.
59. Dunn DT, Newell ML, Ades AE, Peckham CS: Risk of human immunodeficiency virus type 1 transmission through breastfeeding. Lancet 1992; 340:585–588.
60. Lewis P, Nduati R, Kreiss JK, et al: Cell-free human immunodeficiency virus type 1 in breast milk. J Infect Dis 1998; 177:34–39.
61. Leroy V, Newell ML, Dabis F, et al: International multicentre pooled analysis of late postnatal mother-to-child transmission of HIV-1. Lancet 1998; 352:597–600.
62. Miotti PG, Taha TET, Kumwenda NI, et al: HIV transmission through breastfeeding: A study in Malawi. JAMA 1999; 282:744–749.
63. Semba RD, Kumwenda N, Hoover DR, et al: Human immunodeficiency virus load in breast milk, mastitis, and mother-to-child transmission of human immunodeficiency virus type 1. J Infect Dis 1999; 180:93–98.
64. Coutsoudis A, Pillay K, Spooner E, et al: Influence of infant feeding patterns on early mother-to-child transmission of HIV-1 in Durban, South Africa: A prospective cohort study. Lancet 1999; 354:471–476.
65. Tess BH, Rodriguez LC, Newell M-L, et al: Infant feeding and risk of mother-to-child transmission of HIV-1 in Sao Paulo State, Brazil. JAIDS 1998; 19:189–194.
66. Greenberg AE, Nguyen-Dinh P, Mann JM, et al: The association between malaria, blood transfusions, and HIV seropositivity in a pediatric population in Kinshasa, Zaire. JAMA 1988; 259:545–549.
67. Mann JM, Francis H, Davachi F, et al: Human immunodeficiency virus seroprevalence in pediatric patients 2 to 14 years of age at Mama Yemo Hospital, Kinshasa, Zaire. Pediatrics 1986; 78:637.
68. Schacker TW, Hughes JP, Shea T, et al: Biological and virological characteristics of primary HIV infection. Ann Intern Med 1998; 128:613–620.
69. Shearer WT, Quinn TC, LaRussa P, et al: Viral load and disease progression in infants infected with human immunodeficiency virus type 1. N Engl J Med 1997; 336:1337–1342.
70. Abrams EJ, Weedon J, Steketee RW, et al: Association of human immunodeficiency virus (HIV) load early in life with disease progression among HIV-infected infants. J Infect Dis 1998; 178:101–108.

71. Longini IM, Clark WS, Byers RH, et al: Statistical analysis of the stages of HIV infection using a Markov model. Stat Med 1989; 8:831–843.
72. Barnhardt HX, Caldwell MB, Thomas P, et al: Natural history of human immunodeficiency virus disease in perinatally infected children: An analysis from the Pediatric Spectrum of Disease Project. Pediatrics 1996; 97:710–716.
73. Downs AM, Salamina G, Ancelle-Park RA: Incubation of vertically acquired AIDS in Europe before widespread use of prophylactic therapies. JAIDS 1995; 9:297–304.
74. Minkoff HL, Henderson C, Mendez H, et al: Pregnancy outcomes among mothers infected with human immunodeficiency virus and uninfected control subjects. Am J Obstet Gynecol 1990; 163:1598–1604.
75. Alger LS, Farley JJ, Robinson BA, et al: Interactions of human immunodeficiency virus infection and pregnancy. Obstet Gynecol 1993; 82:787–796.
76. Spinillo A, Iasci A, Dal Maso J, et al: The effect of fetal infection with human immunodeficiency virus type 1 on birthweight and length of gestation. Eur J Obstet Gynecol 1995; 57:13–17.
77. Johnstone FD, Raab GM, Hamilton BA: The effects of human immunodeficiency virus infection and drug use on birth characteristics. Obstet Gynecol 1996; 88:321–326.
78. Stratton P, Tuomala RE, Abboud R, et al: Obstetric and newborn outcomes in a cohort of HIV-infected pregnant women: A report from the Women and Infants Transmission Study. JAIDS 1999; 20:179–180.
79. Martin R, Boyer P, Hammill H, et al: Incidence of premature birth and neonatal respiratory disease in infants of HIV-positive mothers. J Pediatr 1997; 131:851–856.
80. Markson LE, Turner BJ, Houchens R, et al: Association of maternal HIV infection with low birth weight. JAIDS 1996; 13:227–234.
81. Chandwani S, Greco MA, Mittal K, et al: Pathology and human immunodeficiency virus expression in placentas of seropositive women. J Infect Dis 1991; 163:1134–1138.
82. Lee B-N, Ordonez N, Popek E, et al: Inflammatory cytokine expression is correlated with the level of human immunodeficiency virus (HIV) transcripts in HIV-infected placental trophoblastic cells. J Virol 1997; 71:3628–3635.
83. The European Collaborative Study: Is zidovudine therapy in pregnant HIV-infected women associated with gestational age and birthweight? AIDS 1998; 13:119–124.
84. Lorenzi P, Spicher VM, Laubereau B, et al: Antiretroviral therapies in pregnancy: Maternal, fetal and neonatal effects. AIDS 1998; 12:F241–F247.
85. Shapiro D, Tuomala R, Samelson R, et al: Antepartum antiretroviral therapy and pregnancy outcomes in 462 HIV-infected women in 1998–1999 (PACTG 367). Paper presented at the Seventh Conference on Retroviruses and Opportunistic Infections. Jan 30–Feb 2, 2000, San Francisco, California.
86. Scott GB, Hutto C, Makuch RW, et al: Survival of children with perinatally acquired human immunodeficiency virus type 1 infection. N Engl J Med 1989; 321:1791–1796.
87. Krasinski K, Borkowsky W, Holzman RS: Prognosis of human immunodeficiency virus infection in children and adolescents. Pediatr Infect Dis J 1989; 8:216–220.
88. Blanche S, Tardieu M, Duliege A-M, et al: Longitudinal study of 94 symptomatic infants with perinatally acquired human immunodeficiency virus infection: Evidence for bimodal expression of clinical and biological symptoms. Am J Dis Child 1990; 144:1210–1215.
89. The French Pediatric HIV Infection Study Group and European Collaborative Study: Morbidity and mortality in European children vertically infected by HIV-1. JAIDS 1997; 14:442–450
90. The European Collaborative Study: Natural history of vertically acquired human immunodeficiency virus-1 infection. Pediatrics 1994; 94:815–819.
91. Tovo PA, de Martino M, Gabiano C, et al: Prognostic factors and survival in children with perinatal HIV-1 infection. Lancet 1992; 339:1249–1253.
92. Diaz C, Hanson C, Cooper ER, et al: Disease progression in a cohort of infants with vertically acquired HIV infection observed from birth: The Women and Infants Transmission Study (WITS). JAIDS 1998; 18:221–228.
93. Italian Register for HIV Infection in Children: Features of children perinatally-infected with HIV-1 surviving longer than 5 years. Lancet 1994; 343:191–195.
94. Galli L, de Martino M, Tovo P-A, et al: Onset of clinical symptoms in children with HIV-1 perinatal infection. AIDS 1995; 9:455–461.
95. Blanche S, Mayaux M-J, Rouzioux C, et al: Relation of the course of HIV infection in children to the severity of the disease in their mothers at delivery. N Engl J Med 1994; 330:308–312.
96. Mayaux M-J, Burgard M, Teglas J-P, et al: Neonatal characteristics in rapidly progressive perinatally acquired HIV-1 disease. JAMA 1996; 275:606–610.
97. Misrahi M, Teglas J-P, N'Go N, et al: CCR5 chemokine receptor variant in HIV-1 mother-to-child transmission and disease progression in children. JAMA 1998; 279:277–280.
98. Rich K, Fowler MG, Mofenson LM, et al: Maternal and infant factors predicting disease progression in human immunodeficiency virus type 1-infected infants. Pediatrics 2000; 105:e8 (URL: http://www.pediatrics.org/cgi/contents/full/105/1/e8).
99. Persaud D, Chandwani S, Rigaud M: Delayed recognition of human immunodeficiency virus infection in preadolescent children. Pediatrics 1992; 90:688–689.

100. Grubman S, Gross E, Lerner-Weiss N, et al: Older children and adolescents living with perinatally acquired human immunodeficiency virus infection. Pediatrics 1995; 95:657–663.
101. Kline MW, Paul ME, Bohannon B, et al: Characteristics of children surviving to 5 years of age or older with vertically acquired HIV infection. Pediatr AIDS HIV Infect Fetus Adolesc 1995; 6:350–353.
102. Nielsen K, McSherry G, Petru A, et al: A descriptive survey of pediatric human immunodeficiency virus-infected long-term survivors. Pediatrics 1997; 99:e4 (URL: *http://www.pediatrics.org/cgi/content/full/99/4/e4*).
103. Johann-Liang R, Cervia JS, Noel GJ: Characteristics of human immunodeficiency virus-infected children at the time of death: An experience in the 1990s. Pediatr Infect Dis J 1997;16:1145–1150.
104. Bamji M, Thea DM, Weedon J, et al: Prospective study of human immunodeficiency virus 1-related disease among 512 infants born to infected women in New York City. Pediatr Infect Dis J 1996;15:891–898.
105. Forsyth BW, Andiman WA, O'Connor T: Development of a prognosis-based clinical staging system for infants infected with human immunodeficiency virus. J Pediatr 1996; 129:648–655.
106. Centers for Disease Control and Prevention: 1994 revised classification system for human immunodeficiency virus infection in children less than 13 years of age. MMWR 1994; 43 (RR-12):1–10.
107. De Martino M, Zappa M, Galli L, et al: Does the classification system fit disease progression in perinatal human immunodeficiency virus infection? Acta Paediatr 1996; 85:724–727.
108. Simonds RJ, Oxtoby MJ, Caldwell B, et al: *Pneumocystis carinii* pneumonia among U.S. children with perinatally acquired HIV infection. JAMA 1993; 270:470–473.
109. Centers for Disease Control and Prevention: 1995 revised guidelines for prophylaxis against *Pneumocystis carinii* pneumonia for children infected with or perinatally exposed to human immunodeficiency virus. MMWR 1995; 44(RR-4):1–11.
110. Thea DM, Lambert G, Weedon J, et al: Benefit of primary prophylaxis before 18 months of age in reducing the incidence of *Pneumocystis carinii* pneumonia and early death in a cohort of 112 human immunodeficiency virus-infected infants. Pediatrics 1996; 97:59–64.
111. Rigaud M, Pollack H, Leibovitz E, et al: Efficacy of primary chemoprophylaxis against *Pneumocystis carinii* pneumonia during the first year of life in infants infected with human immunodeficiency virus type 1. J Pediatr 1994; 125:476–480.
112. Peters V, Bornschlegel K, Brooks A, et al: Evidence for improved outcome in HIV-infected New York City children. Paper presented at the Second Global Conference for the Prevention of HIV Transmission from Mothers to Infants. Sept 1–6, 1999, Montreal, Canada (abstract 205).
113. Working Group on Antiretroviral Therapy: Antiretroviral therapy and medical management of the human immunodeficiency virus-infected child. Pediatr Infect Dis J 1993; 12:513–522.
114. Centers for Disease Control and Prevention: Guidelines for the use of antiretroviral agents in pediatric HIV infection. MMWR 1998; 47(RR-4):1–43.
115. Moore RE, Chaisson RE: Natural history of HIV infection in the era of combination antiretroviral therapy. AIDS 1999; 13:1933–1942.
116. Vittinghoff E, Scheer S, O'Malley P, et al: Combination antiretroviral therapy and recent declines in AIDS incidence and mortality. J Infect Dis 1999; 179:717–720.
117. Canai RB, Spagnuolo M, Cirillo P, et al: Decreased needs for hospital care and antibiotics in children with advanced HIV-1 disease after protease inhibitor-containing combination therapy. AIDS 1999; 13:1005–1006.
118. Gortmaker S, Hughes M, Cervia J, et al: Effect of combination therapy including protease inhibitors on mortality among children and adolescents infected with HIV-1. N Engl J Med 2001; 345:1522–1528.
119. Wanke CA: Epidemiological and clinical aspects of the metabolic complications of HIV infection: The fat redistribution syndrome. AIDS 1999; 13; 1287–1293.
120. Babl FE, Regan AM, Pelton SI: Abnormal body-fat distribution in HIV-1-infected children on antiretrovirals. Lancet 1999; 353:1243–1244.
121. Jaquet D, Levine M, Ortega-Rodriguez E, et al: Clinical and metabolic presentation of the lipodystrophic syndrome in HIV-infected children. AIDS 2000; 14:2123-2128.
122. Brambilla P, Bricalli D, Sala N, et al: Highly active antiretroviral-treated HIV-infected children show fat distribution changes even in absence of lipodystrophy. AIDS 2001; 15:2415–2422.
123. The Italian Register for HIV Infection in Children: Rapid disease progression in HIV-1 perinatally infected children born to mothers receiving zidovudine monotherapy during pregnancy. AIDS 1999; 13:927–933.
124. McSherry GD, Shapiro DE, Coombs RW, et al: The effects of zidovudine in the subset of infants infected with human immunodeficiency virus type 1 (Pediatric AIDS Clinical Trials Group Protocol 076). J Pediatr 1999; 134:717–724.
125. Brocklehurst P, French R: The association between maternal HIV infection and perinatal outcome: A systematic review of the literature and meta-analysis. Br J Obstet Gynecol 1998; 105:836–848.
126. Leroy V, Ladner J, Nyiraziraje M, et al: Effect of HIV-1 infection on pregnancy outcome in women in Kigali, Rwanda, 1992–1994. AIDS 1998; 12:643–650.

127. Taha TE, Kumwenda NI, Broadhead RL, et al: Mortality after the first year of life among human immunodeficiency virus type 1-infected and uninfected children. Pediatr Infect Dis J 1999; 18:689–694.
128. Ryder RW, Nsuami M, Nsa W, et al: Mortality in HIV-1-seropositive women, their spouses and their newly born children during 36 months of follow-up in Kinshasa, Zaire. AIDS 1994; 8:667–672.
129. Lallemant M, Lallemant S, Cheynier D, et al: Mother-child transmission of HIV-1 and infant survival in Brazzaville, Congo. AIDS 1989; 3:643–646.
130. Mmiro F, Ndugwa C, Guay L, et al: Effect of human immunodeficiency virus-1 infection on the outcome of pregnancy in Ugandan women. Pediatr AIDS HIV Infect Fetus Adolesc 1993; 4:67–73.
131. Aiken CGA: HIV-1 infection and perinatal mortality in Zimbabwe. Arch Dis Child 1992; 67:595–599.
132. Semba RD, Miotti PG, Chiphangwi JF, et al: Infant mortality and maternal vitamin A deficiency during human immunodeficiency virus infection. Clin Infect Dis 1995; 21:966–972.
133. Fawzi WW, Msamanga GI, Spiegelman D, et al: Randomized trial of effects of vitamin supplements on pregnancy outcomes and T cell counts in HIV-1-infected women in Tanzania. Lancet 1998; 351:1477–1482.
134. Coutsoudis A, Pillay K, Spooner E, et al: Randomized trial testing the effect of vitamin A supplementation on pregnancy outcomes and early mother-to-child HIV-1 transmission in Durban, South Africa. AIDS 1999; 13:1517–1524.
135. Bloland PB, Wirima JJ, Steketee RM, et al: Maternal HIV infection and infant mortality in Malawi: Evidence for increased mortality due to placental malaria infection. AIDS 1995; 9:721–726.
136. Jean SS, Pape JW, Verdier R-I, et al: The natural history of human immunodeficiency virus infection in Haitian infants. Pediatr Infect Dis J 1999; 18:58–63.
137. Commenges D, Alioum A, Lepage P, et al: Estimating the incubation period of paediatric AIDS in Rwanda. AIDS 1992; 6:1515–1520.
138. Bobat R, Coovadia H, Moodley D, Coutsoudis A: Mortality in a cohort of children born to HIV-1 infected women from Durban, South Africa. S Afr Med J 1999; 89:646–648.
139. Spira R, Lepage P, Msellati P, et al: Natural history of human immunodeficiency virus type 1 infection in children: A five-year prospective study in Rwanda. Pediatrics 1999; 104:e56 (URL: http://www.pediatrics.org/cgi/content/full/104/5/e56).
140. Taha TET, Dallabetta GA, Canner JK, et al: The effect of human immunodeficiency virus infection on birthweight, and infant and child mortality in urban Malawi. Int J Epidemiol 1995; 24:1022–1029.
141. Lucas SB, Peacock SC, Hounnou A, et al: Disease in children infected with HIV in Abidjan, Cote d'Ivoire. BMJ 1996; 312:335–338.
142. Lucas SB, Hounnou A, Peacock CS, et al: The mortality and pathology of HIV disease in a West African city. AIDS 1993; 7:569–579.
143. Vetter KM, Djomand G, Zadi F, et al: Clinical spectrum of human immunodeficiency virus disease in children in a West African city. Pediatr Infect Dis J 1996; 15:438–442.
144. Jean SS, Reed GW, Verdier R-I, et al: Clinical manifestations of human immunodeficiency virus infection in Haitian children. Pediatr Infect Dis J 1997; 16:600–607.
145. Lepage P, Msellati P, Hitimana D-G, et al: Growth of human immunodeficiency type 1-infected and uninfected children: A prospective cohort study in Kigali, Rwanda, 1988 to 1993. Pediatr Infect Dis J 1996; 15:479–485.
146. Bailey RC, Kamenga M, Nsuami MJ, et al: Growth of children according to maternal and child HIV, immunological and disease characteristics: a prospective cohort study in Kinshasa, Democratic Republic of Congo. Int J Epidemiol 1999; 28:532–540.
147. Henderson RA, Miotti PG, Saavedra JM, et al: Longitudinal growth during the first 2 years of life in children born to HIV-infected mothers in Malawi, Africa. Pediatr AIDS HIV Infect Fetus Adolesc 1996; 7:91–97.
148. Drotar D, Olness K, Wiznitzer M, et al: Neurodevelopmental outcomes of Ugandan infants with human immunodeficiency virus type 1 infection. Pediatrics 1997; 100:e5 (URL: http//www.pediatrics.org/cgi/content/full/100/1/e5).
149. Msellati P, Lepage P, Hitimana D-G, et al: Neurodevelopmental testing of children born to human immunodeficiency virus type 1 (HIV-1) seropositive and seronegative mothers: A prospective cohort study in Kigali, Rwanda. Pediatrics 1993; 92: 843–848.
150. Sirisanthana V, Sirisanthana T: Disseminated *Penicillium marneffei* infection in human immunodeficiency virus-infected children. Pediatr Infect Dis J 1995; 14:935–940.
151. Malin AS, Gwanzura LKZ, Klein S, et al: *Pneumocystis carinii* pneumonia in Zimbabwe. Lancet 1995; 346:1258–1261.
152. Jeena PM, Coovadia HM, Chrystal V: *Pneumocystis carinii* and cytomegalovirus infections in severely ill, HIV-infected African infants. Ann Trop Pediatr 1996; 16:361–368.
153. Kamiya Y, Mtitimila E, Graham SM, et al: *Pneumocystis carinii* pneumonia in Malawian children. Ann Trop Pediatr 1997; 1:121–126.
154. Ikeogu MO, Wolf B, Mathe S: Pulmonary manifestations of HIV seropositivity and malnutrition in Zimbabwe. Arch Dis Child 1997; 76:124–128.
155. Chokephaibulkit K, Wanachiwanawin D, Chearskul S, et al: *Pneumocystis carinii* severe pneumonia among human immunodeficiency virus-infected children in Thailand: The effect of a primary prophylaxis strategy. Pediatr Infect Dis J 1999; 18:147–152.

156. Anglaret X, Chene G, Attia A, et al: Early chemoprophylaxis with trimethoprim-sulfamethoxazole for HIV-1-infected adults in Abidjan, Cote d'Ivoire: A randomised trial. Lancet 1999; 353:1463–1468.
157. Madhi SA, Gray GE, Huebner RE, et al: Correlation between CD4+ lymphocyte counts, concurrent antigen skin test and tuberculin skin test reactivity in human immunodeficiency virus type 1-infected and -uninfected children with tuberculosis. Pediatr Infect Dis J 1999; 18:800–805.
158. Mandalakas AM, Guay L, Musoke P: Human immunodeficiency virus status and delayed-type hypersensitivity skin testing in Ugandan children. Pediatrics 1999; 103:490.
159. Mukadi YD, Wiktor SZ, Coulibaly I-M, et al: Impact of HIV infection on the development, clinical presentation and outcome of tuberculosis among children in Abidjan, Cote d'Ivoire. AIDS 1997; 11:1151–1158.
160. Espinal MA, Reingold AL, Perez G, et al: Human immunodeficiency virus infection in children with tuberculosis in Santo Domingo, Dominican Republic: Prevelance, clinical findings and response to antituberculosis treatment. JAIDS 1996; 13:155–159.
161. Chintu C, Bhat G, Luo C, et al: Seroprevalence of human immunodeficiency virus type 1 infection in Zambian children with tuberculosis. Pediatr Infect Dis J 1993; 12:499–504.
162. Luo C, Chintu C, Bhat G, et al: Human immunodeficiency virus type 1 infection in Zambian children with tuberculosis: Changing seroprevalence and evaluation of a thioacetazone-free regimen. Tubercule Lung Dis 1994; 75:110–115.
163. Sassan-Morokro M, de Cock KM, Ackah A, et al: Tuberculosis and HIV infection in children in Abidjan, Cote d'Ivoire. Trans R Soc Trop Med Hygiene 1994; 88:178–181.
164. Chintu C, Luo C, Bhat G, et al: Cutaneous hypersensitivity reactions to thioacetazone in the treatment of tuberculosis in Zambian children infected with HIV-1. Arch Dis Child 1993; 68:665–668.
165. Schaaf HS, Geldenduys A, Gie RP, Cotton MF: Culture-positive tuberculosis in human immunodeficiency virus type 1-infected children. Pediatr Infect Dis J 1998; 17:599–604.
166. Kalyesubula I, Musoke-Mudido P, Marum L, et al: Effects of malaria infection in human immunodeficiency virus type 1-infected Ugandan children. Pediatr Infect Dis J 1997; 16:876–881.
167. Taha TE, Canner JK, Dallabetta GA, et al: Childhood malaria parasitaemia and human immunodeficiency virus infection in Malawi. Trans R Soc Trop Med Hygiene 1994; 88:164–165.
168. Greenberg AE, Nsa W, Ryder R, et al: *Plasmodium falciparum* malaria and perinatally acquired human immunodeficiency virus type 1 infection in Kinshasa, Zaire. N Engl J Med 1991; 325:105–109.
169. Embree JE, Datta P, Stackwi W, et al: Increased risk of early measles in infants of human immunodeficiency virus type 1-seropositive mothers. J Infect Dis 1992; 165:262–267.
170. De Moraes-Pinto MI, Almeida ACM, Kenj G, et al: Placental transfer and maternally acquired neonatal IgG immunity in human immunodeficiency virus infection. J Infect Dis 1996; 173:1077–1084.
171. Cegielski JP, Msengi AE, Dukes CS, et al: Intestinal parasites and HIV infection in Tanzanian children with chronic diarrhea. AIDS 1993; 7:213–221.
172. Chintu C, Luo C, Baboo S, et al: Intestinal parasites in HIV-seropositive Zambian children with diarrhoea. J Trop Pediatr 1995; 41:149–152.
173. Thea DM, St. Louis ME, Atido U, et al: A prospective study of diarrhea and HIV-1 infection among 429 Zairian infants. N Engl J Med 1993; 329:1696–1702.
174. Fawzi WW, Mbise RL, Hertzmark E, et al: A randomized trial of vitamin A supplements in relation to mortality among human immunodeficiency virus-infected and uninfected children in Tanzania. Pediatr Infect Dis J 1999; 18:127–133.
175. Lepage P, Spira R, Kalibala S, et al: Care of human immunodeficiency virus-infected children in developing countries. Pediatr Infect Dis J 1998; 17:581–586.

2

Vertical Transmission of HIV-1: Timing of Transmission and Risk Factors

Jaime Deville and Yvonne Bryson

The epidemiologic pattern of the HIV-1 epidemic in the United States has significantly changed over the last few years. New cases of HIV infection are increasing in women and minority populations, who now represent approximately two thirds of new HIV-1 infections and AIDS cases,[1] as rates decrease among white men.[1-4] African-American men and women have the highest incidence of HIV-1 and AIDS.[1-3] In the United States, more than 65,000 women were living with AIDS at the end of 1999.[5] Seventeen percent of cases of AIDS reported to the Centers for Disease Control and Prevention (CDC) through June of 2000 are in women, of which 78% belong to minority ethnic groups.[6] Between 1992 and 1994, 6000 to 7000 HIV-1–infected women delivered children yearly in the United States.[7] There has been some regional variability, as rising prevalence has been reported in the Southeast and decreasing prevalence in the Northeast. In the absence of effective preventive strategies, 900 to 2500 HIV-infected infants would be born each year.[8,9]

Recently, the understanding of correlates of perinatal transmission have led to the implementation of effective intervention strategies aimed at reducing the transmission of HIV-1 from mother to child. Use of antiretroviral therapy during pregnancy, delivery, and the neonatal period has led to a dramatic decrease in perinatal transmission in the United States, to less than 7%.[10] The CDC published guidelines for the use of antiretroviral therapy in pregnancies, which have been revised as new data became available.[10-12]

Globally, most new cases of HIV-1 infection occur in Africa, Southeast Asia, China, and India, with a growing epidemic in Latin America. In these areas, the current CDC guidelines are generally not feasible because of the lack of resources in many of these developing countries. Therefore, alternative approaches that are both efficacious and cost effective are being evaluated.[13]

Results of several of these recent intervention trials in developing countries have been published and provide additional insights into the relative contribution of different routes of transmission and the variables affecting them. In this chapter, we review available data in the context of these issues.

The next sections examine some of the most salient issues based on current data regarding transmission of HIV-1 from mother to child.

MOTHER-INFANT TRANSMISSION RATES

The rate of perinatal transmission of HIV-1 varies in different regions of the world. In the United States, rates have varied from 15% to 30% in the absence of intervention.[14-16] Several large, prospective studies have confirmed an expected perinatal transmission rate of approximately 25%.[17-19] European studies have reported lower rates of approximately 15%,[20,21] whereas studies in Thailand report rates of 19% to 24%.[22,23] In contrast, African studies have consistently shown higher

29

transmission rates of 40% to 50%.[24,25] These higher rates observed in some early studies might reflect the difficulties in making an early diagnosis of HIV in the face of a high mortality rate in both infected and uninfected infants. More recent studies reflect overall rates of approximately 35%, depending on the duration of breastfeeding, which is nearly universal in the area.[26]

These observed geographic disparities can be explained by various cofactors, most notably breastfeeding, which is known to be a risk factor for transmission.[27] Different modes of delivery, such as cesarean section, or obstetric practices also could alter transmission rates. In addition, specific nutritional deficiencies, lack of adequate prenatal care, and high rates of infections other than HIV-1 may increase the incidence of prematurity, which is, in itself, a risk factor. Additionally, methodologic differences, such as the background of high infant mortality rates and the proportion of mothers with newly acquired or advanced disease,[28] could play a role.[29]

TIMING OF PERINATAL TRANSMISSION OF HIV-1

Overview

There is both direct and indirect evidence for three routes of transmission of HIV from mother to child: in utero, intrapartum, and transmission by breastmilk. Understanding the timing and routes of transmission of HIV is critical for assessment of maternal and infant risk factors for both transmission and disease progression in the infant, since these may differ based on whether the child is a fetus, a premature or full-term infant, or a young child at the time of infection. In addition, the intervention strategies depend on the time of initiation and the effectiveness of the intervention. Of course, perinatal HIV transmission is a multifactorial process, and many factors are probably interrelated. There have been repeated observations that pregnant women who have more clinically advanced disease (AIDS) and lower CD4+ counts, which are also associated with higher levels of HIV plasma viremia and poorer levels of immune control, have a higher risk of transmission.[18, 30–34]

Over the last five years, we have learned more about the relative contributions of the different routes of transmission and factors affecting them. Advances in technology have led to more sensitive techniques for polymerase chain reaction (PCR), allowing a more precise estimate of the timing of transmission and detection of virus in the infant by DNA and RNA PCR–based assays. Early arguments questioned whether the techniques were sensitive enough to pick up infected infants at birth or whether some of the infants identified in the first few weeks of life were truly infected before birth. Although we are continually refining our detection techniques, to date there have been no dramatic differences in the ability to detect HIV at birth using RNA as opposed to DNA PCR–based analysis. Although we now generally accept that in utero transmission occurs, the relative timing of in utero transmission is unknown but believed to be greatest in the third trimester. Studies using molecular techniques for changes in viral genotype or quasispecies diversity have unfortunately not been revealing. There is too little change in HIV quasispecies in cells and plasma to pinpoint transmission during gestation by current techniques.[35,36]

Perhaps the greatest argument and evidence for estimating the timing of transmission comes from intervention studies. We now have numerous studies with various durations of treatment or times of initiation of the intervention, in the mother and in the infant, and subsequent differences in transmission rates. More of the recent studies have obtained early and subsequent neonatal samples to help better determine the timing of transmission. However, intervention focused broadly on all routes of transmission has the greatest effect. The prime example is ACTG protocol 076, in which zidovudine (ZDV) was administered to HIV-1–infected pregnant women as early as 14 weeks' gestation and continued through delivery and given to the infant for 6 weeks. This study also showed that ZDV treatment initiated as late as 34 weeks can still have an impact on in utero transmission. A more recent study by Lallemant and colleagues[37] showed that in utero transmission was significantly reduced by earlier initiation of ZDV at 28 weeks versus 35 weeks (1.6% vs. 5%; $P < .001$). Questions now remain about whether more potent combination treatment (highly active antiretroviral therapy) that rapidly reduces viral load to undetectable levels, in contrast to ZDV monotherapy, may more specifically pinpoint the timing of in utero transmission.

Because the sensitivity and specificity of diagnostic tests varies according to the timing of transmission, it is important to characterize whether infants are infected in utero or intrapartum so that an algorithm for early diagnosis of HIV infection can be established. This also allows for a better estimate of breastfeeding transmission and may also be important for disease prognosis and initiation of therapy in infected infants. A working definition has been proposed and is currently generally accepted for the determination of the timing of HIV infection in the infant.[26,38]

In this chapter, we discuss the current status of the evidence to support the different routes and timing of transmission and the importance of this determination in terms of assessing maternal and infant risk factors for both transmission and prognosis and approaches for intervention. Some of the major lines of evidence for various routes of transmission are shown in Table 2–1.

In Utero Transmission

An infant is considered to have in utero infection if virologic tests (HIV DNA or RNA or culture) are positive within 48 hours of life and subsequent samples are also positive. Mathematical modeling studies suggest that much of this in utero transmission occurs relatively late in gestation.[39] Owing to the risk of contamination with maternal blood, cord blood samples are generally not recommended for diagnostic evaluations. The mechanism for in utero transmission is most likely via transplacental transmission of HIV, enhanced by placental membrane inflammation that could increase the number of infected maternal lymphocytes in the placenta and amniotic fluid,[40,41] or through maternofetal transfusion, especially following placental disruption. Early in utero transmission in the first trimester appears to be a rare event for live-born infants. HIV has been identified in fetal tissues as early as 10 weeks of gestation, in placentas, and in amniotic fluid,[42] but evidence suggests that HIV infection most probably occurs in the later part of the third trimester of pregnancy. A study of 100 fetal thymuses retrieved mainly from mid-trimester abortions of HIV-infected women detected the presence of virus in only 2% of thymuses.[42] Additional studies have indicated that retrieval of virus from HIV-exposed fetuses is not a frequent finding. There is some evidence to suggest that early in utero infection results in a greater number of fetal losses, as shown in a study of early abortions, which reported a relatively high rate of first-trimester abortions for HIV-infected women compared with reported rates among noninfected women in the United States.[43] Another study, in rural Uganda, reported lower fertility rates among HIV-infected women compared with noninfected women, suggesting that early fetal infection with HIV may result in pregnancy loss.[44] Figure 2–1 illustrates some of the factors associated with in utero transmission.

Intrapartum Transmission

Infants are considered to have intrapartum HIV infection if diagnostic test results within the first 48 hours of life are negative but further virologic testing after 48 hours of life yields positive findings in the absence of breastfeeding. Data indicate that virologic tests performed at birth on HIV-exposed infants will identify only 30% to 50% of HIV-infected infants and that the remainder of HIV-infected infants (50–70%) develop evidence of viral infection days to weeks following birth. Infants infected in

Table 2–1
Evidence for In Utero, Intrapartum, and Breastfeeding Transmission of HIV-1

IN UTERO	INTRAPARTUM	BREASTFEEDING
Positive DNA PCR on first 24–48 hours of life	Negative DNA PCR at birth, with subsequent positive results	Isolation of HIV-1 from cell-free breastmilk
Maternal-fetal transfusion (proposed)	Increased risk in first-born twin	HIV DNA detected in colostrum
Identification of HIV-1 in fetal tissue from 10 weeks of gestation	Isolation of HIV-1 in neonatal gastric aspirates	Increased risk of transmission when compared with exclusively bottle-fed infants
Placental membrane inflammation	Increased transmission risk with prolonged rupture of membranes	Breastfeeding was only exposure of HIV-1 infected children
	Decreased transmission with elective cesarean section	

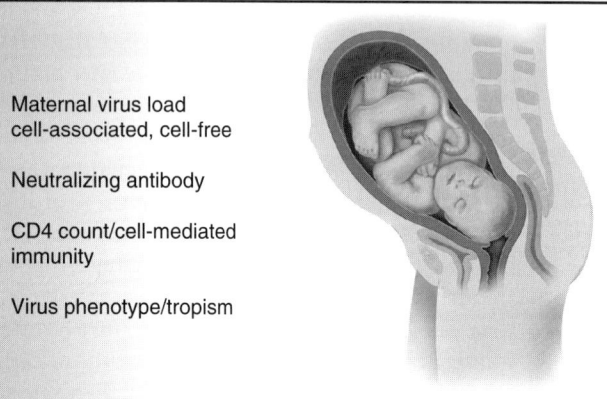
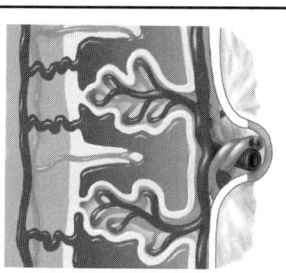

Figure 2–1. In utero transmission of HIV.

utero appear to have a higher risk of rapid disease progression when compared with infants who acquire HIV infection intrapartum.[45–48]

In a study of 271 HIV-infected infants using HIV DNA PCR as the diagnostic test, 38% of infants were positive within 48 hours of life, 93% by 14 days of age, and 96% by 4 weeks of age.[49] A similar study, which used HIV peripheral blood lymphocyte coculture as the virologic method, found virus in 24% of infants during the first week of life, 85% at 1 month, and 91% by 2 months of age.[50] In the absence of breastfeeding, the sensitivity of assays such as HIV DNA PCR, HIV RNA PCR, or HIV peripheral blood lymphocyte coculture approaches 100% by 6 weeks of age.[51,52] Indirect evidence that peripartum transmission is one of the major contributors to perinatal HIV infection comes from data showing that in discordant twins, the first-born twins have a higher risk of infection.[53] In addition, prolonged rupture of membranes also increases transmission risk and elective cesarean sections reduce vertical HIV transmission.[54] Animal models have demonstrated transmission of HIV by oral inoculation,[55] and, in studies of HIV exposed infants, HIV has been isolated from gastric aspirates of infected newborns.[56] Risk factors associated with intrapartum transmission are illustrated in Figure 2–2.

Postpartum Transmission: Role of Breastfeeding

HIV-1 has been isolated from cell-free breastmilk,[57] and HIV DNA has been demonstrated in the majority of milk specimens from HIV-infected mothers. Thus, Ruff and coworkers[58] detected HIV DNA in 70% of milk specimens collected from 47 HIV-seropositive women from 0 to 4 days postpartum, and in about 50% of specimens collected from 6 to 12 months postpartum. Evidence of HIV transmission via breastfeeding has come from reports in which children were exposed to HIV-1 only through breastfeeding[59] and from studies in which breastfed infants had an increased risk of perinatal HIV transmission when compared with children who were bottle-fed.[15, 21, 27, 60]

Although the potential for HIV transmission through maternal milk is clearly evident from these studies, the actual risk for such transmission has been uncertain. Studying a group of mothers with primary HIV infection, Van de Perre and colleagues[61] found that at least 4 of 11 infants (36%) became infected with HIV through breastfeeding. Plasma viral load is known to be high during primary HIV infection,[28] making it difficult to assess the applicability of these data to other stages of HIV

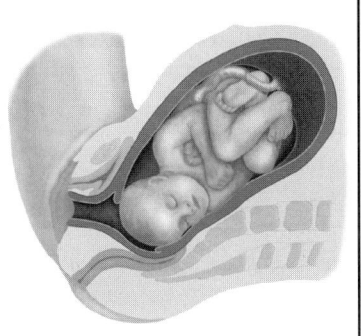
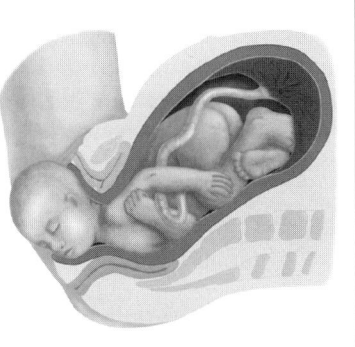

Figure 2–2. Intrapartum transmission of HIV.

infection. In fact, a meta-analysis of five different studies of postnatal transmission reported an excess transmission risk by breastfeeding of 14% for women with established HIV infection, and an excess risk of 29% among women who developed primary infection during the postpartum period.[27]

De Martino and coworkers[62] studied a group of 168 breastfed and 793 bottle-fed children born to seropositive mothers in Italy. Breastfeeding was shown to increase the risk of HIV-1 transmission, with an estimated adjusted odds ratio for 1 day of breastfeeding versus bottle-feeding of 1.19 (95% CI, 1.10–1.28). The odds ratio of transmission increased with the duration of breastfeeding, a finding also reported by Nagelkerke and colleagues.[63]

A recent report by Coutsoudis[64] updated the Durban observational study. Previously reported data described HIV transmission rates of 18.8% in infants aged 3 months who were fed formula and received no breastmilk, 14.6% in infants exclusively breastfed, and 24.1% in infants who had mixed feeds (breastmilk and other liquids/solids). Follow-up data on transmission rates continued to emphasize the superiority of exclusive breastfeeding or formula feeding over mixed feeding. In this study, however, there was no significant difference in HIV transmission rates between infants exclusively breastfed and infants given formula.

The HIV transmission rates at 15 months were 19.4% in formula-fed infants, 24.7% in infants exclusively breastfed and 35.0% in mixed-fed infants. This study was not a randomized controlled trial, but it suggests that early introduction of foods other than breastmilk might create an environment that facilitates transmission of HIV, perhaps by introduction of intestinal pathogens or allergens.

Although breastfeeding has been significantly reduced in HIV-infected mothers in developed countries owing to prenatal screening during pregnancy and use of formula-feeding, acquisition of infection through breastmilk is a major problem in the developing world. The approach to prevention of postnatal breastmilk transmission may involve different strategies. The prolonged risk of infection posed during breastfeeding influences the sensitivity and specificity of diagnostic assays for determination of HIV infection status. Postnatal transmission via lactation is associated with an excess transmission risk of 14% in women with established HIV infection and a 29% excess risk in women who developed primary infection during the postpartum period.[27] The risk of transmission increases with the duration of breastfeeding, although in a nonlinear fashion. A recent study done in Malawi showed that breastfed infants had a 0.7% per month incidence of transmission between 2 and 6 months of age, 0.6% per month for 6- to 11-month-olds and 0.3% per month for 12- to 18-month-olds. The cumulative risk of transmission by breastfeeding was 3.5% at 5 months, 7% at 11 months, and 10.3% at 23 months.[65] Another trial of formula versus breastfeeding in Nairobi showed that two thirds of HIV transmission occurred in the first 6 weeks of life (reflecting mostly in utero and intrapartum transmission), three fourths in the first 6 months, and 84% by 1 year of age (associated with breastfeeding).[66] Therefore, for the developing world, any diagnostic approach that ceases virologic testing at 3 to 4 months of age would be insufficient. Virologic testing under those circumstances must be extended for a longer period of time, and even a negative serologic test result at 18 months might not diagnose subsequent infection of children who continue to be breastfed by HIV-infected women. Strategies to reduce transmission by breastfeeding may include vaccination or use of prolonged antivirals given to the mother or the infant, or both. The estimates for early transmission due to breastfeeding are difficult to assess because of the confounding effect of intrapartum transmission during the first 6 weeks. However, intervention trials that focus on intrapartum transmission in breastfeeding and non-breastfeeding populations should provide additional data. Figure 2–3 illustrates factors associated with breastfeeding transmission.

Correlation Between Transmission Timing and Disease Progression in the Infant

It has been shown that timing of infant infection has a significant prognostic value for long-term outcome. Dickover and coworkers[45] have shown that both the time of infection in fetuses or infants and the pattern and magnitude of HIV-1 viral load during early primary infection have significant prognostic value for long-term outcome. Children who have HIV-1 detected at birth generally have a higher number of copies of viral RNA, faster clinical progression, and a higher rate of mortality. Rapid progressors showed a continued rise in plasma viremia that did not reach a maximum peak until 12 weeks of age and was associated with a profound drop in CD4+ cell count (Fig. 2–4). Infants who were infected intrapartum generally had a lower rate of disease progression and a higher chance of becoming long-term nonprogressors (Fig. 2–5). In contrast with studies of primary viremia in adults, there was no definite "set point," although the lowest HIV RNA levels following primary viremia are at 6 months. This confirms earlier findings by the Mayaux and the French Pediatric HIV Infection Study Groups, which observed an increased risk of rapid progression in infants who had HIV-1 detected at birth or who had high levels of HIV-1 DNA in the first few weeks of life. Shearer and colleagues[67] have also found that

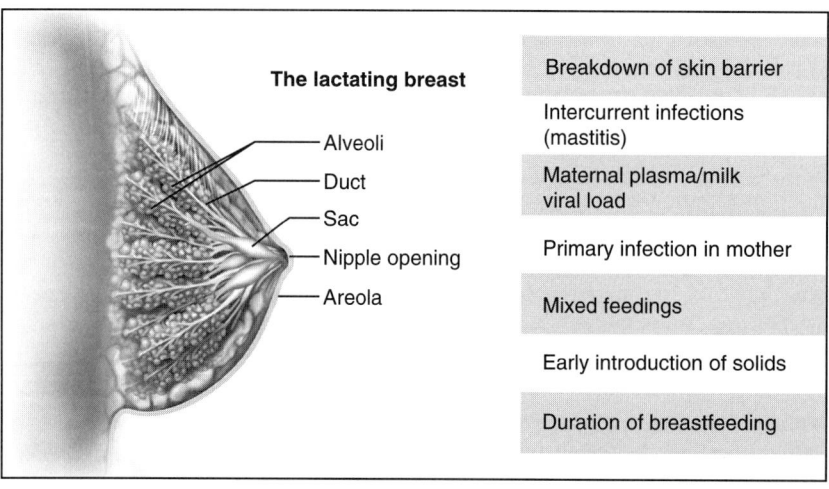

Figure 2–3. Breastfeeding transmission of HIV.

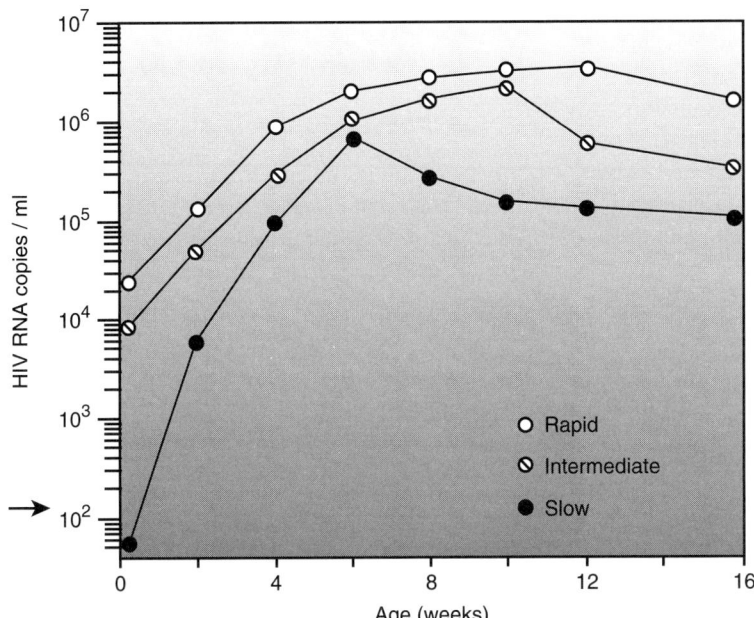

Figure 2–4. Median HIV-1 RNA copy numbers in infected infants over the first 4 months of life.

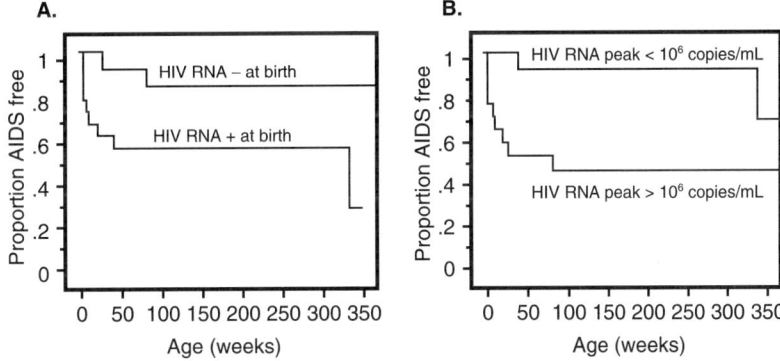

Figure 2–5. Onset of AIDS in infected infants.

children who had HIV-1 RNA present at birth and high levels of plasma HIV RNA in the first few months of life had a higher risk of earlier onset of symptoms, as well as more rapid disease progression, compared with children who did not have HIV-1 DNA detected at birth.

Although it is known that perinatally infected children have very high levels of HIV-1 RNA during the first year of life, some children have a slow drop in HIV-1 RNA levels over years 2 to 5.[50] This is in contrast to adults with primary infection, who show a rapid increase in the early weeks after infection, followed by a rapid decline.[68] In adults, it is known that plasma RNA levels after 120 days are predictive of ultimate disease progression.[69–72]

Primary HIV-1 infection in perinatally infected infants is dependent on multiple factors, including the influence of the timing of infection and the fact that this is occurring in a rapidly growing host with an immature immune system. In addition, virologic factors, including virus tropism coreceptor use and predilection of virus for the fetal thymus, may also be important.[73–75] Transplacental HIV neutralizing antibody may also modify primary infection in infants, as seen in experimental animal models.[76–79] A report by Mofenson and associates found that, in perinatally infected infants older than 1 month of age, baseline HIV-1 RNA levels of more than 100,000 copies/mL in serum were associated with an increased risk of mortality. Shearer has also reported that median HIV-1 RNA levels over the first 2 months of life in perinatally infected infants are predictive of the rate of disease progression.

Therefore, both the timing of transmission and the early virus load are predictors of long-term outcome in perinatally HIV-1–infected infants. As outlined in Figure 2–6, we have developed a hypothetical model of the risk of disease progression in infants based on our current knowledge. This also includes the possibility of aborted or transient infection, which has been reported in rare cases in HIV-exposed infants.[80-83] As depicted in this graph, data suggest that the majority, but not all of the "in utero" infected infants tend to have HIV RNA present at various levels at birth, with higher levels of viremia during the first 16 weeks of life. These rapid progressors have a high risk of AIDS or death by 2 years of age without treatment intervention. The category of slow progressors is more commonly seen in children who have negative viral tests at birth and subsequent viremia at lower levels peaking earlier (6–8 weeks) and slowly decreasing over the first year to 2 years of life. Most recently, our group has reported that HIV envelope diversity as measured by heteroduplex mobility assay during the first 6 months of life was predictive of long-term outcome.[84] It is currently unknown but speculated that the first 6 months of life are critical for the long-term prognosis of disease. This will be important for the development of future treatment strategies based on the time of early infant diagnosis. However, we still have more to learn about the interplay of virologic, immunologic, and genetic factors that predispose infants to rapid or slow progression.

LESSONS FROM INTERVENTION TRIALS

Nonbreastfeeding Trials

Information is available from several recent intervention trials that provides insight into strategies for reduction of intrauterine and intrapartum transmission and new opportunities to assess the relative contributions of various routes of infection. Table 2–2 summarizes results of selected clinical intervention trials. This shows their relative efficacy compared with the timing of initiation of the intervention.

One of the first early observational studies that showed an effect of ZDV on transmission[30] followed 68 mother-infant pairs, with an overall transmission rate of 19% and 10.2% intrauterine infections versus 8.8% intrapartum transmission. This study showed that ZDV given only prenatally and intravenously during delivery to the mother significantly reduced transmission to approximately 8%, a reduction also found in later studies in which only the mother was treated.[22, 85]

Data from ACTG 076[17, 86] showed that in a randomized, placebo-controlled trial of ZDV given during pregnancy, labor, and to the infant for 6 weeks, transmission was reduced by more than 70% in the ZDV arm. The breakdown of the timing of transmission, however, was similar in both arms. In the ZDV arm, 40% of the transmissions were in utero and 60% were intrapartum, compared with 43% versus 57% in the placebo group.

A large, randomized trial of hyperimmune intravenous immunoglobulin (HIVIG) versus intravenous

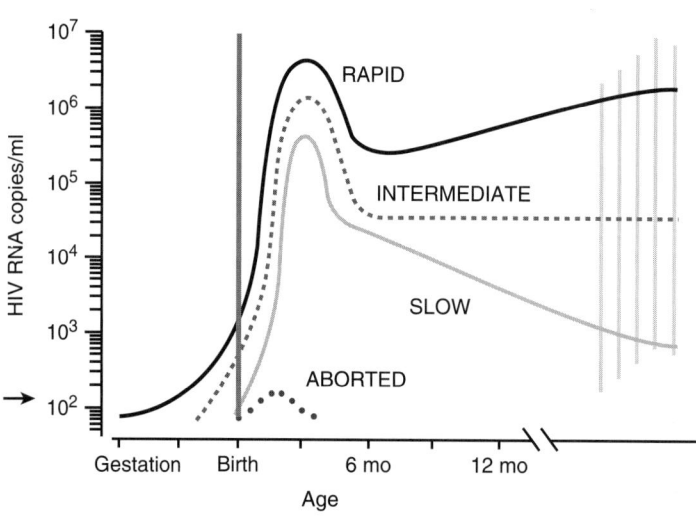

Figure 2–6. Hypothetical model of HIV-1 perinatal infection.

Table 2-2
Trials of Antiretroviral Regimens to Reduce Vertical Transmission of HIV-1

TRIAL	INTERVENTION	Antenatal 14w	Antenatal 28w	Antenatal 36w	Intrapartum Onset of labor Delivery	Postpartum 1w	Infant (Postnatal) Birth 3d 1w 6w	AGE	Placebo (overall)	Intrapartum (if available)	Overall Intrapartum (if available)	EFFICACY, %
Non breastfeeding												
ACTG 076	ZDV	100 mg 5 × day from 14 w			2 mg/kg then 1 mg/kg/hr IV	None	2 mg/kg q6h for 6 w	18 m	26	10.2/15.3	8% 3.3/5	68
ACTG 185	ZDV	100 mg 5 × day from 14 w			2 mg/kg then 1 mg/kg/hr IV	None	2 mg/kg q6h for 6 w	18 m			5% 1.1/3.7	
CDC Thailand	ZDV	None	300 mg q12h from 36 w		300 mg q3h	None	None	3 m	19	6.7/12.2	9% 4.8/4.6	50
BMS 094	ddI	None	200 mg q12h from 34–36 w				120 mg/m² q12h for 6 w	6 w			2%	
	d4T	None	40 mg q12h from 34–36 w				1 mg/kg q12h for 6 w	6 w			4%	
	ddI + d4T	None	200 mg + 40 mg q12h from 34–36 w				120 mg/m² + 1 mg/kg q12h for 6 w	6 w			2%	
	ZDV	None	300 mg q12h from 34–36 w				2 mg/kg q12h for 6 w	6 w			6%	
Thai-Harvard	ZDV		300 mg q12h from 28 w		300 mg bid	None	2 mg/kg q12h for 6 w	6 m			7% Mat long combined IU: 1.6%	
	ZDV		300 mg q12h from 28 w		300 mg bid	None	2 mg/kg q12h for 3 d	6 m			5%	

Table 2-2
Trials of Antiretroviral Regimens to Reduce Vertical Transmission of HIV-1 *Continued*

TRIAL	INTERVENTION	MOTHER Antenatal 14w	28w	36w	Intrapartum Onset of labor	Delivery	Postpartum 1w	INFANT (Postnatal) Birth	3d	1w	6w	AGE	TRANSMISSION RATE, % Placebo (overall)	Intrapartum (if available)	(Overall Intrapartum (if available)	EFFICACY, %
	ZDV	300 mg q12h from 35 w			300 mg bid		None			2 mg/kg q12h for 6 w		6 m		9%	Mat short combined IU: 5.1	
	ZDV	300 mg q12h from 35 w			300 mg bid		None			2 mg/kg q12h for 3 d		6 m		11%		37%
Breastfeeding																
CDC Cote d'Ivoire	ZDV	None		300 mg q12h from 36 w	300 mg q3h		None	None				4 w / 3 m	22% / 26%	4.3/17.4	12% / 16%	4.9/7.3
PETRA*																
Arm A	ZDV+3TC	None		q12h from 36 w	ZDV q3h; 3TC q12h		q12h for 1 w			q12h for 1 w	None	6 w	19%		8%	54%
Arm B	ZDV+3TC	None		ZDV q3h; 3TC q12h	q12h for 1 w		q12h for 1 w			q12h for 1 w	None	6 w			12%	39%
Arm C	ZDV+3TC	None		ZDV q3h; 3TC q12h	None		None					6 w			19%	NS
HIVNET 012	ZDV	None		600 mg then 300 mg q3h	None		None	None				6-8 w			20%	10.3/9.7
	NVP	None		600 mg	None		None	None				6-8 w			12%	8.1/3.7
SAINT	ZDV +3TC	None		ZDV q3h; 3TC q12h	q12h for 1 w		q12h for 1 w	None				6 w			11%	6.6/4.2
	NVP	None		200 mg	200 mg		2 mg/kg	None				6 w			14%	7.7/6.3

ddI, didanosine; d4T, stavudine; NS, not significant; NVP, nevirapine; 3TC, lamivudine; ZDV, zidovudine.
*Maternal antenatal and postpartum doses: ZDV 300 mg, 3TC 150 mg; Intrapartum dose: Arm A: ZDV 300 mg, 3TC 150 mg; Arms B and C: ZDV first dose 600 mg, subsequent doses 300 mg, 3TC 150 mg; Infant dose: ZDV 4 mg/kg, 3TC 2 mg/kg. IP: Intrapartum.

immunoglobulin (IVIG) (ACTG 185) was instituted in HIV-infected women with lower CD4+ T cell counts who were also receiving ZDV. The trial, which included 454 mother-infant pairs, was stopped because of the overall low transmission rate of about 5% and because it would have required a much larger sample size to assess efficacy.[33] Of the 22 infected infants, 5 (23%) had a positive HIV culture at birth, and 17 (77%) were negative. Dry pellets or plasma from birth was available for 13 of the 17 infants; one was DNA PCR positive, all were RNA PCR negative, including the DNA PCR positive infant. On the basis of these data, it could be estimated that 27% of infants were infected in utero and 73% intrapartum.

The results of a randomized, placebo-controlled trial in Thailand have shown that shorter antiretroviral regimens using ZDV at 36 weeks through delivery in the mother only are also efficacious in preventing vertical transmission of HIV-1.[22] In this study, 395 mothers without prior antiretroviral treatment were enrolled. Overall, efficacy analysis shows a 28.6% efficacy for prevention of in utero transmission versus 61.4% efficacy for interruption of intrapartum transmission. In utero transmission in the ZDV group was 4.8%, compared with 6.7% in the placebo group, whereas intrapartum transmission in the ZDV group was 5.2% versus 12.2% in the placebo group. Maternal viral load was significantly reduced by delivery in the ZDV arm, which presumably resulted in reduced exposure of the infant to maternal virus at delivery.[22]

In another recent study (BMS 094) performed in South Africa,[87] investigators compared stavudine (d4T), didanosine (ddI), d4T + ddI, and ZDV given prepartum (start at 34–36 weeks), intrapartum, and postpartum (6 weeks to infant) and enrolled 204 women. Preliminary analysis at 6 weeks shows transmission rates of 4.2%, 1.9%, 2.0%, and 6.3% for each respective arm. This trial is still ongoing but is important in demonstrating that antivirals (other than ZDV) can also reduce transmission. DDI and a combination of ddI and d4T had the greatest effect on maternal virusloadreduction: −0.9 and −1.9 log viral RNA, respectively.

The most recently published data from the Thailand group[37] compared various lengths of regimens of oral ZDV given to the mother or infant, or both, to the standard 076 regimen versions. The four groups were (1) long-long (oral zidovudine 300 mg twice a day from 28 weeks to delivery, with the infant receiving oral zidovudine from birth to week 6); (2) short-short (start at 35 weeks, with the infant receiving zidovudine for the first 3 days of life); (3) short-long (start at 35 weeks, with the infant receiving zidovudine from birth to week 6); (4) and long-short (start at 28 weeks, with the infant receiving zidovudine for the first 3 days of life). The short-short group was discontinued after the first interim analysis, because the transmission rate at that time was 10.5% compared with 4.1% in the long-long group. The study was continued with the other 3 arms.

Transmission rates in the long-long group were not significantly different from transmission rates in the others (6.5% versus 4.7% for the long-short group and 8.6% for the short-long regimen). It is remarkable that the rate of transmission for the short-long group was in between that of the short-short group and that of the groups with longer maternal treatment, suggesting that longer infant regimens are beneficial when the mother gets started on therapy late in the pregnancy but may be irrelevant when maternal treatment is started early in pregnancy. The in utero transmission rate in the two groups with shorter maternal treatment was significantly higher (5.1%) than in the two groups who received longer maternal treatment (1.6%). The finding of a 3.5% differential in transmission rate when treatment is begun 7 weeks earlier confirms the importance of in utero transmission during the earlier part of the third trimester. An important caveat here is the consideration that ZDV may not immediately prevent transmission if the major mechanism of action is the reduction of maternal viral load. The moderate reduction in maternal virus load may take several weeks, and other combination therapies would be more likely to reduce maternal viral load rapidly to low to undetectable levels.

Trials That Allowed Breastfeeding

Recent short-course trials in Africa have allowed breastfeeding of infants because of the high infant mortality rate, cost, and stigma associated with alternative feeding options. In a study of birth canal washing in Blantyre, Malawi,[88] in which 5488 women were enrolled, 570 HIV-exposed infants were followed, and the overall transmission rate was 26%. Using cord blood DNA PCR, the investigators identified that one third of the infected infants (absolute rate 9%) were cord blood positive.

Long-term follow-up of the study population[89] followed 2094 HIV-infected women, who delivered 2157 babies, of whom 1406 had at least one follow-up visit. A total of 405 infants were HIV DNA positive (overall transmission rate, 29%). A total of 135 infants had at least two positive samples (possibly including a cord blood sample) or were infected by breastfeeding (even if there was only one positive sample). Of those, 24 infants were infected in utero and 52 intrapartum. In 16 infants, timing (in utero or intrapartum) could not be established owing to lack of early samples. Forty-three infants were infected via breastfeeding.

A study in Côte d'Ivoire[90] enrolled 280 women and was complementary to the short-course therapy study in Thailand[22] in a breastfeeding population. In utero transmission risks were similar for both groups (4.9% for the ZDV group versus 4.3% for placebo). At 4 weeks, the ZDV group had a 12.2% transmission rate, with an estimated intrapartum transmission of 7.3%, compared with 21.7% overall for the placebo arm (17.4% intrapartum transmission; $P = .05$). By 3 months of age, the transmission rates increased by 3.5% and 3.2% in both treatment and placebo arms (15.9% and 24.9%; $P = .07$). In a recent update of the pooled data from the DITRAME and RETROCI trials,[91] 640 infants were followed for 24 months. Transmission rates at birth were again similar (9.4% for ZDV and 8.6% for placebo). At 6 weeks, rates were 14.1% for ZDV and 23.2% for placebo, at 3 months, 16.4% for ZDV and 25.3% for placebo, and at 24 months, 21.6% for ZDV and 30.3% for placebo). In this study, the initial benefit of antiretroviral therapy was lost with continued breastfeeding.

The PETRA study[92] compared three different treatment regimens, including ZDV/3TC with placebo for prevention of perinatal transmission in three African countries. Arm A included oral drug given from 36 weeks gestation and intrapartum and to mother and infant 1 week after delivery, in arm B intrapartum and postpartum drug was given, arm C used only intrapartum ZDV/3TC. Transmission rates were 8.2% for arm A, 12.3% for arm B, 18.8% for arm C, and 19.1% for placebo. However, updated findings[93] show loss of efficacy at month 24 due to breastfeeding.

Data were presented on all 1457 mothers randomized before the termination of the placebo arm, and statistical comparisons were made between the treatment and placebo arms. Mothers were counseled on the benefits of breastfeeding, and a total of 69% of mothers elected to breast-feed for a mean duration of 24 weeks. Transmission rates for arms A, B, C, and placebo at 24 months were, respectively, 21.3%, 24.9%, 27.8%, and 26.8%.

The HIVNET 012 study, performed in Uganda,[94] compared the efficacy of a single dose of nevirapine (NVP) given at onset of labor and to the infant before 72 hours versus ZDV given at onset of labor and every 3 hours to the mother and ZDV given for 7 days to the infant. Overall, 619 women were enrolled, with transmission rates of 8.1% for NVP versus 10.3% for ZDV at birth, and 11.8% versus 20% at 6 to 8 weeks, suggesting the estimated intrapartum transmission was 3.7% for NVP and 9.7% for ZDV. This study showed surprising efficacy for interruption of intrapartum transmission for NVP and harbored hope for an inexpensive therapeutic alternative in developing countries. However, 1 year later, transmission rates have increased to 15.7% in the NVP arm and to 24.1% in the ZDV arm, again due to breastfeeding.[95] The remaining effect is undoubtedly due to prevention of intrapartum transmission by NVP. A significantly higher proportion of women breastfed their infants up to 6 months of age in the ZDV arm, but NVP efficacy remains superior after controlling for this variable.

The SAINT (South African Intrapartum Nevirapine Trial) study used the same NVP arm as HIVNET 012 and compared the regimen to ZDV/3TC given during labor and to mother and child 1 week after delivery.[96] Transmission rates were similar, showing 14% and 10.8% for the NVP and ZDV/3TC arms, respectively. In utero transmission rates were 7.7% and 6.6% for these respective regimens.

A limitation of the presented data is the lack of available data points between 6 weeks and 24 months in the PETRA study. Knowledge of the timing of transmission might allow clinicians to recommend a specific, acceptable duration of breastfeeding. Detailed analysis of the site-specific data of the interventional trials is required, because the proportion of breastfed infants, as well as maternal and infant mortality data, varied considerably among the study sites. The lack of uniformity and the differences in the cultural circumstances in each of the study centers may confound attempts to draw conclusions regarding recommendations for breastfeeding.

All of these studies help to better define the timing of transmission, as seen in Figure 2–7. This illustrates examples of data obtained from intervention studies and natural history. In utero transmission rates are consistent with the natural history data as seen in the HIVNET 012 trial, in which 8.1% of infants in the NVP arm were infected in utero. Conversely, data from ACTG 076, and the maternal long-therapy (start at 28 weeks) of the Thai-Harvard studies show a significant reduction

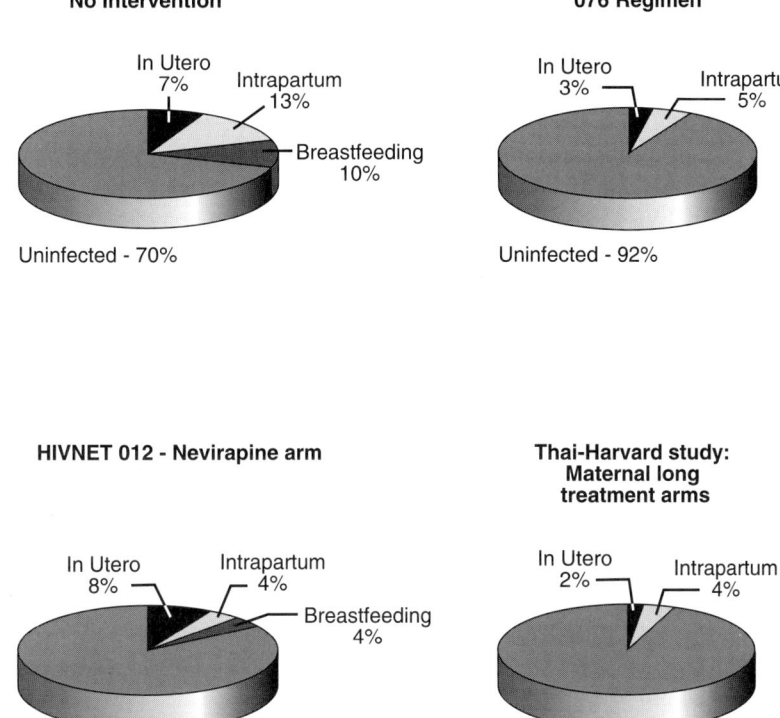

Figure 2–7. Distribution of vertical transmission of HIV-1.

of the in utero transmission rates (3.3% and 1.6%, respectively) It is remarkable that numerous studies agree on the percentage of infants infected intrapartum, as seen in the chart, from an absolute rate of about 13% to a rate of 5% in the ACTG 076 data, 4% in the Thai-Harvard study, and 3.7% in the HIVNET 021 nevirapine arm.

RISK FACTORS

Perinatal transmission is a multifactorial process. Viral, genetic, immune, and clinical factors all play a role. Several reviews and chapters have been published on the subject.[60,97–99] At this time, it is known that women with advanced disease and most probably primary infection during pregnancy have a high risk of transmission. Maternal viral load, not surprisingly, has turned out to be a very consistent, strong predictor of transmission in the majority of studies. Less is known about cervical virus shedding, but this is also considered a potential risk factor for intrapartum transmission during labor and delivery, particularly in light of the correlation with prolonged ruptured membranes and reduction of transmission by elective cesarean section. Other immune factors, such as the presence of autologous neutralizing antibody, have been shown to be protective against transmission in some, but not all, studies.[100–102] Selective transmission of major or minor and multiple HIV quasispecies has been reported in several papers, but the mechanism for this is not clear.[35,103] Our group recently reported that in utero transmitting mothers were more likely to transmit single or multiple major maternal viral variants, whereas those who transmitted intrapartum were more likely to transmit minor variants. These data suggest that different selective pressures may be involved in determining HIV variant transmission, depending on the timing of transmission.[104] Virologic factors such as viral coreceptor use or tropism may also play a role but are less well defined.[105–108] Genetic polymorphisms, which either potentially protect or promote transmission or acquisition, have been recently reported and continue to be investigated.[109–111] It is important to consider the timing of transmission in the evaluation of various risk factors, since the mechanisms for transmission or protection may differ by the route and time of infection of the fetus, neonate, or young infant. Here, we discuss some of the major risk factors.

Maternal Viral Load

Advanced HIV disease in the mother has been associated with increased risk of transmission to the infant.[21,112] The European Collaborative Study[21] found that a CD4+ cell count less than 700 cells/mm^3 was associated with increased risk of maternal-fetal transmission; another study by Mayaux[113] found a 43% transmission rate among women whose CD4+ cell counts were less than 200 cells/mm^3, and mothers with CD4+ counts over 600 cells/mm^3 had a transmission rate of 15%. Progression of HIV disease in children is directly related to severity of maternal HIV disease during pregnancy. Blanche noted a higher death rate during the first 18 months of life in those infants whose mothers had more advanced clinical disease, the presence of p24 antigenemia, lower CD4+ cell count at delivery, or any combination of these factors.[114] Also, some studies have demonstrated that an increased maternal virus load is associated with an increased risk of in utero transmission. Borkowsky[47] observed that mothers with a higher number of infected cells and plasma virus were more likely to have children infected in utero, independently of CD4+ cell counts. In utero transmission, in turn, appears to correlate with an increased rate of disease progression in the infant.[30,45,115–117]

Multiple studies have confirmed the importance of maternal viral load in predicting the risk of HIV transmission to the infant.[47,118,119] Our group studied 92 HIV-seropositive pregnant women and their 97 infants, of whom 20 (21%) were perinatally infected.[32] A maternal viral load over 50,000 copies/mL at delivery was associated with increased transmission: 75% of the 20 mothers that transmitted had viral loads over 50,000 copies/mL as opposed to 4 (5.3%) of the nontransmitters. In contrast, none of the 63 women with viral load less than 20,000 copies/mL transmitted HIV to their infants. Zidovudine was given to 42 mothers during pregnancy, with associated significant decreases in viral load; and none of these women transmitted HIV to the newborn. However, four zidovudine-treated women with persistently high HIV-1 RNA levels gave birth to HIV-infected babies. These data suggest that maternal HIV-1 viral load is an important determinant of perinatal transmission. However, transmission has been reported to occur with undetectable levels of HIV RNA.[18]

The landmark ACTG 076 study also addressed the importance of HIV-1 viral load in predicting the risk of perinatal transmission; this study evaluated the efficacy of zidovudine in the prevention of perinatal transmission of HIV.[18] In this placebo-controlled trial of 402 mother-infant pairs, the rate of transmission of HIV-1 was 7.6% with zidovudine, versus 22.6% in the placebo group ($P < .001$). In the placebo group, a high maternal viral load at study entry (14 weeks of gestation) or at delivery was associated with increased risk of transmission, with a 40% transmission rate in those women with the highest levels of HIV-1 (>15,700 copies/mL on the reverse transcriptase [RT]–PCR assay, and >7530 copies/mL on the branched DNA assay). Of interest, although ZDV was associated with a reduction in perinatal transmission and a median 0.24 log 10 decrease in plasma viral RNA, a reduction in viral RNA from baseline to delivery was not significantly associated with the risk of transmission. Furthermore, ZDV was effective in reducing transmission at all HIV-1 RNA levels. These data suggest that high HIV-1 viral load is most associated with perinatal transmission in untreated women. Further, the ability of ZDV to reduce such transmission is only partially explained by its ability to lower viral load in the mother. It is possible that the effect of ZDV also includes prophylaxis directly to the fetus infant, since this antiretroviral readily crosses the placenta and was also given to the infant for 6 weeks.

Despina and colleagues[120] recently assessed the predictive value of maternal HIV-RNA load in perinatal HIV transmission by performing a meta-analysis of nine cohorts involving 1115 maternal-infant pairs. The overall rate of transmission in untreated women was 21.3%. The HIV-1 viral load was directly correlated with the rate of transmission, rising from a low of 5% in women with fewer than 1000 copies/mL to 15% in those with 1000 to 9999 copies/mL and 37% in those with HIV-RNA levels greater than 10,000 copies/mL (Fig. 2–8). In pregnant women receiving antiretroviral therapy, the perinatal transmission rate was 5% for those with fewer than 1000 copies/mL; 7% for those with viral loads between 1000 and 9999 copies/mL; and 18% for those with greater than 10,000 copies/mL. The risk of transmission, based solely on HIV-1 RNA levels in plasma, appears to be attenuated in women receiving antiretroviral therapy. However, although maternal HIV-RNA levels are quite helpful in predicting the average risk of transmission in a group of women, such information is of more limited use in predicting outcome in individual

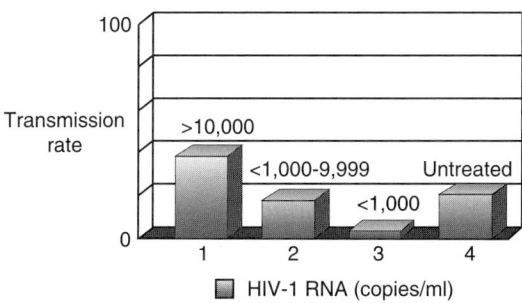

Figure 2–8. Maternal viral load and vertical transmission of HIV-1. (From Despina G, Contopoulos-Loannidis J, Loannidis P: Maternal cell-free viremia in the natural history of perinatal HIV-1 transmissin: A meta-analysis. J Acquir Imm Defic Syndr Hum Retrovirol 1998; 18: 126–135).

patients, since an absolute threshold of safety has not been proven.[34] Another important caveat is that many of the earlier studies, specifically ACTG 076 and the Women and Infants Transmission Study (WITS) did not consistently collect samples to maintain appropriate stability of viral RNA in plasma. Therefore, absolute levels of HIV viral RNA must be interpreted with caution across studies.

Garcia and colleagues[34] measured HIV-1 RNA in 552 pregnant HIV-1–infected women enrolled in WITS. Increasing geometric mean levels of plasma HIV-1 RNA were associated with an increasing risk of transmission on multivariate analysis, higher maternal plasma HIV-1 RNA level, lack of receipt of ZDV therapy according to ACTG protocol 076, low birth weight of the infant, and time from rupture of membranes of delivery greater than 4 hours were all statistically associated with risk of perinatal transmission. This study suggests that while HIV-1 RNA level is highly predictive of transmission, other factors are also important.

Analysis of ACTG 185 showed that maternal viral load was highly predictive of transmission.[33] In this study of 480 pregnant women with advanced HIV-1 disease, all received a minimum of ZDV during pregnancy, and the infants received ZDV for 6 weeks. Half of the women were randomized to receive HIV-1 hyperimmune globulin monthly during pregnancy, and it was given once to the neonates at birth. In this study, baseline HIV RNA at the time of first testing during pregnancy was statistically correlated with perinatal transmission.

At the time of delivery, several factors were associated with increased risk of transmission, including higher maternal HIV-1 RNA levels, higher levels of maternal HIV p24 antibody, and presence of chorioamnionitis. No perinatal transmission occurred among the 84 women who had undetectable HIV RNA (<500 copies/mL) in plasma at baseline, or the 107 women who had undetectable levels at delivery.

These studies indicate that maternal plasma HIV-1 RNA levels are a powerful predictor of HIV-1 transmission. However, obstetric factors are also important, such as prolonged intervals between amniotic membrane rupture and delivery and the presence of chorioamnionitis, which may, in some cases, allow transmission at low HIV RNA levels.

Other Maternal Factors

Although advanced HIV disease in the mother is a major risk factor, additional factors have been associated with an increased chance of perinatal transmission.

Maternal cigarette smoking has been associated with a statistically significant threefold increased risk of perinatal HIV-1 transmission in women with low CD4+ cell counts.[121] Furthermore, mothers who transmitted HIV to their infants were more likely to have clinical chorioamnionitis than those who did not transmit, as demonstrated in a study by Nair and colleagues.[122]

Although use of illicit injection drugs during pregnancy has been associated with an increased risk of perinatal HIV infection, a past history of injection drug use poses no increased risk.[121,123]

Furthermore, geographic origin, educational history, parity, and marital status are not associated with change in risk for transmission.[21,114,122]

Older maternal age, with increasing risk for each 5-year increment over 25 years, has been associated with an increased risk of perinatal transmission,[113] although the majority of studies have not confirmed this relationship.[21, 114, 122]

OBSTETRIC FACTORS

Another major piece of evidence supporting intrapartum or peripartum HIV transmission is the data of increased risk of perinatal infection with prolonged rupture of membranes and decreased risk with elective cesarean section.

Premature Rupture of Membranes

Premature rupture of the membranes has been associated with a higher risk of perinatal HIV transmission, presumably related to increased duration of fetal exposure to infected cervicovaginal secretions. WITS enrolled 525 women who delivered live singleton infants, in whom the serologic status was known. In those mothers whose membranes ruptured more than 4 hours prior to delivery, the rate of perinatal transmission was 25%, versus 14% among those whose membranes ruptured 4 hours or less prior to the time of delivery.[123] This increased risk was independent of the mode of delivery. On multivariate analysis, ruptured membranes for over 4 hours nearly doubled the risk of transmission. Premature rupture was also shown to be a significant factor in predicting perinatal transmission by Burns and colleagues,[121,124] independent of maternal CD4+ cell count. The impact of membrane rupture over 4 hours is also evident among women who have been treated with antiretroviral agents during pregnancy.[123,125]

Mode of Delivery

Initial studies indicated similar rates of HIV transmission in children born after vaginal or cesarean delivery.[15,53,126] However, recent data indicate that elective cesarean section is very effective in reducing perinatal transmission of HIV-1. These discrepancies may be secondary to the fact that elective cesarean section negates the possible influence of premature rupture of the membranes. In addition, the studies were influenced by the inclusion of women who underwent nonelective cesarean section and by the potential bias that some obstetricians may be more or less likely to perform cesarean sections on HIV-infected patients with advanced clinical disease.

The European Collaborative Study, based on 721 children born to 701 mothers, demonstrated that elective cesarean section was associated with a decreased risk of perinatal transmission (relative risk, 0.56); however, these results were not statistically significant.[21] A subsequent report from this group again noted a decreased risk of perinatal HIV transmission after cesarean section.[127] In another study, Duliege and colleagues[128] evaluated data from prospectively identified twins whose mothers were HIV-infected. Among first-born twins, 52% of the transmission risk was found to be related to vaginal delivery.

Read and associates[54] performed a meta-analysis of North American and European studies, each consisting of at least 100 mother-child pairs, to determine the role of elective cesarean section in decreasing perinatal transmission. The primary analysis included data from 8533 mother-child pairs. After adjusting for use of antiretrovirals, maternal disease stage, and infant birth weight, the risk of perinatal transmission was decreased by approximately 50% in those women who underwent elective cesarean section, when compared with other modes of delivery (odds ratio, 0.43; 95% confidence limit, 0.33–0.56). Similar results were found when the control population was limited only to those women with rupture of the membranes immediately prior to delivery. When all cases of cesarean section were compared with all cases of vaginal delivery in this meta-analysis, use of cesarean section remained predictive of decreased risk of transmission, although to a lesser degree compared to elective cesarean section alone.

Among women who did not receive antiretroviral therapy, a transmission rate of 10.4% was documented after elective cesarean section, versus 19% after vaginal delivery.[54] Of importance, use of antiretroviral therapy (mostly ZDV) during pregnancy as well as elective cesarean section resulted in an 87% reduction in perinatal transmission. Among the 196 women who took antiretroviral agents and had an elective cesarean section, the vertical transmission rate was 2%, compared with 7.3% among 1255 mothers on antiretrovirals with other modes of delivery. It is important to note, however, that no maternal virologic data were available from the 15 studies that were included in this meta-analysis, and there was no clear breakdown of in utero versus intrapartum infection in the infants. Further, even though there was clearly a significant association between elective cesarean sections and decrease in perinatal HIV transmission, no conclusions can be drawn about what additional benefit, if any, an elective cesarean section would have in preventing perinatal transmission from mothers with undetectable plasma levels of virus.

A study performed in a French cohort of patients evaluated the association between elective cesarean section and perinatal HIV-1 transmission rates and found a clear benefit only when the cesarean section was performed concomitantly with antiretroviral treatment of the mother.[129] Mandelbrot and colleagues[129] reported a perinatal transmission rate of 17.5% for vaginal deliveries, 15.6% for nonelective cesarean sections, and 17.5% for elective cesarean sections in a group of 1877 women who received no antiretroviral therapy during pregnancy. However, for 872 women who received ZDV treatment during gestation, there was a significant association between mode of delivery and perinatal transmission. Transmission rates were 6.6% for vaginal deliveries, 11.4% for nonelective cesarean sections, and 0.8% for elective cesarean section ($P = .002$) with an odds ratio for elective cesarean section of 0.2 (95% CI, 0.0–0.9). Similar to the Read study,[54] maternal virologic data were not available for analysis in the French study.

The European Mode of Delivery Collaborative study randomized 370 infants born to HIV-infected mothers to either delivery by elective cesarean section (170 infants) or vaginal delivery (200 infants).[54] At 18 months, the rate of HIV transmission to the infants was 1.8% among those born by cesarean section and 10.5% among those assigned to vaginal deliveries. The rate of postpartum complications was small in this study.

Recent data on the rate of infectious complications after surgical deliveries in HIV-infected women are conflicting. WITS reported a morbidity rate associated with elective cesarean delivery of 19%.[130] Morbidity due to infections, including endometritis, wound infections, and urinary tract infections, occurred in 11% of patients undergoing elective cesarean sections and in 21% of those undergoing nonelective cesarean sections. For vaginal deliveries, these rates were 8% for women receiving instrumental assistance and 4% for women with noninstrumented deliveries. ACTG 185 also reported an increased rate of infectious complications in HIV-infected women undergoing surgical deliveries: 26% for elective cesarean sections and 40% for cesarean sections performed after rupture of amniotic membranes.[33] Vaginal deliveries had a lower rate of infectious complications: 13% for spontaneous deliveries and 19% for assisted vaginal deliveries. Of note, in this study, absolute CD4+ cell count did not correlate with an increased rate of infectious complications. These results support a cautious approach, as risks and benefits of surgical procedures must be taken into account when considering elective cesarean sections for HIV-infected women.

The current data do demonstrate a significant advantage to elective cesarean section delivery in HIV-infected mothers when detectable viral load is present. Such a mode of delivery would theoretically be associated with decreased likelihood of microtransfusions of infected blood to the fetus during labor. Also, cesarean section would result in avoidance of direct fetal contact with infected maternal sections in the birth canal. It must be remembered, however, that elective cesarean sections do not prevent in utero infection. Furthermore, the current studies were conducted prior to the advent of highly active antiretroviral therapy.

In terms of vaginally delivered infants, rates of transmission are increased in deliveries in which episiotomy, scalp electrodes, forceps, or vacuum extractors were used, but only in those centers where these procedures are not routinely performed.[21] All of these data support the concept of differences in the timing and routes of infection.

FACTORS RELATED TO THE FETUS

Low birth weight of less than 2500 g,[118,123,131] gestational age less than 34 weeks, and gestational age less than 38 weeks[53,73,118,131] have each been associated with an increased risk of perinatal HIV transmission. This association between prematurity and transmission may be partially a consequence of HIV infection in utero, resulting in abnormalities in fetal development and premature birth. It is known that women with advanced HIV disease are more likely to transmit to their infants and also are more likely to deliver premature infants. Premature infants have less developed immune systems and thus are more susceptible to infection during labor and delivery. Recent studies of this type in HIV-exposed infants have suggested that the rate of intrapartum transmission might be higher among premature babies; this suggests that acquisition of infection occurred because they were born prematurely and not the opposite.[132,133]

The birth order of twins has also been associated with differing risks of infection. Both Goedert[53] and Duliege[128] have shown that the majority of twin pairs are concordant in terms of HIV-1 infection. However, a significantly increased risk of HIV-1 infection is also apparent among first-born ("A") as opposed to second-born ("B") twins, independent of mode of delivery. Thus, as reported by Duliege, HIV-1 infection occurred in 35% of vaginally delivered A twins and only in 15% of vaginally delivered B twins. Twin pairs born by cesarean section delivery showed a risk of HIV infection of 16% among A twins and 8% among B twins.[128] The exact mechanisms for this increased risk in first-born twins are unknown, but it is certainly consistent with the fact that perinatal infection most commonly occurs at the time of delivery.

During the mid-1990s, transient infection was implied when cytotoxic T-lymphocyte responses and virus were detected in the specimens of exposed but uninfected individuals. Attempts to substantiate transient infection of infants using phylogenetic analysis of the specimen purportedly from the infant and of the specimen from the mother demonstrated unrelated viruses or misattribution of specimens to the infant by use of somatic markers in some, but not all, cases.[80,83] Although the virologic data did not support transient infection in many of these cases, an unsolved enigma from these studies was the circumstances that generated cytotoxic T-lymphocytes in some infants. Unlike classic cytotoxic T-lymphocyte responses, antigen-specific interleukin-2 production by lymphocytes is not thought to require infection and could follow exposure to noninfectious antigens. An investigation was recently conducted[134] to evaluate whether HIV-1–specific cell-mediated immune responses may protect infants from HIV-1 infection. Cord blood samples from infants of HIV-1–seropositive women enrolled in a study in Durban, South Africa, and of a control group of seronegative women were tested for in vitro reactivity to a cocktail of HIV-1 envelope peptides (env) using a bioassay measuring interleukin-2 production in a murine cell line. T-helper cell responses to HIV-1 env peptides were detected in 38% of cord blood samples from infants born to HIV-1–seropositive and 0% born to seronegative women ($P = .03$). Among 41 infants who appeared uninfected at 6 months old, 56% had responses to env. These cellular immune responses were not related to whether the infant was breastfed. HIV-1 infection was more common among infants who did not have cord blood HIV-1 antigen-specific interleukin-2 compared with responsive infants ($P = .02$). These findings suggest that protective cell-mediated immune responses from in utero exposure may be a more important mechanism of newborn protection against HIV-1 from viral exposure both in the peripartum period and during breastfeeding. Clearly, further studies in this area are warranted.

CONCLUSIONS

During the past decade, significant advances have been made in both the prevention and the understanding of the timing and factors associated with the risk of vertical transmission of HIV-1. In developed countries, there must be continued emphasis on rapid identification and appropriate treatment of and prophylaxis for HIV-positive women and their infants to maintain or further reduce perinatal HIV transmission. If the infrastructure and public health measures that have been created are not maintained, we will quickly revert to the era in which early maternal diagnosis was the exception and not the rule. Continued vigilance is also necessary to monitor the emergence of antiretroviral resistance to current therapy. Additionally, newer, simpler, and more effective regimens need to be explored, with complete eradication of transmission as an attainable goal.

The growing epidemic in underdeveloped countries is the most urgent challenge, as our intervention strategies are only on the threshold of implementation. We have applied our knowledge of the different timing (routes) and risk factors associated with transmission to rational development of intervention strategies. Shortened, targeted interventions around the time of delivery in the mother and infant have significantly reduced intrapartum transmission, as seen in the HIVNET 012 and SAINT trials. Treatment of the mother in the third trimester has a significant impact on in utero transmission, and future studies may further define when and how in utero transmission occurs. In countries where breastfeeding is necessary due to the lack of acceptable alternate feeding methods, the challenge of reducing transmission by this route remains. Approaches include use of antiretrovirals in the mother or infant, or both, sustained release of antivirals in the infant, and the prospect for an efficacious vaccine. The setting of perinatal (intrapartum and postpartum) transmission of HIV is ideal for the use of HIV vaccines, which could potentially provide long-term protection.

We have made major advances in the area, but much is left to be done. This includes the establishment of national networks and the participation of governments, agencies, pharmaceutical manufacturers, and international investigators to achieve our goal of global eradication of perinatal transmission of HIV.

REFERENCES

1. Centers for Disease Control and Prevention: HIV/AIDS Surveillance Report: Midyear Edition. 1998;10:5–21.
2. Centers for Disease Control and Prevention: HIV/AIDS Surveillance Supplemental Report: Characteristics of persons living with AIDS at the end of 1997. 1999; 5:4–6.
3. Rosenberg P, Biggar R: Trends in HIV incidence among young adults in the United States. JAMA 1998;279:1894–1899.

4. Rosenberg P: Scope of the AIDS epidemic in the United States. Science 1995;270:1372–1375.
5. Centers for Disease Control and Prevention: HIV/AIDS Surveillance Supplemental Report: Characteristics of persons living with AIDS at the end of 1999. 2000;7:1–16.
6. Successful Implementation of Perinatal HIV Prevention Guidelines. MMWR 2001;50:17.
7. CDC. Update: perinatally acquired HIVAIDS-United States, 1997. MMWR 1997;46:1086–1092.
8. Davis SF, Byers RH Jr, Lindegren ML, et al: Prevalence and incidence of vertically acquired HIV infection in the United States. JAMA 1995;274:952–955.
9. Rogers MF, Jaffe HW: Reducing the risk of maternal-infant transmission of HIV: A door is opened. N Engl J Med 1994;331:1222–1223.
10. Centers for Disease Control and Prevention: Public Health Service Task Force recommendations for the use of antiretroviral drugs in pregnant women infected with HIV-1 for maternal health and for reducing perinatal HIV-1 transmission in the United States (published errata appear in MMWR Morb Mortal Wkly Rep 1998;47:287 and 1998;47:315). MMWR Morb Mortal Wkly Rep 1998;47:1–30.
11. Centers for Disease Control and Prevention: Recommendations of the US Public Health Service Task Force on the use of zidovudine to reduce perinatal transmission of human immunodeficiency virus. MMWR 1994;43:1–20.
12. Centers for Disease Control and Prevention: US Public Health Service Task Force recommendations for the use of antiretroviral drugs in pregnant women infected with HIV-1 for maternal health and for reducing perinatal HIV-1 transmission in the United States. MMWR 1998;47:1–30.
13. De Cock KM, Fowler MG, Mercier E, et al: Prevention of mother-to-child HIV transmission in resource-poor countries: Translating research into policy and practice. JAMA 2000;283:1175–1182.
14. Andiman WA, Simpson BJ, Olson B, et al: Rate of transmission of human immunodeficiency virus type 1 infection from mother to child and short-term outcome of neonatal infection. Results of a prospective cohort study. Am J Dis Child 1990;144:758–766.
15. Blanche S, Rouzioux C, Moscato ML, et al: A prospective study of infants born to women seropositive for human immunodeficiency virus type 1: HIV Infection in Newborns French Collaborative Study Group. N Engl J Med 1989;320:1643–1648.
16. Nesheim SR, Lindsay M, Sawyer MK, et al: A prospective population-based study of HIV perinatal transmission. AIDS 1994;8:1293–1298.
17. Connor EM, Sperling RS, Gelber R, et al: Reduction of maternal-infant transmission of human immunodeficiency virus type 1 with zidovudine treatment: Pediatric AIDS Clinical Trials Group Protocol 076 Study Group. N Engl J Med 1994;331:1173–1180.
18. Sperling RS, Shapiro DE, Coombs RW, et al: Maternal viral load, zidovudine treatment, and the risk of transmission of human immunodeficiency virus type 1 from mother to infant: Pediatric AIDS Clinical Trials Group Protocol 076 Study Group. N Engl J Med 1996;335:1621–1629.
19. Pitt J, Brambilla D, Reichelderfer P, et al: Maternal immunologic and virologic risk factors for infant human immunodeficiency virus type 1 infection: Findings from the Women and Infants Transmission Study. J Infect Dis 1997;175:567–575.
20. Italian Multicentre Study: Epidemiology, clinical features, and prognostic factors of paediatric HIV infection. Lancet 1988;2:1043–1046.
21. European Collaborative Study: Risk factors for mother-to-child transmission of HIV-1. Lancet 1992;339:1007–1012.
22. Shaffer N, Roongpisuthipong A, Siriwasin W, et al: Maternal virus load and perinatal human immunodeficiency virus type 1 subtype E transmission, Thailand. Bangkok Collaborative Perinatal HIV Transmission Study Group. J Infect Dis 1999;179:590–599.
23. Shaffer N, Bulterys M, Simonds RJ: Short courses of zidovudine and perinatal transmission of HIV. N Engl J Med 1999;340:1042–1043.
24. Ryder RW, Nsa W, Hassig SE, et al: Perinatal transmission of the human immunodeficiency virus type 1 to infants of seropositive women in Zaire. N Engl J Med 1989;320:1637–1642.
25. Adjorlolo-Johnson G, De Cock KM, Ekpini E, et al: Prospective comparison of mother-to-child transmission of HIV-1 and HIV-2 in Abidjan, Ivory Coast (published erratum appears in JAMA 1994;272:1482). JAMA 1994;272:462–466.
26. Leroy V, Newell ML, Dabis F, et al: International multicentre pooled analysis of late postnatal mother-to-child transmission of HIV-1 infection. Ghent International Working Group on Mother-to-Child Transmission of HIV (published erratum appears in Lancet 1998;352:1154). Lancet 1998;352:597–600.
27. Dunn DT, Newell ML, Ades AE, Peckham CS: Risk of human immunodeficiency virus type 1 transmission through breastfeeding. Lancet 1992;340:585–588.
28. Clark SJ, Saag MS, Decker WD, et al: High titers of cytopathic virus in plasma of patients with symptomatic primary HIV-1 infection. N Engl J Med 1991;324:954–960.
29. Ryder RW, Behets F: Reasons for the wide variation in reported rates of mother-to-child transmission of HIV-1. AIDS 1994;8:1495–1497.
30. Boyer PJ, Dillon M, Navaie M, et al: Factors predictive of maternal-fetal transmission of HIV-1. Preliminary analysis of zidovudine given during pregnancy and/or delivery. JAMA 1994;271:1925–1930.
31. European Collaborative Study: Risk factors for mother-to-child transmission of HIV-1. Lancet 1992;339:1007–1012.

32. Dickover RE, Garratty EM, Herman SA, et al: Identification of levels of maternal HIV-1 RNA associated with risk of perinatal transmission: Effect of maternal zidovudine treatment on viral load. JAMA 1996;275:599–605.
33. Mofenson LM, Lambert JS, Stiehm ER, et al: Risk factors for perinatal transmission of human immunodeficiency virus type 1 in women treated with zidovudine. Pediatric AIDS Clinical Trials Group Study 185 Team. N Engl J Med 1999;341:385–393.
34. Garcia PM, Kalish LA, Pitt J, et al: Maternal levels of plasma human immunodeficiency virus type 1 RNA and the risk of perinatal transmission. Women and Infants Transmission Study Group. N Engl J Med 1999;341:394–402.
35. Contag CH, Ehrnst A, Duda J, et al: Mother-to-infant transmission of human immunodeficiency virus type 1 involving five envelope sequence subtypes. J Virol 1997;71:1292–1300.
36. Rodrigo AG, Mullins JI: Human immunodeficiency virus type 1 molecular evolution and the measure of selection. AIDS Res Hum Retroviruses 1996;12:1681–1685.
37. Lallemant M, Jourdain G, Le Coeur S, et al: A trial of shortened zidovudine regimens to prevent mother-to-child transmission of human immunodeficiency virus type 1. Perinatal HIV Prevention Trial (Thailand) Investigators. N Engl J Med 2000;343:982–991.
38. Bryson YJ, Luzuriaga K, Sullivan JL, Wara DW: Proposed definitions for in utero versus intrapartum transmission of HIV-1. N Engl J Med 1992;327:1246–1247.
39. Rouzioux C, Costagliola D, Burgard M, et al: Estimated timing of mother-to-child human immunodeficiency virus type 1 (HIV-1) transmission by use of a Markov model. The HIV Infection in Newborns French Collaborative Study Group. Am J Epidemiol 1995;142:1330–1337.
40. St. Louis M, Kamenga M, Brown C, et al: Risk for perinatal HIV-1 transmission according to maternal immunologic, virologic, and placental factors. JAMA 1993;269:2853–2859.
41. Van Dyke RB, Korber BT, Popek E, et al: The Ariel Project: A prospective cohort study of maternal-child transmission of human immunodeficiency virus type 1 in the era of maternal antiretroviral therapy. J Infect Dis 1999;179:319–328.
42. Brossard Y, Aubin JT, Mandelbrot L, et al: Frequency of early in utero HIV-1 infection: A blind DNA polymerase chain reaction study on 100 fetal thymuses. AIDS 1995;9:359–366.
43. Langston C, Lewis DE, Hammill HA, et al: Excess intrauterine fetal demise associated with maternal human immunodeficiency virus infection. J Infect Dis 1995;172:1451–1460.
44. Gray RH, Wawer MJ, Serwadda D, et al: Population-based study of fertility in women with HIV-1 infection in Uganda. Lancet 1998;351:98–103.
45. Dickover R, Dillon M, Leung K, et al: Early prognostic indicators in primary perinatal HIV-1 infection: Importance of viral RNA and the timing of transmission on long term outcome. J Infect Dis 1998:375–387.
46. Borkowsky W, Krasinski K, Pollack H, et al: Early diagnosis of human immunodeficiency virus infection in children less than 6 months of age: Comparison of polymerase chain reaction, culture, and plasma antigen capture techniques. J Pediatr 1992;125:345–351.
47. Borkowsky W, Krasinski K, Cao Y, et al: Correlation of perinatal transmission of human immunodeficiency virus type 1 with maternal viremia and lymphocyte phenotypes. J Pediatr 1994;125:345–351.
48. Mayaux MJ, Burgard M, Teglas JP, et al: Neonatal characteristics in rapidly progressive perinatally acquired HIV-1 disease. The French Pediatric HIV Infection Study Group. JAMA 1996;275:606–610.
49. Dunn DT, Brandt CD, Krivine A, et al: The sensitivity of HIV-1 DNA polymerase chain reaction in the neonatal period and the relative contributions of intra-uterine and intra-partum transmission. AIDS 1995;9:F7–F11.
50. McIntosh K, Pitt J, Brambilla D, et al: Blood culture in the first 6 months of life for the diagnosis of vertically transmitted human immunodeficiency virus infection. The Women and Infants Transmission Study Group. J Infect Dis 1994;170:996–1000.
51. Kalish LA, Pitt J, Lew J, et al: Defining the time of fetal or perinatal acquisition of human immunodeficiency virus type 1 infection on the basis of age at first positive culture. Women and Infants Transmission Study (WITS). J Infect Dis 1997;175:712–715.
52. Krivine A, Le Bourdelles S, Firtion G, Lebon P: Viral kinetics in HIV-1 perinatal infection. Lancet 1997;350:493.
53. Goedert JJ, Duliege AM, Amos CI, et al: High risk of HIV-1 infection for first-born twins. The International Registry of HIV-exposed Twins. Lancet 1991;338:1471–1475.
54. The International Perinatal HIV Group: The mode of delivery and the risk of vertical transmission of human immunodeficiency virus type 1—a meta-analysis of 15 prospective cohort studies. N Engl J Med 1999;340:977–987.
55. Baba TW, Koch J, Mittler ES, et al: Mucosal infection of neonatal rhesus monkeys with cell-free SIV. AIDS Res Hum Retrovirus 1994;10:351–357.
56. Nielsen K, Boyer P, Dillon M, et al: Presence of human immunodeficiency virus (HIV) type 1 and HIV-1-specific antibodies in cervicovaginal secretions of infected mothers and in the gastric aspirates of their infants. J Infect Dis 1996;173:1001–1004.
57. Thiry L, Sprecher-Goldberger S, Jonckheer T, et al: Isolation of AIDS virus from cell-free breast milk of three healthy virus carriers. Lancet 1985;2:891–892.
58. Ruff AJ, Coberly J, Halsey NA, et al: Prevalence of HIV-1 DNA and p24 antigen in breast milk and

correlation with maternal factors. J Acquir Immune Defic Syndr 1994;7:68–73.
59. Stiehm ER, Vink P: Transmission of human immunodeficiency virus infection by breast-feeding. J Pediatr 1991;118:410–412.
60. Peckham C, Gibb D: Mother-to-child transmission of the human immunodeficiency virus. N Engl J Med 1995;333:298–302.
61. Van de Perre P, Simonon A, Msellati P, et al: Postnatal transmission of human immunodeficiency virus type 1 from mother to infant. A prospective cohort study in Kigali, Rwanda. N Engl J Med 1991;325:593–598.
62. de Martino M, Tovo PA, Tozzi AE, et al: HIV-1 transmission through breast-milk: Appraisal of risk according to duration of feeding. AIDS 1992;6:991–997.
63. Nagelkerke NJ, Moses S, Embree JE, et al: The duration of breastfeeding by HIV-1-infected mothers in developing countries: Balancing benefits and risks. J Acquir Immune Defic Syndr Hum Retrovirol 1995;8:176–181.
64. Coutsoudis A: Method of feeding and transmission of HIV-1 from mothers to children by 15 months of age: Prospective cohort study from Durban. In: Proceedings of the XIII International AIDS Conference, Durban, South Africa, 2000.
65. Miotti PG, Taha TE, Kumwenda NI, et al: HIV transmission through breastfeeding: a study in Malawi. JAMA 1999;282:744–749.
66. Nduati R, John G, Mbori-Ngacha D, et al: Effect of breastfeeding and formula feeding on transmission of HIV-1: A randomized clinical trial. JAMA 2000;283:1167–1174.
67. Shearer WT, Quinn TC, LaRussa P, et al: Viral load and disease progression in infants infected with human immunodeficiency virus type 1. Women and Infants Transmission Study Group. N Engl J Med 1997;336:1337–1342.
68. Mellors JW, Rinaldo CR, Gupta P, et al: Prognosis in HIV-1 infection predicted by the quantity of virus in the plasma. Science 1996;272:1167–1170.
69. Lefrere JJ, Roudot-Thoraval F, Mariotti M, et al: The risk of disease progression is determined during the first year of human immunodeficiency virus type 1 infection. J Infect Dis 1998;177:1541–1548.
70. Mellors JW, Munoz A, Giorgi JV, et al: Plasma viral load and CD4+ lymphocytes as prognostic markers of HIV-1 infection. Ann Intern Med 1997;126:946–954.
71. Sabin CA, Devereux H, Phillips AN, et al: Immune markers and viral load after HIV-1 seroconversion as predictors of disease progression in a cohort of haemophilic men. AIDS 1998;12:1347–1352.
72. Vlahov D, Graham N, Hoover D, et al: Prognostic indicators for AIDS and infectious disease death in HIV- infected injection drug users: plasma viral load and CD4+ cell count. JAMA 1998;279:35–40.
73. Nahmias AJ, Clark WS, Kourtis AP, et al: Thymic dysfunction and time of infection predict mortality in human immunodeficiency virus-infected infants. CDC Perinatal AIDS Collaborative Transmission Study Group. J Infect Dis 1998;178:680–685.
74. Jamieson BD, Uittenbogaart CH, Schmid I, Zack JA: High viral burden and rapid CD4+ cell depletion in human immunodeficiency virus type 1-infected SCID-hu mice suggest direct viral killing of thymocytes in vivo. J Virol 1997;71:8245–8253.
75. Kourtis AP, Ibegbu C, Nahmias AJ, et al: Early progression of disease in HIV-infected infants with thymus dysfunction (published erratum appears in N Engl J Med 1997;336:595). N Engl J Med 1996;335:1431–1436.
76. Baba TW, Liska V, Hofmann-Lehmann R, et al: Human neutralizing monoclonal antibodies of the IgG1 subtype protect against mucosal simian-human immunodeficiency virus infection. Nat Med 2000;6:200–206.
77. Van Rompay KK, Otsyula MG, Tarara RP, et al: Vaccination of pregnant macaques protects newborns against mucosal simian immunodeficiency virus infection. J Infect Dis 1996;173:1327–1335.
78. Giavedoni LD, Planelles V, Haigwood NL, et al: Immune response of rhesus macaques to recombinant simian immunodeficiency virus gp130 does not protect from challenge infection. J Virol 1993;67:577–583.
79. Lohman BL, Higgins J, Marthas ML, Marx PA, Pedersen NC: Development of simian immunodeficiency virus isolation, titration, and neutralization assays which use whole blood from rhesus monkeys and an antigen capture enzyme-linked immunosorbent assay. J Clin Microbiol 1991;29:2187–2192.
80. Bryson YJ, Pang S, Wei LS, et al: Clearance of HIV infection in a perinatally infected infant. N Engl J Med 1995;332:833–838.
81. Newell ML, Dunn D, De Maria A, et al: Detection of virus in vertically exposed HIV-antibody-negative children. Lancet 1996;347:213–215.
82. Roques PA, Gras G, Parnet-Mathieu F, et al: Clearance of HIV infection in 12 perinatally infected children: clinical, virological and immunological data. AIDS 1995;9:F19–F26.
83. Frenkel LM, Mullins JI, Learn GH, et al: Genetic evaluation of suspected cases of transient HIV-1 infection of infants. Science 1998;280:1073–1077.
84. Dickover R, Bryson Y, Garratty E: Early HIV env gene evolution in perinatally infected infants predicts the rate of disease progression. Paper presented at the 8th Conference on Retroviruses, Chicago, Ill, 2001.
85. Frenkel LM, Wagner LE 2nd, Demeter LM, et al: Effects of zidovudine use during pregnancy on resistance and vertical transmission of human immunodeficiency virus type 1. Clin Infect Dis 1995;20:1321–1326.
86. McSherry GD, Shapiro DE, Coombs RW, et al: The effects of zidovudine in the subset of infants infected with human immunodeficiency virus type-1 (Pediatric

AIDS Clinical Trials Group Protocol 076). J Pediatr 1999;134:717–724.
87. Gray G, McIntyre J, Jikov B, et al: Preliminary efficacy, safety, tolerability and pharmacokinetics of short course regimens of nucleoside analogues for the prevention of mother-to-child transmission (MTCT) of HIV. Abstract TuOrB355. Paper presented at the XIII International AIDS Conference, Durban, South Africa, 2000.
88. Biggar RJ, Mtimavalye L, Justesen A, et al: Does umbilical cord blood polymerase chain reaction positivity indicate in utero (pre-labor) HIV infection? AIDS 1997;11:1375–1382.
89. Biggar RJ, Janes M, Pilon R, et al: Virus levels in untreated African infants infected with human immunodeficiency virus type 1. J Infect Dis 1999;180:1838–1843.
90. Wiktor SZ, Ekpini E, Karon JM, et al: Short-course oral zidovudine for prevention of mother-to-child transmission of HIV-1 in Abidjan, Cote d'Ivoire: A randomised trial. Lancet 1999;353:781.
91. Wiktor S, Leroy V, Ekpini E, et al: 24 month efficacy of short course zidovudine for the prevention of mother-to-child HIV-1 transmission in a breastfeeding population: A pooled analysis of two randomized clinical trials in West Africa. Paper presented at the XIII International AIDS Conference, Durban, South Africa, 2000.
92. Saba J: Interim analysis of early efficacy of three short ZDV/3TC combination regimens to prevent mother to child transmission of HIV-1: The PETRA trial [abstract S7]. Paper presented at the 6th Conference on Retroviruses and Opportunistic Infections, Chicago, Ill, 1999.
93. Gray G: The PETRA Study: Early and late efficacy of three short ZDV/3TC combination regimens to prevent MTCT of HIV-1. Abstract LbOr5. Paper presented at the XIII International AIDS Conference, Durban, South Africa, 2000.
94. Guay LA, Musoke P, Fleming T, et al: Intrapartum and neonatal single-dose nevirapine compared with zidovudine for prevention of mother-to-child transmission of HIV-1 in Kampala, Uganda: HIVNET 012 randomised trial. Lancet 1999;354:795–802.
95. Owor M, Deseyve M, Duefield C, et al: The one year safety and efficacy data of HIVNET 012 trial. Abstract LbOr1. Paper presented at the XIII International AIDS Conference, Durban, South Africa, 2000.
96. Moodley D, McIntyre J, Team SS: Evaluation of safety and efficacy of two simple regimens for the prevention of mother to child transmission (MTCT) of HIV infection: Nevirapine vs lamivudine and zidovudine used in a randomised clinical trial (the SAINT study) [abstract TuOrB356]. Paper presented at the XIII International AIDS Conference, Durban, South Africa, 2000.
97. Bryson YJ: Perinatal HIV-1 transmission: Recent advances and therapeutic interventions. AIDS 1996;10(Suppl 3):S33–42.
98. Newell ML, Gray G, Bryson YJ: Prevention of mother-to-child transmission of HIV-1 infection. AIDS 1997;11:S165–72.
99. Peckham C, Newell ML: Preventing vertical transmission of HIV infection. N Engl J Med 2000;343:1036–1037.
100. Mabondzo A, Narwa R, Roques P, et al: Lack of correlation between vertical transmission of HIV-1 and maternal antibody titers against autologous virus in human monocyte-derived macrophages. J Acquir Immune Defic Syndr Hum Retrovirol 1998;17:92–94.
101. Scarlatti G, Albert J, Rossi P, et al: Mother-to-child transmission of human immunodeficiency virus type 1: Correlation with neutralizing antibodies against primary isolates. J Infect Dis 1993;168:207–210.
102. Husson RN, Lan Y, Kojima E, et al: Vertical transmission of human immunodeficiency virus type 1: Autologous neutralizing antibody, virus load, and virus phenotype. J Pediatr 1995;126:865–871.
103. Wolinsky SM, Wike CM, Korber BT, et al: Selective transmission of human immunodeficiency virus type-1 variants from mothers to infants. Science 1992;255:1134–1137.
104. Dickover R, Garratty E, Plaeger S, Bryson Y: Perinatal transmission of major, minor and multiple maternal HIV variants in utero and intrapartum. J Virol 2001;75:2194–2203.
105. Scarlatti G, Hodara V, Rossi P, Muggiasca L, Bucceri A, Albert J, Fenyo EM. Transmission of human immunodeficiency virus type 1 (HIV-1) from mother to child correlates with viral phenotype. Virology 1993;197:624–629.
106. Kliks SC, Levy JA: Maternal antibody response and maternal-infant HIV-1 transmission. Lancet 1994;343:1364.
107. Ometto L, Zanotto C, Maccabruni A, et al: Viral phenotype and host-cell susceptibility to HIV-1 infection as risk factors for mother-to-child HIV-1 transmission. AIDS 1995;9:427–434.
108. Lathey JL, Tsou J, Brinker K, et al: Lack of autologous neutralizing antibody to human immunodeficiency virus type 1 (HIV-1) and macrophage tropism are associated with mother-to-infant transmission. J Infect Dis 1999;180:344–350.
109. Kostrikis LG: Impact of natural chemokine receptor polymorphisms on perinatal transmission of human immunodeficiency virus type 1. Teratology 2000;61:387–390.
110. Kostrikis LG, Neumann AU, Thomson B, et al: A polymorphism in the regulatory region of the CC-chemokine receptor 5 gene influences perinatal transmission of human immunodeficiency virus type 1 to African-American infants. J Virol 1999;73:10264–10271.
111. Kostrikis LG, Huang Y, Moore JP, et al: A chemokine receptor CCR2 allele delays HIV-1 disease progression and is associated with a CCR5 promoter mutation. Nat Med 1998;4:350–353.

112. Bertolli J, St. Louis ME, Simonds RJ, et al: Estimating the timing of mother-to-child transmission of human immunodeficiency virus in a breast-feeding population in Kinshasa, Zaire. J Infect Dis 1996;174:722–726.
113. Mayaux MJ, Blanche S, Rouzioux C, et al: Maternal factors associated with perinatal HIV-1 transmission: the French Cohort Study: 7 years of follow-up observation. The French Pediatric HIV Infection Study Group. J Acquir Immune Defic Syndr Hum Retrovirol 1995;8:188–194.
114. Blanche S, Mayaux MJ, Rouzioux C, et al: Relation of the course of HIV infection in children to the severity of the disease in their mothers at delivery. N Engl J Med 1994;330:308–312.
115. Rouzioux C, Burgard M, Chaix ML, et al: Human immunodeficiency virus-1 infection in neonates: Correlation of plasma and cellular viremia and clinical outcome. French Pediatric Cohort Study Group. Acta Paediatrica Suppl 1997;421:17–21.
116. Dickover RE, Dillon M, Gillette SG, et al: Rapid increases in load of human immunodeficiency virus correlate with early disease progression and loss of CD4 cells in vertically infected infants. J Infect Dis 1994;170:1279–1284.
117. Stiehm ER, Lambert JS, Mofenson LM, et al: Efficacy of zidovudine and human immunodeficiency virus (HIV) hyperimmune immunoglobulin for reducing perinatal HIV transmission from HIV-infected women with advanced disease: Results of Pediatric AIDS Clinical Trials Group protocol 185. J Infect Dis 1999;179:567–575.
118. Fang G, Burger H, Grimson R, et al: Maternal plasma human immunodeficiency virus type 1 RNA level: A determinant and projected threshold for mother-to-child transmission. Proc Nat Acad Sci U S A 1995;92:12100–121104.
119. Weiser B, Nachman S, Tropper P, et al: Quantitation of human immunodeficiency virus type 1 during pregnancy: Relationship of viral titer to mother-to-child transmission and stability of viral load. Proc Natl Acad Sci U S A 1994;91:8037–8041.
120. Despina G, Contopoulos-Loannidis J, Loannidis P: Maternal cell-free viremia in the natural history of perinatal HIV-1 transmission: A meta-analysis. J Acquir Imm Defic Syndr Hum Retrovirol 1998;18:126–135.
121. Burns DN, Landesman S, Muenz LR, et al: Cigarette smoking, premature rupture of membranes, and vertical transmission of HIV-1 among women with low CD4+ levels. J Acquir Immune Defic Syndr 1994;7:718–726.
122. Nair P, Alger L, Hines S, et al: Maternal and neonatal characteristics associated with HIV infection in infants of seropositive women. J Acquir Immune Defic Syndr 1993;6:298–302.
123. Landesman SH, Kalish LA, Burns DN, et al: Obstetrical factors and the transmission of human immunodeficiency virus type 1 from mother to child. The Women and Infants Transmission Study. N Engl J Med 1996;334:1617–1623.
124. Minkoff H, Burns DN, Landesman S, et al: The relationship of the duration of ruptured membranes to vertical transmission of human immunodeficiency virus. Am J Obstet Gynecol 1995;173:585–589.
125. Simonds RJ, Steketee R, Nesheim S, et al: Impact of zidovudine use on risk and risk factors for perinatal transmission of HIV. Perinatal AIDS Collaborative Transmission Studies. AIDS 1998;12: 301–308.
126. Hutto C, Parks WP, Lai SH, et al: A hospital-based prospective study of perinatal infection with human immunodeficiency virus type 1. J Pediatr 1991;118:347–353.
127. The European Collaborative Study: Caesarean section and risk of vertical transmission of HIV-1 infection. Lancet 1994;343:1464–1467.
128. Duliege AM, Amos CI, Felton S, et al: Birth order, delivery route, and concordance in the transmission of human immunodeficiency virus type 1 from mothers to twins. International Registry of HIV-Exposed Twins. J Pediatr 1995;126:625–632.
129. Mandelbrot L, Le Chenadec J, Berrebi A, et al: Perinatal HIV-1 transmission: Interaction between zidovudine prophylaxis and mode of delivery in the French Perinatal Cohort. JAMA 1998;280:55–60.
130. Read J, Kpamegan E, Tuomala R, et al: Mode of delivery and postpartum morbidity among HIV-infected women: The women and infants transmission study (WITS) [abstract 683]. Paper presented at the 6th Conference on Retroviruses and Opportunistic Infections, Chicago, Ill, 1999.
131. Stratton P, Tuomala RE, Abboud R, et al: Obstetric and newborn outcomes in a cohort of HIV-infected pregnant women: A report of the women and infants transmission study. J Acquir Immune Defic Syndr Hum Retrovirol 1999;20:179–186.
132. Kuhn L, Abrams EJ, Matheson PB, et al: Timing of maternal-infant HIV transmission: Associations between intrapartum factors and early polymerase chain reaction results. New York City Perinatal HIV Transmission Collaborative Study Group. AIDS 1997;11:429–435.
133. Nielsen K, Dillon M, Boyer P, et al: Peripartum risk factors for vertical transmission of HIV. Paper presented at the Conference on Global Strategies for the Prevention of HIV Transmission from Mother to Infant, Washington, D. C., 1997.
134. Kuhn L, Coutsoudis A, Moodley D, et al: T-helper cell responses to HIV envelope peptides in cord blood: Protection against intrapartum and breast-feeding transmission. AIDS 2001;15:1–9.

3 Immunopathogenesis of Pediatric HIV Infection

Stuart E. Starr

Damage to the immune system is one of the most important consequences of pediatric HIV infection. Almost all HIV-infected children eventually develop some degree of immunodeficiency, and those with severe immunologic impairments are more likely to acquire opportunistic infections. HIV infection also activates the immune system, and such activation may have a variety of consequences.

Mechanisms responsible for immunodeficiency in HIV-infected children have not been delineated fully. HIV replication in certain types of immune cells may lead to their destruction, but since few cells are infected in vivo, the profound immunodeficiency that develops in many untreated children may involve mechanisms that do not require replication of the virus. Apoptosis, also known as programmed cell death, may be responsible for loss of immune cells in lymphoid organs, including thymus, lymph nodes, and spleen. Inadequate production of naive T lymphocytes also may contribute to immunodeficiency in HIV-infected children.

HIV-specific cell-mediated immune responses, particularly those mediated by cytotoxic T lymphocytes (CTL), appear to play a major role in control of HIV replication. If such responses are reduced, as a result of HIV-specific mechanisms or general immaturity or attrition of the immune system, HIV may replicate to higher levels, thus exposing additional cells of the immune system to HIV virions and proteins. Initiation of combination antiretroviral therapy during the first few months of life can lead to preservation of the immune system, but cell-mediated HIV-specific immune responses do not appear, and HIV antibodies fall to undetectable levels, suggesting that HIV antigens have been eliminated by the therapy. In both adults and children, combination antiretroviral therapy leads to partial immune reconstitution. Naive T cells, which have greater potential to reconstitute the immune system than memory T cells, appear sooner and attain higher levels in children than in adults. HIV-specific cell-mediated immunologic responses, thought to be necessary for long-term control of virus replication, are not detected in most HIV-infected children and adults.

In this chapter, immunologic impairments in HIV-infected children, putative mechanisms responsible for such impairments, and immunorestorative effects of antiretroviral therapy will be reviewed.

ROLE OF IMMATURITY OF THE IMMUNE SYSTEM

HIV infection of the fetus and newborn occurs in the setting of an immature immune system.[1] Fetal T lymphocytes probably have a limited repertoire of antigen-specific receptors until late in gestation, and thus may not recognize HIV antigens. Fetal and neonatal T lymphocytes are impaired in their ability to produce certain cytokines, particularly interferon-γ. This impairment may contribute to reduced ability to generate or amplify HIV-specific CTL. In addition, diminished expression of

CD40 ligand by fetal and neonatal T lymphocytes may contribute to impaired or delayed provision of help to B lymphocytes for the production of antibodies to HIV and other pathogens.

Feeble immune responses to HIV in the fetus and newborn may allow more rapid and extensive virus replication than in older hosts. In addition, certain fetal and neonatal cells, including monocyte-macrophages and CD8+ lymphocytes, are more susceptible to HIV infection in vitro than corresponding adult cells.[2,3] Such increased susceptibility may contribute to the high viral loads detected in neonates.

EFFECT OF HIV INFECTION ON LYMPHOCYTE SUBPOPULATIONS

The major effects of pediatric HIV infection on the immune system, summarized in Table 3–1, are discussed in this section and in Section 5. Effects are shown according to stage of infection; however, in infants with rapidly progressive disease, "late" effects may appear as early as the first year of life.

Peripheral Blood Lymphocytes

Depletion of circulating CD4+ cells was the earliest recognized immunologic consequence of HIV infection in children. CD4+ cell depletion provides a useful indicator of severity of HIV infection, since the incidence of disease progression, as manifested by opportunistic infections and other complications, correlates with number and percentage of CD4+ lymphocytes.[4–6] These CD4+ lymphocyte parameters also constitute the basis for the current definition of immunologic categories for HIV-infected children.[7] Interpretation of CD4+ cell parameters requires comparison to age-matched control subjects. Currently, normal values for CD4+ cell number and percentage are based on studies of uninfected children born to HIV-infected mothers or small cohorts of unexposed healthy children.[8,9] Based on such data, absolute numbers of circulating lymphocytes, including CD4+ lymphocytes, have been found to be higher in infants and young children than in adults and to decline over the first few years of life. CD4+ percentage varies less by age than by absolute CD4+ cell counts. A study now in progress, sponsored by the Pediatric AIDS Clinical Trials Group (PACTG), will provide more definitive data on lymphocyte subpopulations in healthy children who have not been exposed to HIV.

In untreated children with HIV infection, depletion of circulating CD4+ cells may appear within the first year or two of life or occur much later. Children who develop very low CD4+ lymphocyte counts during the first year of life have a shortened life expectancy.[5]

Over the first 24 months of life, circulating CD8+ lymphocyte counts are similar or slightly higher in most HIV-infected infants compared with age-matched control subjects.[10] During the first 6 months of life, approximately 15% of HIV-infected infants have absolute counts of both CD4+ and CD8+ cells that are less than the fifth percentile for uninfected age-matched control subjects.[11] Total CD8+ cell counts have been reported to be similar[12] or significantly higher[13,14] in HIV-infected children compared with age-matched control subjects. HIV-infected adolescents 13 to 19 years of age have higher CD8+ cell counts than uninfected age-matched control subjects.[15,16]

CD4+ and CD8+ lymphocytes are classified further as naive or memory cells, based on phenotypical markers that can be easily detected by flow cytometry. Naive cells express the CD45 isoform known as CD45RA. When naive T cells encounter antigen and proliferate, a different CD45 isoform known as CD45RO appears and CD45RA disappears. In general, CD45RA+ and CD45RO+ T cell populations are mutually exclusive. CD45RO+ T cells may occasionally revert to a CD45RA phenotype, but such revertant cells are thought to represent a relatively minor fraction of the total CD45RA+ population, particularly in children who are undergoing active thymopoiesis.

In several studies, naive and memory subpopulations of CD4+ and CD8+ lymphocytes were enumerated in HIV-infected children and adolescents, and the results were compared to those obtained in uninfected age-matched control subjects. HIV-infected children maintain normal ratios of CD4+ naive and memory cells, even when the absolute number of CD4+ cells is reduced.[17,18] Similar results were reported for HIV-infected adolescents.[15,16] In contrast, CD8+ memory cells were increased, while CD8+ naive cells were decreased in HIV-infected children compared with uninfected control subjects,[12,14] a pattern also observed in HIV-infected adults.[19] HIV-infected adolescents with CD4+ cell counts of less than 200 cells/mm^3, 200 to 499 cells/mm^3, and greater than 500 cells/mm^3 had reduced, comparable, or elevated numbers of CD8+ naive cells, respectively, compared to age-matched uninfected control subjects.[16] Of particular importance, at each of the CD4+ strata,

Table 3–1
Major Effects of Pediatric HIV Infection on the Immune System

STAGE OF INFECTION	STRUCTURAL CHANGES	CELLULAR EFFECTS	FUNCTIONAL EFFECTS
Early	Thymitis	Polyclonal stimulation of B cells	Generation of HIV-specific antibodies and cytotoxic T lymphocytes
	Lymph node hyperplasia	Activation of T cells	Decreased lymphocyte proliferation to recall antigens
		Expansion of CD8+ cell clones	Impaired production of antibodies to vaccine antigens
		Increased apoptosis of T cells	Decreased ability to produce type 1 cytokines
		?Reduced ability to generate naive T cells	Decreased neutrophil chemotaxis and killing
Late	Thymic involution	All of above, plus:	All of above, plus:
	Lymph node depletion	CD4+ cell depletion	Decreased lymphocyte proliferation to alloantigens and mitogens
		Naive CD8+ cell depletion	

HIV-infected adolescents had higher numbers of CD8+ naive cells compared with HIV-infected adults.[19]

Markers of T cell activation, such as HLA-DR and CD38, are expressed on a higher percentage of lymphocytes, particularly CD8+ cells, of HIV-infected children and adolescents compared with uninfected age-matched control subjects.[10,13–15,17,20]

Thymus and Lymph Nodes

A spectrum of thymic pathologic changes, ranging from mild to severe depletion of lymphocytes in the cortex and medulla, epithelial injury, and decreased or absent Hassall corpuscles, has been seen in HIV-infected fetuses and newborns.[21,22] Similar changes were noted, with calcification of Hassall corpuscles in some cases, in autopsy specimens from children who died of AIDS.[23] Thymus biopsy specimens obtained at the time of open lung biopsy in HIV-infected children showed thymitis, precocious involution, or involution mimicking thymic dysplasia.[24] Thymitis, thought to be an early manifestation of HIV infection, possibly developing in response to thymic epithelial injury, was the most common finding. Since these studies involved a limited number of specimens, the incidence of thymic damage in HIV-infected children remains to be determined.

Certain strains of HIV may have greater tropism for immature thymocytes and therefore greater potential to produce thymic damage.[25] As a result of such damage, the ability of the thymus to produce naive T lymphocytes may be impaired (see later).

Morphologic changes in peripheral lymphoid tissue (tonsils and lymph nodes) also have been described.[26] Follicular hyperplasia is the earliest manifestation of HIV infection in lymph nodes of infected children. At a later stage, follicular fragmentation can be seen with beginning loss of germinal centers and the follicular dendritic cell network. In children with end-stage disease, complete loss of lymph node structure, including germinal centers, is a common finding.

POSSIBLE MECHANISMS RESPONSIBLE FOR LOSS OR EXPANSION OF LYMPHOCYTE SUBPOPULATIONS

A number of mechanisms may play a role in the loss or expansion of certain lymphocyte populations in HIV-infected children.

Direct Effects of HIV Infection on CD4+ Lymphocytes

Since HIV is capable of infecting CD4+ lymphocytes, some loss of CD4+ cells might be attributable to death of infected cells. However, only a small fraction of CD4+ lymphocytes are infected with HIV, making it unlikely that loss of CD4+ lymphocytes can be explained entirely by this mechanism. Since HIV usually does not infect CD8+ lymphocytes, loss of cells within this subpopulation must occur through other mechanisms.

Role of Apoptosis

Several groups reported that CD4+ and CD8+ lymphocytes of HIV-infected children undergo programmed cell death, also known as apoptosis, at a more rapid rate than lymphocytes from age-matched uninfected children.[27,28] Additional studies showed that apoptotic lymphocytes were mainly CD45RO+ memory cells that expressed the activation marker HLA-DR, suggesting that HLA-DR+ lymphocytes may be more susceptible to apoptosis.[29] In addition, a higher percentage of lymphocytes from HIV-infected children expressed CD95, a key molecule involved in apoptosis,[28,30] and CD95-expressing lymphocytes were more susceptible to CD95-mediated apoptosis.[30] In addition, CD4+ and CD8+ lymphocytes from HIV-infected children have decreased expression of CD28, a costimulatory molecule that is associated with protection from apoptosis.[31] Taken together, these observations suggest that CD4+ and CD8+ lymphocytes from HIV-infected children are more susceptible to apoptosis owing to activation and differential expression of certain surface molecules. Most of the lymphocytes that undergo apoptosis are not infected with HIV, thus making apoptosis a mechanism by which massive numbers of CD4+ and CD8+ lymphocytes could be destroyed in HIV-infected individuals.[32] Interaction of gp120 on an infected cell with CD4+ on an uninfected cell may initiate the process of apoptosis.[33]

Decreased Generation of T Lymphocytes

Hematopoietic progenitor cells of HIV-infected individuals were shown to have reduced ability to produce colonies in vitro.[34] Such impairment of stem cell function could contribute to decreased generation of prethymic lymphocyte precursors, as well as other hematopoietic cells, in HIV-infected children.

HIV infection also might interfere with T lymphocyte development in the thymus. Several mechanisms could be involved, including destruction of thymic epithelium or of specific subpopulations of thymocytes. The end result might be decreased production of naive CD4+ and CD8+ cells. Although mature CD8+ lymphocytes are not susceptible to HIV infection, thymic precursors of mature CD8 lymphocytes are susceptible to HIV infection,[35] which may explain low CD8+ counts in some HIV-infected infants.

Limited data exist on the contribution of thymic damage to the immunopathogenesis of HIV infection. Progress in this field has been limited by the lack of a reliable assay to measure thymic function or damage in HIV-infected individuals. Infected infants thought to have thymic dysfunction on the basis of having CD4+ and CD8+ cell counts below the fifth percentile for age had significantly greater mortality over the first 2 years of life than infants with higher cell counts.[11,36] Infants with low cell counts who were infected in utero had a worse prognosis than those infected at the time of birth. Interpretation of these results is complicated by uncertainty about the relationship of low CD4+ and CD8+ cell counts to thymic function in the HIV-infected children studied. In addition, these observations were made prior to the advent of highly active antiretroviral therapy, which has improved the prognosis for HIV-infected children, including those with low CD4+ cell counts at the onset of therapy (see later). Thymic volume as determined by magnetic resonance imaging correlates with CD4+ lymphocyte count and with the percentage and absolute number of naive CD4+ cells in HIV-infected children.[37] In addition, the ability of peripheral blood mononuclear cells to proliferate in response to tetanus antigen is directly proportional to thymic volume. These results suggest that thymic function is essential for maintenance of CD4+ cell number and function in HIV-infected children. It must be pointed out, however, that a correlation between thymic volume and function has not been established, and that early damage to the thymus may not be accompanied by loss of volume. Alternatively, loss of thymic volume and circulating CD4+ cells may occur independently in children infected with certain strains of HIV or with higher levels of viral replication.

Role of Clonal Expansion

Clones of CD8+ CTL capable of killing HIV-infected target cells may be expanded in HIV-infected children. The exact mechanisms responsible for generation of CD8+ CTL have not been defined, but cytokines produced by T helper 1 (Th1) CD4 cells appear to be essential. Production of such cytokines in vivo may lead to proliferation of HIV-specific CD8+ CTL clones. If sufficient numbers of CD8+ CTLs are produced, the total CD8 cell count may rise, as has been observed in some HIV-infected children and adolescents. Since CD8+ CTLs have a memory phenotype and also bear activation markers, the increase in memory and activated CD8+ cells may be attributable in part to increased numbers of CD8+ CTL.

Role of T Lymphocyte Turnover

To understand better the dynamics of T cell production and destruction in HIV-infected individuals, T cell turnover has been studied in adults using a variety of techniques, including detection of Ki67, a nuclear antigen found in proliferating cells, and incorporation of a stable isotope, deuterated glucose, into DNA of lymphocytes. In a study of Ki67 expression in lymphocyte subsets, turnover of CD4+ cells appeared to be increased approximately twofold in HIV-infected adults, while that of CD8+ cells was increased sixfold.[38] In vivo studies of incorporation of deuterated glucose into lymphocyte DNA have given similar results.[39] Taken together, these results suggest moderate rates of CD4+ cell destruction and replacement in HIV-infected individuals, in contrast to massive generation and destruction of CD8+ cells, many of which may be CTL. T cell turnover has not been studied to date in HIV-infected children or adolescents.

IMPAIRED IMMUNOLOGIC FUNCTION IN HIV-INFECTED CHILDREN

As discussed earlier, HIV infection causes major changes in lymphocyte numbers and phenotype. In addition, HIV infection may deleteriously affect the function of various components of the immune system, including antigen-presenting cells, T lymphocytes, B lymphocytes, natural killer (NK) cells, and neutrophils. As a result, host immune responses against HIV are weakened and, in the absence of antiretroviral therapy, ultimately fail, allowing HIV to replicate at even higher levels.

Lymphocyte Proliferation Responses

Decreased CD4+ helper lymphocyte function is thought to play a central role in the immunodeficiency associated with HIV infection, since these cells provide essential cytokines for both B cell development and generation of CTL. Lymphocyte proliferation to various antigens has been used as an in vitro measure of CD4+ helper function. HIV-infected children demonstrate progressive loss in ability to mount lymphocyte proliferation responses against certain antigens. In a prospective study, impaired responses to *Candida albicans,* diphtheria, and tetanus were detected in some children younger than 1 year of age, and the frequency of impaired responses increased over the next 3 years.[40] Loss of ability to respond to antigens has been detected in children with normal as well as reduced CD4+ cell counts, suggesting that loss of memory CD4+ cells is not the only mechanism involved.[41]

Most HIV-infected children also have poor lymphoproliferative responses to HIV antigens. This observation may be explained by an early loss of ability to respond to antigens in general, but HIV-specific mechanisms may be involved as well. Inability of T lymphocytes to proliferate in response to HIV antigens may represent a key immunologic deficiency in HIV infection, since robust virus-specific helper T cell responses appear to play a major role in recovery from other virus infections.

HIV-infected children may also lose the ability to respond to alloantigens and mitogens such as phytohemagglutinin, pokeweed, and *Staphylococcus* A.[42,43] Most children who fail to respond to alloantigens and mitogens have advanced HIV disease or CD4+ cell counts less than 200 cells/mm^3, but some have higher counts.[43] Loss of ability to respond to these stimuli suggests a greater degree of immunodeficiency and increased susceptibility to opportunistic infections.

Limited information is available on mechanisms responsible for impaired lymphoproliferative responses in HIV-infected children. In some cases, responses to specific antigens such as tetanus can be restored in vitro by the addition of exogenous interleukin-1 or interleukin-2, suggesting that antigen-responsive memory cells are not depleted but rather proliferate poorly owing to decreased production of cytokines.[44]

Ability to respond to specific recall antigens also can be determined with the use of delayed type hypersensitivity skin testing. Most HIV-infected children with greater than 25% CD4+ cells are able to respond to one or more recall antigens, such as *Candida albicans*, mumps, and tetanus.[45] Children with less than 15% CD4+ cells are more likely to be anergic against these antigens. The relative sensitivity and specificity of lymphocyte proliferation assays and DTH reactions in HIV-infected children have not been defined.

Cytokine Production

HIV-infected children develop major perturbations in ability to produce cytokines essential for certain immune functions. Cytokines can be divided into those that stimulate T lymphocytes (type 1 cytokines) and those that stimulate B lymphocytes (type 2 cytokines). Cytokines are produced by both lymphocytes and monocytes. Two major classes of cytokine-producing CD4 lymphocytes have been described: helper type 1 (Th1) and helper type 2 (Th2). Th1 lymphocytes produce type 1 cytokines, including interleukin-2 and interferon-γ, whereas Th2 lymphocytes produce type 2 cytokines such as interleukin-4, interleukin-5, interleukin-6, and interleukin-10. Macrophages produce interleukin-10, a type 2 cytokine, and interleukin-12, a type 1 cytokine.

Initial studies of in vitro cytokine production in HIV-infected children suggested that production of interleukin-2 and interferon-γ was reduced, while production of type 2 cytokines interleukin-4 and interleukin-10 was increased as compared with uninfected age-matched control subjects.[46,47] The authors proposed that HIV-infected children undergo a shift in cytokine production from predominantly type 1 to predominantly type 2, and that this shift contributes to disease progression. Subsequent studies by other groups confirmed decreased production of type 1 cytokines, including interleukin-2, interleukin-12, and interferon-γ, in HIV-infected children but did not confirm increased production of type 2 cytokines.[48–50]

Another approach has been to measure cytokine levels in the serum of HIV-infected children. In one study, elevated levels of interleukin-6 and tumor necrosis factor-α, but not interleukin-4, were detected in HIV-infected children as compared with uninfected control subjects, and interleukin-6 levels correlated with levels of IgG and IgA.[51] In another study, serum interleukin-2 levels were elevated in most HIV-infected children who had little or no evidence of immune impairment but were significantly lower in infected children in whom immunodeficiency was present.[52]

Taken together, these results suggest that the ability to produce type 1 cytokines is progressively lost in HIV-infected children. Loss of ability to produce these cytokines may explain, at least in part, the reduced lymphocyte proliferation and CTL responses noted in some HIV-infected children. Overproduction of certain cytokines, particularly interleukin-6 and tumor necrosis factor-α, may contribute to some manifestations of HIV infection in children, either through direct effects of these cytokines or through their ability to upregulate HIV replication.[53] Most of the data accumulated to date do not support a shift from production of type 1 to type 2 cytokines in HIV-infected children.

Cytotoxicity

Cytotoxic T Lymphocytes

The activity of CTLs can be measured using fresh peripheral blood mononuclear cells (sometimes referred to as direct or primary CTL activity) or peripheral blood mononuclear cells (PBMC) incubated with HIV antigens and interleukin-2 for 2 to 3 weeks. Such in vitro stimulation allows CTL precursors to develop cytotoxic capability. In HIV-infected individuals, CTL activity has been detected against a number of HIV structural or regulatory proteins, including Env, Gag, Pol, and Nef.

Direct CTL activity has been detected in a minority of HIV-infected children but is present in some young infants.[54,55] In contrast, such activity is detected readily in untreated HIV-infected adults. The inability of most HIV-infected children to develop direct CTL activity has not been explained adequately. CTL precursors can be demonstrated in HIV-infected children, but in most studies such precursors have been detected regularly only in children 12 months of age or older.[55,56] When present, CTL precursors are detected at frequencies similar to those observed in HIV-infected adults.[56]

Delayed and weak CTL responses in HIV-infected children may explain the higher viral loads noted in children compared with adults, as well as the more rapid progression of disease in some HIV-infected children. In some studies, detection of broad CTL activity against multiple HIV proteins correlated with higher CD4+ cell counts and lower viral loads.[57] In contrast, the early presence of precursor CTL activity did not prevent disease progression in HIV-infected infants.[58]

Natural Killer Cell Activity

Natural killer (NK) cell–mediated cytotoxicity against HIV-infected targets has been measured in both HIV-infected and uninfected children of various ages. In healthy term neonates, the magnitude of NK cell–mediated cytotoxicity against HIV-infected targets was similar to that detected in healthy adults.[59] In contrast, premature neonates had significantly lower levels of NK cell–mediated cytotoxicity against HIV-infected targets compared with term neonates.[60] In HIV-infected children 15 to 54 months of age, NK cell–mediated lysis of tumor (K562) cells was reduced significantly compared with age-matched, uninfected children.[61] Similarly, NK cell counts and lytic activity were reduced in HIV-infected adolescents compared with age-matched control subjects, and these changes appeared to occur at early stages of disease (SD Douglas, personal communication).

Antibody-Dependent Cellular Cytotoxicity

Cord blood NK cells are deficient in their ability to mediate antibody-dependent cellular cytotoxicity (ADCC) against HIV-infected targets.[59] HIV-infected children have impaired ADCC activity against CD4+ cells expressing HIV antigens.[62] Furthermore, sera from HIV-infected children inhibited ADCC against HIV-infected targets mediated by adult PBMC, suggesting that factors capable of blocking ADCC may be present in the sera of some infected children.

CD8-Mediated Suppression of HIV Replication in CD4+ cells

Walker and colleagues[63] first described the ability of CD8+ cells to inhibit replication of HIV in CD4+ cells via a noncytotoxic mechanism. CD8+ cells produce a soluble, not yet identified factor, that mediates inhibition of HIV replication in CD4+ cells. CD8-mediated suppression of HIV replication has been demonstrated in HIV-infected children by a number of investigators.[64–66] In the largest study of this phenomenon to date, Pollack and associates[64] detected CD8-mediated suppression in 11 of 16 HIV-infected infants during the first year of life. Infants with demonstrable suppression had lower viral loads and higher CD4+ percentages at 1 year of age than those who did not.

Furthermore, infants with CD8-mediated suppression survived longer than those who lacked this activity. Others have detected CD8-mediated suppression in older children who have progressed to AIDS, suggesting that this mechanism is not sufficient to prevent disease progression.[66]

Expansion of CD4+ and CD8+ Lymphocytes with Restricted T Cell Receptor Genes

CD4+ and CD8+ lymphocytes express T cell receptors (TCRs) that are encoded by genes produced through somatic recombination. As a result, multiple TCR families, with diverse sequences and antigenic specificity, appear during T cell development. Such TCR families can be detected by flow cytometry using panels of monoclonal antibodies or using molecular techniques to identity variable sequences within the complement-determining region 3 (CDR3), a region that is directly involved in recognition of peptide-HLA complexes.

Lymphocytes from healthy children and adults express most known TCR families, and each family represents a small proportion of the total repertoire. Several studies have demonstrated expansions of CD8+ cells expressing one or more TCR Vα or Vβ families in HIV-infected children.[67–69] Different TCR families were expanded in different children, with no apparent propensity for particular families. In one of these studies, expansion of two or more CD8+ cell TCR Vβ families correlated with a higher percentage of CD4+ cells and more robust lymphocyte proliferation responses against recall antigens.[68] Since expanded CD8+ cell populations may contain CTL, these results may indicate a positive correlation between CTL activity and helper T cell function. Expansions in CD4 cell TCR Vβ families have been detected as well, but their significance has not been established.[69]

Depletions within TCR Vβ families also have been described in HIV-infected adults,[70] as well as HIV-infected children.[71] The existence of a large pool of naive T cells, plus the ability to generate new T cells in the thymus, may help to avert such depletions in HIV-infected children.

Antibody Production

Hyperimmunoglobulinemia and Production of Autoantibodies

Hyperimmunoglobulinemia is commonly observed in HIV-infected children who have not yet received antiretroviral therapy.[72,73] The increased levels of IgG, IgM, IgA, or IgE detected in such children do not appear to have a deleterious effect, but children with hyperimmunoglobulinemia may produce autoantibodies that cause specific manifestations. Such autoantibodies may be directed against platelets, neutrophils, erythrocytes, or lymphocytes and may cause autoimmune disorders such as thrombocytopenia or neutropenia. HIV-infected children with hyperimmunoglobulinemia may have impaired ability to produce antibodies to recall antigens and neoantigens, because their B lymphocytes are in a state of chronic activation. Hyperimmunoglobulinemia is thought to be the consequence of a direct effect of HIV on B lymphocytes. Overproduction of Th2 cytokines may contribute to hyperimmunoglobulinemia in some HIV-infected children. Hypogammaglobulinemia has been described in a small number of HIV-infected children. The mechanisms responsible for low levels of immunoglobulins in these children have not been defined.

HIV-Specific Antibodies

Neutralizing antibodies to HIV have been detected in some HIV-infected children, and their presence may correlate with slower disease progression. In one of the first studies of this type, neutralizing antibodies were detected in 12 HIV-infected children with stable disease, but in only one of 12 children with progressive disease.[74] These results were confirmed in larger subsequent studies.[75–77] In contrast, levels of enzyme-linked immunosorbent assay antibodies were not significantly higher in HIV-infected children with stable disease compared with those with progressive disease.

ADCC antibodies attach to HIV epitopes on HIV-infected cells and then bind to Fc receptor on NK cells, thus allowing NK cells to mediate ADCC against target cells expressing HIV antigens. Infants born to HIV-infected women have detectable levels of HIV-specific ADCC antibodies of the IgG class, consistent with transplacental passage of maternal antibodies. Levels of HIV-specific ADCC antibodies are similar in exposed, uninfected infants and in those who acquire HIV infection, suggesting that such antibodies cannot prevent perinatal transmission.[58,78]

Over the first year of life, ADCC antibodies fall and then rise progressively from 12 to 36 months. Lack of production of ADCC antibodies during the first year of life may contribute to the high viral loads that are maintained in infants for the first few years of life.[78]

Some studies have shown a relationship between ADCC antibody titers and HIV disease status in

HIV-infected children, with less disease progression in children with higher levels of antibodies.[75,76] Other investigators found similar mean ADCC antibody titers in rapid and slow progressors and thus failed to confirm a relationship between ADCC antibodies and disease status.[78]

Antibodies to Other Antigens

HIV-infected children respond poorly to a number of antigens contained in standard pediatric vaccines. Several groups have noted that HIV-infected infants respond poorly to immunization with hepatitis B vaccine. For example, Rutstein and coworkers reported that only 30% of infected children developed protective levels of antibodies to hepatitis B after receiving three immunizations, compared with 92% of HIV-exposed, but not infected, infants.[79] Responses to diphtheria, tetanus, and pertussis vaccine have been determined by a number of investigators. Response rates to the diphtheria component of this vaccine ranged from 80% to 86% after the primary series and 80% to 83% after the booster dose.[40] Importantly, only 50% of infants maintained protective levels 6 to 36 months after the booster dose.[40] Response rates to the tetanus component of diphtheria, tetanus, and pertussis vaccine have been variable, with response rates of 54% to 100% after the primary series and 69% to 90% after the booster dose.[40] Most of the immunized children maintained protective antibody levels for 6 to 30 months after the booster dose. HIV-infected infants do not respond as well as uninfected infants to the primary series of conjugate *Haemophilus influenzae* type B vaccine, but protective antibody titers develop in most after a booster dose.[80, 81] In the majority of children who receive the primary series and booster, protective levels of antibodies persist for at least 24 months after the booster.[81] Of HIV-infected children given the measles, mumps, and rubella vaccine at 12 to 15 months of age, 25% to 80% develop protective levels of antibody to the measles component.[82–84] Responders may experience a more rapid decline of measles antibody titers than uninfected children.

Taken together, these results indicate that HIV-infected children have an impaired ability to produce and maintain antibodies to pediatric vaccines. Furthermore, this impaired ability appears early in life, as illustrated by the reduced responses to hepatitis B vaccine given at birth, 1 to 2 months, and 6 months of age.

Defective humoral immunity has also been demonstrated in a small number of HIV-infected children immunized with the T cell–dependent neoantigen bacteriophage phiX 174.[85] These children also had decreased lymphocyte proliferation responses to staphylococcal Cowan A, a specific B cell mitogen, and failed to develop protective levels of pneumococcal antibodies after immunization with unconjugated pneumococcal vaccine. Since the response to this vaccine is primarily B cell–dependent, these results, taken together, suggest that HIV-infected children have intrinsic B lymphocyte defects.

Neutrophil Function

Impaired neutrophil function in HIV-infected children may contribute to the increased frequency of bacterial infections, including pneumonia, sinusitis, and sepsis. In one study, neutrophil chemotaxis was reduced in asymptomatic HIV-infected children and increased in those with symptomatic HIV infection, suggesting that decreased chemotaxis may predispose asymptomatic HIV-infected children to bacterial infections.[86] The increased chemotaxis observed in symptomatic HIV-infected children may be due to exposure to high levels of cytokines such as tumor necrosis factor-α. More importantly, neutrophils from both asymptomatic and symptomatic children demonstrated decreased bactericidal activity against *Staphylococcus aureus* in vitro. In another study, 6 of 13 children with symptomatic HIV infection had bactericidal activity that ranged from 10% to 60% of normal.[87] Such decreased bactericidal activity could explain the increased incidence of bacterial infections in HIV-infected children. In one study, superoxide production appeared to be normal,[86] but in a subsequent study in which different stimulants were used, neutrophil superoxide production was decreased in asymptomatic HIV-infected children regardless of CD4+ cell count.[88] In addition, monocyte superoxide production was reduced in those with CD4 cell counts less than 400 cells/mm^3. These results suggest that neutrophil, and possibly monocyte, function is impaired in HIV-infected children and may contribute to the increased frequency of bacterial infections.

ROLE OF EARLY THERAPY IN PRESERVATION OF IMMUNE FUNCTION

Since HIV infection causes progressive damage to the immune system, early therapy that controls viral replication effectively might limit the extent of immunodeficiency. This hypothesis was tested in PACTG 356, a study in which HIV-infected infants were started on highly active retroviral therapy (HAART) with three or four antiretroviral drugs in combination, prior to 3 months of age.[89] Thirteen of the infants enrolled in this trial attained plasma HIV-1 RNA levels of fewer than 400 copies/mL that were sustained for at least 48 weeks. In these infants, the percentage of peripheral blood CD4+ counts remained (11 infants) or returned (2 infants) to normal for age. In addition, the percentage of CD4+ naive cells remained at appropriate levels for age. A subset of these infants who were tested for lymphocyte proliferation responses after viral suppression had been achieved. All responded well to pokeweed mitogen and tetanus antigen. Two infants who received pediatric immunizations developed antibodies to hepatitis B, tetanus, *Haemophilus influenzae* type B, and varicella-zoster virus. Taken together, these data suggest that immunologic function was preserved in these infants as a result of early therapy. Interestingly, these infants generally failed to respond to HIV antigens in lymphocyte proliferation assays and did not have detectable HIV-specific CTL responses. In addition, all but one infant became seronegative for HIV as determined by enzyme-linked immunosorbent assay and Western blot assay. This failure to develop HIV-specific lymphoproliferative responses may reflect the reduced ability of young infants to develop such immunologic responses to a number of viruses, including cytomegalovirus[90, 91] and measles.[92] An age-related inability to develop CTL activity cannot explain the lack of HIV-specific CTL responses in infants in whom viral production was controlled, since infants enrolled in PACTG 356, who were virologic nonresponders and had detectable levels of plasma HIV RNA, developed HIV-specific CTL activity after 6 months of age.

IMMUNE RECONSTITUTION AFTER ANTIRETROVIRAL THERAPY

With the recent availability of HAART with potent combinations of antiretrovirals, the degree of immune reconstitution achieved in different patient populations has become a major research focus. In one of the first studies of immune reconstitution in adults, Autran and coworkers[93] reported that administration of combination antiretroviral therapy consisting of zidovudine, dideoxycytidine, and ritonavir to HIV-infected adults was associated with the appearance of increased numbers of memory (CD45RO+) CD4+ cells during the first 4 months of therapy, followed by increased numbers of naive CD4+ cells (defined as CD45RA+CD62L+) by 12 months.

Among patients receiving chemotherapy for cancer, the ability to regenerate naive CD4+ cells, as well as total CD4+ cells, correlates inversely with age, with patients older than 15 years of age having diminished regenerative activity.[94] Similarly, in bone marrow transplant recipients, absolute numbers of naive T cells at 1 year after transplantation correlate inversely with age.[95] These age-related differences in regenerative ability have been attributed to decreased thymic function in adults compared with children. Thus, the failure of HIV-infected adults to develop normal levels of naive and total CD4+ cells after HAART also may be due, at least in part, to age-related thymic deficiency. The smaller pool of post-thymic naive T cells available for expansion in adults compared to children may also play a role. Interestingly, age-related differences have not been found for the reconstitution of CD8+ cells, and CD8+ cell regeneration does not appear to be thymic dependent.

Based on these observations, infants and children and perhaps adolescents would be expected to achieve more complete immune reconstitution after HAART than adults. Naive cells are likely to appear earlier and in greater numbers in children than in adults, and naive cell function, for instance responses to neoantigens, may appear earlier and be more vigorous in children.

Limited data are available on the effects of HAART on lymphocyte subpopulations in HIV-infected children. In addition, differences in baseline characteristics of study populations, antiretroviral regimens, assays used to characterize immune responses, and statistical methods make it difficult to compare the results of published studies. Despite these limitations, several overall conclusions can be made. CD4+ cell number and percentage rise in most children receiving HAART. These rises tend to be of greater magnitude in children who had low CD4+ counts at baseline and in children who achieve viral suppression, although rises in CD4+ cell counts can be detected in some children who fail to achieve suppression or who develop detectable levels of plasma HIV RNA after achieving undetectable levels.

The initial rise in CD4 cells after initiation of HAART involves primarily CD45RO+ memory cells and may be due to redistribution of CD4+ cells from peripheral sites, such as lymph nodes, to the peripheral circulation.[96] In contrast to results obtained in HIV-infected adults, increased numbers of CD4+ naive cells appear early after initiation of HAART in children.[71, 97–99] In one study, CD4+ naive cells appeared after 4 weeks of HAART, and the number of naive cells continued to rise through at least 24 weeks.[98] In this study, children younger than 6 years of age had the highest increase in all lymphocyte populations. Similarly, in another study, recovery rates for naive, memory, and total CD4+ cell were higher in children younger than 3 years of age as compared with older children, and the recovery rates in younger children were 10- to 40-fold higher compared with recovery rates in adults.[97] Even in severely immunocompromised children with advanced disease and 6% or less CD4+ cells, impressive increases in CD4+ percentage and absolute counts were observed after initiation of HAART, and 70% of the reconstituted CD4+ cells were naive.[100] Furthermore, in one study in which thymic volume was assessed by nuclear magnetic resonance imaging, rises in total and naive CD4+ cells correlated with increases in thymic volume.[71] Taken together, these results suggest that children do have greater potential for reconstitution of thymic-derived naive CD4+ lymphocytes than adults. Support for this suggestion is provided by a recent study in which HIV-infected children who achieved profound and sustained viral suppression after receiving antiretroviral therapy demonstrated increased thymic function, as determined by quantification of T cell receptor rearrangement excision circles (TRECs) in peripheral blood.[101] T cells that have recently emigrated from the thymus contain greater numbers of TRECs, compared with T lymphocytes that have undergone multiple cell divisions. Therefore, determining the number of TRECs per 100,000 CD4+ cells provides an estimate of the ability of the thymus to produce naive T cells.

Limited information is available on the effects of HAART on immunologic function in HIV-infected children. In a study of 25 HIV-infected children who received stavudine, lamivudine, and indinavir, the proportion of children with at least one positive lymphoproliferative response increased significantly when responses to tetanus, *Aspergillus fumigatus* and *Candida albicans* were determined after 12 months of therapy.[102] The magnitude of positive lymphoproliferative responses also increased with therapy. In PACTG 338, among HIV-infected children who received a protease inhibitor–containing antiretroviral combination, the percentage with lymphocyte proliferation responses to *Candida albicans* increased from baseline to week 48, although the difference did not achieve statistical significance.[103] In contrast, lymphoproliferative responses to tetanus did not improve over this time.

Since responses to recall antigens are mediated by memory cells, it is not surprising that lymphoproliferative responses to recall antigens improve as CD4+ memory cell counts rise. The contrasting response to *Candida albicans* and tetanus in PACTG 338 might reflect differences in natural exposure to antigens, since subjects were more likely to be exposed to *Candida albicans* than to tetanus toxin. It is not yet known whether rises in CD4+ naive cell number correlate with ability to respond to neoantigens. In a PACTG study currently in progress, responses to hepatitis A vaccine, a neoantigen for most children, will be determined after initiation of HAART.

Although improved responses to some recall antigens have been documented in HIV-infected children after initiation of HAART, such children generally do not respond to HIV antigens in lymphocyte proliferation assays. Also, in HIV-infected children with viral suppression after receiving HAART, the frequency of HIV-1–specific CTL responses declines.[104] Since strong HIV-specific lymphoproliferative and CTL responses are detected in long-term nonprogressors (see later) and are thought to contribute to control of viral replication, it is of concern that these responses are deficient in most HIV-infected children who have received HAART.

The above-mentioned studies on immune reconstitution in HIV-infected children receiving HAART have provided much useful information, but it is unclear whether rises in T cell subpopulations are due to increased production or decreased destruction of CD4 and CD8 cells. Although the proportion of CD8+ cells expressing activation markers is reduced after initiation of HAART in HIV-infected children,[103] the effect of HAART on apoptosis remains controverial.[99, 105] Better understanding of the mechanisms involved in reconstitution would contribute to the development of new strategies. For example, if incomplete immune reconstitution were attributable to decreased ability to generate naive cells, strategies to enhance or replace thymic function might be considered. On the other hand, if destruction of T cells through apoptosis and other mechanisms is found to hamper reconstitution, strategies to reduce cell loss through such mechanisms should be considered. Studies of turnover of CD4+ and CD8+ naive and memory cells before and after HAART are needed to resolve these issues. The long-term effects of HAART on immune reconstitution in HIV-infected children also remain to be determined.

LONG-TERM NONPROGRESSORS

A small group of HIV-infected individuals, designated as long-term nonprogressors, remain healthy and maintain normal CD4+ cell counts for at least 10 years without taking antiretroviral therapy. A comparable group of HIV-infected children has not been described. In one study, among perinatally HIV-infected children who were at least 8 years old (range, 8–15 years), 20% had never had an AIDS-defining condition and had absolute CD4+ lymphocyte counts of greater than 500 cells/mm^2, but 82% of these children had received antiretroviral therapy.[106] Preliminary studies indicated that such children may have more robust HIV antibody production and HIV-specific CTL activity than children with rapid progression.[107] Detailed studies on long-term nonprogressing HIV-infected children could shed light on mechanisms contributing to relative preservation of the immune system in such children. Such information would be useful for the development of immunotherapeutic approaches for HIV-infected children.

REFERENCES

1. Wilfert CM, Wilson C, Luzuriaga K, et al: Pathogenesis of pediatric human immunodeficiency virus type 1. J Infect Dis 1994;170:286–292.
2. Ho W-Z, Lioy J, Song L, et al: Infection of cord blood monocyte-derived macrophages with human immunodeficiency virus type 1. J Virol 1992;66:573–579.
3. Yang LP, Riley JL, Carroll RG, et al: Productive infection of neonatal CD8+ T lymphocytes by HIV-1. J Exp Med 1998;187:1139–1144.
4. McKinney RE, Wilfert CM: Lymphocyte subsets in children younger than 2 years old: Normal values in a population at risk for human immunodeficiency virus infection and diagnostic and prognostic application to infected children. Pediatr Infect Dis J 1992;11:639–644.
5. Chirmule N, Lesser M, Gupta A, et al: Immunologic characteristics of HIV-infected children: Relationship to age, CD4 counts, disease progression, and survival. AIDS Res Hum Retroviruses 1995;10: 1209–1219.
6. Mofenson LM, Korelitz J, Meyer WA, et al: The relationship between serum human immunodeficiency virus type 1 (HIV-1) RNA level, CD4 lymphocyte percent, and long-term mortality risk in HIV-1 infected children. J Infect Dis 1997;175:1029–1038.
7. 1994 Revised Classification System for Human Immunodeficiency Virus Infection in Children Less Than 13 Years of Age. MMWR 1994;43:1–10.
8. The European Collaborative Study: Age-related standards for T lymphocyte subsets based on uninfected children born to human immunodeficiency virus-1 infected women. Pediatr Infect Dis J 1992;11: 1018–1026.
9. Denny T, Yogev R, Gelman R, et al: Lymphocyte subsets in healthy children during the first 5 years of life. JAMA 1992;267:1484–1488.
10. Rich KC, Brambilla D, Pitt J, et al: Lymphocyte phenotyping in infants: Maturation of lymphocyte subpopulations and the effects of HIV infection. Clin Immunol Immunopath 1997;85:273–281.
11. Nahmias AJ, Clark WS, Kourtis AP, et al: Thymic dysfunction and time of infection predict mortality in human immunodeficiency virus-infected infants. J Infect Dis 1998;178:680–685.
12. Rabin RL, Roederer M, Maldonado Y, et al: Altered representation of naive and memory CD8 T cell subsets in HIV-infected children. J Clin Invest 1995;95:2054–2060.
13. Ibegbu C, Spira TJ, Nesheim S, et al: Subpopulations of T and B cells in perinatally HIV-infected and non-infected age-matched children compared with those in adults. Clin Immunol Immunopath 1994;71:27–32.
14. Schlesinger M, Peters V, Jiang JD, et al: Increased expression of activation markers on CD8 lymphocytes in children with human immunodeficiency virus-1 infection. Pediatr Res 1995;38:390–396.
15. Douglas SD, Rudy B, Muenz L, et al: Peripheral blood mononuclear cell markers in antiretroviral therapy naive HIV-infected and high risk HIV seronegative adolescents. AIDS 1999;13:1629–1635.
16. Douglas SD, Rudy B, Muenz L, et al: T-lymphocyte subsets in HIV-infected and high-risk HIV-uninfected adolescents: Retention of nave T lymphocytes in human immunodeficiency virus-infected adolescents. Arch Pediatr Adolesc Med 2000;154: 375–380.
17. Plaeger-Marshall S, Isacescu V, O'Rourke S, et al: T cell activation in pediatric AIDS pathogenesis: Three-color immunophenotyping. Clin Immunol Immunopath 1994;71:19–26.
18. Sleasman JW, Aleixo LF, Morton A, et al: CD4+ memory T cells are the predominant population of HIV-1-infected lymphocytes in neonates and children. AIDS 1996;10:1477–1484.

19. Roederer M, Dubs JG, Anderson MT, et al: CD8 naive T cell counts decrease progressively in HIV-infected adults. J Clin Invest 1995;95:2061–2066.
20. Jennings C, Rich K, Siegel JN, et al: A phenotypic study of CD8+ lymphocyte subsets in infants using three-color flow cytometry. Clin Immunol Immunopath 1994;71:8–13.
21. Rosenzweig M, Clark DP, Gaulton GN: Selective thymocyte depletion in neonatal HIV-1 thymic infection. AIDS 1993;7:1601–1605.
22. Langston C, Lewis DE, Hammill HA, et al: Excess intrauterine fetal demise associated with maternal human immunodeficiency virus infection. J Infect Dis 1995;172:1451–1460.
23. Joshi VV, Oleske JM: Pathologic appraisal of the thymus gland in acquired immunodeficiency syndrome in children. Arch Pathol Lab Med 1985;109:142–146.
24. Joshi VV, Oleske JM, Saad S, et al: Thymus biopsy in children with acquired immunodeficiency syndrome. Arch Pathol Lab Med 1986;110:837–842.
25. Uittenbogaart CH, Anisman DJ, Jamieson BD, et al: Differential tropism of HIV-1 isolates for distinct thymocyte subsets in vitro. AIDS 1996;10:F9–F16.
26. Sei S, Akiyoshi H, Bernard J, et al: Dynamics of virus versus host interaction in children with human immunodeficiency virus type 1 infection. J Infect Dis 1996; 173:1485–1490.
27. Launer RP, Hüttner S, Buisson M, et al: T-cell death by apoptosis in vertically human immunodeficiency virus-infected children coincides with expansion of CD8+/interleukin-2 receptor-/HLA-DR+ T cells: Sign of a possible role for herpes viruses as cofactors? Blood 1995;86:1400–1407.
28. McCloskey TW, Oyaizu N, Bakashi S, et al: CD95 expression and apoptosis during pediatric HIV infection: Early upregulation of CD95 expression. Clin Immunol Immunopath 1998;87:33–41.
29. McCloskey TW, Bakshi S, Than S, et al: Immunophenotypic analysis of peripheral blood mononuclear cells undergoing in vitro apoptosis after isolation from human immunodeficiency virus-infected children. Blood 1998;92:4230–4237.
30. Böhler T, Bäumler C, Herr I, et al: Activation of the CD95 system increases with disease progression in human immunodeficiency virus type 1-infected children and adolescents. Pediatr Infect Dis J 1997;16:754–759.
31. Niehues T, Ndagijimana J, Horneff G, et al: CD28 expression in pediatric human immunodeficiency virus infection. Pediatr Res 1998;44:265–268.
32. Finkel TH, Tudor-Williams G, Banda NK, et al: Apoptosis occurs predominantly in bystander cells and not in productively infected cells of HIV- and SIV-infected lymph nodes. Nat Med 1995;1:129–134.
33. Casella CR, Finkel TH: Mechanisms of lymphocyte killing by HIV. Curr Opin Hematol 1997;4:24–31.
34. Nielsen SD, Ersbøll AK, Mathiesen L, et al: Highly active antiretroviral therapy normalizes the function of progenitor cells in human immunodeficiency virus-infected patients. J Infect Dis 1998;178:1299–1305.
35. Gaulton GN, Scobie JV, Rosenzweig M: HIV-1 and the thymus. AIDS 1997;11:403–413.
36. Koutis AP, Ibegbu C, Nahmias AJ, et al: Early progression of disease in HIV-infected infants with thymus dysfunction. N Engl J Med 1996;335:1431–1436.
37. Vigano A, Vella S, Principi N, et al: Thymus volume correlates with the progression of vertical HIV infection. AIDS 1999;13:F29–F34.
38. Sachsenberg N, Perelson AS, Yerly S, et al: Turnover of CD4+ and CD8+ T lymphocytes in HIV-1 infection as measured by Ki67 antigen. J Exp Med 1998;187:1295–1303.
39. Hellerstein M, Hanley MB, Cesar D, et al: Directly measured kinetics of circulating T lymphocytes in normal and HIV-1 infected humans. Nat Med 1999;5:83–88.
40. Borkowsky W, Rigaud M, Krasinski K, et al: Cell-mediated and humoral immune responses in children infected with human immunodeficiency virus during the first four years of life. J Pediatr 1992;120:371–375.
41. Petersen J, Church J, Gomperts E, et al: Lymphocyte phenotype does not predict immune function in pediatric patients infected with human immunodeficiency virus type 1. J Pediatr 1989;115:944–948.
42. Johnson JP, Hebel R, Shinaberry R: Lymphoproliferative responses to mitogen and antigen in HIV-infected children. AIDS Res Hum Retroviruses 1991;7:781–786.
43. Roilides E, Clerici M, DePalma L, et al: Helper T-cell responses in children infected with human immunodeficiency virus type 1. J Pediatr 1991;118:724–730.
44. Petersen JM, Weinberg KI, Annett G, et al: Correction of antigen-specific T-lymphocyte function by recombinant cytokines in children infected with human immunodeficiency virus type 1. J Pediatr 1992;121:565–568.
45. Raszka WV, Moriarity RA, Ottolini MG, et al: Delayed-type hypersensitivity skin testing in human immunodeficiency virus-infected pediatric patients. J Pediatr 1996;129:245–250.
46. Vigano A, Principi N, Villa ML, et al: Immunologic characterization of children vertically infected with human immunodeficiency virus, with slow or rapid disease progression. J Pediatr 1995; 126:368–374.
47. Vigano A, Balotta C, Trabattoni D, et al: Virologic and immunologic markers of disease progression in pediatric HIV infection. AIDS Res Hum Retroviruses 1996;12:1255–1262.
48. Hyjek E, Lischner HW, Hyslop T, et al: Cytokine patterns during progression to AIDS in children with perinatal HIV infection. J Immunol 1995;155:4060–4071.
49. Lee B-N, Lu J-G, Kline MW, et al: Type 1 and type 2 cytokine profiles in children exposed to or infected with vertically transmitted human immunodeficiency virus. Clin Diag Lab Med 1996;3:493–499.

50. Than S, Hu R, Oyaizu N, et al: Cytokine pattern in relation to disease progression in human immunodeficiency virus-infected children. J Infect Dis 1997; 175:47–56.
51. Rautonen J, Rautonen N, Martin NL, et al: Serum interleukin-6 concentrations are elevated and associated with elevated tumor necrosis factor-a and immunoglobulin G and A concentrations in children with HIV infection. AIDS 1991;5:1319–1325.
52. Johann-Liang R, Cervia J, Noel GJ: Endogenous interleukin-2 serum levels in children infected with human immunodeficiency virus. Clin Infect Dis 1997;25:1233–1236.
53. Poli G, Bressler P, Kinter AL, et al: Interleukin 6 induces human immunodeficiency virus expression in infected monocytic cells alone and in synergy with tumor necrosis factor by transcriptional and post-transcriptional mechanisms. J Exp Med 1990;172:151–158.
54. Luzuriaga K, Koup RA, Pikora CA, et al: Deficient human immunodeficiency virus type 1-specific cytotoxic T cell responses in vertically infected children. J Pediatr 1991;119:230–236.
55. Luzuriaga K, Holmes D, Hereema A, et al: HIV-1-specific cytotoxic T lymphocyte responses in the first year of life. J Immunol 1995;154:433–443.
56. McFarland EJ, Harding PA, Luckey D, et al: High frequency of gag- and envelope-specific cytotoxic T lymphocyte precursors in children with vertically acquired human immunodeficiency virus type 1 infection. J Infect Dis 1994;170:766–774.
57. Buseyne F, Burgard M, Teglas JP, et al: Early HIV-specific cytotoxic T lymphocytes and disease progression in children born to HIV-infected mothers. AIDS Res Hum Retroviruses 1998;14:1435–1444.
58. Pikora CA, Sullivan JL, Panicali D, et al: Early HIV-1 envelope-specific cytotoxic T lymphocyte responses in vertically infected infants. J Exp Med 1997;185:1153–1161.
59. Jenkins M, Mills J, Kohl S: Natural killer cytotoxicity and antibody-dependent cellular cytotoxicity of human immunodeficiency virus-infected cells by leukocytes from human neonates and adults. Pediatr Res 1993;33:469–474.
60. Merrill JD, Sigaroudinia M, Kohl S: Characterization of natural killer and antibody-dependent cellular cytotoxicity of preterm infants against human immunodeficiency virus-infected cells. Pediatr Res 1996;40:498–503.
61. Bonagura VR, Cunningham-Rundles SL, Schuval S: Dysfunction of natural killer cells in HIV-infected children with or without *Pneumocystis carinii* pneumonia. J Pediatr 1992;121:195–201.
62. Ziegner U, Campbell D, Weinhold K, et al: Deficient antibody-dependent cellular cytotoxicity against human immunodeficiency virus (HIV)-expressing target cells in perinatal HIV infection. Clin Diag Lab Med 1999;6:718–724.
63. Walker CM, Moody DL, Stites DP, et al: CD8+ T lymphocytes can control HIV infection *in vitro* by suppressing virus replication. Science 1986;234:1563–1566.
64. Pollack H, Zhan M-X, Safrit JT, et al: CD8+ T-cell-mediated suppression of HIV replication in the first year of life: Association with lower viral load and favorable early survival. AIDS 1997;11:F9–F13.
65. Levy JA, Hsueh F, Blackbourn DJ, et al: CD8 non-cytotoxic antiviral activity in human immunodeficiency virus-infected and -uninfected children. J Infect Dis 1998;177:470–472.
66. Salimi B, Yogev R, Kabat W, et al: CD8+ T cell-mediated suppression of human immunodeficiency virus replication in older children with acquired immunodeficiency syndrome. Pediatr Infect Dis J 2000;19:109–113.
67. Halapi E, Gigliotti D, Hodara V, et al: Detection of CD8 T-cell expansions with restricted T-cell receptor V gene usage in infants vertically infected by HIV-1. AIDS 1996;10:1621–1626.
68. Than S, Kharbanda M, Chitnis V, et al: Clonal dominance patterns of CD8 T cells in relation to disease progression in HIV-infected children. J Immunol 1999;162:3680–3686.
69. Soudeyns H, Champagne P, Holloway CL, et al: Transient T cell receptor β-chain variable region-specific expansions of CD4+ and CD8+ T cells during the early phase of pediatric human immunodeficiency virus infection: Characterization of expanded cell populations by T cell receptor phenotyping. J Infect Dis 2000;181:107–120.
70. Connors M, Kovacs JA, Krivat S, et al: HIV infection induces changes in CD4+ T-cell phenotype and depletions within the CD4+ T-cell repertoire that are not immediately restored by antiviral or immune-based therapies. Nat Med 1997;3:533–540.
71. Vigano A, Vella S, Saresella M, et al: Early immune reconstitution after potent antiretroviral therapy in HIV-infected children correlates with the increase in thymus volume. AIDS 2000;14:251–261.
72. Scott GB, Buck BE, Leterman JG, et al: Acquired immunodeficiency syndrome in infants. N Engl J Med 1984;310:76–81.
73. Bernstein LJ, Krieger BZ, Novick B, et al: Bacterial infection in the acquired immunodeficiency syndrome of children. Pediatr Infect Dis 1985;4:472–475.
74. Robert-Guroff M, Oleske JM, Connor EM, et al: Relationship between HTLV-III neutralizing antibody and clinical status of pediatric acquired immunodeficiency syndrome (AIDS) and AIDS-related complex. Pediatr Res 1987;21:547–550.
75. Ljunggren K, Moschese V, Broliden P-A, et al: Antibodies mediating cellular cytotoxicity and neutralization correlate with a better clinical stage in children born to human immunodeficiency virus-infected mothers. J Infect Dis 1990;161:198–202.
76. Broliden K, Sievers E, Tovo PA, et al: Antibody-dependent cellular cytotoxicity and neutralizing

activity in sera of HIV-1-infected mothers and their children. Clin Exp Immunol 1993;93:56–64.

77. Robert-Guroff M, Roilides E, Muldoon R, et al: Human immunodeficiency virus (HIV) type 1 strain MN neutralizing antibody in HIV-infected children: Correlation with clinical status and prognostic value. J Infect Dis 1993;167:538–546.

78. Pugatch D, Sullivan JL, Pikora CA, et al: Delayed generation of antibodies mediating human immunodeficiency virus type 1-specific antibody-dependent cellular cytotoxicity in vertically infected infants. J Infect Dis 1997;176:643–648.

79. Rutstein RM, Rudy B, Codispoti C, et al: Response to hepatitis B immunization by infants exposed to HIV. AIDS 1994;8:1281–1284.

80. Kale KI, King JC, Fraley JJ, et al: The immunogenicity of *Haemophilus influenzae* type b conjugate (HbOC) vaccine in human immunodeficiency virus-infected and uninfected infants. Pediatr Infect Dis J 1995;14:350–353.

81. Rutstein RM, Rudy BJ, Cnaan A: Response of human immunodeficiency virus-exposed and infected infants to *Haemophilus influenzae* type b conjugate vaccine. Arch Pediatr Adolesc Med 1996;150:838–841.

82. Krasinski K, Borkowsky W: Measles and measles immunity in children infected with human immunodeficiency virus. JAMA 1989;261:2512–2516.

83. Brena AE, Cooper ER, Cabral HJ, et al: Antibody response to measles and rubella vaccine by children with HIV infection. J Acquir Immune Defic Syndr 1993;6:1125–1129.

84. Al-Attar I, Reisman J, Muehlmann M, et al: Decline of measles antibody titers after immunization in human immunodeficiency virus-infected children. Pediatr Infect Dis J 1995;14:149–151.

85. Bernstein LJ, Ochs HD, Wedgewood RJ, et al: Defective humoral immunity in pediatric acquired immune deficiency syndrome. J Pediatr 1985;107:352–357.

86. Roilides E, Mertins S, Eddy J, et al: Impairment of neutrophil chemotactic and bactericidal function in children infected with human immunodeficiency virus type 1 and partial reversal after in vitro exposure to granulocyte-macrophage colony-stimulating factor. J Pediatr 1990;117:531–540.

87. Shearer WT, Kline MW, Abramson SL, et al: Recombinant human gamma interferon in human immunodeficiency virus-infected children: Safety, CD4+-lymphocyte count, viral load, and neutrophil function (AIDS Clinical Trials Group Protocol 211). Clin Diag Lab Immunol 1999;6:311–315.

88. Dorenbaum A, Shearer WT, Abramson SL: Phagocytic cell superoxide production in children with HIV infection. Pediatr AIDS HIV Infect 1993;4:215–221.

89. Luzuriaga K, McManus M, Catalina M, et al: Early therapy of vertical human immunodeficiency virus type 1 (HIV-1) infection: Control of viral replication and absence of persistant HIV-1-specific immune responses. J Virol 2000;74:6984–6991.

90. Gehrz RC, Marker SC, Knorr SO, et al: Specific cell-mediated immune defect in active cytomegalovirus infection of young children and their mothers. Lancet 1977;2:844–847.

91. Starr SE, Tolpin MD, Friedman HM, et al: Impaired cellular immunity to cytomegalovirus in congenitally infected children and their mothers. J Infect Dis 1979;140:500–505.

92. Gans HA, Maldonado Y, Yasukawa LL et al: IL-12, IFN-γ, and T cell proliferation to measles in immunized infants. J Immunol 1999;162:5569–5575.

93. Autran B, Carcelain G, Li TS, et al: Positive effects of combined antiretroviral therapy on CD4+ T cell homeostasis and function in advanced HIV disease. Science 1997;277:112–116.

94. Mackall CT, Fleisher TA, Brown MR, et al: Age thymopoiesis and CD4+ T-lymphocyte regeneration after intensive chemotherapy. N Engl J Med 1995;332:143–149.

95. Weinberg K, Annett GM, Kashyap A, et al: The effect of thymic function on immunocompetence following bone marrow transplantation. Bone Marrow Transplant 1995;1:18–23.

96. Bucy RP, Hockett RD, Derdeyn CA, et al: Initial increase in blood CD4+ lymphocytes after HIV antiretroviral therapy reflects redistribution from lymphoid tissues. J Clin Invest 1999;103:1391–1398.

97. Cohen Stuart JWT, Slieker WAT, Rijkers GT, et al: Early recovery of CD4+ T lymphocytes in children on highly active antiretroviral therapy. AIDS 1998;12:2155–2159.

98. Sleasman JW, Nelson RP, Goodenow MM, et al: Immunoreconstitution after ritonavir therapy in children with human immunodeficiency virus infection involves multiple lymphocyte lineages. J Pediatr 1999;134:597–606.

99. Böhler T, Walcher J, Hölzl-Wenig, et al: Early effect of antiretroviral combination therapy on activation, apoptosis and regeneration of T cells in HIV-1-infected children and adolescents. AIDS 1999;13:779–789.

100. Essajee SM, Kim M, Gonzalez C, et al: Immunologic and virologic responses to HAART in severely immunocompromised HIV-1-infected children. AIDS 1999;13:2523–2532.

101. Douek DC, Koup RA, McFarland RD, et al: Effect of HIV on thymic function before and after antiretroviral therapy in children. J Infect Dis 2000;181:1479–1482.

102. Vigano A, Dally L, Bricalli D, et al: Clinical and immuno-virologic characterization of the efficacy of stavudine, lamivudine, and indinavir in human immunodeficiency virus infection. J Pediatr 1999;135:675–682.

103. Borkowsky W, Stanley K, Douglas SD, et al: Immunologic response to combination nucleoside analogue plus protease inhibitor therapy in stable

antiretroviral therapy-experienced HIV-infected children. J Infect Dis 2000;182:96–103.
104. Spiegel HML, DeFalcon E, Ogg GS, et al: Changes in frequency of HIV-1-specific cytotoxic T cell precursors and circulating effectors after combination antiretroviral therapy in children. J Infect Dis 1999;180:359–368.
105. Chougnet C, Fowke KR, Mueller BU, et al: Protease inhibitor and triple-drug therapy: Cellular immune parameters are not restored in pediatric AIDS patients after 6 months of treatment. AIDS 1998;12:2397–2406.
106. Nielsen K, McSherry G, Petru A, et al: A descriptive survey of pediatric immunodeficiency virus-infected long-term survivors. Pediatrics 1997;99:e4.
107. Martin N, Koup R, Kaslow R, et al: Workshop on perinatally acquired human immunodeficiency virus infection in long-term surviving children: A collaborative study of factors contributing to slow disease progression. AIDS Res Hum Retroviruses 1996;12:1565–1570.

4

Identification and Treatment of the HIV-Infected Pregnant Woman

*Howard L. Minkoff and
Traci C. Burgess*

Over the last decade, there have been dramatic changes in the standards of care for HIV-infected pregnant women. These changes occurred shortly after, and at times concurrent with, evolving standards for the care of nonpregnant, HIV-infected persons. That standard of care is now built on powerful new therapeutic regimens and diagnostic and treatment protocols that are increasingly complex. Therapies that can dramatically reduce transmission of the virus to children and substantially improve the prognosis of women are now readily available in the United States. Globally, however, the social, political, and financial burdens associated with the treatment of pregnant women remain overwhelming. To bring the recent therapeutic advances to bear in the care of women in the United States and abroad, women's health care providers must take an active role. Public health agencies and professional organizations have stressed that role of obstetricians and primary care providers, noting that it includes identifying and managing seropositive women. In pursuing that role and in attempting to ensure the best possible outcomes for their patients, primary care providers caring for these women must stay abreast of the rapidly expanding diagnostic and therapeutic tools that are becoming available. An understanding of these treatment strategies requires a basic familiarity with current concepts of HIV pathogenesis. This chapter therefore depends on readers' understanding of HIV virology and pathophysiology, which are described elsewhere in this text. It is on that understanding that we can build strategies, described herein, for the obstetric care of, and antiretroviral therapy for, HIV-infected pregnant women.

IDENTIFICATION

Tests for the detection of the antibody to HIV became available for clinical use in the United States in 1985. The two methods most frequently used remain an enzyme-linked immunosorbent assay for initial screening and then a Western blot test for confirmation. These tests all use antigens derived from disrupted whole virus. The published sensitivity and specificity of the combined tests are about 99%. A small number of test results (15%–20%) from low-risk patients are indeterminate and remain so even if the test is repeated over many months. Individuals recently infected may also have indeterminate results, but repeat tests in 6 months usually reveal a positive Western blot reaction. The patient's final results are considered positive only if *both* the enzyme-linked immunosorbent assay and the Western blot test yield positive results (as currently constructed, rapid test results are not based on Western blot results). If an individual is indeterminate, polymerase chain reaction testing can be used to detect virus and make a final assignation.

The first rapid test for HIV was approved by the Food and Drug Administration (FDA) in 1992.

Other tests have since been developed and are in use internationally. These rapid tests are colorimetric assays that respond in 10 minutes when exposed to the patient's sera. The intensity of the color reflects the quantity of circulating antibody.[1] This test does not require a complex laboratory or additional personnel. Its complexity can be equated to a urine pregnancy test. Field testing in developing countries and in the United States has found the test to be easy to administer and accurate.[2-4] Some laboratories run enzyme-linked immunosorbent assays alone as a means of rapid testing. The Centers for Disease Control and Prevention (CDC) demonstrated the rationale for this test using a decision analysis based on the 2.5 million individuals in 1995 that had standard HIV testing in publicly funded sites. The routine algorithm included a follow-up appointment for the patient approximately 2 weeks later for the test results. Statistics for those sites revealed that 25% of these patients with a positive test and 33% of patients with a negative test result did not return for their post-test counseling and results.[4] Using the results of all the tests performed in that year and the return rate of those patients, the mathematical model found that if the rapid test had been used, almost 700,000 more individuals would have learned of their HIV status, and 2 million people who learned of a negative test result would not have needed to return for a second visit. In that population, approximately 8300 HIV-negative people would have received a preliminary false-positive result out of the 2.1 million people tested. This equates to a 0.4% false-positive rate, which is similar to that found with standard testing.[4] The predictive value of the test depends on the prevalence of HIV in the population being tested. Most communities have a relatively low number of individuals testing positive for HIV. For those communities, the rapid test will have a low positive predictive value (46%–88% in the CDC's series) and a very high negative predictive value. Thus, the suggested algorithm is that when a rapid test result is negative, no further testing is required. However, a positive rapid test result would need confirmation.[4] In the setting of intrapartum testing, decisions regarding the immediate use of zidovudine (ZDV) or nevirapine to reduce transmission must often be made before confirmatory test results are available.

Based on these findings, and after much debate, the CDC revised previous recommendations on rapid screening tests and began to advocate their use. The settings where rapid testing may be most appropriate include the labor and delivery room for maternal intrapartum and immediate postpartum infant evaluation, rapid evaluations, and occupational or recent suspected exposure.[1] Although the cost of the actual rapid test may be more expensive than the standard testing regimen, when medical and societal costs are evaluated, it appears that not only is rapid HIV testing convenient and preferred by clients, it is also cost efficient.[5] Recently, New York State implemented a policy that requires the offer of a rapid test to all women in labor whose HIV status is unknown and the *mandatory* testing of all infants whose mother's HIV status is unknown and who refuse rapid testing during labor. However, the best way to avoid the possibility of a false-positive test result associated with rapid testing technologies is to obtain a woman's HIV status with traditional testing (and confirmation) during the prenatal period.

In fact, HIV testing should be recommended to *all* prenatal patients. Traditional teaching has been that the test should be obtained with pretest counseling and documented patient consent. More recently, the Institute of Medicine and others have suggested that a program of informed right of refusal might be a reasonable alternative. Even with such an approach, however, pretest counseling should be provided to all patients and should include the following information:

- Spectrum of HIV disease and relationship to AIDS
- Modes of HIV transmission
- What the HIV antibody test is and the implications of a negative or positive test result
- The importance of knowing one's HIV status with regard to pregnancy and perinatal transmission
- Risk-reduction behaviors, both sexual and drug-related

Counseling is useful, regardless of the woman's decision to be tested. Such counseling provides an opportunity to educate patients about behaviors that may put them at risk for HIV infection or any other sexually transmitted disease and to discuss risk-reduction practices. This information can be imparted through clinician-patient discussion, by the use of written educational materials or videotapes, or by some combination of these methods. The particular mix depends on the clinical setting and the prevalence of HIV in the community. The counseling session can generally be performed in a relatively brief period of time (5 minutes), such that even busy clinicians can include it as a part of their routine practice at a first prenatal visit. Patients should be counseled about HIV and offered the antibody test as early in their pregnancy as possible. Ideally, the test should be performed when the patient is contemplating pregnancy in the preconception time period. Pretest counseling and patients' decisions about testing should be documented in the medical record. Attempts to selectively offer the test only to women who acknowledge risk behaviors inevitably fail to identify large numbers of infected women, since individuals do not routinely acknowledge behaviors that are not socially sanctioned.[6] Federal legislation has mandated that all states must document that they have increased the number of women tested and reduced the number of children tested or they will lose federal funds earmarked for AIDS care. As noted, the Institute of Medicine has recommended that universal HIV testing with patient notification become a routine component of prenatal care throughout the nation. The American Academy of Pediatrics and the American College of Obstetricians and Gynecologists published a joint statement in July 1999 strongly supporting this recommendation.[7]

It is critical that all patients whose test results are positive be given a comprehensive post-test counseling session. The post-test session should cover the implications of the patient's positive HIV antibody test result, a brief review of HIV infection and how it is transmitted (and not transmitted), discussion of "safer sex" and "safer needle use" if appropriate, and the implications of HIV infection during pregnancy. The most important information to share with the patient is the dramatically improved prognosis for the woman, with appropriate care, and her ability to reduce mother-to-child transmission of HIV to as low as 2% if she accepts appropriate interventions.

Studies of seropositive women's reproductive decisions have shown that women frequently do not choose to terminate the pregnancy and that decisions about abortion are often independent of serostatus.[8,9] However, many of those studies are old and date back to the early years of the HIV epidemic. Now that interventions to reduce transmission are available, it is even more unlikely that HIV infection will be a critical determinant of the decision to continue or terminate a pregnancy.

The primary goals of identifying the HIV-positive pregnant woman are twofold: maintain maternal health and minimize fetal risks. First and foremost, with knowledge of serostatus the patient can undergo HIV-specific medical evaluation to allow appropriate assessment of her current immunologic and virologic condition with the intent of optimizing her care and maintaining her in the best possible health. This effort would include the initiation of pharmacologic therapy, as will be discussed later in the chapter. Second, appropriate efforts can be directed at decreasing the transmission of the virus to the infant (see Chapters 2 and 5).

Finally, as noted earlier, rapid screening tests have become a potential strategy for testing in pregnancy. The potential importance of that approach was highlighted recently. Wade and colleagues,[10] in New York, were able to demonstrate that pharmaceutical intervention, even if not begun until the intrapartum or immediate newborn period, could have a salutary effect on transmission. In their series, they found that the transmission rate of HIV among women who received antepartum, intrapartum, and neonatal ZDV was 6.1%. For women who received intrapartum and neonatal ZDV it was 10.0%, and in those instances in which only the neonate received therapy (within the first 48 hours) it was 9.3%. When therapy was begun on or later than the third day of life, the rate of transmission was 18.4%. When no therapy was received, the transmission rate was 26.6%. The logical extension of these findings was that women whose HIV status were unknown when they came to a hospital in labor could still be the beneficiaries of treatments designed to reduce rates of maternal-to-child HIV transmission if their status could be expeditiously determined. Given the coincidence of HIV infection and drug use, it is not uncommon for HIV-infected women to have had little or no prenatal care, making intrapartum testing and therapy an important consideration. These strategies are realistic considerations because, as discussed previously, rapid screening tests are now available.[1]

INTERACTION OF HIV DISEASE AND PREGNANCY

Several investigators have studied the effect of HIV disease on pregnancy outcomes. Most such reports have not found significant effects. In one study, follow-up of 31 asymptomatic seropositive pregnant women and their infants showed that the prevalence of premature delivery, fetal growth retardation, and early neonatal disease was comparable to that in pregnant seronegative women with similar drug use status. Other authors, when comparing 50 asymptomatic seropositive pregnant women and 64 seronegative control subjects reported that, except for an increased incidence of spontaneous abortion in the seropositive group, a difference attributed to the small sample size, there were no differences in pregnancy outcome.[11,12] However, they did note that the incidence of prematurity and low birth weight infants in both groups of intravenous drug users was about twice that recorded in the general population. In a study that included both drug users and non–drug users,[13] it was reported that when comparing HIV-infected pregnant women and matched control subjects there were no differences in birth weight, gestational age, or other outcome parameters. All of these reports came from the developed world. In contrast, some reports from the developing world have shown a disproportionate number of adverse outcomes in pregnancies among HIV-infected women. In a report on 466 HIV-infected women in Zaire, an increased rate of premature births, low birth weight, and neonatal death was noted when compared with 606 HIV-uninfected women.[14] In these populations, the findings may be related to the general health of the women under study. The Zaire population had a significantly greater number of women with AIDS, who may be most prone to adverse perinatal events.

Concern has been raised not only about the effects of HIV on pregnancy outcomes but also about the effects of pregnancy on HIV disease. Pregnancy is associated with perturbations in the immune system, and it is one of several examples of the sexual dimorphism of the immune response. Most investigators agree that there is a decrease in cell-mediated immunity during pregnancy, which is probably mediated through an altered T helper cell–to–T suppressor cell ratio. Other factors contributing to the immunosuppression of pregnancy may be increased levels of total steroids and other pregnancy-specific plasma proteins and hormones such as human chorionic gonadotropin (HCG), alpha-fetoprotein, and pregnancy-associated α_2-glycoprotein.[15]

Partially in response to these concerns, many authors have assessed the relationship of HIV serostatus and pregnancy to lymphocyte subset changes. In a study of 416 pregnant HIV-1 infected women and an age- and parity-matched HIV-seronegative group of 407 pregnant women, Temmerman[16] reported that CD4+ percentage was lower postpartum than antenatally in both HIV-seropositive and HIV-seronegative women. The differences in changes during pregnancy in CD4+ and CD8+ cell counts and ratios between HIV-1 seropositive and seronegative women were not statistically significant. In an analysis of prospectively collected immunologic and clinical data from 145 women seen in Edinburgh between 1985 and 1992, Brettle[17] reported that there were differences between marker paths of women according to risk activity; women who had acquired HIV from drug use had a higher level of absolute CD4+ cells, CD4+ percentage and total lymphocytes at seroconversion than those who had acquired HIV via heterosexual intercourse, whereas immunologic markers declined more steeply in the former group. There was no evidence that pregnancy, either before or after seroconversion, had an adverse effect on marker paths of HIV disease, however. Bigger and associates[18] showed that the direction of immunologic changes seen in HIV-positive mothers was the same as that in HIV-negative, pregnant control subjects, except that drops in CD4+ counts were 10% to 20% greater among seropositive women.

Burns reported on a cohort of 192 HIV-1 infected women and 148 seronegative women who had lymphocyte subset analysis during pregnancy and the postpartum period.[19] Consistent with prior reports that CD4+ levels decline during pregnancy and return to normal postpartum, these authors reported that percentage levels increased between the third trimester and 12 months postpartum among HIV-1 seronegative women (1.98%; $P = .04$). However, CD4+ levels declined steadily during pregnancy and postpartum among seropositive women (-1.57%, $P = .02$, between the third trimester and 12 months postpartum; -2.65%, $P = .0004$ between 2 and 24 months postpartum), demonstrating that HIV disease continues to progress during pregnancy. In fact, the rate of decline during pregnancy was twofold to threefold greater than in the postpartum period, but power considerations prevented these differences from being statistically significant. CD8+ levels increased at or near delivery and declined to baseline between 2 and 6 months postpartum in both seronegative and seropositive women, although only the declines were statistically significant in both groups (−2.66%, $P = .004$; and −2.02%, $P = .02$, respectively).

Finally, Tuomala and colleagues[20] reported on total, CD4+, and CD8+ lymphocytes during pregnancy and at 1 year follow-up among HIV-infected women in the Women and Infants Transmission Study. Assessments were made in each of 226 women during pregnancy and 1 year postpartum and in each of 100 nonpregnant women during 1 year of follow-up. Trends over time were compared between pregnant women with and without multiple covariates. There was a mean increase of 2.76 per week in the CD4+ cell count during pregnancy ($P = .04$). No other characteristics changed significantly during pregnancy. The mean CD4+ and CD8+ cell counts, the CD8+ percentage, and the total lymphocyte count and percentage increased immediately post delivery. During the first postpartum year, there were statistically significant declines in the absolute CD4+ and CD8+ cell counts, the relative CD4+ and CD8+ percentages, and the total lymphocyte count and percentage. The rate of change for CD4+ and CD8+ counts, but not for CD4+ percentage was less during 1 year in the nonpregnant cohort than in the first postpartum year, and the CD8+ percentage increased in the nonpregnant women. A wide variability in trends of all measurements during pregnancy was seen. The authors concluded that there were no *clinically* significant changes during pregnancy or the postpartum period in any of the lymphocyte parameters they assessed. These data, meticulously collected and eloquently analyzed, are perhaps the strongest evidence to date that any effect of pregnancy on immunologic parameters is marginal, at most.

Although the data cited are compatible with the thesis that pregnancy has minimal immunologic effects, at the beginning of the epidemic there was fear that there might be clinical effects. In one of the earliest reports on HIV infection among pregnant women it was noted that among 34 HIV-positive mothers followed-up for a mean of 27.8±21.6 months, 15 had developed AIDS or AIDS-related complex.[21] This was higher than the expected progression of the disease in nonpregnant patients and suggested that pregnancy was responsible for the acceleration of the women's illness. However, a definitive conclusion could not be drawn from that report, since the mothers were identified through the birth of a child who developed AIDS so that these findings may have been representative of those in a cohort of women with advanced immunocompromise. Indeed, evidence has been presented that suggests that the course of illness in a child relates to the stage of maternal illness, with the infant's risk of death correlated inversely with the mother's CD4+ count and directly with her p24 antigen level at delivery.[22] Subsequently, several controlled studies have been reported in which HIV-positive mothers have been prospectively evaluated. Schaeffer and colleagues[23] followed 32 HIV-positive women and 40 HIV-negative women during pregnancy and for 6 months following delivery, and observed no clinical progression of illness during pregnancy among seropositive women. However, 9% of patients developed signs of clinical deterioration during postpartum observation. The authors believed that pregnancy had only a minor effect on the course of HIV disease.

Other investigators have failed to show any evidence of progression of disease during pregnancy.[24] In a follow-up of 88 postpartum patients, MacCallum and colleagues[25] were unable to demonstrate any adverse effect of pregnancy on the course of HIV disease. Similarly, in a study of 23 pregnant patients followed for 2 years following delivery, compared with matched seropositive nonpregnant control subjects, no significant differences were observed in the number of opportunistic infections between the two groups.[26]

In a prospective study from Bordeaux, France, 57 women who completed a pregnancy during the course of their HIV infection were compared with 114 HIV-infected women who never conceived.[27] The two groups were matched on CD4+ lymphocyte count, age, and year of HIV diagnosis. The main outcome measures were death, occurrence of a first AIDS-defining event, and a drop of the CD4+ below 200/mm^3. The mean follow-up period in pregnant women was 61 months from HIV diagnosis (median CD4+ at entry 455/mm^3) and 54 months from beginning of pregnancy. Nonpregnant women were followed for 50 months since HIV diagnosis (median CD4+ 460/mm^3). The proportion of asymptomatic women at entry in the study was 51 of 57 (90%) in pregnant and 87 of 114 (76%) in nonpregnant women. No significant difference was observed in the two groups with regard to the different end points studied, even after adjustment for other prognostic variables. Adjusted hazards ratio (pregnant/nonpregnant) were 0.92 for death (95% CI, 0.40–2.12), 1.02 for occurrence of a first AIDS-defining event (95% CI, 0.48–2.18), and 1.20 for drop in CD4+ count to less than 200/mm^3 (95% CI, 0.63–2.27). Recently, the results of the Italian seroconversion cohort were reported.[28] In a group of 331 women followed from the time of seroconversion, pregnant women (38 were pregnant at the time of seroconversion and 31 became pregnant after seroconversion) did not experience a more rapid rate of progression of disease even when adjusting for age, exposure group, CD4+ cell count, or use of treatment.

At present, a significant biologic influence of pregnancy on the course of HIV disease has not been documented. The available evidence suggests that pregnancy may exert only a minor influence on the progression of disease. However, given the demonstrated benefits of highly active antiretroviral therapy (HAART) on the course of HIV disease, any effect of pregnancy on access to treatment could have an adverse impact on disease progression in the future.

MANAGEMENT OF THE PREGNANCIES OF HIV-INFECTED WOMEN

As noted in the introduction, two key goals direct the management of pregnancies in HIV-infected women: vouchsafing the health of the mother and minimizing the rate of transmission to the neonate. The latter issue is covered in some detail in Chapter 5, and we touch on it only insofar as it is a consideration in the choice of pharmaceutical care of the woman. In this section, we focus on strategies to keep the woman in optimal health during her pregnancy.

To provide optimal care to the HIV-infected woman, the obstetrician must monitor the patient's immunologic and virologic status and then use the results of that monitoring to choose an appropriate and safe therapeutic regimen. The latter step in turn depends on an understanding of the various regimens available and any considerations unique to pregnancy.

Monitoring Maternal Status

Appropriate prenatal care is the cornerstone of good maternal and neonatal outcome. For all pregnant patients, antepartum visits serve as a means of detection of potential medical and social issues. This is especially true for the HIV-positive pregnant patient. The evaluation of an HIV-infected pregnant woman should reflect the fact that HIV is a sexually and perinatally transmitted virus. Those risk factors associated either with HIV acquisition or with immunocompromise should be assessed. Routine testing should occur for gonorrhea, syphilis, *Chlamydia* infection, hepatitis B, and hepatitis C. *Mycobacterium tuberculosis* screening should be performed by purified protein derivative skin testing. A positive purified protein derivative test result in an HIV-infected patient is 5 mm or greater 2 to 3 days after the intradermal injection. If the patient has a current or past positive purified protein derivative test result or is anergic, a chest radiograph should be obtained once she is in the second trimester. A lead apron can be used to further decrease the minimal risk of fetal exposure. If, on Papanicolaou testing, there is evidence of dysplasia, colposcopy should be performed by an experienced colposcopist. Although routine *Toxoplasma gondii* antibody testing has fallen out of favor as a screening test in the low-risk pregnant population, baseline studies should be obtained in the HIV-infected pregnant female. If an HIV-infected woman with evidence of past infection with *Toxoplasma* experiences substantial immunocompromise, the infection can "reactivate" and can pose a threat to both the mother and the fetus.

When a patient presents for antepartum care with a newly diagnosed HIV infection, CD4 levels and the viral load measurements are important baseline studies to perform. For patients with established infections predating the current pregnancy, these studies need not be repeated if they were performed within the last 3 months.[29] Knowing this information will help in the appraisal of the woman's immune function, the progression or stabilization of her disease, in clinical decision making regarding the most appropriate treatment, and in monitoring the patient's response to her treatment.[30] Current consensus is that treatment should be initiated early and aggressively to attain the most benefit. The U.S. division of the International AIDS Society recommended initiating therapy when the HIV-positive patient has a viral load of 5000 copies/mL plasma or greater or a CD4+ count below 500/mm^3 and the patient is able to consent to long-term treatment.[31] This approach is valid for all HIV-infected individuals, including those who are pregnant. Aggressive treatment requires a multidrug regimen. There are few remaining indications for monotherapy. Perhaps the only indication would be a pregnant patient who, if not pregnant, would be on no medication based on her immunologic and virologic study findings. In that case, the woman would benefit from the use of ZDV after the first trimester, as established in the ACTG 076 protocols.[32]

Once treatment has begun, viral load studies should be assessed in 4 to 6 weeks and then every 3 months once a stable regimen is chosen. In comparing test results over time, there will be better concordance between tests if the same assay and laboratory are used when following a patient. Otherwise, the clinician may not be able to distinguish a true difference from the standard variability of various tests. A third-trimester HIV RNA sample is particularly important for planning the mode of delivery (see Chapter 5). When the viral load is greater than 1000 copies/mL, there should be a discussion with the patient regarding the potential benefit of cesarean section in decreasing perinatal transmission. These recommendations may change with additional data regarding perinatal transmission in the HAART era.

Monitoring is not only necessary to guide antiretroviral therapy, it is also part of the approach to management of opportunistic infections. Management includes the prevention, identification, and treatment of opportunistic infections. Pregnancy should not interfere with the vigorous use of standard prophylactic and therapeutic modalities. The time to institute various prophylactic regimens is based on the woman's immune status. Specific treatments are discussed in the section on medications.

Choice of Medications

The use of antiretroviral medications should reflect an understanding of viral dynamics. Studies of the viral kinetics of HIV have demonstrated high rates of viral turnover with an associated predilection to mutation. Evidence suggests that despite the seemingly successful suppression of *detectable* viral particles, the virus remains in a reservoir within the body.[33,34] Currently, the approach to treatment of HIV is long-term therapy with multidrug regimens designed to keep viral replication quiescent, as mentioned earlier. The therapeutic principle behind the use of drug combinations is to attack or target the virus at various sites in the duplication process, thereby slowing the development of new viable virions.[35] The goal in using these medications in the pregnant patient is to create a regimen that is potent yet has the least toxicity and complexity possible, to achieve low morbidity, improved survival, and the least likelihood for perinatal transmission. Adherence to a multidrug regimen is essential to reduce the rate at which resistance develops. This requires a commitment on the part of the patient and ongoing education and encouragement on the part of the provider. Informed counseling must include discussions regarding the efficacy of the regimen, its effect on the patient's quality of life, and the potential for future drug resistance should adherence slip.[30] It is a key responsibility of the obstetrician to assure appropriate therapy for HIV infection during pregnancy.

The classes of antiretrovirals are nucleoside reverse transcriptase inhibitors, non-nucleoside reverse transcriptase inhibitors, and protease inhibitors. The synopsis of drugs and their use in pregnancy, which is presented subsequently, is derived and updated from a more expanded discussion published elsewhere.[36]

Nucleoside analogues block the action of reverse transcriptase, the enzyme that converts the RNA genome of HIV-1 into DNA in an infected cell. Zidovudine, Didanosine, Zalcitabine, Stavudine, Lamivudine (Epivir), and abacavir are examples of reverse transcriptase inhibitors. They are briefly described in the following sections.

Nucleoside Analogues

Zidovudine (ZDV, AZT, Retrovir)

Zidovudine, the first antiretroviral agent approved, inhibits viral reverse transcriptase by preventing the phosphodiester linkages necessary for nucleic acid replication. Approval by the FDA was based on the results of a double-blind study that showed that, over 6 months of follow-up, progression of disease, including death, occurred more frequently among the patients who received placebo than among those who received 1500 mg ZDV per day.[37] A subsequent AIDS Clinical Trials Group (ACTG) study demonstrated that lower doses of ZDV could provide the same benefit with far fewer side effects.[38] Similar studies examining the effect of ZDV in patients with only moderately advanced HIV disease have demonstrated benefit during relatively short follow-up.[39] As a result of these and other data, a National Institute of Allergy and Infectious Diseases panel subsequently made the recommendation that ZDV monotherapy be initiated when patients' CD4+ cell counts dropped below 500 cells/mm^3.[40]

Over time, additional data related to ZDV use began to accrue that, although demonstrating delayed progression of disease in the short term, failed to demonstrate a clear-cut survival benefit.[41] Data from the Concorde Trial released in 1994 suggested that the benefit of ZDV use did not exceed approximately 3 years. This finding did not support early intervention with ZDV for people with CD4+ counts above 500 cells/mm^3.[42] Subsequent studies have confirmed a lack of benefit from ZDV use beyond 2 or 3 years, a finding attributable, at least in part, to the development of viral resistance.

The currently recommended dose is 100 mg orally every 4 hours, five times a day. Many clinicians prescribe 200 mg every 8 hours for convenience and, in pregnant patients, 300 mg twice a day. The main adverse effect of ZDV is bone marrow suppression. Blood counts must be monitored carefully during its use, particularly if other potential bone marrow suppressive agents are administered concomitantly. Other important side effects include fever, myopathy, lactic acidosis, and hypersensitivity reactions.

The long-term consequences of ZDV when utilized solely during pregnancy to reduce perinatal transmission are not known, but concerns include potential mutagenic and carcinogenic effects, possible teratogenicity, and possible effects on neurodevelopment and on the reproductive system.[43] Part of the theoretical margin of safety of ZDV is based on the fact that ZDV triphosphate inhibits human cellular DNA polymerase only at concentrations much higher than those required to inhibit HIV polymerase. However, gamma DNA polymerase, which is required for mitochondrial replication, may be inhibited by ZDV at concentrations nearer to those that can be achieved in vivo, raising concerns regarding possible effects on tissues with high mitochondrial content (such as hepatic and cardiac tissue).[43] The only prospective study of HIV-infected children demonstrated no effect of ZDV therapy on cardiac function.[44]

Zidovudine has been shown to be a mutagen in vitro, and, in a mammalian in vitro cell transformation assay, ZDV was positive at concentrations of 0.5 micrograms/mL or greater.[45] Noninvasive squamous epithelial vaginal tumors were produced in 3% to 12% of rats and mice after prolonged, continuous exposure to dosages equivalent to three to 24 times the estimated human exposure at the recommended therapeutic dosage. Since rodents excrete metabolites of ZDV in urine and soil the vaginal vault with micturition, these studies may not be predictive of human experience. Reproductivity and fertility studies in animals have demonstrated no adverse effects of ZDV on either the fertility of male or female rats or the reproductive capacity of their offspring.[46] ZDV administered to mice early in gestation was associated with an embryo toxic effect and fetal resorptions[47]; however, ZDV administered at or beyond midgestation had no detectable effect on the fetus.[48] Although some animal models have suggested an increased risk of transplacental carcinogenicity, most subsequent work has not replicated those findings, and current guidelines continue to advocate the prenatal use of ZDV.

Although most studies of ZDV administered to pregnant animals have not demonstrated teratogenicity, in one study in which pregnant rats were administered toxic doses of ZDV during organogenesis (i.e., equivalent to approximately 50 times the recommended daily clinical dose, based on relative body surface area), developmental malformations and skeletal abnormalities were found in 12% of fetuses.[49] ZDV is assigned pregnancy category C status by the FDA.

In humans, observational studies involving small numbers of subjects have not revealed excess malformations with antenatal ZDV use.[50-53] In ACTG Protocol 076, the incidence of congenital malformations was similar for ZDV and placebo recipients. However, because ZDV was not administered until after 14 weeks of gestation in this study, the potential teratogenicity of ZDV administered during the first trimester cannot be assessed. Reported follow-up of the 076 cohort[54] revealed no neurodevelopmental compromise among the HIV-exposed group. Similarly, in a report from the Antiretroviral Pregnancy Registry maintained by the Wellcome Foundation and Hoffman-LaRoche in conjunction with the CDC, no increase in the risk of congenital abnormalities above the expected rate for all pregnancies was observed among infants born to 121 prospectively registered HIV-infected women who received ZDV during pregnancy, nor was there any unusual pattern of birth defects.[55]

Concerns have been raised that use of ZDV during pregnancy could be associated with the development of ZDV-resistant virus, which may lessen the drug's therapeutic benefit for the woman when it is needed for her own health. The development of resistance is a particular risk in the setting of ZDV monotherapy. Further, many therapeutic regimens have been shown to be less efficacious in treating ZDV-experienced, as opposed to ZDV-naive, patients. However, patients with early-stage HIV disease rarely develop ZDV-resistant strains before they have received 18 to 24 months of continuous therapy.[56] After discontinuation of ZDV therapy, an increase in ZDV-susceptible isolates has been observed in some patients who had ZDV-resistant isolates while they were receiving ZDV, although resistance to ZDV has been reported to persist for more than a year after therapy was discontinued.[57,58] Thus, the development of ZDV-resistant viral strains secondary to transient ZDV use during pregnancy remains a theoretical concern. These concerns may be somewhat mitigated, however, given the current recommendations regarding multidrug therapy.

Didanosine (ddI; Videx)

The FDA approved didanosine (ddI) for the treatment of advanced HIV infection and prolonged prior therapy for HIV infection as well as advanced infection and ZDV intolerance or significant clinical or immunologic deterioration during ZDV treatment. The drug is administered according to patient body weight (≥60 kg, 200 mg twice daily; <60 kg, 125 mg twice daily). ddI should be taken on an empty stomach to prevent gastric degradation before absorption. Elimination is primarily renal. Its most important side effects are pancreatitis and peripheral neuropathy.[59] The former has been fatal in some cases.

Early studies suggested that ddI monotherapy was a reasonable alternative to ZDV in those patients who were ZDV experienced, perhaps after as little as 16 weeks of ZDV use.[42]

Limited information is available regarding the use of this agent in pregnancy. Administration of ddI prior to midtrimester abortion in two HIV-positive women demonstrated no pregnancy-related alteration in drug kinetics. Placental passage of ddI was documented both in that study and using perfused term human placental cotyledons.[60,61] Medline and Reprotox searches failed to locate published studies on possible adverse reproductive effects of ddI. According to the manufacturer (Bristol Laboratories, Evansville, Ind), this agent did not produce adverse fertility or fetal effects in rats and rabbits at doses up to 12 and 14 times the human dose (calculated based on plasma levels). There was some reported toxicity to nursing rat pups, however, noting decreased weight and food intake at the doses used.

Zalcitabine (ddC; Hivid)

The FDA originally approved zalcitabine (ddC) as monotherapy for advanced HIV infection and intolerance or progression of disease with ZDV. It was also approved for use in combination with ZDV in selected patients whose CD4+ count is less than $300/mm^3$. The recommended dosage is 0.75 mg orally every 8 hours. The primary side effect is peripheral neuropathy which, like that seen with didanosine, appears to be dose related. Pancreatitis may also occur. Subsequent data have failed to support a role for this, or any other, drug as monotherapy for HIV infection.

In pharmacokinetic studies using titrated ddC in pregnant monkeys, label is found in the fetus, with the total drug exposure approximately half that of the mother.[62] ddC is concentrated in the fetal kidney and a relatively small proportion (20% of the fetal blood concentration) reaches the brain. Teratology testing has been conducted in mice with maternal doses as high as 2000 mg/kg/day, doses at which maternal toxicity was present.[63] Developmental toxicity was seen at 1000 mg/kg/day and consisted of decreased fetal weight and skeletal defects. There was an evident decreasing trend in developmental toxicity at lower dose levels, and it is unclear whether the "no effect" level for developmental toxicity is 200 mg/kg/day or 400 mg/kg/day.

Late fetal rat thymuses in culture show inhibition of proliferation and differentiation of lymphoid cells when exposed to ddC at concentrations as low as 10 μM (about 100 times the concentrations achieved with therapeutic doses).[64] There appears to be a cytotoxic effect on the thymocytes, with relative sparing of the epithelium.

Unpublished studies reported by the manufacturer (Roche Laboratories, Nutley, NJ) indicate no impairment in rat fertility at plasma concentrations more than 200 times those achieved in humans. Embryo lethality was observed at this high dose.

The manufacturer of ddC has, as have the manufacturers of many antiretrovirals, established a pregnancy registry to monitor the outcome of pregnancies that include exposure to ddC.

Stavudine (d4T; Zerit)

Stavudine (d4T) is suggested for use when there is advanced HIV infection and intolerance to ZDV, ddI, and ddC or when there is significant clinical or immunologic deterioration on those therapies. The recommended dosage for patients weighing more than 60 kg is 40 mg orally twice daily. For patients weighing less than 60 kg, 30 mg orally twice daily is recommended. There is substantial renal clearance of d4T, although the metabolism of the drug is poorly understood. The main side effect is peripheral neuropathy.

Studies demonstrate that monotherapy with stavudine in zidovudine-experienced patients is associated with an elevation in the CD4+ count.[65] Others suggest the antiviral efficacy of stavudine may be compromised by prior treatment with zidovudine.[66] Interestingly, stavudine use seems less likely to incur viral resistance than does monotherapy with any of the other currently available nucleoside analogues,[67] although the clinical implications of this finding are unclear.

Exposure of early embryos to concentrations of 10 µM inhibited progression to the blastocyst state.[68] This drug did not impair fertility in rats given more than 200 times the human dose on a serum concentration basis. Teratology studies in rats and rabbits with about 400 and 183 times the human serum concentrations, respectively, did not show an increase in birth defects. At the top dose in rats, there was a small increase in neonatal mortality and minor skeletal ossification delay. These changes are consistent with general toxicity.

Lamivudine (3TC; Epivir)

Lamivudine (3TC) is a synthetic nucleoside analogue that differs from ddI by the presence of a sulfur atom instead of a methylene group at the 3″ position of the ribose ring. It has potent antiviral activity against HIV-1, including ZDV-resistant strains,[69] and is also very active against hepatitis B.[70] It is a weak inhibitor of human cellular polymerases and has a very favorable side effect profile when compared with other currently available antiretroviral agents.

Lamivudine is rapidly absorbed after oral administration and has 80% bioavailability, with a plasma half life of 2 to 4 hours. It is administered to patients as 150 mg capsules twice daily by mouth.

Side effects include diarrhea, headache, nausea, and abdominal pain, all of which are usually mild and transient. 3TC is eliminated renally, and dosage adjustments in patients with impaired renal function are recommended. Studies conducted in Europe and the United States have demonstrated that sustained CD4+ increases and HIV RNA plasma load decreases are achievable when 3TC is combined with ZDV in patients with moderately depressed CD4+ cell counts.[71] Smaller European studies suggest that the combination is also efficacious in patients with severely depressed CD4+ counts.[72] When administered as monotherapy or in combination with ZDV, viral resistance develops rapidly to 3TC associated with a mutation at codon 184.[73] Despite this finding, the mutation appears to confer viral sensitivity to ZDV and may account for the combination's efficacy.[74] 3TC is currently indicted for use in combination for ZDV. There are no specific stages of immunosuppression associated with HIV infection for which this recommendation is made.

Studies conducted in pregnant rats and rabbits at doses 130 and 160 times higher, respectively, than those administered to humans have demonstrated no evidence of harm to the fetus. Some evidence of early embryo lethality was seen in the rabbit at doses similar to those produced by the usual adult dose and higher, but there was no indication of this effect in the rat at orally administered doses up to 130 times the usual adult dose. Studies in pregnant rats and rabbits showed that lamivudine is transferred to the fetus through the placenta. In the rat, lamivudine concentrations are somewhat higher in breastmilk than in plasma. There are no adequate and well-controlled studies in pregnant women.

Nucleoside analogue drugs have been shown to interfere with DNA polymerase, thus disturbing replication and causing the dysfunction of mitochondrial DNA. This toxicity occurs in patients who have been on long-term therapy with these agents and appears to be reversible when the medications are discontinued. There may be a genetic predisposition to this side effect.[75] A French review by Blanche reported on eight cases of infants exposed to nucleoside analogues (ZDV and 3TC) during the perinatal period who developed sequelae related to mitochondrial dysfunction. These children were not HIV positive. In this series, there were two deaths, three patients with moderate symptoms, and three patients with laboratory abnormalities.[76] These findings have not been seen in other large databases of children under study following in utero and neonatal exposure to nucleoside analogues, but further evaluation of these living children for mitochondrial dysfunction is in progress.[77] If mitochondrial disruption is a side effect of this class of medication, one must balance the risks and benefits of its use. Given that this side effect appears to be rare (and if more frequent than suspected, likely reversible) and that the benefits of reduced perinatal HIV transmission are very significant, at this time these agents continue to be administered and the children closely studied.

Abacavir (ABC; Ziagen)

Abacavir is the first guanosine analogue HIV-1 reverse transcriptase inhibitor that is clinically available. It is a very potent nucleoside analogue and is safe and well tolerated. Long-term studies have not yet been completed. The common side effects are mild to moderate headache, lymphadenopathy, musculoskeletal chest pain, neck stiffness, hematuria, nausea, rash, and fever. It can be taken with or without food. When coadministered with ZDV or 3TC, there are no clinically significant interactions.[78] The dosage is 600 mg orally once daily or 300 mg twice daily. No studies have been conducted in pregnant women or infants, and the FDA pregnancy category of this drug is C.

Protease Inhibitors

Protease inhibitors act by blocking aspartate protease, which is the enzyme that HIV-1 uses to cleave functional core proteins from precursors. They prevent viral protease, to which they bind, from cleaving the gag-pol polypeptide (the product of the transcription and translation of the HIV-1 *gag* and *pol* genes) into individual viral proteins.[79,80] Many scientists consider this class of drug the most active available antiretroviral agents. Saquinavir, ritonavir, indinavir, and nelfinavir are the currently available agents.

Saquinavir (Invirase)

The recommended dose of saquinavir is 600 mg by mouth three times daily. Mild diarrhea, abdominal discomfort, and nausea have been the most significant reported side effects. Laboratory markers of disease activity such as CD4+ cell count and plasma viral load determinations have shown the beneficial effects of this drug in combination with ZDV as well as with ZDV and ddC.[81] These changes have tended to revert to baseline over time, consistent with the development of drug-resistant strains.

The bioavailability of this drug is quite poor and is improved only slightly with the administration of food. It is hepatically metabolized by cytochrome p450. Other drugs that act to induce or inhibit this enzyme system may interact adversely with saquinavir. Efforts are being directed toward improving drug bioavailability that may enhance antiviral activity. A gel cap with better bioavailability has come on the market.

In regard to potential fetal effects, according to the manufacturer, carcinogenicity studies in rats and mice have not yet been completed. Mutagenicity and genotoxicity studies, with and without metabolic activation where appropriate, have shown that saquinavir has no mutagenic activity in vitro in either bacterial (Ames test) or mammalian cells (Chinese hamster lung V79/HPRT test). Saquinavir does not induce chromosomal damage in vivo in the mouse micronucleus assay or in vitro in the unscheduled DNA synthesis test. Fertility and reproductive performance were not affected in rats at plasma exposures up to five times those achieved in humans at the recommended dose.

Saquinavir is a category B drug. Reproduction studies conducted with saquinavir in rats have shown no embryo toxicity or teratogenicity at plasma exposures up to five times those achieved in humans at the recommended dose or in rabbits at plasma exposures four times those achieved at the recommended clinical dose. Studies in rats indicated that exposures to saquinavir from late pregnancy through lactation at plasma concentrations up to five times those achieved in humans at the recommended dose had no effect on the survival or growth and development of offspring.

Ritonavir (Norvir)

Ritonavir is well absorbed orally and reaches plasma concentrations well above those necessary for in vitro inhibition of virus. In two short-term studies conducted in the United States, Europe, and Australia, ritonavir as monotherapy in patients with wide-ranging CD4+ counts was found to be a potent inhibitor of viral replication, suppressing viral plasma load by a little over 1 log and increasing CD4+ cell counts by 100 to 200 cells/mm^3.[82–84] At doses less than the currently recommended 600 mg twice daily these effects tended to diminish over time. In a randomized double-blind study of patients with CD4+ counts less than 100 cells/mm^3 and at least 9 months of antiretroviral therapy, death or progression to other markers of disease were significantly lower in the group that received ritonavir.[85]

Ritonavir is available as 100 mg capsules, and six must be taken at each dosing. Gastrointestinal disturbances are a problem with ritonavir, although they can be mitigated by slow escalation of doses at the onset of therapy, which may also help to achieve higher steady-state serum levels, since the drug induces its own metabolism. Circumoral paresthesias have also been noted. An area of concern is the extensive potential for drug interactions with ritonavir. It has a high affinity for several cytochrome p450 isoforms and may significantly increase the levels of other drugs metabolized by this enzyme system. Ritonavir is primarily metabolized by the liver. Very little of unchanged drug or its metabolites appear in the urine. Ritonavir must be refrigerated and protected from exposure to light.

Ritonavir is a category B drug. It produced no effects on fertility in rats at drug exposures approximately 40% (male) and 60% (female) of those achieved with therapeutic dosages. Higher dosages were not feasible due to hepatic toxicity.

No treatment-related malformations were observed when ritonavir was administered to pregnant rats or rabbits. Developmental toxicity observed in rats (early resorptions, decreased fetal body weight, and ossification delays and developmental variations) occurred at a maternal exposure equivalent to approximately 30% of that achieved with the therapeutic dose. A slight increase in the incidence of cryptorchidism was also noted in rats at an exposure approximately 22% of that achieved with the proposed therapeutic dose.

In rabbits, developmental toxicity (resorptions, decreased litter size, and decreased fetal weights) occurred at a maternally toxic dosage equivalent to 1.8 times the proposed therapeutic dose based on a body surface area conversion factor. There are, however, no adequate and well-controlled studies in pregnant women.

Indinavir (Crixivan)

Indinavir is available as 200 mg and 400 mg capsules. The recommended daily dosage is 800 mg every 8 hours. Absorption is adversely affected by meals, and so the drug should be administered without food. Metabolism of indinavir is predominantly hepatic, and excretion is via the gastrointestinal tract. Indinavir's approval by the FDA was based solely on data that, to that date, had appeared only in abstract form.[72,73] In one study, indinavir alone or in combination with ZDV in antiretroviral agent–naive patients with a mean CD4+ count of 145 caused an increase in CD4+ count (100 cells/mm^3) and a decrease in serum viral RNA (1 log). Of note, approximately one third of patients receiving indinavir either alone or in combination had serum RNA levels below the limit of detection of the assay. A similar study in patients with a higher mean CD4+ count at enrollment yielded similar results.

In a study of antiretroviral-experienced patients randomized to receive indinavir, ZDV, 3TC, each alone, or all three drugs together, the triple-drug therapy had a greater effect on serum viral load while the triple-drug therapy and indinavir alone had comparable effects on CD4+ counts. More than 85% of subjects on triple-drug therapy in this study had suppression of viral load below the threshold of detection at 24 weeks of therapy. An additional study examining indinavir in combination with ZDV/ddI has yielded similar results.

The most significant adverse effect reported with indinavir use has been nephrolithiasis. In addition, because of its effects on isoforms of the cytochrome p450 system, coadministration of indinavir with drugs also metabolized by these enzymes should be performed with extreme caution. Rifampin and ketoconazole may decrease indinavir levels, whereas levels of terfenadine, astemizole, cisapride, triazolam, and midazolam may increase when indinavir is administered.

Indinavir is a category C drug. Developmental toxicity studies performed in rats and rabbits (at doses comparable to or slightly greater than human exposure) revealed no evidence of teratogenicity. Treatment-related increases over controls in the incidence of supernumerary ribs (at exposures at or below those in humans) and of cervical ribs (at exposures comparable to or slightly greater than those in humans) were seen in rats. No treatment-related external, visceral, or skeletal changes were observed in rabbits. In both species, no treatment-related effects on embryonic or fetal survival or fetal weight were observed. In utero exposure to indinavir was significant in rats. There are no adequate and well-controlled studies in pregnant women.

There may also be important nonteratogenic effects. Hyperbilirubinemia has occurred among adults during treatment with indinavir. Although indirect bilirubin would be cleared through the placenta during pregnancy, it is unknown whether indinavir administered to the mother in the perinatal period will exacerbate physiologic hyperbilirubinemia in neonates.

Nelfinavir

Nelfinavir is a newer agent and had been granted FDA pregnancy category B status. The drug is well tolerated, with gastrointestinal upset being the most common side effect. Placental and breastmilk passage is unknown in humans. Commonly, it is given as first-line therapy orally, 750 mg three times a day with ZDV and 3TC, with a favorable response.[86] Its efficacy has also been established when used in a dose of 1250 mg twice daily instead of three times a day.[87]

Amprenavir

Amprenavir is a new protease enzyme inhibitor that can be administered twice daily with or without food. To date, its use has been as a part of combination regimens, and it may show promise as salvage therapy when resistance develops with other protease enzymes.[88]

Non-Nucleoside Analogues

This category of antiviral medications also inhibits reverse transcriptase, thus blocking the replication of HIV. These agents are selective for HIV-1 reverse transcriptase enzyme. They are for use as a part of combination therapy. When used alone, they are associated with the development of drug-resistant viral strains.

Nevirapine

Nevirapine is an FDA pregnancy category C drug. Through its interaction with the cytochrome p450 system, similar to efavirenz, it may induce the metabolism of other medications, including protease inhibitors. A trial was performed in Uganda using nevirapine in an abbreviated regimen at the onset of labor (see Chapter 5). Further studies are in progress with this drug and its role in decreasing perinatal transmission of HIV.[89]

Delavirdine

Delavirdine is an FDA category C drug and is yet to be evaluated in pregnant HIV-infected women.

Efavirenz

Efavirenz is a new non-nucleoside reverse transcriptase inhibitor that is prescribed once daily. It induces the cytochrome p450 system and may interact with other medications that are metabolized by the liver. It is currently recommended that this agent *not* be used in pregnant patients because of malformations in the monkey model.[90] However, this drug can be used in the pregnant woman without other treatment alternatives when the potential benefit justifies potential risks.

Choice of Regimen

The current standard of care is to use HAART for those patients whose immunologic or virologic circumstance warrants antiretroviral therapy.[30,36] Perhaps the simplest regimen to use is ZDV 300 mg twice daily, 3TC 150 mg twice daily, and nelfinavir 1250 mg twice daily. Changes in regimen are based on toxicities and virologic response. Management should be in consultation with an expert in HIV disease.

Currently, there are insufficient data to justify the substitution of any agent for ZDV in most circumstances. Even if there is evidence of ZDV resistance, which might make therapy for the prevention of mother-to-child transmission seem futile, ZDV might still have a role. The demonstration of transmission of escape mutants from mother to child[79] suggests that an individual ZDV-susceptible virus might be transmitted even if the predominant strains in the mother are not susceptible. Further research is needed to see whether there is advantage to combination therapy as part of a strategy to prevent transmission of resistant strains. If the mother is intolerant of ZDV, it may be reasonable to consider using an alternative agent, which could potentially reduce viral load during the antepartum period, and then adding ZDV for the intrapartum period (depending on the type of toxicity experienced by the mother) and neonatal period. Alternatively, nevirapine could be added in the intrapartum period (see Chapter 5).

In sum, pregnant women should be the beneficiaries of any clinical advantage offered by new regimens and should not be restricted to single-drug therapy. However, the continued use of the public health service panel's recommended ZDV regimen as part of any therapeutic strategy should be ensured.

Antiretroviral medications are only one part of the clinician's pharmaceutical armamentarium. Medications are also available for the prevention and treatment of opportunistic infections. If the CD4+ count is found to be less than 200 cells/mm^3 at any time, the patient is at risk for developing *Pneumocystis carinii* pneumonia, and prophylaxis is required. First-line therapy is trimethoprim-sulfamethoxazole double strength. This therapy will coincidentally serve as effective prophylaxis against *Toxoplasma gondii*. If the CD4+ count falls below 100 cells/mm^3, rifabutin prophylaxis for *Mycobacterium avium* should be given. If the CD4+ count falls below 50 cells/mm^3 there is a risk of cryptococcal infection and fluconazole prophylaxis is recommended. Vaccinations for hepatitis A and B, *Pneumococcus* infection, viral influenza, and *Haemophilus influenzae* B infection should be considered and may be used in pregnant patients. There is controversy regarding the use of viral vaccines in pregnant women, as there may be an induction of a transient HIV viremia that may have an associated risk of fetal transmission. If the HIV-positive pregnant woman develops an opportunistic infection, a specialist in the management of HIV disease should be consulted. Recently, there has been some suggestion that if the CD4+ level climbs above 200 cells/mm^3 in response to HAART and remains there for 6 months, discontinuation of prophylaxis can be considered.

OBSTETRIC ISSUES

Other than the issues discussed, there are only a few aspects of routine prenatal care that require modification in the setting of HIV infection. For example, amniocentesis, which is a procedure that is frequently performed during the course of a pregnancy for genetic and therapeutic indications and for the determination of fetal lung maturity, may have a different benefit-to-burden ratio in this setting. The HIV-infected woman must weigh the benefits and burdens of the information to be gathered and its impact on pregnancy management against its potential for facilitating HIV transmission to the fetus. In most circumstances, specialists would advise against this invasive procedure. Attention to nutrition, psychosocial well-being, and the maintenance of a healthy lifestyle are also beneficial for these patients. Successful models of prenatal care often require a multidisciplinary approach to patient management so that all aspects of the patient's (and her family's) health are addressed. When exemplary prenatal care is combined with state-of-the-art HIV care, the prognoses for mother and child can be remarkably better than they were just a few years ago.

REFERENCES

1. Kane B: Rapid testing for HIV: Why so fast? Ann Intern Med 1999;131:481–483.
2. Asihene P, Kline R, Moss M, Carella A, Quinn T: Evaluation of rapid test for detection of antibody to human immunodeficiency virus type 1 and 2. J Clin Microbiol 1994;32:1341–1342.
3. Mitchell SW, Mboup S, Mingle J, et al: Field evaluation of alternative HIV test: Strategy with rapid immunobinding assay and as agglutination assay. Lancet 1991;33:1328–1331.
4. Update: HIV counseling and testing using rapid test—U.S. 1995. MMWR 1955;47:211–215.
5. Kassler WJ, Dillon BA, Haley C, Jones WK, Goldman A: On-site, rapid testing with same day results and counseling. AIDS 1997;11:1045–1051.
6. Landesman S, Minkoff HL, Holman S, et al: Serosurvey of human immunodeficiency virus infection in parturients. JAMA 1987;258:2701.
7. American Academy of Pediatrics and American College of Obstetricians and Gynecologists: Joint statement of the American Academy of Pediatrics and the American College of Obstetricians and Gynecologists. Pediatrics 1999;104(1 Pat 1):128.
8. Sunderland A, Minkoff HL, Handte J, et al: The influence of serostatus on women's reproductive decisions. Obstet Gynecol 1992;79:1027.
9. Selwyn DA, Carter RJ, Shoenbaum EE, et al: Knowledge of HIV antibody status and decisions to terminate pregnancy among intravenous drug users. JAMA 1989;261:2567.
10. Wade NA, Birkhead GS, Warren GL, et al: Abbreviated regimens of zidovudine prophylaxis and perinatal transmission of the human immunodeficiency virus. N Engl J Med 1998;339:1461–1463.
11. Johnstone FD, McCallum L, Brettle R, et al: Does HIV infection affect the outcome of pregnancy. BMJ 1988;296:467.
12. Johnstone FD, McCallum L, Brettle R, et al: Does HIV infection affect the outcome of pregnancy? BMJ 1988;296:467.
13. Minkoff HL, Henderson C, Mendez H, et al: Pregnancy outcomes among mothers infected with human immunodeficiency virus and uninfected control subjects. Am J Obstet Gynecol 1990; 163:1598–1604.

14. Ryder RW, Nsa W, Hassig SE, et al: Perinatal transmission of the human immunodeficiency virus type 1 to infants of seropositive women in Zaire. N Engl J Med 1989;320:1637–1642.
15. Weinberg ED: Pregnancy-associated depression of cell-mediated immunity. Rev Infect Dis 1984;6:814.
16. Temmerman M, Nageklkerke N, Bwayo J, et al: HIV-1 and immunologic changes during pregnancy: A comparison between HIV-1 seropositive and HIV-1 seronegative women in Nairobi, Kenya. AIDS 1995;9:1057–1060.
17. Brettle RP, Raab GM, Ros A, et al: HIV infection in women: Immunologic markers and the influence of pregnancy. AIDS 1995;10:1177–1184.
18. Biggar RJ, Pahava S, Minkoff HL, et al: Immunosuppression in pregnant women infected with human immunodeficiency virus. Am J Obstet Gynecol 1989;161:1239–1244.
19. Burns D, Nourjah P, Minkoff H, et al: Changes in CD4 and CD8 cells levels during pregnancy and postpartum in women seropositive and seronegative for human immunodeficiency virus-1. Am J Obstet Gynecol 1996;174:1461–1468.
20. Tuomala RE, Kalish LA, Zorilla C, et al: Changes in total CD4+ and CD8+ lymphocytes during pregnancy and one year post partum in HIV infected women. Obstet Gynecol 1997;89:967–974.
21. Nossal GJV: Current concepts. Immunology: The basic components of the immune system. N Engl J Med 1987;316:1320.
22. Blanche S, Mayaux MJ, Rouzioux C, et al: Relation of the course of HIV infection in children to the severity of the disease in their mothers at delivery. N Engl J Med 1994;330:308–312.
23. Schaefer A, Grosch-Woerner, Friedman I, et al: The effect of pregnancy on the natural course of HIV disease. Paper presented at the Fourth International Conference on AIDS, Stockholm, 1988. Abstract No. 4039.
24. Minkoff HL, Nanda D, Menez R, et al: Pregnancies resulting in infants with acquired immunodeficiency syndrome or AIDS related complex. Obstet Gynecol 1987;69:285.
25. MacCallum LR, France AJ, Jones ME, et al: The effects of pregnancy on progression of HIV disease. Paper presented at the Fourth International Conference on AIDS, Stockholm, 1988. Abstract No. 4032.
26. Berrebi A, Puel J, Granjean H, Herne F, Pontonnier G: The influence of pregnancy on the evolution of HIV infection. Paper presented at the Fourth International Conference on AIDS, Stockholm, 1988. Abstract No. 4041.
27. Hocke C, Morlat P, Chene G, et al: Prospective cohort study of the effect of pregnancy on the progression of human immunodeficiency virus infection. Obstet Gynecol 1995;86:886–891.
28. Alliegro MB, Dorrucci M, Phillips AN, et al: Incidence and consequences of pregnancy in women with known duration of HIV infection. Arch Intern Med 1997;157:2585–2590.
29. Birkhead GS (ed): Prevention of Perinatal HIV Transmission Clinical Guidelines: Management of Pregnant Women and Infants. New York State Department of Health AIDS Institute, 1999.
30. Carpenter CC, Fischl MA, Hammer SM, et al: Antiretroviral therapy for HIV infection in 1998: Updated recommendations of the international AIDS society—USA panel. JAMA 1998;280:78–84.
31. Carpenter CC, Fischl MA, Hammer SM, et al: Antiretroviral therapy for HIV infection in 1997: Updated recommendations of the international AIDS society—USA panel. JAMA 1997;277:1962–1969.
32. Connor EM, Sperling RS, Gelber R, et al: Reduction of maternal-infant transmission of human immunodeficiency virus type 1 with zidovudine treatment. N Engl J Med 1994;331:1173–1180.
33. Wong JK, Hezareh M, Gunthard H, et al: Recovery of replication-competent HIV despite prolonged suppression of plasma viremia. Science 1997;278:1291–1295.
34. Finzi D, Hermankova M, Pierson T, et al: Identification of a reservoir for HIV-1 in patients on highly active antiretroviral therapy. Science 1997;278:1295–1300.
35. Bartlet JG, Moore RD: Improving HIV therapy. Scientific American 1998;279(1):84–93.
36. Minkoff H, Augenbraun M: Antiretroviral therapy of the pregnant women. Am J Obstet Gynecol 1997;176:478–489.
37. Fischl M, Richman D, Grieco M, et al: The efficacy of ZDV in the treatment of patients with AIDS and AIDS-related complex: A double blind placebo controlled trial. N Engl J Med 1987;317:185–191.
38. Fischl M, Parker C, Pettinelli C, et al: A randomized controlled trial of reduced daily dose of ZDV in patients with acquired immunodeficiency syndrome. The AIDS Clinical Trials Group. N Engl J Med 1990;323:1009–1014.
39. Fischl M, Richman D, Hansen N, et al: The safety and efficacy of zidovudine (AZT) in the treatment of subjects with mildly symptomatic human immunodeficiency virus type 1 (HIV) infection: A double blind placebo controlled trial. The AIDS Clinical Trials Group. Ann Intern Med 1990;112:727–737.
40. Sande M, Carpenter C, Cobbs G, et al: Antiretroviral therapy for adult HIV-infected patients: Recommendations from a state-of-the-art conference. JAMA 1993;270:2582–2589.
41. Hamilton J, Hartigan P, Simberkoff M, et al: A controlled trial of early versus late treatment with ZDV in symptomatic human immunodeficiency virus infection: Results of the Veterans Affairs

Cooperative Study. N Engl J Med 1992; 326:437–443.
42. Concorde Coordinating Committee: Concorde: MRC/ANRS randomized double blind controlled trial of immediate and deferred ZDV in symptom free HIV infection. Lancet 1994;343:871–878.
43. U.S. Public Health Service Task Force: Recommendations on the use of zidovudine to reduce perinatal transmission of HIV. MMWR 1994;43:1–15.
44. Lipschultz SE, Orav EJ, Sanders SP, et al: Cardiac structure and function in children with human immunodeficiency virus infection treated with zidovudine. N Engl J Med 1992;327:1260–1265.
45. Ayers KM: Preclinical toxicology of zidovudine: An overview. Am J Med 1988;85(suppl 2A):186–188.
46. Physicians' Desk Reference, 48th ed. Montvale, NJ, Medical Economics Data Production Company, 1994, pp 742–749.
47. Toltzis P, Marx CM, Kleinman N, et al: Zidovudine-associated embryonic toxicity in mice. J Infect Dis 1991;163:1212–1218.
48. Toltzis P, Mourton T, Magnuson T: Effect of zidovudine on preimplantation murine embryos. Antimicrob Agents Chemother 1993;37:1610–1613.
49. Burroughs Wellcome Company: Comprehensive information for investigators: retrovir (July 1993). Research Triangle Park, NC, Burroughs Wellcome, 1993.
50. O'Sullivan MJ, Boyer PJJ, Scott GB, et al: The pharmacokinetics and safety of zidovudine in the third trimester of pregnancy for women infected with human immunodeficiency virus and their infants: Phase I ACTG study (protocol 082). Am J Obstet Gynecol 1993;168:1510–1516.
51. Watts DH, Brown ZA, Tartaglione GT, et al: Pharmacokinetic disposition of zidovudine during pregnancy. J Infect Dis 1991;163:226–232.
52. Ferrazin A, de Maria A, Gotta C, et al: Zidovudine therapy of HIV-1 infection during pregnancy: Assessment of the effect on the newborns. J Acquir Immune Defic Syndr Hum Retrovirol 1993; 6:376–379.
53. Boyer PJJ, Dillon M, Navaie M, et al: Factors predictive of maternal-fetal transmission of HIV-1: Preliminary analysis of zidovudine (ZDV) given during pregnancy and/or delivery. JAMA 1994;271:1925–1930.
54. Connor E, Sperling R, Shapiro D, et al: Long-term effect of ZDV exposure among uninfected infants born to HIV-infected mothers in AIDS clinical trials group 076. Proc ICAACX 1995;205:1.
55. Centers for Disease Control and Prevention: Birth outcomes following zidovudine therapy in pregnant women. MMWR 1994;43:409, 415–416.
56. Richman DD, Grimes JM, Lagakos SW: Effect of stage of disease and drug dose on zidovudine susceptibilities of isolates of human immunodeficiency virus. J Acquir Immune Defic Syndr Hum Retrovirol 1990;3:743–746.
57. Hirsch MS, Aquila RT: Therapy for human immunodeficiency virus infection. N Engl J Med 1993;328:1686–1695.
58. Smith MS, Koerber KL, Pagano JS: Long-term persistence of zidovudine resistance mutations in plasma isolates from human immunodeficiency virus type 1 of dideoxyinosine-treated patients removed from zidovudine therapy. J Infec Dis 1994;169:184–188.
59. Schindzielorz A, Pike I, Daniels M, et al: Rates and risk factors for adverse events associated with didanosine in the expanded access program. Clin Infect Dis 1994;19:1076–1083.
60. Pons JC, Boubon MC, Taburet AM, et al: Fetoplacental passage of 2'3'-dideoxyinosine. Lancet 1991;337:732.
61. Bawdon R, Sobhi S, Dax J: The transfer of anti-human immunodeficiency virus nucleoside compounds by the term human placenta. Am J Obstet Gynecol 1992;167:1570–1574.
62. Silkker W Jr, Lipe GD, Ali SF, et al: Placenta transfer and fetal distribution of 3H-ddC in the monkey. Teratology 1992;45:457–458.
63. Lindstrom P, Harris M, Hoberman AM, et al: Developmental toxicity of 2'3'-dideoxycytidine (DDC) in mice. Toxicologist 1990;10:124.
64. Foerster M, Kastner U, Neubert R: Effect of six virustatic nucleoside analogues on the development of fetal rat thymus in organ culture. Arch Toxicol 1992;66:688–699.
65. Nightingale S: From the Food and Drug Administration. JAMA 1994;272:582.
66. Barry M, Mulcahy F, Merry C, et al: Pharmacokinetics and potential interactions amongst antiretroviral agents used to treat patients with HIV infection. Clin Pharmacokinet 1999;36:289–304.
67. Lin P, Samanta H, Rose R, et al: Genotypic and phenotypic analysis of human immunodeficiency virus type 1 isolates for patients on prolonged stavudine therapy. J Infect Dis 1994;170:1157–1160.
68. Toltzis P, Mourton T, Magnuson T: Comparative embryonic cytotoxicity of antiretroviral nucleosides. J Infect Dis 1994;169:1100–1102.
69. Merril D, Moonis M, Chou T, Hirsch M: Lamivudine or stavudine in 2- and 3-drug combinations against human immunodeficiency type 1 replication in vitro. J Infect Dis 1996;173:355–364.
70. Dienstag J, Perillo R, Schiff E, et al: A preliminary trial of lamivudine for chronic hepatitis B infection. N Engl J Med 1995;333:1657–1661.
71. Eron J, Benoit S, Jemsek J, et al: Treatment with lamivudine, zidovudine or both in HIV-positive patients with 200–500 CD4 cells per cubic millimeter. N Engl J Med 1995;333:1662–1669.
72. Michelet C, Ruffault A, Arvieux C, et al: 3TC + ZDV in patients with CD4 under 50/mm^3: A phase II

study. Paper presented at the 3rd Conference on Retroviruses and Opportunistic Infections, Washington, DC, 1996.
73. Schuurman R, Nijhuis M, van Leeuwen R, et al: Rapid changes in human immunodeficiency virus type 1 RNA local and appearance of drug-resistant virus populations in persons treated with lamivudine (3TC). J Infect Dis 1995;171:1411–1419.
74. Larder B, Kemp S, Harrigan P: Potential mechanism for sustained antiretroviral efficacy of AZT-3TC combination treatment. Science 1995;269:696–699.
75. Brinkman K, Ter Hofstede HJM, Burger DM, et al: Adverse effects of reverse transcriptase inhibitors: Mitochondrial toxicity as common pathway. AIDS 1998;12:1735–1744.
76. Blanche S, Tardieu M, Rustin P, et al: Persistent mitochondrial dysfunction and perinatal exposure to antiretroviral nucleoside analogues. Lancet 1999;354:1084–1089.
77. Smith ME and the U.S. Nucleoside Safety Review Working Group: Ongoing nucleoside safety review of HIV-exposed children in the U.S. studies. Paper presented at the Second Conference on Global Strategies for the Prevention of HIV Transmission from Mothers to Infants, September 1–6, 1999, Montreal, Canada. Abstract 096.
78. Wang LH, Chittick GE, McDowell JA: Single-dose pharmacokinetics and safety of abacavir, zidovudine, and lamivudine administered alone and in combination in adults with human immunodeficiency virus infection. Antimicrob Agents Chemother 1999;43:1708–1715.
79. Ezzel C: Emergence of the protease inhibitors: A better class of AIDS drugs? J NIH Res 1996;8:41–45.
80. McQuade TJ, Tomasseli AG, Liu L, et al: A synthetic HIV-1 protease inhibitor with antiviral activity arrests HIV-1 like particle maturation. Science 1990;247:454–456.
81. Collier A, Coombs R, Schoenfeld D, et al: Treatment of human immunodeficiency virus infection with saquinavir, zidovudine and zalcitibine. N Engl J Med 1996;334:1011–1017.
82. Danner S, Carr A, Leonard J, et al: A short term study of the safety pharmacokinetics and efficiency of ritonavir, an inhibitor of HIV-1 protease. N Engl J Med 1995;333:1528–1533.
83. Markowitz M, Saag M, Powderly W, et al: A preliminary study of ritonavir, an inhibitor of HIV-1 protease, to treat HIV-1 infection. N Engl J Med 1995;333:1543–1549.
84. Mathez D, Truchis P, Gorin I, et al: Ritonavir, AZT, ddC as a triple combination in AIDS patients. Paper presented at the Third Conference on Retroviruses and Opportunistic Infections, Washington, DC, 1996.
85. Cameron B, Heath-Chiozzi M, Kravcik S, et al: Prolongation of life and prevention of AIDS in advanced immunodeficiency with ritonavir. Paper presented at the Third Conference on Retroviruses and Opportunistic Infections, Washington, DC, 1996.
86. Powderly WG, Tebas P: Nelfinavir, a new protease inhibitor, early clinical results. AIDS 1999;13 (Suppl 1): S41–48.
87. Jarvis B, Faulds D: Nelfinavir: A review of its therapeutic efficacy in HIV infection. Drugs 1998; 56:147–167.
88. Gatell J: Coming therapies: Amprenavir. Int J Clin Pract Suppl 1999;103:42–44.
89. Guay LA: Intrapartum and neonatal single-dose nevirapine compared with zidovudine for prevention of mother-to-child transmission of HIV-1 in Kampala, Uganda: HIVNET 012 randomised trial. Lancet 1999;354:795–802.
90. Ruiz N: Clinical history of efavirenz. Int J Clin Pract Suppl 1999;103:3–7.

5

Perinatal HIV: Obstetric Issues

Ruth E. Tuomala

Obstetric care of HIV-infected pregnant women centers on defining and utilizing the appropriate initial and ongoing medical and obstetric evaluations and management to minimize perinatal transmission of HIV and maximize both the health of the pregnant woman and the outcome of the pregnancy. Defining appropriate care requires knowledge of (1) risk factors for vertical transmission of HIV; (2) the impact of HIV infection on the outcome of pregnancy; (3) the impact of pregnancy on the health of HIV-infected women; (4) treatment and prevention of opportunistic illnesses; and (5) the principles of use of antiretroviral therapy both in HIV-infected adults and during pregnancy. Both perinatal transmission of HIV and the use of antiretroviral therapy are discussed in detail elsewhere in this book. Information that pertains directly to obstetric management is reviewed in this chapter.

RISK FOR PERINATAL HIV TRANSMISSION: STRATEGIES TO MINIMIZE TRANSMISSION

The pathophysiology of vertical transmission of HIV-1 is multifactorial, and several factors that have an impact on the transmission risk have been defined.[1] Some risk factors that have been associated with vertical transmission can be modified by appropriate treatment both during the pregnancy and prior to pregnancy in women planning to become pregnant.

The major risk factor for perinatal transmission of HIV that has emerged is maternal peripheral viral load. Data on risk factors for transmission derived from early observational studies suggested that the risk for vertical transmission was affected by the stage of maternal illness, as suggested by increasing maternal age, as well as immune function as measured by CD4+ absolute cell count and percentage. More recent data have suggested that maternal viral load is more strongly correlated with transmission than is CD4+ cell count.[2-4]

In women who are receiving either no antiretroviral therapy (ART) or monotherapy, initial maternal viral load and viral load at the time of delivery are directly related to the risk for vertical transmission.[2,3] There appears to be an increasing risk for transmission with increasing titer of viral load,[3] regardless of antiretroviral use.[4] Although there is no level below which lack of transmission is guaranteed, the risk for transmission at viral load levels below 1000 copies/mL by RNA–polymerase chain reaction (PCR) appears to be very low, in some series approximating 2%.[4-8] Although there have been no clinical trials that have looked directly at the impact of lowering viral load during the course of pregnancy on relative risk for vertical transmission, current obstetric management emphasizes the aggressive use of ART during pregnancy to minimize viral load and achieve nondetectable levels by the time of delivery. In addition, preconception counseling of HIV-infected women who are of childbearing age includes the desirability of attaining a nondetectable viral load through the use of ART prior to conception, regardless of decisions about the long-term use of antiretroviral agents for overall health reasons.

Appropriate use of ART is independently correlated with the risk for perinatal HIV transmission. In 1994, the Pediatric AIDS Clinical Trials Group study 076 showed that the use of antenatal, intrapartum, and neonatal zidovudine decreases vertical transmission by approximately two thirds.[9] In clinical use, the three-part zidovudine monotherapy regimen utilized in study 076 achieves rates of perinatal HIV transmission in the 5% to 10% range,[10-12] regardless of viral load. Studies of shortened antepartum and neonatal courses of zidovudine and of intrapartum and neonatal nevirapine in developing and mid-developed countries have shown protection against vertical transmission of somewhat lesser magnitudes.[13-16] No protection against transmission is achieved with the use of intrapartum therapy alone.[17]

Recent observations have shown that the use of antepartum combination ART plus intrapartum and neonatal ART is associated with the lowest rates for perinatal HIV transmission. As has been shown for zidovudine, the use of such combination therapy appears to have an effect separate from its effect on viral load.[4,18,19] Optimal obstetric management in developed countries includes the use of combination antiretroviral therapy during pregnancy along with intrapartum and neonatal zidovudine.

There are some risk factors for vertical transmission of HIV that can be modified either during the time course of pregnancy or prior to conception if discussed during preconception counseling. Among these are cigarette smoking, illicit drug use, and unprotected sexual intercourse with multiple partners during pregnancy.[20-25] The presence of sexually transmitted diseases, including bacterial vaginosis, is similarly amenable to treatment, although less strongly implicated in vertical transmission. In addition, two risk factors independently associated with vertical transmission in multiple studies, preterm gestational age at delivery and chorioamnionitis, can potentially be decreased if not eliminated through targeted interventions.[25-28] Obstetric management of HIV-infected pregnant women should also include strategies to screen for and impact upon these factors.

IMPACT OF PREGNANCY ON OUTCOME OF HIV INFECTION

Initial reports describing pregnancy in HIV-infected women centered around descriptions of morbidity and mortality due to AIDS-defining conditions newly diagnosed during pregnancy as well as small case series suggesting high rates of development of complications during pregnancy or the postpartum period. These reports raised concerns that the immunologic changes associated with pregnancy could accelerate disease progression in HIV-infected women. Subsequent data from multiple observational studies have failed to demonstrate a consistent influence of pregnancy on the course of HIV clinical, immunologic, or virologic progression, and studies that have followed women for many years postpartum have failed to show a negative impact of pregnancy on health.[29-33] It appears that the general rate of clinical progression of disease in women is similar to that in men when adjusted for comparable medical care.[34-37]

The effect of pregnancy on immunologic and virologic parameters is incompletely understood. During pregnancy, there is an increase in the total white blood cell count and total polymorphonuclear leukocyte count and a decrease in the absolute number and percentage of lymphocytes.[38-40] Most observations have suggested an alteration in the absolute CD4+ cell count during pregnancy, with a decrease early in gestation followed by an increase in count later during pregnancy.[40-47] However, changes in the CD4+ cell count during pregnancy appear to be highly variable across individuals.[42] Postpartum, changes in the CD4+ cell count are thought to reflect physiologic changes related to delivery and the end of pregnancy. There does not appear to be any long-term, pregnancy-related decline in CD4+ cell count or in measures of immune function.[42-44,48,49] The CD4+ cell percentage is stable during pregnancy and the immediate postpartum period[50] and probably a better reflection of the immunologic stage of HIV-infection during pregnancy.

It is unclear whether pregnancy affects viral load. One observational study documented an increase in plasma HIV-1 RNA levels by 6 months postpartum, unrelated to antiretroviral use patterns.[51] This has suggested to some that there may be suppression in viral load during pregnancy. Specific evidence of such is lacking. Regardless of potential pregnancy-related effects on CD4+ count or viral load, any significant changes in these parameters during pregnancy should prompt thorough evaluation and consideration of any appropriate changes in HIV-related therapy.

EFFECT OF HIV INFECTION ON THE OUTCOME OF PREGNANCY

Infection with HIV-1 has not been convincingly associated with spontaneous abortion prior to 20 weeks of gestation, intrauterine fetal death, stillbirths, or fetuses with congenital anomalies.[52,53] Temmerman and coworkers[54] suggested an association between HIV infection and early spontaneous abortion in a comparison between women presenting with pregnancy loss prior to 20 weeks of gestation and women with viable pregnancies. Kumer and coworkers,[55] in a comparison between HIV-infected and uninfected pregnant women also reported a higher rate for both spontaneous abortion and intrauterine fetal death in the HIV-infected women with symptomatic disease. Langston and coworkers[56] demonstrated HIV infection by in situ hybridization in tissues from 7 of 14 pathologic specimens from HIV-infected women with early fetal loss. In addition, thymic abnormalities were noted. It was postulated that transmission of HIV to the fetoplacental unit early in pregnancy resulted in both inflammation and fetal thymic dysfunction that resulted in disruption of pregnancy and immunologic rejection of the fetus. Although studies subsequent to these have failed to show associations between HIV infection and early pregnancy loss, it is reasonable to ensure pregnancy viability with ultrasonography performed early during pregnancy of HIV-infected women.

Multiple studies have suggested that HIV-infected women do have an increase in preterm deliveries and low birth weight, intrauterine growth retarded, or small for gestational age infants.[57–61] Preterm birth and low birth weight rates for HIV-infected pregnant women in the United States in the 20% range have been observed.[61–63] These are higher than rates suggested for general obstetric populations.[63–67] Some studies that have controlled for multiple risk factors for adverse pregnancy outcome have found that adverse pregnancy outcomes are more related to the presence of risk factors unrelated to HIV infection.[68–74] Two studies, using multivariate analysis, suggested that adverse pregnancy outcome is associated with factors specifically related to HIV infection and with more broad risk factors for adverse pregnancy outcome present at relatively high frequencies in the populations of HIV-infected women who were studied.[62,75] Some studies have specifically linked degree of immunosuppression with increased risk for adverse pregnancy outcome.[26,27,62,76,77] Similar to studies of adverse pregnancy outcome in general obstetric populations, receipt of good prenatal care[75,78] and good nutrition[77] have been shown to decrease adverse pregnancy outcomes in HIV-infected pregnant women. In addition to encouraging prenatal care for HIV-infected women, during pregnancy HIV-infected women need to have close monitoring and management to maximize pregnancy outcome.

The majority of studies that have analyzed the effect of HIV infection on pregnancy outcome have been conducted in HIV-infected women receiving either no antepartum ART or monotherapy. There have been no definitive data by which to judge the effect of combination antiretroviral therapy on pregnancy outcome. A high risk of preterm delivery (33%) was reported in a retrospective Swiss cohort of 30 HIV-infected women who received combination antiretroviral therapy during pregnancy, 13 of whom received combination therapy with protease inhibitors and 17 of whom did not receive protease inhibitors.[79]

A combined analysis of the European Collaborative Study and the Swiss Cohort Study found a significant increase in preterm delivery associated with combination therapy without and with protease inhibitors (odds ratios, 1.8 and 2.6, respectively), after adjustment for maternal CD4+ cell count and injecting drug use.[80] Although preterm delivery rates in the European study for women receiving no therapy or monotherapy were similar to rates reported in other U.S. cohorts, rates in women who received combination therapy without and with protease inhibitors (22% and 29%, respectively) were somewhat higher.

There has been no definitive study of the effect of individual or combination antiretroviral agents on the outcome of pregnancy. In addition, the safety profile for most antiretroviral agents during pregnancy for the pregnant woman and for her fetus is not known. The benefits of combination

ART in decreasing vertical transmission of HIV are substantial, and the use of highly active antiretroviral therapy (HAART) is important in terms of tangible benefits to health for many pregnant women. Appropriate care for pregnant HIV-infected women should include the use of combination ART. However, it is equally necessary during obstetric care to approach the unknown with caution and intensively monitor for potential adverse effects of therapies on pregnancy outcome, on the pregnant woman, and on the fetus.

INITIAL EVALUATION AND MANAGEMENT

HIV-infected women who are pregnant come to the attention of medical care providers during the antenatal time period either knowing that they were HIV-infected prior to pregnancy or because they are identified as being HIV-infected during pregnancy, largely due to prenatal screening. Approximately 50% to 60% of women know they were HIV-infected pre-pregnancy, and 40% to 50% of women become aware of their infection status during the pregnancy. Some HIV-infected women who give birth are identified only during the postpartum period, often because of newborn screening.[81] Lack of knowledge of HIV status during pregnancy can occur because of poor or nonexistent prenatal care or because of lack of testing during the prenatal period, either because women refuse to be tested or because health care providers do not appropriately offer testing. Identification of HIV status may still occur because an HIV-infected woman presents during pregnancy with an AIDS-defining illness or only through identification of a symptomatic HIV-infected infant.

Multidisciplinary Approach

Pregnancy in HIV-infected women requires multidisciplinary management. It is typical that medical care of HIV-infected women during pregnancy, including antiretroviral therapy, be managed both by obstetric providers and primary care or infectious disease specialists knowledgeable about HIV infection. If a woman has been newly diagnosed as being HIV-infected during the pregnancy, immediate referral to such a health care professional needs to be instituted. If a woman has prior knowledge of HIV infection, adequacy of medical care appropriate to circumstances of obstetric care needs to be determined. In some instances, collaborative care between HIV providers and obstetricians can be easily arranged. In others, HIV medical care within the same health care plan as obstetric care needs to be arranged at least for the duration of the pregnancy.

Women who are newly identified as HIV infected during pregnancy need to have extensive counseling about HIV infection. Additional considerations may include arranging for evaluation of sexual partners and children. All women need to be counseled about risks for vertical transmission of HIV, pregnancy-specific issues related to HIV care and antiretroviral therapy, and the need for comprehensive obstetric care. A major focus of counseling should be on the importance to pregnancy outcome of good adherence to prenatal care and planning appropriate prenatal care. Referral of all pregnant HIV-infected women to a perinatal obstetrician or center with special expertise in the care of HIV infection during pregnancy should be strongly considered. At least one study has suggested improved outcome with such referral.[78]

Needs for psychological, financial, and social supports should be assessed and referrals initiated as necessary. If questions of abuse of alcohol, illicit drugs, or cigarettes are determined, then appropriate referral needs to be made for counseling and comprehensive management. Many HIV-infected pregnant women require referral for services that can assist with financial help for medical services, medication procurement, and assistance with transportation and child care to attend necessary health care visits, and assessment for mental health assessment and domestic violence.

Staging of HIV Infection

Initial evaluation during pregnancy should be directed toward gathering all data necessary to be able to determine the stage of HIV infection and status of maternal health at the onset of pregnancy as well as screening for underlying conditions that could affect vertical transmission to the infant, outcome of pregnancy, and medication toxicity. Women who already know they are HIV infected need to have a complete history of antiretroviral and other HIV-associated therapies determined, including current use and tolerance of medications. Some HIV-infected women become pregnant only after preconception consultation and counseling. In these instances, health care providers may need to familiarize themselves with all of the historical and recent data and provide much more discreet initial counseling and focused laboratory evaluation. Preconception counseling for HIV-infected women of reproductive age and potential has been recommended by the U.S. Public Health Service and the American College of Obstetricians and Gynecologists.[82,83]

In addition to clinical staging, all women should have lymphocyte subset profiles and plasma HIV RNA measurements obtained as early in pregnancy as possible. For all women, but in particular for the newly diagnosed, viral load and lymphocyte subsets provide information that is essential to determine an individual's risk for disease progression and need for antiretroviral and other HIV-specific therapies.[84–86] Baseline laboratory studies relevant for both clinical staging and evaluation of potential medication toxicities that should be obtained, including a complete blood cell count, platelet count, liver function tests, renal function tests, and electrolytes.

Opportunistic Infections

Serologic status to cytomegalovirus, toxoplasmosis, and varicella-zoster virus should be assessed by obtaining antibody testing, unless antibody status is already known. Complications due to cytomegalovirus and toxoplasmosis are AIDS-defining conditions, and baseline titers can be helpful in assessing symptoms. No increased risk for vertical transmission of toxoplasmosis or cytomegalovirus in HIV-infected pregnancies has been reported. Although the presence of antibodies predating the pregnancy usually precludes serious fetal infection with these agents, fetal cytomegalovirus and toxoplasmosis infection have both been reported in HIV-infected women with preexisting antibodies who are severely immunosuppressed.[87–92] Women who are varicella-zoster antibody negative should receive both varicella-zoster immunoglobulin, in cases of exposure, and prophylactic acyclovir at the onset of any symptoms of disease to decrease disease severity.

All women should be screened for tuberculosis with appropriate skin testing. Mofenson and associates[93] have documented a 14% rate of either prior or newly diagnosed evidence of tuberculosis in a cohort of HIV-infected pregnant women. All women with a positive PPD result should have a chest radiograph. High rates of anergy have been noted.[94] In case of a negative PPD finding, chest radiography should be performed if the patient is at high epidemiologic risk for contact with tuberculosis or in the case of unexplained or persistent respiratory symptoms.

Women who are HIV infected have a higher rate than non-HIV-infected women of past exposure to sexually transmitted diseases[95] and increased prevalence of syphilis, genital herpes simplex virus, human papillomavirus (HPV), including oncogenic HPV, and hepatitis B and C.[96–101]

All women need to be screened for syphilis. There is an increase in biologically false-positive serologic test results for syphilis in patients with HIV infection.[102] Positive results confirmed by a treponemal specific test such as a fluorescent treponemal antibody absorption test or microhemagglutination assay–*Treponema pallidum* should be evaluated, along with the history of previous test results and treatment. If appropriate, a lumbar puncture can be done to exclude neurosyphilis, in particular if the duration of titer and adequacy of previous therapy for coexisting syphilis in an HIV-infected person cannot be determined.

At the initial visit, a history of prior lesions suggestive of genital herpes and a history of exposure to genital herpes or sexual partners with genital herpes should be ascertained. In addition to being more prevalent in HIV-infected women, genital herpes simplex can manifest with atypical or persistent ulcers. There appears to be an increased risk for reactivation of genital herpes as CD4+ cell counts decrease,[98,100] including of previously asymptomatic disease. All genital tract ulcers that appear during pregnancy, even in women with no prior history of herpes, need to be evaluated for the possibility of herpes simplex virus.

No specific laboratory screening for HPV is currently indicated for all HIV-infected women. However, because HIV-infected women are at increased risk for cervical disease associated with HPV,[103–108] and because HIV-infected women have a higher prevalence of abnormal Pap smears and cervical dysplasia, all women should have Pap smears performed early in pregnancy. Although there is no evidence that pregnancy affects the occurrence or progression of cervical lesions, if abnormalities in Pap smear are noted during pregnancy, appropriate evaluation and Pap smears should be repeated during pregnancy as indicated.

Coinfection with both hepatitis B and hepatitis C is frequent. In particular, rates of coinfection with hepatitis C of 30% to 50% have been documented in HIV-infected adults. Coinfection with hepatitis C has been associated with significant morbidity, including more severe liver disease, cirrhosis, and higher rates of mortality in HIV-infected adults.[109,110] Hepatotoxicity of HIV-associated medications may be of particular concern with the coexistence of chronic hepatitis. In addition, several studies have now documented greater rates for vertical transmission of both HIV and hepatitis C virus in coinfected pregnant women. Rates for vertical transmission of HIV are higher in women who are coinfected with hepatitis C,[111] and rates for hepatitis C transmission are increased in particular with concomitant HIV infection of the infant.[112] Unless their status is already known, all women should have screening for hepatitis B with hepatitis B surface antigen testing and for hepatitis C by hepatitis C antibody. If screens are positive, or in cases of known positivity, liver function tests should be performed. In the case of positive hepatitis C antibody, hepatitis C RNA-PCR should be done.

Assessments for infection with *Chlamydia trachomatis*, *Neisseria gonorrhea*, or trichomonas and bacterial vaginosis should be performed on all patients. It is not clear whether women with previous knowledge of their HIV infection have increased prevalence of these sexually transmitted diseases. Early studies demonstrated that all four infections are seen in similar to increased rates in HIV-infected women as compared with other women attending gynecologic and obstetric clinics.[37,99,113] Recent observations have suggested that after diagnosis of HIV infection, women are more likely to have protected intercourse in general and that sexually transmitted diseases such as chlamydial infection and gonorrhea are less prevalent.[95,114] Any diagnosed infection should be treated. Treatment is indicated to prevent complications for the infant of chlamydial and gonococcal disease. Although treatment of trichomonas and bacterial vaginosis in routine obstetric populations has not been shown to decrease the risk for adverse outcome of pregnancy, treatment in women with bacterial vaginosis who are also at increased risk for adverse pregnancy outcomes has been shown to improve the outcome of the index pregnancy.[115]

All women should have an early ultrasonogram to establish the integrity of the pregnancy early in the course of obstetric care, in particular prior to making pregnancy-specific HIV management decisions. In addition, prior to starting ART in women who are therapy naive, there should be some assurance of normal fetal development up to that point in gestation.

HIV-infected pregnant women should receive all immunizations routinely recommended for HIV-infected adults. All HIV-infected pregnant women should receive appropriate influenza vaccine, and newly diagnosed women should receive pneumococcal vaccine and *Haemophilus influenzae* type B vaccine. In addition, hepatitis B–negative women should receive hepatitis B vaccine.

ANTIRETROVIRAL THERAPY

For many women, the recommendation to initiate antiretroviral therapy for the first time is made during pregnancy. For HIV-infected adults in general, decisions about recommending initiation of therapy are individualized according to symptoms, baseline viral load, and CD4+ count.[86] Currently, there are no absolute recommendations for the use of antiretroviral therapy. Rather, the decision to recommend and initiate antiretroviral therapy in adults takes into account the strength of data available by which to judge the impact of therapy on prevention of morbidity, progression of disease, and occurrence of death as well as the potential for antiretroviral toxicities and viral resistance with long-term use of ART. For some adults comparatively early in the course of illness, clinical trials have demonstrated no clear-cut clinical benefits to initiation of antiretroviral therapy. In these instances, delaying therapy may not only prevent medication-related side effects and morbidities but also preserve options for antiretroviral therapy in the future as it becomes more crucial to long-term outcome. During pregnancy, however, the use of antiretroviral agents should be recommended to all HIV-infected women for the substantial benefit of decreasing vertical transmission.

When to Begin Treatment

In general, prior to starting ART, recommendations for the long-term use of ART specific to health outcome should be made, and the woman should decide whether she will begin ART during pregnancy that will be continued postpartum for her own health. Long-term ART is typically recommended for all HIV-infected adults who are symptomatic and for those with CD4+ cell counts of less than 200 cells/mm or viral loads of greater than 50,000 to 100,000 copies/mL.[86] Some clinicians and guidelines use a CD4+ cell count of less than 350 cells/mm to initiate therapy or a high rate of CD4+ cell decline, i.e., greater than 100 cells/mm per year.[86,116] When ART is begun for maternal health, the use of HAART, including a minimum of three antiretroviral agents, should always be recommended, because HAART has been associated with long-term beneficial response and delayed or lesser development of viral resistance compared with less intense therapy. If antiretroviral therapy is to be used primarily for prevention of vertical infection, according to current guidelines, in select cases of very low or nondetectable viral loads, monotherapy with zidovudine can be utilized.

The choice of antiretroviral agents to be used during pregnancy should be similar to the choice in nonpregnant adults. The relative efficacy and toxicity of most combination regimens, including those containing protease inhibitors, non-nucleoside reverse transcriptase inhibitors (NNRTI), and multiple nucleoside reverse transcriptase inhibitors (NRTI), during pregnancy is currently unknown. As part of combination therapy, however, if not precluded by history of toxicity, zidovudine should be included because of the large body of data indicating its efficacy in preventing vertical transmission.

Issue of Fetal Toxicities

To date, there have been no congenital syndromes or specific fetal malformations associated with the use of antiretroviral therapy during the first trimester of pregnancy. Therefore, if an HIV-infected woman enters into pregnancy on antiretroviral therapy, discontinuation of ART during pregnancy is not generally recommended. In addition, women who are initiating antiretroviral therapy for maternal health reasons should consider starting therapy immediately during pregnancy, including during the first trimester. Two specific antiretroviral agents should be avoided during pregnancy, in particular during the first trimester. Efavirenz and hydroxyurea have both been associated with teratogenic effects in animals. Efavirenz has been associated with teratogenic effects including anencephaly anophthalmia and microphthalmia in rhesus monkeys at drug levels similar to those seen in humans. Hydroxyurea has been demonstrated to have potent teratogenic effects in multiple animal species.[117–120] Women who are receiving either drug as part of HAART should be advised to discontinue its use when pregnancy occurs or if pregnancy is planned; alternative regimens should be prescribed.

If the nausea and vomiting of early pregnancy prevent adherence to appropriate ART dosing, new ART should not be initiated and prior ART should be stopped to prevent the occurrence of viral resistance, which is enhanced by intermittent medication administration. When vomiting has ceased to be a problem or is adequately treated, ART should then be reinitiated.

Goals of Therapy

The goal for ART during pregnancy is to achieve a nondetectable viral load. If a woman on ART has a nondetectable viral load at the first prenatal visit, viral load assessment should be repeated every trimester, at a minimum. If ART is being initiated or changed in the presence of a detectable viral load, repeat viral load measurements should be timed according to ART management, as described for nonpregnant adults, to assess the virologic response.[86] In most cases, viral load becomes undetectable by 16 to 20 weeks after initiation of therapy. Failure of viral load to decrease, or an increase in viral load despite therapy, may be due to viral resistance or subtherapeutic medication levels either because of alterations in pharmacokinetics during pregnancy or lack of adherence to ART regimens. The presence of viral resistance should be assessed and the ART regimen changed as necessary to achieve virologic suppression. In cases in which medication intolerance or social circumstances make adherence to medication regimens impossible, hospitalization for directly observed therapy and treatment of side effects has been shown to be a strategy that can be employed to achieve an optimal decrease in viral load.

Maternal Toxicities

Monitoring for routinely described toxicities of antiretroviral therapy should take place during pregnancy. Many NRTIs have been associated with bone marrow suppression and hepatotoxicity. The use of zidovudine during pregnancy has been associated with anemia.[9] Complete blood cell counts, including platelet counts and liver function tests, should be followed throughout pregnancy in women receiving ART. In addition, the obstetric care provider should be aware of some special considerations in the use of ART during pregnancy.

Nucleoside reverse transcriptase inhibitors have been associated with the occurrence of lactic acidosis and hepatic steatosis in adults.[121–123] The mechanism of this relatively rare but potentially fatal syndrome may be related to mitochondrial toxicity and dysfunction.[124] Although all NRTIs have been implicated with the occurrence of this toxicity, d4T (stavudine) is the NRTI that has been most strongly associated with lactic acidosis.[125–127] There have been reports of the lactic acidosis syndrome occurring during the third trimester of pregnancy, with maternal death occurring during pregnancy or postpartum in women who were receiving the combination of d4T and ddI (didanosine) along with other antiretroviral agents during pregnancy.[128,129] Some cases were also complicated by fetal death. Initial reports were in women who were on the combination of these two agents prior to and during the entire pregnancy. It is not known whether pregnancy enhances the occurrence or severity of this potential complication of NRTI use. Initial manifestations of the lactic acidosis syndrome may include nonspecific gastrointestinal symptoms, including nausea, vomiting, diarrhea, anorexia, and abdominal pain, plus malaise and weakness. The syndrome also includes hepatomegaly, liver dysfunction, metabolic acidosis, respiratory distress, and death. Laboratory abnormalities may include elevated lactic acid levels, anion gap, elevated transaminases, and increases in amylase, lipase, creatine phosphokinase, and lactate dehydrogenase. Discontinuation of antiretroviral therapy has resulted in resolution of the syndrome.[123,125] There needs to be a high degree of suspicion for this syndrome in pregnant women receiving NRTIs. Third-trimester toxicity monitoring should include liver function tests and electrolyte measurements. Early, nonspecific symptoms should prompt evaluation, including liver function tests and amylase, electrolytes, and blood lactate levels, and discontinuation of potential offending agents as necessary. The use of the combination of d4T and ddI during pregnancy should be avoided whenever possible.

Protease inhibitor therapy has been associated with hyperglycemia in adults, including worsening of preexisting diabetes and new onset of glucose intolerance.[130–133] It is not known whether pregnancy-induced diabetes occurs with greater frequency in women who are receiving protease inhibitors during pregnancy. Because of this potential, women who are receiving protease inhibitors should be screened for diabetes early during pregnancy and should have repeat screening during the pregnancy, and serum glucose levels should be obtained whenever glucosuria or symptoms of diabetes are newly noted. In general, protease inhibitor therapy that is successfully controlling viral load should not be discontinued because of hyperglycemia. In the case of either newly diagnosed or preexisting diabetes, blood sugar levels should be closely monitored and therapy adjusted accordingly.

Nevirapine is the NNRTI used most frequently during pregnancy. Severe and, in some cases, fatal hepatotoxicity has been reported to occur in adults receiving nevirapine as part of combination antiretroviral therapy used either for treatment of HIV infection or for postexposure prophylaxis.[134–137] It is not known whether hepatotoxicity is enhanced due to pregnancy. Women begun on nevirapine during pregnancy should have liver function monitored frequently and also at the occurrence of any nonspecific or specific symptoms possibly related to hepatotoxicity.

Pediatric Toxicities

Animal data have shown the midlife occurrence of squamous cell tumors of the vagina, lung, skin, and liver in rats exposed to zidovudine in utero. Human reports have thus far failed to demonstrate congenital abnormalities or toxicities in infants who were exposed to zidovudine in utero and observed through early childhood.[137–139] In addition, French researchers have reported eight cases of a mitochondrial syndrome, including neurologic manifestations and pancreatitis, five of which were associated with death, occurring in infants who had in utero exposure to either zidovudine monotherapy or to the combination of zidovudine and 3TC (lamivudine).[140] An analysis of more than 20,000 pregnancies followed in U.S. cohorts failed to show any deaths due to mitochondrial syndrome.[141] Although no definitive long-term toxicities of in utero exposure have been determined, in utero exposure to antiretroviral therapy needs to become a permanent part of the infant medical record so that symptomatology can be assessed accordingly and, if delayed toxicities are discovered, infants can be appropriately screened.

Management of Opportunistic Infections and HIV-Related Conditions

There are no data to suggest that HIV-infected women are at any greater risk from or have any different presentation of opportunistic infections during pregnancy. Nonetheless, it should be recognized that AIDS-associated conditions can occur during pregnancy, and all diagnostic tests are performed as necessary. In addition, other conditions at increased prevalence in HIV-infected women need to considered. Prophylaxis against and treatment for opportunistic and other infections should be provided for HIV-infected pregnant women.[142]

Indications for therapy of cytomegalovirus disease are the same during pregnancy as in nonpregnant adults. However, ganciclovir and foscarnet have been found to be embryotoxic and teratogenic in animal modes, and their use during pregnancy has been very limited.[143] In non-HIV-infected women, the occurrence of in utero infection with cytomegalovirus is approximately 1% to 2%. The risk for infection and the severity of disease sequelae are much higher in cases in which primary maternal infection occurs during pregnancy. The risk for transmission to the fetus is increased among HIV-infected pregnant women and has been reported to be 4.5%.[144] Cases of symptomatic, congenital cytomegalovirus infection have been reported in infants born to HIV-infected women who are seropositive prior to pregnancy.[92] However, the risk of this occurrence is thought to be low and probably is much less than in the case of primary infection occurring during pregnancy.

Case reports have documented the occurrence of in utero transmission of toxoplasmosis with reactivation of preexisting, chronic disease in HIV-infected pregnant women.[87,145] Nonetheless, the risk of in utero transmission in women who are seropositive is low.[88,89] Therefore, routine fetal evaluation is not warranted in these women. However, if findings suggestive of in utero toxoplasmosis are found on routine ultrasonographic examination, such as hydrocephalus, intracerebral calcifications, or unexplained growth retardation, the fetus and pregnancy should be assessed regardless of maternal serostatus. In the case of symptomatic reactivation of toxoplasmosis during pregnancy, ultrasonography of the fetus looking for signs of toxoplasmosis should be performed, and pediatricians should be notified to assess the infant for congenital toxoplasmosis upon birth.

Treatment of active tuberculosis during pregnancy should be the same as for a nonpregnant adult, although the experience during pregnancy with most second-line drugs used to treat drug-resistant tuberculosis is limited. There is evidence that isoniazid-associated hepatotoxicity may occur more frequently and be more severe during pregnancy.[146] Therefore, when isoniazid is used either as a sole agent for newly diagnosed positive tuberculin test or as part of multidrug regimen for treatment of active tuberculosis, liver function tests should be checked on a regular basis during pregnancy. Fluoroquinolones have been noted to cause arthropathy in immature animals, and their use is not routinely recommended during pregnancy. They should be used in the treatment of drug-resistant tuberculosis only when necessary. Streptomycin has been associated with eighth nerve toxicity in infants who are exposed in utero, so its use should also be avoided when possible.

Women who are HIV infected have greater rates of lower genital tract colonization with *Candida* as well as higher rates of symptomatic candidiasis during pregnancy.[147] There is no evidence that colonization needs to be treated. Symptomatic disease can be treated using either topical antifungal medications or fluconazole. Recurrent symptomatic candidiasis can be successfully prevented using fluconazole; however, in the lack of other invasive candidal infections, local suppressive therapy may be a more reasonable option. Women who are receiving chronic fluconazole either for suppression of vulvovaginal candidiasis or for the treatment or prevention of esophageal or systemic candidiasis should have liver function tests during pregnancy.

Primary herpes during pregnancy or severe manifestations of recurrent disease should be treated with acyclovir. In addition, frequent recurrences of genital herpes may warrant suppressive therapy. Because of the relatively large experience with use during pregnancy, acyclovir is preferred to valacyclovir or famciclovir. In non-HIV-infected pregnant women, there is evidence that the use of suppressive acyclovir late in pregnancy can prevent lesions of genital herpes and thus reduce the need for cesarean delivery for prevention of transmission to the neonate.[148,149] Although efficacy in

HIV-infected women has not been tested, a similar strategy may be used.

Genital warts have been described to undergo increased growth during pregnancy in non-HIV-infected women. The influence of pregnancy on genital warts in HIV-infected women is not known. It is not necessary to treat genital warts during pregnancy, but if treatment is indicated during pregnancy because of symptoms or large size, genital warts should be treated with bichloracetic and trichloracetic acid as well as ablative therapies, including excision. Podophyllin should not be used during pregnancy, because podophyllin use has been associated with an increased risk of fetal death in animals as well as the potential for neurotoxicity.

Chronic hepatitis B and chronic hepatitis C infection are usually not treated during pregnancy, because the safety of therapies for chronic hepatitis during pregnancy is not well established. There is no good evidence that pregnancy exacerbates activity of chronic hepatitis. However, an increase in hepatitis C RNA-PCR levels during the third trimester of pregnancy has been reported. In HIV-infected women, as in other women, risk for vertical transmission of hepatitis C virus is associated with hepatitis C viral load.[112,150] Therefore, hepatitis C RNA-PCR levels should be repeated during the third trimester to assist in determining the risk for vertical transmission of hepatitis C.

During pregnancy, active management of conditions associated with increased risk for transmission should be considered. HIV-infected women should be urged to stop smoking and offered both behavior modification and pharmacologic intervention to assist with smoking cessation. Sexually transmitted diseases, including gonorrhea, chlamydia trachomatis, trichomonas, and bacterial vaginosis should be treated. Although all women who are abusing illicit drugs during pregnancy should be entered into drug treatment programs, in addition to methadone maintenance, withdrawal from drugs should be considered an option as possible.

OBSTETRIC MANAGEMENT

Amniocentesis and Other Antepartum Invasive Procedures

The invasive procedure most commonly performed during pregnancy prior to parturition is amniocentesis. Typical reasons for performing amniocentesis include prenatal diagnosis, determination of fetal lung maturity, diagnosis of intra-amniotic infection, and evaluation of potential isoimmunization, fetal hydrops, or fetal infection of nonbacterial origin. Amniocentesis performed for prenatal diagnosis is most often performed at 15 to 20 weeks of gestation. Amniocentesis to determine fetal lung maturity or intra-amniotic infection is more typically done during the third trimester. For evaluation of isoimmunization, hydrops, or fetal infection, amniocenteses may be performed any time after approximately 20 weeks of gestation and may be performed only once or on multiple occasions.

There is a theoretical possibility that amniocentesis could cause transmission of HIV from an infected woman to the fetus. This could occur by directly inoculating maternal blood from the needle tip into the fetus; however, amniocentesis is performed under ultrasonographic guidance and it is not common for fetal injury to occur. Of greater concern is the possibility that HIV in the maternal bloodstream could be carried into the amniotic fluid via the needle or if subclinical bleeding in the placenta or membrane-placenta interface occurs due to needle puncture. Infected amniotic fluid could then infect the fetus as it is swallowed or as it bathes mucous membranes.

There are few data by which to judge the actual risk for fetal HIV infection through amniocentesis. Towers and associates[151] reported seven HIV-infected women receiving no antiretroviral therapy who underwent a total of 10 amniocentesis procedures with no sequelae of fetal infection. However, both Mandelbrot and colleagues[152] and Tess and colleagues[153] did find associations between amniocentesis and perinatally transmitted HIV infection. Mandelbrot did not examine amniocentesis specifically but found a rate for perinatal HIV infection of 36% among neonates whose mothers underwent either amniocentesis or amnioscopy, a procedure involving a larger gauge needle, at some time during pregnancy. In a multivariate analysis of risk factors for perinatal transmission, invasive procedures (amniocentesis plus four other procedures) were associated with a statistically significant increase in transmission (RR, 2.08 [1.02–4.25]). In a multivariate logistic regression analysis of risk factors for perinatal transmission among 434 infants born to

HIV-infected women, Tess found that third-trimester amniocentesis was associated with a significantly increased risk for transmission (OR, 4.1; 95% CI, 1.2–13.5). The vast majority of women in both the Mandelbrot and the Tess study were not receiving antiretroviral agents. Conclusions that can be drawn from both studies are limited by lack of information concerning the timing of and indications for amniocentesis and by lack of information concerning maternal viral load. It is likely that the risk for perinatal HIV transmission associated with performing amniocentesis is intimately associated with maternal peripheral blood viral load at the time of the procedure as well as maternal antiretroviral therapy. With low viral load, transmission risk is also probably quite low.

It is prudent to avoid performing amniocentesis in HIV-infected women whenever possible. In some instances, however, amniocentesis may be uniquely beneficial, as in the indication of prenatal diagnosis or management of isoimmunization or hydrops. When undergoing amniocentesis, women should be counseled about the potential risk for transmission. If the need for amniocentesis is anticipated, efforts should be made to minimize viral load prior to the procedure.

The risk of perinatal HIV transmission associated with other antepartum procedures, including chorionic villus sampling, cervical cerclage, and external cephalic version, are unknown. There are no data by which to judge the efficacy in prevention of transmission of intravenous zidovudine or single-dose nevirapine at the time of procedures.

Antepartum Fetal Assessment

Although no specific teratogenesis has been described for the use of any antiretroviral agent or combination of agents, a second-trimester ultrasonographic screen for fetal structural development should be performed on all women who have received antiretroviral therapy in the first half of pregnancy. In addition, third-trimester antepartum assessment of fetal well-being is indicated for most pregnancies in HIV-infected women. This is both because of concerns relevant to the possibility of adverse outcome of pregnancy due to HIV infection and because the impact on placental function and fetal well-being is not known for most antiretroviral agents. Such assessment includes ultrasonograms obtained every 4 to 6 weeks for amniotic fluid volume and fetal growth and weekly nonstress tests or biophysical profiles after 32 weeks of gestation. Interpretation and management of these tests should be identical to interpretation and management in non-HIV-infected women.

Labor and Delivery Management: Cesarean Section

Data from two prospective cohort studies, a large 15-study meta-analysis, and a controlled clinical trial of elective cesarean section, are consistent and show that women who receive no ART or zidovudine monotherapy have a significant decrease in vertical transmission with elective cesarean section as compared with other routes of delivery.[154–157] Elective cesarean section is defined as cesarean section performed prior to the onset of labor or ruptured membranes; other routes of delivery include vaginal delivery and nonelective cesarean section. The risk for vertical HIV transmission in women receiving zidovudine for the prevention of transmission plus elective cesarean section has been shown by two studies to be approximately 2%.[154,155] In addition, the use of elective cesarean section to prevent vertical HIV transmission has been demonstrated to be cost effective in three separate analyses.[158–160] The efficacy of elective cesarean section to achieve further reductions in vertical HIV transmission among women receiving combination ART or among women with undetectable viral loads, who already have a low rate of transmission, is unknown but is thought to be of no to minimal benefit.

The American College of Obstetricians and Gynecologists has recommended that mode of delivery be discussed with all HIV-infected pregnant women, including the potential advantages of elective cesarean section in prevention of vertical transmission among subgroups of pregnant women.[161] Cesarean section is associated with greater risks for maternal complications than is vaginal delivery, however, including both infectious complications and the need for blood transfusions.[73,162–165]

It is probable that HIV-infected pregnant women, in particular those with the lowest CD4+ cell counts, have an increased risk for peripartum obstetric bacterial infections. The incidence of both histologic and clinical chorioamnionitis appears to be high and increased over that seen in HIV-negative women.[28,162,166,167] Ladner has suggested that there is no increase in the rate of chorioamnionitis if lower genital tract infections, in particular sexually transmitted diseases, are controlled during pregnancy.[60] In addition, an increased rate of postpartum infectious complications, including fever, endometritis, wound infection, and sepsis, has been observed.[73,162–164]

In a large cohort of HIV-infected women, Read and colleagues[165] demonstrated a 15% rate for postpartum morbidity among women undergoing cesarean delivery. A significant increase in fever, urinary tract infection, and combined morbidities was seen in women undergoing elective cesarean section. A significant increase in endometritis was seen in association with nonelective cesarean section. Similarly, Watts and associates[166] found higher rates for endometritis, wound infection, and risk for transfusion among HIV-infected women undergoing cesarean section compared with those undergoing vaginal delivery. The association between stage of maternal HIV infection and occurrence of postpartum complications is not clear. Semprini[163] suggested that postpartum complications were increased with immunosuppression, and Read and associates[165] found a decreased risk for postpartum complications with lower HIV-RNA-PCR levels. However, in a population of women receiving ART during pregnancy, no clear association between immunologic stage of disease and postpartum complications was seen.[166]

Currently, elective cesarean section is recommended as the route of delivery that minimizes vertical transmission of HIV among HIV-infected women who are receiving no antiretroviral therapy or monotherapy during pregnancy and among HIV-infected women who have a detectable peripheral viral load. Because of concerns for maternal complications, elective cesarean section is not routinely recommended as a means to decrease vertical transmission of HIV for women who are receiving combination ART and have viral loads of less than 1000 copies/mL.

A viral titer should be obtained at 34 to 36 weeks of gestation to assist in decision making about route of delivery. If elective cesarean section is planned, it should be scheduled for 38 weeks of gestation to avoid the onset of labor in most women. Appropriate antiretroviral therapy, including at least 3 hours of intravenous zidovudine, should be administered prior to the cesarean section. Because of the risk for postpartum complications, the use of perioperative antimicrobial prophylaxis should be considered. If labor or ruptured membranes occurs prior to the time of scheduled cesarean section, the potential advantages to cesarean section in decreasing transmission are lost, and vaginal delivery may be considered.

There are special considerations for labor management in HIV-infected women who are undergoing vaginal delivery. Multiple cohort studies of HIV-infected pregnant women have demonstrated increased risk for vertical transmission of HIV with increasing duration of ruptured membranes.[20,25,168,169] However, these studies did not control for maternal viral load and were among women on no antiretrovirals or monotherapy. It has been assumed that the increase in transmission seen with increased duration of ruptured membranes is due in part to contact with virus in the lower genital tract. In addition, early observations suggested that vertical transmission might be increased with invasive peripartum procedures that increased the possibilities of contact with maternal blood, including the use of fetal scalp electrode.[170] Whether there is additive risk for transmission due to increased duration of ruptured membranes or invasive obstetric procedures among women on HAART and among those with very low viral loads has not been determined. However, the risk for shedding of lower genital tract virus in these women is decreased, and the overall risk for vertical transmission of HIV is quite low. Nevertheless, routine artificial rupture of membranes and use of fetal scalp electrodes should be avoided in HIV-infected pregnant women during labor. If spontaneous rupture of membranes occurs, active management of labor to achieve expeditious vaginal delivery may be considered. In very circumscribed conditions, cesarean section may be performed in cases in which very long duration of ruptured membranes is anticipated. Because of concerns for increased rates of amnionitis in addition to postpartum complications, the use of peripartum antibiotics may be considered, in particular for women who are at high risk for bacterial infection due to immunosuppression. If maternal fever occurs, broad-spectrum antibiotics should always be initiated.

If preterm labor or premature rupture of the membranes in a preterm gestation occur, management should be initiated that would be appropriate for any pregnant woman. In general, considerations of potential prematurity for the fetus should dictate management.

Peripartum Antiretroviral Therapy

Antepartum antiretroviral therapy should be continued throughout the course of labor and delivery. Intravenous zidovudine should be administered according to the regimen studied during PACTG study 076. It should be initiated at the onset of labor or at the time of ruptured membranes. In the case of preterm labor or preterm premature rupture of membranes, intravenous zidovudine should be administered for the time period during which there is a possibility of delivery. Zidovudine and d4T should not be administered together because of potential pharmacologic antagonism, so options for women receiving oral d4T as part of their antenatal therapy include continuation of oral d4T during labor without intravenous zidovudine, or withholding of the oral d4T during the period of intravenous administration during labor.

Screening for HIV Infection at the Time of Labor or Postpartum

There is evidence that rates for prenatal screening for HIV infection have increased markedly since initial U.S. Public Health Service recommendations for counseling and testing of pregnant women.[171] However, experience with mandatory newborn screening in New York State suggests that substantial numbers of HIV-infected women are not aware of their status during pregnancy.[172] Women may not be tested because they do not recognize themselves to be at risk for infection or because of an incomplete approach to screening on the part of the health care provider. In addition, women at the highest risk for being HIV infected because of personal habits involving drug use may not be identified because of refusal to be tested or because of poor or no prenatal care.[173–175]

Some experts advocate HIV screening for women whose status is not known at the time of presentation for delivery. McNeeley demonstrated that 30% of all infected infants were born to women whose HIV status was not known at the time of birth, suggesting that testing during labor could potentially decrease perinatal HIV infection because of the ability to provide postexposure prophylaxis to the neonate.[176] Grobman[177] suggested that such an approach could be cost-saving both because of the decrease in pediatric HIV disease and because of improved outcome for women who might thus be diagnosed earlier in the course of the disease. Webber[178] demonstrated an 85% acceptance rate for HIV testing during labor. Feasibility of screening during labor or immediately postpartum is dependent on rapid availability of results plus the ability to deliver appropriate care to HIV-positive women and at-risk infants identified through this approach.[179]

Breastfeeding

HIV can be transmitted to an uninfected infant through breastfeeding. Although the exact risk for transmission through breastfeeding is not known, current estimates are approximately 15%.[180,181] Infection can be transmitted at all times of postnatal life, although increased frequency of transmission with colostrum and during the first few weeks of life has been suggested.[182] Factors that increase risk for transmission through breastfeeding include mastitis and bleeding nipples. In industrialized countries, where risks for major infant morbidity from infectious illnesses are small, avoidance of all breastfeeding among HIV-infected women is recommended and is the norm. In developing countries, the risk of infant morbidity and mortality from infection, in particular diarrheal diseases, is high and can be decreased through breastfeeding. Therefore, HIV-infected women routinely breastfeed their infants. The relative impact of transmission of HIV through breastfeeding and morbidity and mortality due to other infections in formula-fed infants in developing countries is not known. However, recent studies have suggested that mixed feeding, intermittently using both breastfeeding and formula-feeding, is associated with a very high risk for transmission of HIV and should not be supported.[183]

Postpartum Management

Postpartum, HIV-infected pregnant women should be provided with necessary prescriptions to continue HIV-specific therapies, including antiretroviral agents as appropriate. Observations have suggested that women who are HIV infected are at risk for high rates of noncompliance with their own health care and with the use of HIV-specific therapies, including antiretroviral therapy, postpartum. Appropriate liaisons with HIV health care professionals should be made during pregnancy and facilitated during the postpartum period by obstetric care providers. In conjunction with HIV care providers, all postpartum women should be provided with adequate reproduction counseling and contraception as desired.

REFERENCES

1. Mofenson LM: Mother-child HIV-1 transmission. Obstet Gynecol Clin 1997;24:750–784.
2. Mofenson LM, Lambert JS, Stiehm ER, et al: Risk factors for perinatal transmission of human immunodeficiency virus type 1 in women treated with zidovudine. N Engl J Med 1999;34:385–393.
3. Garcia PM, Kalish LA, Pitt J, et al: Maternal levels of plasma human immunodeficiency virus type 1 RNA and the risk of perinatal transmission. N Engl J Med 1999;34:394–402.
4. Cooper ER, Charurat M, Mofenson L, et al: Combination antiretroviral strategies for the treatment of pregnant HIV-1 infected women and prevention of perinatal HIV-1 transmission. J Acquir Immun Defic Syndr 2002;29:484–494.
5. Mandelbrot L, Landreau-Mascaro A, Rekacewicz C, et al: Lamivudine-zidovudine combination for prevention of maternal-infant transmission of HIV-1. JAMA 2001;285:2083–2093.
6. McGowan JP, Crane M, Wiznia AA, Blum S: Combination antiretroviral therapy in human immunodeficiency virus-infected pregnant women. Obstet Gynecol 1999;94:641–646.
7. Mayaux MJ, Dussaix E, Isopet J, et al: Maternal virus load during pregnancy and the mother-to-child transmission of human immunodeficiency virus type 1: the French Perinatal Cohort Studies. J Infect Dis 1997;175:172–175.
8. The European Collaborative Study: Maternal viral load and vertical transmission of HIV-1: An important factor but not the only one. AIDS 1999; 13:1377–1385.
9. Connor EM, Sperling RS, Gelber R, et al: Reduction of maternal-infant transmission of human immunodeficiency virus type 1 with zidovudine treatment. N Engl J Med 1994;331:1173–1180.
10. Cooper ER, Nugent RP, Diaz C, et al: After AIDS Clinical Trial 076: The changing pattern of zidovudine use during pregnancy, and the subsequent reduction in vertical transmission of human immunodeficiency virus in a cohort of infected women and their infants. J Infect Dis 1996;174:1207–1211.
11. Fiscus SA, Adimora AA, Schoenbach VJ, et al: Perinatal HIV infection and the effect of zidovudine therapy on transmission in rural and urban counties. JAMA 1996;275:1483–1488.
12. Wade NA, Birkhead GS, Warren BL, et al: Abbreviated regimens of zidovudine prophylaxis and perinatal transmission of the human immunodeficiency virus. N Engl J Med 1998;339:1409–1414.
13. Shaffer N, Chauchoowong R, Mock PA, et al: Sort-course zidovudine for perinatal HIV-1 transmission in Bangkok, Thailand: A randomized controlled trial. Lancet 1999;353:773–780.
14. Lallemant M, Jourdain G, Kim S, et al: A trial of shortened zidovudine regimens to prevent mother-to-child transmission of human immunodeficiency virus type 1. N Engl J Med 2000;343:982–991.
15. Dabis F, Msellati P, Meda N, et al: 6-month efficacy, tolerance, and acceptability of a short regimen of oral zidovudine to reduce vertical transmission of HIV in breastfed children in Cote d'Ivoire and Burkina Faso: A double-blind placebo-controlled multicentre trial. Lancet 1999;353:786–792.
16. Guay LA, Musoke P, Fleming T, et al: Intrapartum and neonatal single-dose nevirapine compared with zidovudine for prevention of mother-to-child transmission of HIV-1 in Kampala, Uganda: HIVNET 012 randomized trial. Lancet 1999;354:795–802.
17. Saba J, on behalf of the PETRA Trial Study Team: Interim analysis of early efficacy of three short ZDV/3TC combination regimens to prevent mother-to-child transmission of HIV-1: The PETRA trial (abstract S-7). Paper presented at the Sixth Conference on Retroviruses and Opportunistic infections, Chicago, Illinois, January 1999.
18. Melvin AJ, Burchett SK, Watts DH, et al: Effect of pregnancy and zidovudine therapy on viral load in HIV-1 infected women. J Acquir Immune Defic Syndr Hum Retrovirol 1997;14:232–236.
19. Shapiro DE, Sperling RS, Coombs RW: Effect of zidovudine on perinatal HIV-1 transmission and maternal viral load. Lancet 1999;354:156.
20. Burns DN, Landesman S, Muenz LR, et al: Cigarette smoking, premature rupture of membranes and vertical transmission of HIV-1 among women with low CD4+ levels. J Acquir Immune Defic Syndr Hum Retrovirol 1994;7:718–726.
21. Turner BJ, Hauck WW, Fanning R, Markson LE: Cigarette smoking and mother-child HIV transmission. J Acquir Immune Defic Syndr Hum Retrovirol 1997;14:327–337.
22. Rodriquez EM, Mofenson LM, Chang B-H, et al: Association of maternal drug use during pregnancy with maternal HIV culture positivity and perinatal HIV transmission. AIDS 1996;10:273–282.
23. Bulterys M, Landesman S, Burns DN, et al: Sexual behavior and injection drug use during pregnancy and vertical transmission of HIV-1. J Acquir Immune Defic Syndr Hum Retrovirol 1997; 15:76–82.
24. Matheson PB, Thomas PA, Abrams EJ, et al: Heterosexual behavior during pregnancy and perinatal transmission of HIV-1. AIDS 1996;10:1249–1256.

25. Landesman SH, Kalish LA, Burns DN, et al: Obstetrical factors and the transmission of human immunodeficiency virus type 1 from mother to child. N Engl J Med 1996;334:1617–1623.
26. Ryder RW, Nsa W, Hassig SE, et al: Perinatal transmission of the human immunodeficiency virus type 1 to infants of seropositive women in Zaire. N Engl J Med 1989;320:1637–1642.
27. Newell ML, Dunn DT, Peckham CS, et al: Vertical transmission of HIV-1: Maternal immune status and obstetric factors. The European Collaborative Study. AIDS 1996;10:1675–1681.
28. St. Louis ME, Kamenga M, Brown C, et al: Risk for perinatal HIV-1 transmission according to maternal immunologic, virologic, and placental factors. JAMA 1993;269:2853–2859.
29. Deschamps MM, Pape JW, Desvarieux M, et al: A prospective study of HIV-seropositive asymptomatic women of childbearing age in a developing country. J Acquir Immune Defic Syndr Hum Retrovir 1993;6:446–451.
30. Berrebi A, Kobuch WE, Puel J, et al: Influence of pregnancy on human immunodeficiency virus disease. Eur J Obstet Gynecol 1990;37:211–217.
31. Saada M, LeChenadec J, Berrebi A, et al: Pregnancy and progression to AIDS: Results of the French prospective cohorts. AIDS 2000;14:2355–2360.
32. Weisser M, Rudin C, Battegay M, et al: Does pregnancy influence the course of HIV infection? Evidence from two large Swiss cohort studies. J Acquir Immune Defic Syndr Hum Retrovir 1998;117:404–410.
33. Alliegro MB, Dorrucci MD, Phillips AN, et al: Incidence and consequences of pregnancy in women with known duration of HIV infection. Arch Int Med 1997;157:2585–2590.
34. Cozzi Lepri A, Pezzotti P, Dorrucci M, et al: HIV disease progression in 854 women and men infected through injecting drug use and heterosexual sex and followed for up to nine years from seroconversion. Italian Seroconversion Study. BMJ 1994;309:1537–1542.
35. Turner BJ, Markson LE, McKee LJ, et al: Health care delivery, zidovudine use, and survival of women and men with AIDS. J Acquir Immune Defic Syndr Hum Retrovir 1994;7:1250–1262.
36. Bastian L, Bennett CL, Adams J, et al: Differences between men and women with HIV-related *Pneumocystis carinii* pneumonia: Experience from 3,070 cases in New York City in 1987. J Acquir Immune Defic Syndr Hum Retrovir 1993;6:617–623.
37. Cu-Uvin S, Flanigan TP, Rich JD, et al: Human immunodeficiency virus infection and acquired immunodeficiency syndrome among North American women. Am J Med 1996;101:316–322.
38. Pitkin RM, Witte DL: Platelet and leukocyte counts in pregnancy. JAMA 1979;242:2696–2698.
39. Valdimarsson H, Mulholland C, Fridriksdottir V, Coleman DV: A longitudinal study of leucocyte blood counts and lymphocyte response in pregnancy: A marked early increase of monocyte-lymphocyte ratios. Clin Exp Immunol 1983;53:437–443.
40. Brettle RP, Raab GM, Ross A, et al: HIV infection in women: Immunological markers and the influence of pregnancy. AIDS 1998;9:1177–1184.
41. Biggar RJ, Pahwa S, Minkoff H, et al: Immunosuppression in pregnant women infected with human immunodeficiency virus. Am J Obstet Gynecol 1989;161:1239–1244.
42. Tuomala RE, Kalish LA, Zorilla C, et al: Changes in total, CD4+, and CD8+ lymphocytes during pregnancy and 1 year postpartum in human immunodeficiency virus-infected women. The Women and Infants Transmission Study. Obstet Gynecol 1997;89:967–974.
43. Miotti PG, Liomba G, Dallabetta GA, et al: T-lymphocyte subsets during and after pregnancy: Analysis in human immunodeficiency virus 1-infected and uninfected Malawian mothers. J Infect Dis 1992;165:146–149.
44. Temmerman M, Nagel Kerke N, et al: HIV-1 immunological changes during pregnancy: A comparison between HIV-1 seropositive and HIV-1 seronegative women in Nairobi, Kenya. AIDS 1995;9:1057–1060.
45. Barnett MA, Learmonth RP, Pihl E, Wood EC: T-helper lymphocyte depression in early human pregnancy. J Reprod Immunol 1983;5:55–57.
46. Degenne D, Canepa S, Lecomte C, et al: Serial study of T-lymphocyte subsets in women during very early pregnancy. Clin Immunol Immunopathol 1988;48:187–191.
47. Canapa S, Horowitz R, Degenne D, et al: Correlation of plasma hormone levels and peripheral circulating lymphocyte subpopulations during human pregnancy. Immunol Lett 1984;8:159–163.
48. Mikyas Y, Aziz N, Harawa N, et al: Immunologic activation during pregnancy: Serial measurement of lymphocyte phenotype and serum activation molecules in HIV-infected and uninfected women. J Reprod Immunol 1997;33:157–170.
49. Lindgren S, Martin C, Anzen B, et al: Pattern of HIV viraemia and CD4 levels in relation to pregnancy in HIV-1 infected women. Scand J Infect Dis 1996;28:425–433.
50. Kidd PG, Cheng SC, Paxton H, et al: Prediction of CD4 count from CD4 percentage: Experience from three laboratories. AIDS 1993;7:933–940.
51. Cao Y, Drogstad P, Korber BT, et al: Maternal HIV-1 viral load and vertical transmission of infection: The Ariel Project for the prevention of HIV transmission from mother to infant. Nature Med 1997;3:549–552.
52. Qazi QH, Sheikh TM, Fikrig S: Lack of evidence for craniofacial dysmorphism in perinatal HIV infection. J Pediatr 1988;112:7–12.
53. European Collaborative Study: Perinatal findings in children born to HIV-infected mothers. Br J Obstet Gynaecol 1994;101:136–141.

54. Temmerman M, Lopita MI, Sanhvi HC, et al: The role of maternal syphilis, gonorrhoea, and HIV-1 infections in spontaneous abortion. Int J STD AIDS 1992;3:418–422.
55. Kumar RM, Uduman SA, Khurrana AK, et al: Impact of maternal HIV-1 infection on perinatal outcome. Int J Gynecol Obstet 1995;49:137–143.
56. Langston C, Lewis DE, Hammill HA, et al: Excess intrauterine fetal demise associated with maternal human immunodeficiency virus infection. J Infect Dis 1995;172:1451–1460.
57. Chamiso D: Pregnancy outcome in HIV-1 positive women in Gandhi Memorial Hospital, Addis Ababa, Ethiopia. East Afr Med J 1996;73:805–809.
58. Temmerman M, Chomba EN, Ndinya-Achola J, et al: Maternal human immunodeficiency virus-1 infection and pregnancy outcome. Obstet Gynecol 1994; 83:495–500.
59. Alger LS, Farley JJ, Robinson BA, et al: Interactions of human immunodeficiency virus infection and pregnancy. Obstet Gynecol 1993; 82:787–796.
60. Ladner J, Leroy V, Hoffman P, et al: Chorioamnionitis and pregnancy outcome in HIV-infected African women. J Acquir Immun Defic Syndr 1998; 18:293–298.
61. Martin R, Boyer P, Hammill H, et al: Incidence of premature birth and neonatal respiratory disease in infants of HIV-positive mothers. J Peds 1997; 131:851–856.
62. Stratton P, Tuomala RE, Abboud R, et al: Obstetric and newborn outcomes in a cohort of HIV-infected pregnant women: A report of the Women and Infants Transmission Study. J Acquir Immun Defic Syndr 1999; 20:179–186.
63. Turner BJ, McKee LJ, Silverman NS, et al: Prenatal care and birth outcomes of a cohort of HIV-infected women. J Acquir Immune Defic Syndr Hum Retrovirol 1996; 12:259–267.
64. Goldenberg RL, Rouse DJ: Prevention of premature birth. N Engl J Med 1998; 339:313–320.
65. Singh GK, Yu SM: Adverse pregnancy outcomes: Differences between US- and foreign-born women in major US racial and ethnic groups. Am J Public Health 1996; 86:837–843.
66. Shiono PH, Klebanoff MA: Ethnic differences in preterm and very preterm delivery. Am J Public Health 1986; 76:1317–1321.
67. Adams MM, Read JA, Rawlings JS, et al: Preterm delivery among black and white enlisted women in the United States Army. Obstet Gynecol 1993; 81:65–71.
68. Lambert J, Watts H, Mofenson L, et al: Risk factors for preterm birth, low birth weight, and intrauterine growth retardation in infants born to HIV-infected pregnant women receiving zidovudine. AIDS 2000; 14:1389–1399.
69. Minkoff HL, Henderson C, Mendez H, et al: Pregnancy outcomes among mothers infected with human immunodeficiency virus and uninfected control subjects. Am J Obstet Gynecol 1990; 163:1598–1604.
70. Bulterys M, Chao A, Munyemana S, et al: Maternal human immunodeficiency virus-1 infection and intrauterine growth: A prospective cohort study in Butare, Rwanda. Pediatr Infect Dis J 1994; 13:94–100.
71. Bucceri A, Luchini L, Rancillo L, et al: Pregnancy outcome among HIV positive and negative intravenous drug users. Eur J Obstet Gynecol Reprod Biol 1997; 72:169–174.
72. Johnstone FD, Raab GM, Hamilton BA: The effect of human immunodeficiency virus infection and drug use on birth characteristics. Obstet Gynecol 1996; 88:321–326.
73. Sprauve ME: Substance abuse and HIV pregnancy. Clin Obstet Gynecol 1996; 39:316–332.
74. Brocklehurst P, French R: The association between maternal HIV infection and perinatal outcome: A systematic review of the literature and meta-analysis. Br J Obstet Gynecol 1998; 105:836–848.
75. Markson LE, Turner BJ, Houcheno R, et al: Association of maternal HIV infection with low birth weight. J Acquir Immune Defic Syndr Hum Retrovirol 1996; 13:227–234.
76. Fawzi WW, Msamanga GI, Spiegelman D, et al: Randomised trial of effects of vitamin supplements on pregnancy outcomes and T cell counts in HIV-1 infected women in Tanzania. Lancet 1998; 351:1477–1482.
77. Turner BJ, Newschaffer CJ, Cocroft J, et al: Improved birth outcomes among HIV-infected women with Enhanced Medicaid Prenatal Care. Am J Publ Health 2000; 90:85–91.
78. Kumar RM, Udaman SA, Khurrana AK: Impact of maternal HIV-1 infection on perinatal outcome. In J Gynaecol Obstet 1995; 49:137–143.
79. Lorenzi P, Spicher VM, Laubereau B, et al: Antiretroviral therapy in pregnancy: Maternal, fetal and neonatal effects. AIDS 1998; 12:F241–F247.
80. The European Collaborative Study and the Swiss Mother and Infant HIV Cohort Study: Combination antiretroviral therapy and duration of pregnancy. AIDS 2000; 14:2913–2920.
81. McNeeley DF, Laroche L, Bhutra S, et al: Newborn screening for human immunodeficiency virus infection in the Bronx, NY, and evolving public health policy. Am J Perinatol 1999; 16:503–507.
82. Centers for Disease Control and Prevention: Recommendations for use of antiretroviral drugs in pregnant HIV-1 infected women for maternal health and interventions to reduce perinatal HIV-1 transmission in the United States. MMWR Morbid

Mortal Wkly Rep 1998; 45:RR-5 (and updates *http:www.hivatis.org*).
83. American College of Obstetricians and Gynecologists Technical Bulletin. Preconceptional Care. Number 205, May 1995.
84. Mellors JW, Rinaldo CR, Gupta P, et al: Prognosis in HIV-1 infection predicted by the quantity of virus in plasma. Science 1996; 272:1167–1170.
85. Mellors JW, Munoz A, Giorgi JV, et al: Plasma viral load and CD4+ lymphocytes as prognostic markers of HIV-1 infection. Ann Intern Med 1997; 126:946–954.
86. Yeni PG, Hammer SM, Carpenter CCJ: Antiretroviral treatment for adult HIV infection in 2002: Updated recommendations of the International AIDS Society–USA Panel. JAMA 2002; 288:222–235.
87. Mitchell CD, Erlich SS, Mastrucci MT, et al: Congenital toxoplasmosis occurring in infants perinatally infected with human immunodeficiency virus 1. Pediatr Infect Dis J 1990; 9:512–518.
88. Minkoff H, Remington JS, Holman S, et al: Vertical transmission of *Toxoplasma* by human immunodeficiency virus-infected women. Am J Obstet Gynecol 1997; 176:555–559.
89. European Collaborative Study and Research Network on Congenital Toxoplasmosis: Low incidence of congenital toxoplasmosis in children born to women infected with human immunodeficiency virus. Eur J Obstet Gynecol Reprod Biol 1996; 68:93–96.
90. Marty P, Bongain A, Rahal A, et al: Prenatal diagnosis of severe fetal toxoplasmosis as a result of toxoplasma reactivation in an HIV-1 seropositive woman. Prenat Diagn 1994; 14:414–415.
91. Mussi-Pinhata MM, Yamamoto AY, Figueiredo LTM, et al: Congenital and perinatal cytomegalovirus infection in infants born to mothers infected with human immunodeficiency virus. J Pediatr 1998; 132:285–290.
92. Shewebke K, Henry K, Balfour HH Jr, et al: Congenital cytomegalovirus infection as the result of nonprimary cytomegalovirus disease in a mother with acquired immunodeficiency syndrome. J Pediatr 1995; 126:293–295.
93. Mofenson LM, Rodriguez EM, Hershow R, et al: *Mycobacterium tuberculosis* infection in pregnant and nonpregnant women infected with HIV in the Women and Infants Transmission Study. Arch Intern Med 1995; 155:1066–1072.
94. Eriksen NL, Helfgott AW: Cutaneous anergy in pregnant and nonpregnant women with human immunodeficiency virus. Infect Dis Obstet Gynecol 1998; 6:13–17.
95. Minkoff HL, Eisenberger-Matiyahu D, Feldman J, et al: Prevalence and incidence of gynecologic disorders among women infected with human immunodeficiency virus. Am J Obstet Gynecol 1999; 180:824–836.
96. Fennema JS, van Ameijden EJ, Coutinho RA, van den Hoek AA: HIV, sexually transmitted diseases and gynaecologic disorders in women: Increased risk for genital herpes and warts among HIV-infected prostitutes in Amsterdam. AIDS 1995; 9:1071–1078.
97. Hitti J, Watts DH, Burchett DK, et al: Herpes simplex virus seropositivity and reactivation at delivery among pregnant women infected with human immunodeficiency virus-1. Am J Obstet Gynecol 1997; 177:450–454.
98. Augenbraun M, Feldman J, Chirgwin K, et al: Increased genital shedding of herpes simplex virus type 2 in HIV-seropositive women. Ann Intern Med 1995; 123:845–847.
99. Lindsay MK, Adefris W, Willis S, Klein L: The risk of sexually transmitted diseases in human immunodeficiency virus-infected parturients. Am J Obstet Gynecol 1993; 169:1031–1035.
100. LaGuardia KD, White MH, Saigo PE, et al: Genital ulcer disease in women infected with human immunodeficiency virus. Am J Obstet Gynecol 1995; 172(2 Pt 1):553–562.
101. Chirgwin KE, Feldman J, Augenbraun M, et al: Incidence of venereal warts in human immunodeficiency virus-infected and uninfected women. J Infect Dis 1995; 172:235–238.
102. Augenbraun MH, Dehovitz JA, Feldman J, et al: Biological false-positive syphilis test results for women infected with human immunodeficiency virus. Clin Infect Dis 1994; 19:1040–1044.
103. Fruchter RG, Maiman M, Sillman FH, et al: Characteristics of cervical intraepithelial neoplasia in women infected with the human immunodeficiency virus. Am J Obstet Gynecol 1994; 171:531–537.
104. Klein RS, Ho GY, Vermund SH, et al: Risk factors for squamous intraepithelial lesions on PAP smear in women at risk for human immunodeficiency virus infection. J Infect Dis 1994; 170:1404–1409.
105. Miotti PB, Dallabetta GA, Daniel RW, et al: Cervical abnormalities, human papillomavirus, and human immunodeficiency virus infections in women in Malawi. J Infect Dis 1996; 173:714–717.
106. Wright TC Jr, Ellerbrock TV, Chaisson MA, et al: Cervical intraepithelial neoplasia in women infected with human immunodeficiency virus: Prevalence, risk factors and validity of Papanicolaou smears. New York Cervical Disease Study. Obstet Gynecol 1994; 84:591–597.
107. Klevens RM, Fleming PL, Mays MA, Frey R: Characteristics of women with AIDS and invasive cervical cancer. Obstet Gynecol 1996; 88:269–273.
108. Fruchter RG, Maiman M, Sedlis A, et al: Multiple recurrences of cervical intraepithelial neoplasia in women with the human immunodeficiency virus. Obstet Gynecol 1996; 87:338–344.

109. Dodig M, Tavill AS: Hepatitis C and human immunodeficiency virus coinfections. J Clin Gastroenterol 2000; 33:367–374.
110. Bonacini M, Puoti M: Hepatitis C in-patients with human immunodeficiency virus infection: Diagnosis, natural history, meta-analysis of sexual and vertical transmission, and therapeutic issues. Arch Intern Med 2000; 160:3365–3373.
111. Hershow RC, Riester KA, Lew J, et al: Increased vertical transmission of human immunodeficiency virus from hepatitis C virus-coinfected mothers. J Infect Dis 1997; 176:414–420.
112. Thomas DL, Villano SA, Riester KA, et al: Perinatal transmission of hepatitis C virus from human immunodeficiency virus type 1-infected mothers. Women and Infants Transmission Study. J Infect Dis 1998; 177:1480–1488.
113. Laga M, Manoka A, Kivuvu M, et al: Non-ulcerative sexually transmitted diseases as risk factors for HIV-1 transmission in women: Results from a cohort study. AIDS 1993; 7:395–412.
114. Greenblatt RM, Bacchetti P, Barkan S, et al: Lower genital tract infections among HIV-infected and high-risk uninfected women: Findings of the Women's Interagency HIV Study (WIHS). Sex Transm Dis 1999; 26:143–151.
115. Hauth JC, Goldenberg RL, Andrews WW, et al: Reduced incidence of preterm delivery with metronidazole and erythromycin in women with bacterial vaginosis. N Engl J Med 1995; 333:1732–1736.
116. Montaner JSG, Hogg RS, Yip B, et al: Diminished effectiveness of antiretroviral therapy among patients initiating therapy with CD4+ T cell counts below 200/mm^3. Paper presented at the 13th International AIDS Conference, Durban, South Africa, 2000, Abstract LbPeB7050.
117. Chaube S, Murphy ML: The effects of hydroxyurea and related compounds on the rat fetus. Cancer Res 1966; 26:1448–1457.
118. Ferm V: Severe developmental malformations. Arch Pathol 1966; 81:174–177.
119. Khera K: A teratogenicity study on hydroxyurea and diphenylhydantoin in cats. Teratology 1979; 20:447–452.
120. Wilson JG, Scott WJ, Ritter EF, Fradkin R: Comparative distribution and embryotoxicity of hydroxyurea in pregnant rats and rhesus monkeys. Teratology 1975; 11:169–178.
121. Fortgang IS, Belitsos PC, Chaisson RE, Moore RD: Hepatomegaly and steatosis in HIV-infected patients receiving nucleoside analog antiretroviral therapy. Am J Gastroenterol 1995; 90:1433–1436.
122. terHofstede HJ, de Marie S, Foudraine NA, et al: Clinical features and risk factors of lactic acidosis following long-term antiretroviral therapy: 4 fatal cases. Int J STD AIDS 2000; 11:611–616.
123. Lonergan JT, Behling C, Pfander H, et al: Hyperlactatemia and hepatic abnormalities in 10 human immunodeficiency virus-infected patients receiving nucleoside analogue combination regimens. Clin Infect Dis 2000; 31:162–166.
124. Kakuda TN: Pharmacology of nucleoside and nucleotide reverse transcriptase inhibitor-induced mitochondrial toxicity. Clin Ther 2000; 22:685–708.
125. Miller KD, Cameron M, Wood LV, et al: Lactic acidosis and hepatic steatosis associated with use of stavudine: Report of four cases. Ann Intern Med 2000; 133:192–196.
126. Mokrzycki MH, Harris C, May H, et al: Lactic acidosis associated with stavudine administration: A report of five cases. Clin Infect Dis 2000; 30:198–200.
127. Gerald Y, Maulin L, Yazdanpanah Y, et al: Symptomatic hyperlactatemia: An emerging complication of antiretroviral therapy. AIDS 2000; 14:2723–2730.
128. Bristol-Myers Squibb Company: Healthcare provider important drug warning letter. January 5, 2001.
129. Luzzati R, Del Bravo P, Di Perri G, et al: Riboflavin and severe lactic acidosis [letter]. Lancet 1999; 353:901–902.
130. Visnegarwala F, Krause KL, Musher DM: Severe diabetes associated with protease inhibitor therapy. Ann Intern Med 1997; 127:947.
131. Eastone JA, Decker CF: New-onset diabetes mellitus associated with use of protease inhibitor. Ann Intern Med 1997; 127:948.
132. Mulligan K, Grunfeld C, Tai VW, et al: Hyperlipidemia and insulin resistance are induced by protease inhibitors independent of changes in body composition in patients with HIV infection. J Acquir Immune Defic Syndr 2000; 23:35–43.
133. Dube M: Metabolic complications of antiretroviral therapies. AIDS Clin Care 1998; 10:41–48.
134. Piliero PJ, Purdy B: Nevirapine-induced hepatitis: A case series and review of the literature. AIDS Reader 2001; 11:379–382.
135. Martinez E, Polanco JL, Arnaiz JA, et al: Hepatotoxicity in HIV-1-infected patients receiving nevirapine-containing antiretroviral therapy. AIDS 2001; 15:1261–1268.
136. Centers for Disease Control and Prevention: Serious adverse events attributed to nevirapine regimens for post exposure prophylaxis after HIV exposure-worldwide, 1997–2000. MMWR Morbid Mortal Wkly Rep 2001; 49:1153–1156.
137. Antiretroviral Pregnancy Registry. PharmaResearch Corporation, Wilmington, NC. January 1989-July 2001.
138. Culnane M, Fowler MG, Lee SS, et al: Lack of long-term effects of in utero exposure to zidovudine among uninfected children born to HIV-infected women. JAMA 1999; 281:151–157.

139. Hanson IC, Antonelli TA, Sperling RS, et al: Lack of tumors in infants with perinatal HIV-1 exposure and fetal/neonatal exposure to zidovudine. J Acquir Immune Defic Syndr Hum Retrovirol 1999; 20:463–467.
140. Blanche S, Tardieu M, Rustin P, et al: Persistent mitochondrial dysfunction and perinatal exposure to antiretroviral nucleoside analogues. Lancet 1999; 354:1084–1089.
141. The Perinatal Safety Review Working Group: Nucleoside exposure in the children of HIV-infected women receiving antiretroviral drugs: Absence of clear evidence for mitochondrial disease in children who died before 5 years of age in five United States cohorts. J Acquir Immune Defic Syndr Hum Retrovirol 2000; 25:261–268.
142. 2001 USPHS/IDSA Guidelines for the Prevention of Opportunistic Infections in Persons Infected with HIV. http:/www.hivatis.org. Posted November 28, 2001.
143. Chahoud I, Bochert G, Stahlmann R: Teratogenic effect of ganciclovir in rats. Teratology 1997; 55:40.
144. Kovacs A, Schluchter M, Easley K, et al: Cytomegalovirus infection and HIV-1 disease progression in infants born to HIV-1-infected women. N Engl J Med 1999; 341:77–84.
145. Dunn D, Wallon M, Peyron F, et al: Mother-to-child transmission of toxoplasmosis: Risk estimates for clinical counseling. Lancet 1999; 353: 1829–1833.
146. Franks AL, Binkin NJ, Snider DE, et al: INH hepatitis among pregnant and nonpregnant Hispanic patients. Public Health Rep 1989; 104:151–155.
147. Burns DN, Tuomala R, Chang BH, et al: Vaginal colonization or infection with *Candida albicans* in human immunodeficiency virus-infected women during pregnancy and the postpartum period. The Women and Infants Transmission Study Group. Clin Infect Dis 1997; 24:201–210.
148. Scott LL, Sanchez PJ, Jackson GL, et al: Acyclovir suppression to prevent cesarean delivery after first-episode genital herpes. Obstet Gynecol 1996; 87:69–73.
149. Braig S, Luton D, Sibony O, et al: Acyclovir prophylaxis in late pregnancy prevents recurrent genital herpes and viral shedding. Eur J Obstet Gynecol Reprod Biol 2001; 96:55–58.
150. Yeung LTF, King SM, Roberts EA: Mother-to-infant transmission of hepatitis C virus. Hepatol 2001; 34:223–229.
151. Towers CV, Deveikis A, Asrat T, et al: A "bloodless cesarean section" and perinatal transmission of the human immunodeficiency virus. Am J Obstet Gynecol 1998; 179:708–714.
152. Mandelbrot L, Mayaux M, Bongain A, et al: Obstetrics: Obstetric factors and mother-to-child transmission of human immunodeficiency virus type 1: The French perinatal cohorts. Am J Obstet Gynecol 1996; 175:661–667.
153. Tess BH, Rodrigues LC, Newell ML, et al: Breastfeeding, genetic, obstetric and other risk factors associated with mother-to-child transmission of HIV-1 in Sao Paulo State, Brazil. Sao Paulo Collaborative Study for Vertical Transmission of HIV-1. AIDS 1998; 12:513–520.
154. The International Perinatal HIV Group: The mode of delivery and the risk of vertical transmission of human immunodeficiency virus type 1: A meta-analysis of 15 prospective cohort studies. N Engl J Med 1999; 340:977–987.
155. The European Mode of Delivery Collaboration: Elective caesarean section versus vaginal delivery in prevention of vertical HIV-1 transmission: A randomized clinical trial. Lancet 1999; 353:1035–1039.
156. Kind C, Rudin C, Siegrist CA, et al: Prevention of vertical HIV transmission: Additive protective effect of elective cesarean section and zidovudine prophylaxis. AIDS 1998; 12:205–210.
157. Mandelbrot L, LeChenadec J, Berrebi A, et al: Perinatal HIV-1 transmission: Interaction between zidovudine prophylaxis and mode of delivery in the French Perinatal Cohort. JAMA 1998; 280:55–60.
158. Chen KT, Sell RL, Tuomala RE: Cost-effectiveness of elective cesarean delivery in human immunodeficiency virus-infected women. Obstet Gynecol 2001; 97:161–168.
159. Mrus JM, Goldie SJ, Weinstein MC, Tsevat J: The cost-effectiveness of elective Cesarean delivery for HIV-infected women with detectable HIV RNA during pregnancy. AIDS 2000; 14:2543–2552.
160. Halpern MT, Read JS, Ganoczy DA, Harris DR: Cost-effectiveness of cesarean section delivery to prevent mother-to-child transmission of HIV-1. AIDS 2000; 14:691–700.
161. ACOG Committee Opinion No. 234. Vertical Transmission of HIV Infection. May, 2000.
162. Gichangi PB, Nyongo AO, Temmerman M: Pregnancy outcome and placental weights: Their relationship to HIV-1 infection. East Afr Med J 1993; 70:85–89.
163. Semprini AE, Castagna C, Ravizzi M, et al: The incidence of complications after cesarean section in 156 HIV-positive women. AIDS 1995; 9:913–917.
164. Bulterys M, Chao AM, Dushimimana A, et al: Fatal complications after cesarean section in HIV-infected women. AIDS 1996; 10:923–924.
165. Read JS, Tuomala R, Kpamegan E, et al: Mode of delivery and postpartum morbidity among HIV-infected women. J Acquir Immun Defic Syndr 2001; 26:236–245.
166. Watts DH, Lambert JS, Stiehm ER, et al: Complications according to mode of delivery

among human immunodeficiency virus-infected women with CD4 lymphocyte counts of ≤ 500/ml. Am J Obstet Gynecol 2000; 183:100–107.
167. Popek EJ, Korber BT, Merrit L, et al: Acute chorioamnionitis and duration of membrane rupture correlates with vertical transmission of HIV-1. Abstract presented at the 3rd National Conference on Human Retroviruses and Related Infections. Washington, DC, 1997.
168. Minkoff H, Burns DN, Landesman S, et al: The relationship of the duration of ruptured membranes to vertical transmission of human immunodeficiency virus. Am J Obstet Gynecol 1995; 173:585–589.
169. The International Perinatal HIV Group: Duration of ruptured membranes and vertical transmission of HIV-1: A meta-analysis from 15 prospective cohort studies. AIDS 2001; 15:357–368.
170. Boyer PJ, Dillon M, Navaie M, et al: Factors predictive of maternal-fetal transmission of HIV-1: Preliminary analysis of zidovudine given during pregnancy and/or delivery. JAMA 1994; 271:1925–1930.
171. Lindegren ML, Byers RH Jr, Thomas P, et al: Trends in perinatal transmission of HIV/AIDS in the United States. JAMA 1999; 282:531–538.
172. Birkhead GS, Chang HG, Smith PF, et al: Consented testing of newborns and childbearing women for human immunodeficiency virus through a newborn metabolic screening program. Am J Obstet Gynecol 2000; 183:245–251.
173. Krasinski K, Borkowski W, Bebenroth D, Moore T: Failure of voluntary testing for human immunodeficiency virus to identify infected parturient women in a high-risk population [letter]. N Engl J Med 1988; 318:185.
174. Ellerbrock T, Harrington PE, Bush TJ, et al: Risk of HIV infection among pregnant crack cocaine users in a rural community. Obstet Gynecol 1995; 86:400–404.
175. Abeni DD, Porta D, Perucci CA: Deliveries, abortion, and HIV-1 infection in Rome, 1989-1994. The Lazio AIDS Collaborative Group. Eur J Epidemiol 1997; 13:378–380.
176. McNeeley DF, Laroche L, Bhutra S, et al: Newborn screening for human immunodeficiency virus infection 1 in the Bronx, NY, and evolving public health policy. Am J Perinatol 1999; 16:503–507.
177. Grobman WA, Garcia PM: The cost-effectiveness of voluntary intrapartum rapid human immunodeficiency virus testing for women without adequate prenatal care. Am J Obstet Gynecol 1999; 180:1062–1071.
178. Webber MP, Demas P, Enriquez E, et al: Pilot study of expedited HIV-1 testing of women in labor at an inner-city hospital in New York City. Am J Perinatol 2001; 18:49–57.
179. Rotheram-Borus MJ, Newman PA, Etzel MA: Effective detection of HIV. J Acquir Immun Defic Syndr 2000; 25:S105–S114.
180. Newell ML: Infant feeding and HIV-1 transmission. Lancet 1999; 354:442–443.
181. Van De Perre P: Breast milk transmission of HIV-1 laboratory and clinical studies. Ann N Y Acad Sci 2000; 918:122–127.
182. John GC, Richardson VA, Nduati RW, et al: Timing of breast milk HIV-1 transmission: A meta-analysis. East Afr Med J 2001; 78:75–79.
183. Nduati R, John G, Mbori-Ngacha D, et al: Effect of breastfeeding and formula feeding on transmission of HIV-1: A randomized clinical trial. JAMA 2000; 283:1167–1174.

6

Diagnostic Methods for Infants Born to HIV-Infected Women

Paul Palumbo

The diagnosis of HIV infection among newborns and infants born to HIV-infected mothers has posed a unique challenge to clinicians. This challenge is similar to that posed by other perinatal infections and results from the fact that all exposed infants will have detectable, maternally acquired antibody specific for the pathogen in question but only a fraction of exposed infants will be truly infected. The diagnostic approach employed through much of the 1980s consisted of monitoring the decay of passively acquired antibody in the infant. The loss of detectable HIV-specific antibody by 18 to 24 months of age was (and still is) considered evidence of noninfection. This approach was necessary and adequate during the mid-1980s, but the advent of therapeutic and prophylactic options and the general desire to reduce the "waiting period" stimulated the development and implementation of assays that directly detect HIV or its components (Table 6–1). This chapter focuses on the historical perspective of diagnostic assays, current practice, and strategies in development targeting remaining problem areas.

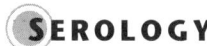SEROLOGY

HIV antibody detection assays were developed very rapidly once HIV was identified and propagated in cell culture.[1–4] These consisted largely of enzyme immunoassays (EIA)[5,6] and have been documented to be very effective for screening at-risk populations.[7] As with many screening assays, false-positive results occur with an increasing rate as the risk for

Table 6–1
HIV Diagnostic Approaches

TEST	UTILITY/COMMENTS
Serology (enzyme immunoassay; Western blot)	Rapid; inexpensive
	Used for individuals > 2 years of age
DNA PCR (targets proviral DNA within cells)	Rapid; sensitive; moderately expensive
	Primarily used for infants < 2 years of age
RNA PCR (targets plasma virus)	Rapid; sensitive; moderately expensive
	Used for recent (acute) infection and when DNA PCR is not available
p24 Antigen	Rapid; inexpensive
	Sensitivity and specificity limited
Viral culture	Sensitive but costly in time and resources

PCR, polymerase chain reaction.

infection in a population decreases. This has been effectively managed by confirming any specimen that is repeatedly reactive in an EIA with a Western blot assay. The latter portrays the HIV protein specificity of the antibody response. Minimum specific criteria have been established regarding "banding patterns" required to confirm a diagnosis.[8–10] This serologic algorithm (EIA finding confirmed by Western blot assay) remains the current standard for the diagnosis of HIV infection in older children and adults. False-positive results have been observed in a number of settings, including recent immunization, infection with viruses of the herpes class or influenza, autoimmune diseases, highly transfused individuals, and certain hematologic malignancies. False-negative results can occur when testing is performed prematurely, such as during acute infection before a detectable immune response, and in the setting of hypo- or agammaglobulinemia. In the acute infection setting, virus may be detectable in clinical specimens (by plasma RNA polymerase chain reaction [PCR], for instance) before an immune response is detectable.

Assays configured to detect HIV-specific IgM have not proven diagnostically useful, as with many other congenital infections, because of problems with nonspecificity and reaction with rheumatoid factor. Several laboratories have developed HIV-specific IgA assays that have excellent specificity and whose sensitivity is acceptable after about 6 months of age.[11–16] Before 6 months of age, however, performance deteriorates to the point where the assay is not indicated. HIV-specific IgA EIAs have potential appeal in situations in which cost and technologic expertise are limiting factors. The reliance on direct viral detection assays in infancy within developed countries has limited interest in the commercial development and deployment of IgA diagnostic assays.

DIRECT DETECTION OF HIV OR ITS COMPONENTS

DNA Polymerase Chain Reaction

The PCR is a recent technologic achievement (1986) that earned its developer a Nobel prize.[17, 18] The assay targets a specific genetic region of DNA for enzymatic amplification, copying the nucleic acid target literally billions of times. PCR has had enormous impact on both applied and basic science and is a central feature in the detection and quantitation of HIV in clinical specimens.

Diagnostic DNA PCR is configured to detect a small section of the proviral DNA present within infected mononuclear cells. Specificity is obtained by synthesizing small DNA probes made up of about 20 nucleotides (oligonucleotide), which will hybridize to the complementary HIV DNA target. Most HIV DNA PCR assays target a small portion of the *gag* gene, about 200 nucleotides in length, which is relatively conserved (nonvariable) among different viral quasispecies. The two DNA probes bracket the ends of this double-stranded DNA gag target region, one specific for each strand. Mononuclear cells from a blood specimen are isolated either by red blood cell lysis of whole blood or by means of Ficoll-Hypaque density gradient centrifugation. Approximately 125,000 mononuclear cells are subjected to membrane lysis and proteolysis. A PCR assay consists of the exposed cellular genetic material in combination with a probe pair, deoxynucleotides (DNA building blocks), a nucleic acid copying enzyme (*Thermus aquaticus* or Taq polymerase), and the appropriate buffer. The actual reaction is performed in a very small volume—usually 0.05 to 0.1 mL—in a programmable heat block, which allows rapid temperature changes in a cyclic fashion. A single cycle of PCR is composed of (1) denaturation of the target DNA ("melting" into single strands) at 95 to 100°C; (2) annealing or hybridization of the oligonucleotide probe to the gag gene target at 56°C; and (3) extension or copying of the DNA target using the probe as the starting point (72°C). After the first cycle, an exact doubling of any initial target should have occurred. By repeating this cyclic process 30 to 35 times, billions of copies will theoretically be synthesized.

A central feature of PCR is the Taq polymerase, which is a temperature-stable enzyme derived from the thermophilic bacterium *Thermus aquaticus*. This enzyme is able to withstand the repetitive temperature extremes and maintain function. Detection of the PCR "amplicons" is accomplished by hybridization to probes fixed to a solid phase and subsequent EIA-like enzymatic reactions, leading to a visibly detectable color change.

In the context of extensive amplification, microaerosols created by the simple opening of reaction tubes pose a significant specimen-to-specimen contamination hazard—the bane of PCR laboratories. Techniques have been designed to minimize or eliminate such contamination.[19, 20] One method is the physical separation of the different phases of PCR—sample preparation, PCR set-up, amplification, and detection. A second complementary approach is to use the nucleotide uracil in place of thymidine and the addition of the enzyme uracil-*N*-glycosylase to the initial PCR reaction. Any contaminating PCR product from a previous reaction will contain uracil and will be degraded by uracil-*N*-glycosylase. Current DNA PCR assays can reliably and reproducibly detect HIV with a sensitivity of 1 to 10 copies of HIV target per reaction.

False-positive or indeterminate results do occur on occasion and are the basis of the requirement for two positive assays from independent blood samplings before a diagnosis of infection can be established. Laboratory investigations focused on the source of these false-positive findings have almost universally implicated contamination of the specimen in question with exogenous virus or a mislabeling phenomenon.[21,22]

The first application and analyses of DNA PCR for infant HIV diagnosis were reported in 1988–89.[23–25] The assay has subsequently gained considerable favor, to the point that it is the diagnostic method of choice in the developed world. Supporting this position are reasonable cost, short turnaround time, and desirable sensitivity and specificity. Many studies employing large cohorts have evaluated the use of PCR, but their results are difficult to compare because of the inherent heterogeneity of both the early assays and the cohorts studied. Studies of high quality, however, have been in general agreement, as supported and documented in a meta-analysis.[26] Sensitivity and specificity of 95% and 97%, respectively, for specimens collected among infants older than 1 month of age were reported in one large North American study.[27] For HIV-infected newborns younger than 1 month of age, and especially in the first 2 weeks of life, only 30% to 50% will have detectable proviral DNA within circulating mononuclear cells by DNA PCR or by any other detection assay.[28] These newborns with initially negative assay findings who convert within a few weeks are thought to be in an "incubation" period, in which the virus is slowly replicating in fixed tissue, and have not established infection within the circulating compartment to any appreciable extent.

An empirical working definition distinguishes in utero from peripartum mother-to-infant HIV transmission by the pattern of detection: those who have detectable infection within the first 48 hours of life are considered to be infected in utero whereas those with a delayed pattern of detection are most likely to have been infected around the time of delivery.[29] Although this definition has considerable appeal and support within the research community, it is a hypothesis that has never been rigorously proven.

Current newborn testing recommendations using DNA PCR are as follows:

- 0–48 hours
- 14 days (optional)
- 1 month
- 2 months
- 4 months

If all assay findings are negative and at least two assays are from beyond the newborn period, the infant is considered to be uninfected. Assay findings at two individual time points must be positive to establish the diagnosis of HIV infection.

HIV Culture

Cocultivation techniques were those initially used for the identification of the LAI/HTLV IIIb strains as the causative agent of AIDS.[1,2] Where accessible in research laboratories, cell culture was relied upon for the diagnosis of exposed infants through much of the 1980s and early 1990s.[30,31] This was the gold standard, in addition to serology performed from 18 to 24 months of age, against which DNA PCR was directly compared for diagnostic utility.

In vitro cultivation of human cells for the isolation of HIV is a cocultivation technique in that equal numbers of mononuclear cells from an individual to be tested and from an uninfected donor are mixed. Mononuclear cells are typically isolated from whole blood by Ficoll-Hypaque gradient centrifugation and prestimulated with phytohemagglutinin for optimal yields. Generally, 1 to 5 million cells from donor and test subjects are mixed and cultured in a flask for as long as 28 days. Twice weekly, culture supernatant is sampled and subjected to p24 antigen detection and the flask renewed with an aliquot of fresh media. Two sequential time point samplings must be positive for p24 antigen for a culture to be considered positive. A cell culture assay sample is incubated for at least 28 days before being considered negative. The majority of positive specimens will become detectably positive by 7 to 14 days. Qualitative and quantitative as well as microculture formats are available.

Although cell culture possesses an equivalent diagnostic performance profile compared with DNA PCR, it is not as universally available and is considerably more expensive and time consuming. Recently, there has been renewed interest in culture from the perspective of evaluating residual viral infectivity among individuals who have successfully suppressed viral replication (plasma RNA measurements are nondetectable) with antiretroviral regimens.[32–34] Continued interest in cell culture remains in research circles where viral phenotypic characteristics may be a focus of study. Enhanced cell culture methods have utilized any number of the following approaches: increased cell input number; concentration of CD4+ and depletion of CD8+ lymphocytes; and specific stimulation with antibodies to CD3+ and CD28+ cells. These techniques purport to increase the chances for positive cultures in the context of very low numbers of infected cells and will possibly be used more frequently in the future to monitor the suppressed patient. It is currently unknown whether enhanced culture techniques would accelerate the time to positivity or the age at which newborns might be definitively diagnosed. Since increased cell input number is a cornerstone of these techniques, it does not seem likely that they will be applied routinely to infant diagnostics.

p24 Antigen

The p24 antigen is a structural protein of the viral core. The p24 antigen assay employs an enzyme immunoassay format in which antibody to p24 antigen is fixed to a solid phase (e.g., a latex bead or the plastic well of a microtiter plate). When a liquid sample is incubated with this solid-phase antibody, it captures any p24 antigen present. After an incubation period, the solid phase is extensively washed and any captured p24 antigen can be detected with a labeled second antibody specific for p24 antigen. This relatively simple EIA format allows for the sensitive detection of an HIV protein and can be quantitated.

This assay does not perform reliably among newborn and infant populations, as many have high levels of maternal HIV-specific antibody that complexes with the p24 antigen. These antigen-antibody complexes can interfere with detection of p24 antigen by the EIA. To resolve this problem, techniques have been devised that dissociate immune complexes before subjecting a specimen to the p24 EIA. Among these are dissociation with acid[35, 36] and by means of simple boiling.[37–39] While not perfect, these preparatory immune complex dissociating treatments markedly enhance performance. Regardless, limitations remain for the prospects of infant diagnosis using the p24 antigen assay, chief of which are limited sensitivity relative to culture and PCR and false-positive findings in the first few days to week of life. The technique remains relatively inexpensive and marginally reliable after the first month of life and maintains usefulness in discrete situations. However, if performance is optimized, it would be an ideal candidate for infant diagnostics as well as disease monitoring in developing countries.

Plasma RNA

Several assays have been developed for the quantitation of plasma virion RNA, in particular, reverse transcriptase PCR,[40,41] branched DNA assay,[42] and nucleic acid sequence based amplification.[43] These tools have desirable performance characteristics[44–47] and have proven remarkably predictive of response to therapy and future clinical course. As such, they have become a universal clinical tool in developed countries. Owing to their widespread dissemination and accessibility, they have also been used for infant diagnosis with the prediction that they would compare favorably with DNA PCR.

Early studies did in fact document the early detection of plasma RNA among HIV-infected newborns and infants, in some cases earlier by days or weeks than DNA PCR.[48–51] Studies among adults with acute infection also documented the early detection of plasma RNA, before a detectable immune response. One nagging concern about using RNA assays for diagnosis is that the assays have been configured for sensitive quantitation in known HIV-infected populations and not for qualitative detection in a diagnostic setting. False-positive results are a real possibility, especially when the plasma RNA results fall in the low quantitative range (e.g., below 1–10 thousand copies/mL). Manufacturers are in the process of developing qualitative RNA detection assays not only for use as a diagnostic assay but also for the purpose of monitoring infected individuals on potent viral suppressive regimens for breakthrough viral replication. In the meantime, standard quantitative plasma RNA assays will continue to be used for infant diagnostics. Care should be exercised when results are in the low quantitative range.

ADDITIONAL DIAGNOSTIC ISSUES AND DEVELOPMENTS

The remarkable genetic diversity of HIV has a direct impact on HIV diagnostic approaches in many ways. Within any given infected individual, subtle genetic variation among the panoply of coexistent virions has been described as the "quasispecies" nature of HIV. For diagnosis or quantitation using molecular techniques such as PCR, regions of relative genetic stability (such as the region of the *gag* gene generally employed for DNA PCR) must be targeted to optimize accuracy.

In the context of a larger, global scale, HIV exists in many family branches, or clades. Within each clade, genetic variation is minimal while between-clade variation can be estimated at several percent. At least eight clades have been documented to date within the clinically relevant M group of HIV-1, with additional representatives being identified on a regular basis. By far the most prevalent clade in the United States is clade B, which has been the primary target for commercial amplification assays. It became clear very early with molecular-based assays that rely on genetic detection of HIV that many non-clade B infections were either not detected or quantitated accurately with the clade-B focused kits.[52–56] In the United States, imported cases of non-clade B may not be detected—for example in the case of newborn diagnosis in which DNA PCR is utilized—or quantitation of plasma virus may be spuriously low. In regions of the world where non-clade B predominates, the problems are magnified many-fold. All commercial kit manufacturers now offer products with primers that have been designed to identify a broad spectrum of HIV clades.[57–61] In some cases, Food and Drug Administration (FDA) approval and broad usage in the United States is pending.

An area of current interest and development is that of rapid diagnostic testing. The traditional serologic approach to diagnosis among older children and adults and the viral detection approach favored for newborns and infants require several days to weeks in assay turnaround time. There are a number of scenarios in which this is clearly inadequate. One example is in a sexually transmitted disease or other clinic in which a follow-up visit cannot be ensured. Relevant to the focus of this chapter, a disturbingly high proportion of pregnant women receive little or no prenatal care, with their first significant medical community interaction being the onset of labor and admission to an hospital obstetric unit. In this setting, rapid diagnosis is very appealing and would support rapid intervention regarding HIV transmission prevention measures.[62] Some medical centers have already instituted rapid serologic diagnosis of pregnant women with unknown HIV infection status, and a number of clinical studies are currently addressing methodologic issues, such as identifying optimal assays or combinations, developing optimal approaches to maternal interaction during this sensitive time, and evaluating optimal intervention strategies.

A large number of rapid serologic assays have been developed, of which only one is currently FDA-approved for use in the United States (Single Use Diagnostic System HIV-1 Test or SUDS; Murex Corp, Norcross, GA). These assays generally use small volumes of blood obtained by finger stick or venipuncture; some are designed for saliva or urine. The easiest employ self-contained devices for use in the medical office or at bedside and have simple color-coded readouts. Some have the potential disadvantage of requiring some technical processing, such as centrifugation, which might limit broad usage. The most rapid require as little as 5 to 15 minutes to perform. Either single assay or simultaneous dual assay formats may ultimately prove to possess the ideal combination of sensitivity, specificity, and ease of use. This is likely to be a rapidly developing area in the near future.

Collection of small blood specimens as dried spots on filter paper (Guthrie cards) from newborns and young infants for diagnostic purposes is a time-honored method. The method has been extensively evaluated for both HIV serology and direct detection of HIV DNA or RNA with very encouraging results. Once the specimen has dried, it is very stable for long periods of time at ambient temperatures with simple storage in sealed plastic bags. This methodology has been validated for detection of proviral DNA by PCR[63–68] and for cell-free RNA[69] in blood specimens. Predictably, this diagnostic and monitoring approach has considerable appeal for field trials and situations in which limited technology and resources preclude refrigeration and complicated processing steps. Whether dried blood spots become routinely employed in the United States as screening for genetic and metabolic disease of the newborn remains to be determined.

With the advent of multidrug antiretroviral treatment being administered to large segments of the HIV-infected population, drug resistance and the transmission of drug-resistant virus has become a major concern. Reports of primary infection with drug-resistant virus have generally ranged from 5% to 10%, and possibly higher, among adults.[70–74] The rate is probably lower in the setting of mother-infant transmission, given that a substantial portion of pregnant women have received limited or no antiretroviral medication. Studies are ongoing to determine the prevalence of antiretroviral resistance among pregnant women, a rate that predictably will change over time in parallel with drug usage. It may be advisable to consider antiretroviral resistance testing for any newly infected individual—newborn, child, or adult—to assist in devising optimal treatment regimens.

Recent developments in defining host susceptibility characteristics regarding infection and disease progression are likely to be transmitted to clinical practice in the near future. Certain HLA alleles have been associated with altered risk for infection and disease progression,[75–79] but the picture is far from complete, and it is highly likely that multiple alleles, singly and in combination, will have an impact on host susceptibility. Genetic polymorphisms in the chemokine receptor genes (coreceptors with CD4+ for HIV infection of human cells) and their natural ligands have been clearly associated with susceptibility to both infection and disease progression.[80–85] There will undoubtedly be many more additions to host susceptibility factors, which together may ultimately portray a comprehensive risk profile. Implementation of host susceptibility analyses will certainly provide a challenge to clinicians, ethicists, and society at large.

References

1. Barre-Sinoussi F, Chermann JC, Rey F, et al: Isolation of a T-lymphotropic retrovirus from a patient at risk for acquired immune deficiency syndrome (AIDS). Science 1983;220:868–871.
2. Gallo RC, Sarin PS, Gelmann EP, et al: Isolation of human T-cell leukemia virus in acquired immune deficiency syndrome (AIDS). Science 1983;220:865–867.
3. Gallo RC, Salahuddin SZ, Popovic M, et al: Frequent detection and isolation of cytopathic retroviruses (HTLV-III) from patients with AIDS and at risk for AIDS. Science 1984;224:500–503.
4. Levy JA, Hoffman JD, Kramer SM, et al: Isolation of lymphocytopathic retroviruses from San Francisco patients with AIDS. Science 1984;224:840–842.
5. Kalyanaraman VS, Cabradilla CD, Getchell JP, et al: Antibodies to the core protein of lymphadenopathy-associated virus (LAV) in patients with AIDS. Science 1984;225:321–323.
6. Sarngadharan MG, Popovic M, Bruch L, et al: Antibodies reactive with human T-lymphotropic retroviruses (HTLV-III) in the serum of patients with AIDS. Science 1984;224:506–508.
7. Constantine NT: Serologic tests for the retroviruses: Approaching a decade of evolution [editorial]. AIDS 1993;7:1–13.
8. Centers for Disease Control and Prevention: Interpretation and use of the Western blot assay for serodiagnosis of human immunodeficiency virus type 1 infections. JAMA 1989;262:3395–3397.
9. Interpretation and use of the Western blot assay for serodiagnosis of human immunodeficiency virus type 1 infections. MMWR Morb Mortal Wkly Rep 1989;38:1–7.
10. Interpretive criteria used to report Western blot results for HIV-1-antibody testing—United States. MMWR Morb Mortal Wkly Rep 1991;40:692–695.
11. Connor E, Wang Z, Stephens R, et al: Enzyme immunoassay for detection of human immunodeficiency virus-specific immunoglobulin A antibodies. J Clin Microbiol 1993;31:681–684.
12. McIntosh K, Comeau AM, Wara D, et al: The utility of IgA antibody to human immunodeficiency virus type 1 in early diagnosis of vertically transmitted infection. National Institute of Allergy and Infectious Diseases and National Institute of Child Health and Human Development Women and Infants Transmission Study Group. Arch Pediatr Adolesc Med 1996;150:598–602.
13. Kline MW, Lewis DE, Hollinger FB, et al: A comparative study of human immunodeficiency virus culture, polymerase chain reaction and anti-human immunodeficiency virus immunoglobulin A antibody detection in the diagnosis during early infancy of vertically acquired human immunodeficiency virus infection. Pediatr Infect Dis J 1994;13:90–94.
14. Quinn TC, Kline RL, Halsey N, et al: Early diagnosis of perinatal HIV infection by detection of viral-specific IgA antibodies. JAMA 1991;266:3439–3442.
15. Martin NL, Levy JA, Legg H, et al: Detection of infection with human immunodeficiency virus (HIV) type 1 in infants by an anti-HIV immunoglobulin A assay using recombinant proteins. J Pediatr 1991;118:354–358.
16. Weiblen BJ, Lee FK, Cooper ER, et al: Early diagnosis of HIV infection in infants by detection of IgA HIV antibodies. Lancet 1990;335:988–990.
17. Mullis K, Faloona F, Scharf S, et al: Specific enzymatic amplification of DNA in vitro: The polymerase chain reaction. Cold Spring Harb Symp Quant Biol 1986;51:263–273.
18. Saiki RK, Scharf S, Faloona F, et al: Enzymatic amplification of beta-globin genomic sequences and restriction site analysis for diagnosis of sickle cell anemia. Science 1985;230:1350–1354.
19. Kwok S, Higuchi R: Avoiding false positives with PCR. Nature 1989;339:237–238.
20. Jackson JB, Drew J, Lin HJ, et al: Establishment of a quality assurance program for human immunodeficiency virus type 1 DNA polymerase chain reaction assays by the AIDS Clinical Trials Group. ACTG PCR Working Group, and the ACTG PCR Virology Laboratories. J Clin Microbiol 1993;31:3123–3128.

21. Frenkel LM, Mullins JI, Learn GH, et al: Genetic evaluation of suspected cases of transient HIV-1 infection of infants. Science 1998;280:1073–1077.
22. Palumbo P, Skurnick J, Lewis D, Eisenberg M: PCR analysis of HIV-seronegative, heterosexual partners of HIV-infected individuals. J Acquir Immune Defic Syndr Hum Retrovirol 1995;10:436–440.
23. Rogers MF, Ou CY, Rayfield M, et al: Use of the polymerase chain reaction for early detection of the proviral sequences of human immunodeficiency virus in infants born to seropositive mothers. New York City Collaborative Study of Maternal HIV Transmission and Montefiore Medical Center HIV Perinatal Transmission Study Group. N Engl J Med 1989;320:1649–1654.
24. Laure F, Courgnaud V, Rouzioux C, et al: Detection of HIV1 DNA in infants and children by means of the polymerase chain reaction. Lancet 1988;2:538–541.
25. Ou CY, Kwok S, Mitchell SW, et al: DNA amplification for direct detection of HIV-1 in DNA of peripheral blood mononuclear cells. Science 1988;239:295–297.
26. Owens DK, Holodniy M, McDonald TW, Scott J, Sonnad S: A meta-analytic evaluation of the polymerase chain reaction for the diagnosis of HIV infection in infants. JAMA 1996;275:1342–1348.
27. Bremer JW, Lew JF, Cooper E, et al: Diagnosis of infection with human immunodeficiency virus type 1 by a DNA polymerase chain reaction assay among infants enrolled in the Women and Infants' Transmission Study. J Pediatr 1996;129:198–207.
28. Dunn DT, Brandt CD, Krivine A, et al: The sensitivity of HIV-1 DNA polymerase chain reaction in the neonatal period and the relative contributions of intra-uterine and intra-partum transmission. AIDS 1995;9:F7–11.
29. Bryson YJ, Luzuriaga K, Sullivan JL, Wara DW: Proposed definitions for in utero versus intrapartum transmission of HIV-1. N Engl J Med 1992;327:1246–1247.
30. Jackson JB, Coombs RW, Sannerud K, et al: Rapid and sensitive viral culture method for human immunodeficiency virus type 1. J Clin Microbiol 1988;26:1416–1418.
31. Alimenti A, O'Neill M, Sullivan JL, Luzuriaga K: Diagnosis of vertical human immunodeficiency virus type 1 infection by whole blood culture. J Infect Dis 1992;166:1146–1148.
32. Chun T, Stuyver L, Mizell SB, et al: Presence of an indicible HIV-1 latent reservoir during highly active antiretroviral therapy. Proc Nat Acad Sci U S A 1997;94:13193–13197.
33. Finzi D, Hermankova M, Pierson T, et al: Identification of a reservoir for HIV-1 in patients on highly active antiretroviral therapy. Science 1997;278:1295–1300.
34. Wong JK, Hezareh M, Gunthard HF, et al: Recovery of Replication-Competent HIV Despite Prolonged Suppression of Plasma Viremia. Science 1997;278:1291–1295.
35. Nishanian P, Huskins KR, Stehn S, Detels R, Fahey JL: A simple method for improved assay demonstrates that HIV p24 antigen is present as immune complexes in most sera from HIV-infected individuals. J Infect Dis 1990;162:21–28.
36. Quinn TC, Kline R, Moss MW, et al: Acid dissociation of immune complexes improves diagnostic utility of p24 antigen detection in perinatally acquired human immunodeficiency virus infection. J Infect Dis 1993;167:1193–1196.
37. Schupbach J, Boni J: Quantitative and sensitive detection of immune-complexed and free HIV antigen after boiling of serum. Virol Methods 1993;43:247–256.
38. Schupbach J, Boni J, Tomasik Z, et al: Sensitive detection and early prognostic significance of p24 antigen in heat-denatured plasma of human immunodeficiency virus type 1-infected infants. Swiss Neonatal HIV Study Group. J Infect Dis 1994;170:318–324.
39. Schupbach J, Flepp M, Pontelli D, et al: Heat-mediated immune complex dissociation and enzyme-linked immunosorbent assay signal amplification render p24 antigen detection in plasma as sensitive as HIV-1 RNA detection by polymerase chain reaction. AIDS 1996;10:1085–1090.
40. Piatak M Jr, Saag MS, Yang LC, et al: High levels of HIV-1 in plasma during all stages of infection determined by competitive PCR. Science 1993;259:1749–1754.
41. Mulder J, McKinney N, Christopherson C, et al: Rapid and simple PCR assay for quantitation of human immunodeficiency virus type 1 RNA in plasma: Application to acute retroviral infection. J Clin Microbiol 1994;32:292–300.
42. Pachl C, Todd JA, Kern DG, et al: Rapid and precise quantification of HIV-1 RNA in plasma using a branched DNA signal amplification assay. J Acquir Immune Defic Syndr Hum Retrovirol 1995;8:446–454.
43. Kievits T, van Gemen B, van Strijp D, et al: NASBA isothermal enzymatic in vitro nucleic acid amplification optimized for the diagnosis of HIV-1 infection. J Virol Methods 1991;35:273–286.
44. Lin HJ, Myers LE, Yen-Lieberman B, et al: Multicenter evaluation of quantification methods for plasma human immunodeficiency virus type 1 RNA. J Infect Dis 1994;170:553–562.
45. Yen-Lieberman B, Brambilla D, Jackson B, et al: Evaluation of a quality assurance program for quantitation of human immunodeficiency virus type 1 RNA in plasma by the AIDS Clinical Trials Group virology laboratories. J Clin Microbiol 1996;34:2695–2701.
46. Vandamme AM, Schmit JC, Van Dooren S, et al: Quantification of HIV-1 RNA in plasma: Comparable results with the NASBA HIV-1 RNA QT and the AMPLICOR HIV monitor test. J Acquir Immune Defic Syndr Hum Retrovirol 1996;13:127–139.
47. Coste J, Montes B, Reynes J, et al: Comparative evaluation of three assays for the quantitation of human

immunodeficiency virus type 1 RNA in plasma. J Med Virol 1996;50:293–302.
48. Palumbo PE, Kwok S, Waters S, et al: Viral measurement by polymerase chain reaction-based assays in human immunodeficiency virus-infected infants. J Pediatr 1995;126:592–595.
49. Steketee RW, Abrams EJ, Thea DM, et al: Early detection of perinatal human immunodeficiency virus (HIV) type 1 infection using HIV RNA amplification and detection. New York City Perinatal HIV Transmission Collaborative Study. J Infect Dis 1997;175:707–711.
50. Delamare C, Burgard M, Mayaux MJ, et al: HIV-1 RNA detection in plasma for the diagnosis of infection in neonates. The French Pediatric HIV Infection Study Group. J Acquir Immune Defic Syndr Hum Retrovirol 1997;15:121–125.
51. Cunningham CK, Charbonneau TT, Song K, et al: Comparison of human immunodeficiency virus 1 DNA polymerase chain reaction and qualitative and quantitative RNA polymerase chain reaction in human immunodeficiency virus 1-exposed infants. Pediatr Infect Dis J 1999;18:30–35.
52. Jackson JB, Piwowar EM, Parsons J, et al: Detection of human immunodeficiency virus type 1 (HIV-1) DNA and RNA sequences in HIV-1 antibody-positive blood donors in Uganda by the Roche AMPLICOR assay. J Clin Microbiol 1997;35:873–876.
53. Alaeus A, Lidman K, Sonnerborg A, Albert J: Subtype-specific problems with quantification of plasma HIV-1 RNA. AIDS 1997;11:859–865.
54. Nkengasong JN, Kalou M, Maurice C, et al: Comparison of NucliSens and Amplicor monitor assays for quantification of human immunodeficiency virus type 1 (HIV-1) RNA in plasma of persons with HIV-1 subtype A infection in Abidjan, Cote d'Ivoire. J Clin Microbiol 1998;36:2495–2498.
55. Parekh B, Phillips S, Granade TC, et al: Impact of HIV type 1 subtype variation on viral RNA quantitation. AIDS Res Hum Retroviruses 1999;15:133–142.
56. Holguin A, de Mendoza C, Soriano V: Comparison of three different commercial methods for measuring plasma viraemia in patients infected with non-B HIV-1 subtypes. Eur J Clin Microbiol Infect Dis 1999;18:256–259.
57. Alaeus A, Lilja E, Herman S, et al: Assay of plasma samples representing different HIV-1 genetic subtypes: An evaluation of new versions of the amplicor HIV-1 monitor assay. AIDS Res Hum Retroviruses 1999;15:889–894.
58. Michael NL, Herman SA, Kwok S, et al: Development of calibrated viral load standards for group M subtypes of human immunodeficiency virus type 1 and performance of an improved AMPLICOR HIV-1 MONITOR test with isolates of diverse subtypes. J Clin Microbiol 1999;37:2557–2563.
59. Pasquier C, Sandres K, Salama G, et al: Using RT-PCR and bDNA assays to measure non-clade B HIV-1 subtype RNA. J Virol Methods 1999;81:123–129.
60. Chew CB, Herring BL, Zheng F, et al: Comparison of three commercial assays for the quantification of HIV-1 RNA in plasma from individuals infected with different HIV-1 subtypes. J Clin Virol 1999;14:87–94.
61. Abravaya K, Esping C, Hoenle R, et al: Performance of a multiplex qualitative PCR LCx assay for detection of human immunodeficiency virus type 1 (HIV-1) group M subtypes, group O, and HIV-2. J Clin Microbiol 2000;38:716–723.
62. HIV Counseling and Testing Using Rapid Tests. MMWR Morbid Mortal Wkly Rep 1998;47:211–215.
63. Cassol SA, Lapoint N, Salas T, et al: Diagnosis of vertical HIV-1 transmission using the PCR and dried blood spot specimens. J Acquir Immune Defic Syndr Hum Retrovirol 1992;5:113–119.
64. Cassol S, Salas T, Gill MJ, et al: Stability of dried blood spot specimens for detection of HIV DNA by PCR. J Clin Microbiol 1992;30:3039–3042.
65. Cassol S, Butcher A, Kinard S, et al: Rapid screening for early detection of mother-to-child transmission of human immunodeficiency virus type 1. J Clin Microbiol 1994;32:2641–2645.
66. Comeau AM, Hsu HW, Schwerzler M, et al: Identifying human immunodeficiency virus infection at birth: Application of polymerase chain reaction to Guthrie cards. J Pediatr 1993;123:252–258.
67. Comeau AM, Pitt J, Hillyer GV, et al: Early detection of human immunodeficiency virus on dried blood spot specimens: Sensitivity across serial specimens. Women and Infants Transmission Study Group. J Pediatr 1996;129:111–118.
68. Comeau AM, Su X, Muchinsky G, et al: Quality-controlled pooling strategies for nucleic-acid based HIV screening: Using PCR as a primary screen on dried blood spot specimens in population studies. Paper presented at the Fifth Conference on Retroviruses and Opportunistic Infections, Chicago, Ill, 1998.
69. Cassol S, Cormier PR, Hillyer GV, et al: Dried blood spots (DBS) for monitoring HIV-1 RNA load in neonates and infants. Paper presented at the Fifth Conference on Retroviruses and Opportunistic Infections, Chicago, Ill, 1998.
70. Salomon H, Wainberg MA, Brenner B, et al: Prevalence of HIV-1 resistant to antiretroviral drugs in 81 individuals newly infected by sexual contact or injecting drug use. Investigators of the Quebec Primary Infection Study. AIDS 2000;14:F17–23.
71. Boden D, Hurley A, Zhang L, et al: HIV-1 drug resistance in newly infected individuals. JAMA 1999;282:1135–1141.
72. Yerly S, Kaiser L, Race E, et al: Transmission of antiretroviral-drug-resistant HIV-1 variants. Lancet 1999;354:729–733.
73. Little SJ, Daar ES, D'Aquila RT, et al: Reduced antiretroviral drug susceptibility among patients with primary HIV infection. JAMA 1999;282:1142–1149.
74. Welles SL, Pitt J, Colgrove R, et al: HIV-1 genotypic zidovudine drug resistance and the risk of

maternal-infant transmission in the women and infants transmission study. The Women and Infants Transmission Study Group. AIDS 2000;14:263–271.
75. Kaslow RA, Carrington M, Apple R, et al: Influence of combinations of human major histocompatibility complex genes on the course of HIV-1 infection. Nat Med 1996;2:405–411.
76. Keet IP, Tang J, Klein MR, et al: Consistent associations of HLA class I and II and transporter gene products with progression of human immunodeficiency virus type 1 infection in homosexual men. J Infect Dis 1999;180:299–309.
77. MacDonald KS, Embree J, Njenga S, et al: Mother-child class I HLA concordance increases perinatal human immunodeficiency virus type 1 transmission. J Infect Dis 1998;177:551–556.
78. Mann DL, Garner RP, Dayhoff DE, et al: Major histocompatibility complex genotype is associated with disease progression and virus load levels in a cohort of human immunodeficiency virus type 1-infected Caucasians and African Americans. J Infect Dis 1998;178:1799–1802.
79. Carrington M, Nelson GW, Martin MP, et al: HLA and HIV-1: Heterozygote advantage and B*35-Cw*04 disadvantage. Science 1999;283:1748–1752.
80. Kostrikis LG, Neumann AU, Thomson B, et al: A polymorphism in the regulatory region of the CC-chemokine receptor 5 gene influences perinatal transmission of human immunodeficiency virus type 1 to African-American infants. J Virol 1999;73: 10264–10271.
81. Kostrikis LG, Huang Y, Moore JP, et al: A chemokine receptor CCR2 allele delays HIV-1 disease progression and is associated with a CCR5 promoter mutation. Nat Med 1998;4:350–353.
82. Misrahi M, Teglas JP, N'Go N, et al: CCR5 chemokine receptor variant in HIV-1 mother-to-child transmission and disease progression in children. French Pediatric HIV Infection Study Group. JAMA 1998; 279:277–280.
83. Smith MW, Dean M, Carrington M, et al: Contrasting genetic influence of CCR2 and CCR5 variants on HIV-1 infection and disease progression. Hemophilia Growth and Development Study (HGDS), Multicenter AIDS Cohort Study (MACS), Multicenter Hemophilia Cohort Study (MHCS), San Francisco City Cohort (SFCC), ALIVE Study. Science 1997;277:959–965.
84. Liu H, Chao D, Nakayama EE, et al: Polymorphism in RANTES chemokine promoter affects HIV-1 disease progression. Proc Natl Acad Sci U S A 1999;96: 4581–4585.
85. Winkler C, Modi W, Smith MW, et al: Genetic restriction of AIDS pathogenesis by an SDF-1 chemokine gene variant: ALIVE Study, Hemophilia Growth and Development Study (HGDS), Multicenter AIDS Cohort Study (MACS), Multicenter Hemophilia Cohort Study (MHCS), San Francisco City Cohort (SFCC). Science 1998;279:389–393.

7

Prophylactic Antiretroviral Treatment of HIV Infection in Neonates

Ross McKinney

The use of perinatal antiretroviral prophylaxis has profoundly affected the state of the HIV epidemic in children in the United States. Whereas infants born to an HIV-infected woman once had a 25% to 30% chance of being infected themselves, that proportion has been decreased dramatically through the use of antiretroviral therapy in the mother and infant. The combination of aggressive antiretroviral therapy in the pregnant woman, cesarean section in some cases, and neonatal antiretroviral therapy may be able to reduce the transmission rates to nearly zero. In fact, the largest barrier to achieving the theoretically achievable near-zero transmission rate has been women who are not recognized to be HIV infected antenatally. The failures in recognition occur both because some women do not present for prenatal care, and because some physicians do not uniformly offer screening for HIV infection to pregnant women.

This chapter discusses the theoretical concepts behind perinatal prophylaxis and early treatment and considers data from clinical trials performed to date.

THEORETICAL BASIS OF PERINATAL PROPHYLAXIS

There is no doubt that perinatal antiretroviral prophylaxis works, which is fortunate, since there are still many questions surrounding the mechanisms by which HIV is transmitted from mother to infant. In particular, there are many unresolved questions about the means by which the virus moves from the mother to the child, both in utero and intrapartum.

To begin at a cellular level, HIV initiates infection through the attachment of gp120 to the CD4 molecule on the surface of a susceptible T cell or monocyte/macrophage. Secondary attachment to one of the chemokine receptors (CXCR4 or CCR5) ensues, and the virus fuses with the cell surface. Once intracellular, the viral capsid releases the two virus RNA strands and their attached reverse transcriptase enzymes into the cytoplasm, and transcription of a DNA copy off the RNA template begins. After the DNA copies are complete, they are carried to the cell nucleus, where they are integrated into the host chromosome. At that point, the cell is permanently HIV infected, and any intervention that is given will be to affect an already infected cell, rather than to prevent infection. Protease inhibitors act to inhibit the processing of proteins synthesized off RNA transcripts from the integrated proviral DNA. As a class of drugs, they may be important to limit the contagiousness of an already infected cell, as well as to decrease the amount of virus circulating in a pregnant women's blood and by so doing reduce neonatal exposure, but they are not truly useful as prophylaxis at an individual cellular level.

There are several steps in the virus life cycle at which intervention is theoretically possible, and attempts have been made to intervene at several of those critical points (Fig. 7–1). The first critical step is virus attachment. This step can be ablated in vitro through the use of neutralizing antibodies against HIV. Another antiattachment strategy is the use of

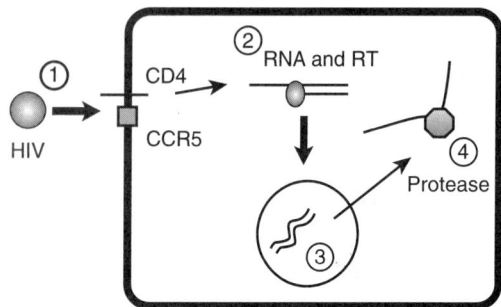

Figure 7–1. Potential prophylactic interventions at a cellular level. This figure depicts a CD4 positive lymphocyte and steps at which intervention against HIV infection could take place. (1) Blockage of the attachment and entry of HIV. Potential therapies include monoclonal antibodies to gp120 and CD4, chemokine inhibitors, and fusion inhibitors; (2) interference with reverse transcription of the viral RNA; (3) blockage of integration of virus into host DNA or transcriptional regulation (still theoretical); (4) protease inhibitor therapy to block assembly and release of new viral particles.

soluble CD4+ molecules, which, if given in sufficient quantity, could saturate the gp120 virus attachment proteins before they are able to latch on to cellular CD4+ molecules. Unfortunately, intravenous immunoglobulin with high neutralization titers against HIV was not able to affect perinatal transmission rates, particularly when coadministered with antiretroviral therapy (PACTG Study 185).[1] Soluble CD4+ had inadequate activity as a therapeutic agent, and development was stopped. The most recently developed drug with an effect on virus attachment and entry is T-20, a small peptide that is able to inhibit fusion of the virus envelope with the cell membrane, and thus to inhibit virus entry. It has not been studied in perinatal transmission models yet.

After the reverse transcriptase makes a single-stranded DNA copy of the virus RNA, the RNA is cleaved off the new DNA template. As noted earlier, once the DNA provirus is integrated, the cell (and host) is infected. Reverse transcriptase inhibitors can work at the level of transcriptional initiation (the non-nucleoside reverse transcriptase inhibitors) or at the DNA elongation step (nucleoside reverse transcriptase inhibitors). Both categories have been shown to be effective as prophylactic agents.

Although it has not been proved, it seems probable that the reverse transcriptase inhibitors are effective, in part, because they slow the process of reverse transcription. The cellular cytoplasm has many RNAses, which degrade RNA molecules. These RNAses will destroy the HIV RNA if it is not transcribed within a short time frame. Anything that delays RNA transcription increases the probability that the RNA will be destroyed before being copied.

In animal model systems, the most prophylactically effective reverse transcriptase inhibitors have been nucleotides rather than nucleosides. Cellular enzymes must phosphorylate nucleosides, such as zidovudine or lamivudine, for the drugs to be active. In contrast, nucleotides such as PMPA and adefovir dipivoxil are already phosphorylated and thus more swiftly able to be active. This property is probably most important around a single HIV exposure, when speed of activity is most essential.

Once there is integration of the proviral DNA, the cell is infected. There may be a minor role for protease inhibitors in slowing the process of spread of HIV from one cell to the next, or perhaps in limiting the infectivity of maternal cells (if a cellular mechanism is responsible for perinatal transmission). The major role of the protease inhibitors is on the maternal side, in decreasing the maternal viral load. Limitation of infection at a cellular level is more likely to be affected by reverse transcriptase inhibitors than protease inhibitors.

The elements of successful prophylaxis can be considered from both the cellular level and the organism level. Optimal prophylaxis includes decreasing the quantity of maternal virus and hence the degree of exposure of the infant. In regard to the infant, the ideal is to maintain therapeutic antiretroviral drug levels in utero, to have an adequate level at the time of delivery, and to maintain therapeutic concentrations for the first few weeks of life. To accomplish these goals, studies of antiretroviral pharmacokinetics are necessary in pregnant women, since pregnancy may have effects on clearance mechanisms and the volume of distribution of a drug.

Questions about in utero drug levels cannot be answered directly in infants, since sampling through the placenta would introduce the possibility of infecting the infant through introduction of maternal blood. Simian models are probably the best system available to answer questions about in utero pharmacokinetics. Several studies have been done on newborn infants to answer questions about drug levels immediately after delivery. Those will be considered later in this chapter.

ANIMAL MODELS OF EARLY ANTIRETROVIRAL TREATMENT

The primary animal model for vertical transmission of HIV has been the use of simian immunodeficiency virus (SIV) in rhesus macaques. The animals can be virus infected either through an oral or subcutaneous route. SIV is not identical to HIV and so is not a precise mimic. For example, there is very little vertical transmission of SIV from the mother macaque to her infant, which is the reason artificial inoculation is required. To further emulate the biology of HIV, chimeras composed of elements of HIV and SIV, referred to as SHIVs, have been constructed and used in animal model studies. The macaque system has the advantage that it can be studied very carefully, and the animals have a complete AIDS-like disease, including development of immunodeficiency. The largest disadvantages are the scarcity and expense of primates like macaques. The number of subjects studied is always small, and statistical conclusions can rarely be drawn.

The simian model has proved to be useful. As an example, the prophylactic and therapeutic effects of zidovudine (ZDV) were tested in an SIV-rhesus macaque model prior to the publication of the ACTG 076 trial.[2] Four 3-month-old macaques were inoculated with SIVmac (macaque SIV), then treated with 50 mg/kg of zidovudine every 8 hours. Two animals were treated 2 hours before inoculation, two not until 6 weeks later. All animals were given ZDV for 6 to 10 weeks. The two pretreated macaques did not get infected, the two treated later did. In the latter two monkeys, the ZDV had no obvious effect on the course.

In addition to prevention of transmission, the other important theme of simian research has been the question of whether treatment soon after infection is beneficial in the long term. This question is difficult to answer in patients, given the infrequency with which the time of infection is known and the inability to intervene around that time point. However, macaques are nearly ideal for this type of investigation. For example, Martin and coworkers[3] began ZDV 1, 8, 24, or 72 hours after inoculating animals with SIV. Treatments were continued for 28 days, and findings were compared with those from control subjects. Animals treated earlier had a delayed development of persistent antigenemia and slower progression in CD4+ decline. This model is very relevant to pediatrics, since the one human situation in which the time of infection is known with some certainty is vertical transmission. A similar theme in pediatric research has been the question of early, aggressive antiretroviral treatment and whether that approach can lead to long-term benefits for the child.

One class of drugs, the nucleotide reverse transcriptase inhibitors (PMPA, PMEA, and adefovir dipivoxil), has shown particularly great potential as prophylactic agents in macaque models. PMPA has been demonstrated to be effective when therapy is begun 48 hours before, 4 hours before, 4 hours after, and 24 hours after SIV inoculation. All control animals were infected, whereas none of the PMPA-treated ones were.[4]

Further refinements of the PMPA system in macaques have shown that even two doses of PMPA may be sufficient for prophylaxis.[5] Eight newborn macaques were inoculated orally with SIV within 3 days of life. Four animals were given PMPA 4 hours before the SIV inoculation and a second dose 24 hours later. The other animals were untreated. The control animals became infected; the PMPA-treated animals did not.

The macaque model has also been used to compare treatment regimens. Macaques were given either ZDV or PMEA.[6] The investigators began the treatment before inoculation with SIV and continued it for 4 weeks. PMEA was able to prevent acute SIV infection, and ZDV-treated animals had a decrease in virus load. Unfortunately, there have been some concerns about toxicities with the nucleotide analogues, so their development has been slowed.

CLINICAL EXPERIENCE OF PERINATAL ANTIRETROVIRAL TREATMENT

Several different strategies have been tried to decrease the rate of mother-to-infant HIV transmission, and only one of these has clearly succeeded. Two different approaches to blocking entry of the virus have failed—HIV-specific immunoglobulin and soluble CD4—as did an attempt to block transmission through the use of chlorhexidine vaginal washes. Vaccines have yet to establish efficacy, and only the use of reverse transcriptase inhibitors has been demonstrated to work.

To review historically, the suggestion that zidovudine treatment of the pregnant woman and child should be attempted was initially made by Dr. Catherine Wilfert at a Surgeon General's Meeting on HIV transmission. From the beginning, the concept of giving a pregnant woman anti-HIV therapy was very controversial, given the lack of proven benefit and the potential for harmful effects to the growing fetus. Nevertheless, the pediatric component of the AIDS Clinical Trials Group organized ACTG 076, a placebo-controlled study of zidovudine administered to the mother during pregnancy and labor and then to the infant after birth. ACTG study 049 was performed in preparation for ACTG 076 and consisted of a pharmacokinetic evaluation of intravenous and oral zidovudine in infants.[7] ACTG 049 included 32 symptom-free infants younger than 3 months of age born to HIV-infected women. Seven of the 32 infants ultimately proved to be infected. Each infant received a single intravenous dose of ZDV, then 4 to 6 weeks of oral drug. Clearance of ZDV increased with age (from 10.9 mL/min/kg in young infants to 19.0 mL/min/kg in older infants), producing a shorter serum half-life in the older infants. In contrast, bioavailability decreased with age. The ultimate recommendation was for oral dosing of 2 mg/kg every 6 hours for infants less than 2 weeks old, and 3 mg/kg for infants older than 2 weeks.

Another important preparatory step was to evaluate ZDV pharmacokinetics in pregnant women.[8–10] From these studies, it became clear that ZDV could be used safely in pregnant women, at least short term, and that ZDV crossed the placenta well. Thus, ZDV is present in the infant during the birth process if the mother has been adherent with her ZDV regimen or treated intravenously.

ACTG 076 enrolled patients between April 1991 and December 1993. The study took a "best shot" approach, which is to say that it was believed that the use of zidovudine during pregnancy, labor, and after delivery provided the optimal chance of showing a difference between the transmission rates in treated and untreated pregnancies. Consideration was given to a factorial design (an independent randomization of the in utero strategy and the postnatal strategy), but this was discarded in order to be certain that some strategy worked. ZDV was given to pregnant women at a dose of 100 mg every 4 hours, five times a day (the night dose was to be skipped). In retrospect, this was an incredibly difficult schedule, and very few women are likely to have achieved high-level adherence. Because there were concerns about gastric emptying, during labor ZDV was infused intravenously. The intravenous dose was an initial 2 mg/kg bolus, followed by a continuous infusion of 1 mg/kg/hr thereafter. Finally, the infants were treated with 2 mg/kg every 6 hours for 6 weeks, beginning 8 to 12 hours after birth.

The success of PACTG 076 was profound and, at the time, quite surprising. Four hundred infants were considered in the final study analysis, 200 of whom received ZDV, 200 of whom received placebo. The only significant problem was transient anemia in the newborns, which resolved after conclusion of the 6-week neonatal treatment regimen. The benefits were in prevention of transmission. The transmission rate in the placebo recipients was 27.5% (95% CI, 21.2–34.1%), for the ZDV patients 7.9% (95% CI, 4.1–11.7%). The difference was highly statistically significant ($P < .001$), and the study was stopped before its planned duration because of the positive effect.

The success of PACTG 076 provoked consideration of several important possibilities. The first new goal was to improve on the regimen, increasing the proportion of children protected. The second was to simplify the regimen, if possible, since the scheme was expensive, complicated, and clearly beyond the resources available in the developing world, where most vertical HIV transmission occurs. Third was to isolate those variables that predicted success or failure in regard to prevention of transmission, and to use that knowledge to improve the understanding of the pathogenesis of transmission.

Evaluation of laboratory data and outcomes from PACTG 076 demonstrated that the most significant risk factor for transmission was the maternal viral load.[11] Among women who were not ZDV treated, the highest quartile for HIV-1 RNA at study entry had a 42% transmission rate. In contrast, the same quartile of ZDV-treated women had a transmission rate of 13%. At all levels of viral load, ZDV had a beneficial effect on transmission rates. Infection rates were also higher with lower maternal CD4+ counts, with a 41% transmission rate in placebo-treated mothers with 200 to 349 CD4+ cells, versus a 9.7% rate in ZDV-treated women with the same CD4+ counts.

All analyses of factors affecting transmission in PACTG 076 were constrained by the very small number of HIV-infected infants in the ZDV-treated group (15 infants). Nevertheless, in a multivariate analysis, the only factor that could be identified as affecting transmission rates in the ZDV treatment group is mother's pretreatment viral load. In the untreated group, CD4+ cell counts were also significant.

On the basis of the PACTG 076 results, a firm recommendation was made, and is still made, that the mother should receive ZDV as perinatal prophylaxis regardless of her viral load.[12] This guideline may be adapted if the mother cannot tolerate ZDV, or if she is on stavudine (since ZDV and stavudine are mutually inhibitory). In addition, current investigations point toward the use of combination therapies, and the critical nature of ZDV itself relative to other aspects of antiretroviral therapy is not known.

In regard to improving the prophylactic regimen, prospective trials have been performed in the United States, Europe, Africa, and Asia. The next large trial performed in the United States, PACTG 185, evaluated the effect of supplementing the PACTG 076 regimen with regular infusions of human immunoglobulin chosen for their high titers of anti-HIV neutralizing antibodies (HIVIg).[13] The comparison was standard intravenous immunoglobulin. The study was performed in women with relatively advanced HIV disease, with CD4+ counts of less than 500/µL (22% <200/µL) and many with previous experience with ZDV. In both study arms, the rate of transmission was approximately 5%, and no effect of HIVIg could be ascertained. Women with lower CD4+ counts at entry had higher transmission rates: 10% transmission for women with CD4+ counts less than 200/µL, 3.6% for women with counts of 200/µL or greater.

Data from ongoing studies such as PACTG 247 suggest that the current transmission rates may be even lower, roughly 2% to 3%, among women who are identified and offered treatment (personal communication). This low rate makes it very difficult to design clinical trials in the United States or Europe to evaluate better treatments if transmission rate is the critical variable. One large efficacy trial, PACTG 316, evaluated the effect of adding one dose of maternal and one dose of infant nevirapine to whatever regimen the mother is taking. However, despite the large sample population in the study, it lacked the statistical power needed to ascertain a difference between the regimens. In addition, a large proportion of the transmissions occurred in utero, a point before perinatal prophylaxis would have been started.

Most prospective studies of efficacy will need to be performed in countries where the transmission rates are higher than in the United States or Europe. There are difficult ethical issues in performing research on therapies that may not ultimately be available in that country.[14, 15] In addition, there is the thorny problem of using a comparative strategy that is less than state of the art, even if the state of the art will never be available in a country because of cost or complexity.

One alternative approach to evaluating less than the complete PACTG 076 regimen is to perform a retrospective analysis. Two large retrospective studies have been reported, from New York and North Carolina.[16,17] In the New York study, 939 HIV-exposed infants were assessed.[16] When prophylactic treatment was begun prenatally, the transmission rate was 6.1%. When started intrapartum, the rate was 10.0%. If ZDV was started in the infant within 48 hours of delivery, the transmission rate was 9.3%. However, if ZDV was not started until after 48 hours, the transmission rate jumped to 18.4%, and in the absence of prophylaxis, to 26.6%.

The experience in North Carolina was similar to that in New York.[17] The study evaluated data from 568 HIV-exposed infants. The transmission rate if all three prophylactic steps were taken (prenatal, intrapartum, postpartum) was only 3.1%. Without the intrapartum infusion, the rate was similar at 2.9%. If only prenatal and intrapartum ZDV was used, the rate was 5%. With intrapartum and postpartum ZDV, the rate was 10.7%. Neonatal ZDV alone (used in only 15 children) led to a transmission rate of 26.7%, but there were wide 95% confidence intervals (7.8–55%). Finally, among women and infants who did not receive prophylaxis at all, the transmission rate was 30.9%.

Allowing for the small sample in the postnatal-only group in North Carolina, the trends are similar. ZDV prophylaxis seems to be most effective when the entire regimen is followed, but ZDV given shortly after birth probably still has a beneficial effect.

Several important studies of more limited regimens have been completed in Asia and Africa. The first important study was performed in Thailand, where non-breastfeeding HIV-infected women were given ZDV (300 mg orally twice daily) beginning at the 36th week of gestation and during labor (300 mg every 3 hours). Infants were not treated.[18] Transmission decreased from 19% in the placebo group to 9% in the ZDV group.

Several studies in Africa have further clarified shorter courses of perinatal prophylaxis. The PETRA study involved breastfeeding HIV-infected women.[19,20] Combination ZDV/lamivudine (3TC) was administered in different patterns to women and infants, as shown in Table 7–1. The results of PETRA are remarkable for several reasons. First, short-course ZDV/3TC, beginning at the onset of labor, without infant ZDV/3TC, had no apparent utility. In contrast, the same short course when paired with 7 days of postpartum ZDV/3TC (maternal and infant) appears to have provided benefit. There may have been a slight further gain by beginning maternal treatment at the 36th week of gestation, but in this study that gain was not very big.

Table 7–1
PETRA Trials of Three Approaches to Perinatal Prophylaxis Using Zidovudine and Lamivudine

MOTHER'S SCHEDULE	INFANT'S SCHEDULE	TRANSMISSION RATE, % (RISK REDUCTION RELATIVE TO PLACEBO, %)
Week 36 of gestation to 1 week postpartum	7 days	8.6 (-50)
Onset of labor to 1 week postpartum	7 days	10.8 (-37)
Onset of labor to delivery	None	17.7 (+3)
Placebo	None	17.2

The other important lesson from PETRA was the critical need for valid comparison arms. As noted earlier, there has been considerable controversy regarding whether to perform antiretroviral trials in underdeveloped nations, and then whether to include placebo controls. Had PETRA been done using historical controls, the predicted transmission rate would probably have been between 25% and 40%. As the study evolved, the transmission rate in the placebo arm was an unusually low 17.2%. This value is sufficiently different from that of historical controls that it would have been interpreted as a therapeutic success, although in reality there was little effect. In the case of the placebo, there is no chance that this result would have been confused with a real but less successful regimen, but in the case of short-course ZDV/3TC alone it might have been. Thus, valid controls remain a critical part of studies in the evolving nature of clinical practice.

The simplest strategy to date for perinatal prophylaxis has been the use of a single dose of nevirapine in the mother, one dose in the infant, as used in HIVNET 012.[21] This study, performed in breast-feeding women in Uganda, used a single 200 mg oral dose of nevirapine at the onset of labor. Nevirapine has a long half-life and induces its own metabolism, and as result the first dose is able to maintain serum concentrations through the duration of most women's labor. Babies were given 2 mg/kg of nevirapine at 48 to 72 hours of life. This simple two-dose regimen was compared to a short regimen of ZDV given during labor and for 1 week to the infant. While this control ZDV regimen appears similar to arms 2 and 3 of the PETRA Trial (see Table 7–1), the efficacy was not ideal, with a transmission rate of 21%. The nevirapine arm was more successful, with 12% transmission, an almost 50% reduction.

Two important advantages of nevirapine are its low cost and its relative safety. It can be administered to women over the short term with little likelihood of a serious reaction. This is very important, since in most African countries the cost of screening for HIV infection is greater than the price would be for universal administration of nevirapine in pregnancy. In addition, many women would prefer not to know their HIV status, since no effective treatments are available. However, it has been reported that nevirapine resistance mutations (K103N) can be selected after as little as a single dose of the drug.[22] This may have implications both for the care of HIV-infected women given nevirapine if antiviral drugs ever do become available, and for the effectiveness of subsequent rounds of prophylaxis. In addition, women with resistant virus may transmit it to their sexual partners, generally decreasing the community-wide effectiveness of nevirapine and other non-nucleoside reverse transcriptase inhibitors.

UNRESOLVED ISSUES

The standard of care for pregnant women infected with HIV is to use combination regimens to optimize reduction in viral load. In general, protease inhibitors appear to be safe during pregnancy, and so are used routinely. The non-nucleoside reverse transcriptase inhibitors are used more often late in pregnancy, owing to concerns about either severe rashes (nevirapine) or birth defects such as those seen when pregnant macaques were treated with efavirenz. Nucleoside reverse transcriptase inhibitors have generally been considered safe, but there have been reports of profound mitochondrial dysfunction, even after limited exposure to nucleoside reverse transcriptase inhibitors.

The initial reports of mitochondrial problems came from France.[23] A group of eight uninfected infants were exposed to nucleoside analogues in utero or perinatally. Two infants developed severe neurologic disease, thought to be related to mitochondrial dysfunction, and died. It is known that the nucleoside analogues inhibit the mitochondrial gamma DNA polymerase. This property can result in mitochondrial DNA depletion and dysfunction.[12, 24] Thus, the French clinical observations have pathophysiologic correlates. However, a review of several combined databases, including that of the Pediatric AIDS Clinical Trials Group, accumulated information on 353 deaths among 20,000 children who may have been exposed to antiretroviral drugs. There were no deaths that appeared to be mitochondrial in origin. However, the issue continues to be evaluated. If the mitochondrial issue turns out to be a real problem, unless the incidence is very high, it would still be outweighed by the benefits of preventing vertical HIV transmission. At some point, selection of drugs that minimize mitochondrial problems might be advantageous, as long as they are therapeutically efficacious.

Transmission of antiretroviral resistant virus is another unresolved problem that provides more challenges than current data can resolve. There have been numerous reports of resistant virus being transmitted from mother to child. In one case, reported by Johnson and coworkers, a neonate's virus was demonstrably resistant to nearly all antiretroviral drugs, probably as a result of her mother's intermittent adherence and sequential monotherapy over several years.[25] In the Woman and Infants Treatment Study (WITS), isolates from 85 HIV-infected infants born between 1989 and 1994 were studied.[26] Twenty-six infants were exposed to ZDV in utero. Fifty-three percent of the infants (45/85) had isolates with at least one ZDV resistance mutation. Of those isolates, 80% had mutations at codon 215, associated with high-level ZDV resistance. Twenty-nine percent had mutations at four or more resistance-associated sites. In short, the level of resistance is high enough that the era of simple monotherapy for perinatal prophylaxis appears to have passed.

Another unresolved issue is breastfeeding. Breastfeeding contributes a significant risk of HIV infection above that of perinatal and in utero transmission. In the United States, very few HIV-infected women breastfeed, so the issue has not been pressing. However, in much of the world, particularly Africa, breastfeeding is the norm, and there is thus a prolonged period of HIV risk. No studies yet address an adequate strategy to prevent transmission in this situation, although suppressing the mother's viral load as far as possible is probably the only achievable goal. It might also be possible to use nevirapine in a prolonged fashion in the at-risk infant, since it has a long half-life and resistance will not develop in the uninfected infant. As long as the mother's virus does not develop non-nucleoside reverse transcriptase inhibitor resistance, nevirapine could work to inhibit transmission to the infant.

PHARMACOKINETICS AND DOSING OF DRUGS USED IN PERINATAL PROPHYLAXIS

There is relatively little information about the dosing of antiretroviral drugs in the perinatal period, particularly for premature infants. Immaturity of the kidneys and liver decreases drug clearance for most agents, prolonging the serum half-live, and a relatively neutral gastric pH means that some drugs are not well absorbed. Since it is critical for prophylaxis that drug concentrations be in the therapeutic range, more research is urgently needed in this area. However, neonatal pharmacology is difficult, with constraints including limited blood volumes, problems in vascular access for blood sampling, and rapidly changing metabolic capabilities. Guidelines for neonatal and perinatal drug dosing are provided in a regularly updated form by the AIDS Clinical Trials Information Service at *www.hivatis.org*

The best established dosing is for zidovudine. ZDV clearance in children is slow because of immature glucuronidation. As a result, the neonatal half-life is longer, and dosing is downwardly adjusted. Dosing guidelines are presented in Table 7–2. In premature infants, the liver is even more immature, so smaller doses are given, farther apart in time.

Lamivudine (3TC) also has fairly well established dosing in newborns. As with ZDV, clearance is delayed, so the dosage is reduced. In this case, the neonatal 3TC dose is half the dose in older children.

Nevirapine pharmacokinetics in newborns have also been studied. Nevirapine autoinduces its own metabolism, and so the initial dose always has a prolonged half-life. Since neonatal enzyme systems are immature, its half-life is particularly prolonged in newborns. A single dose may provide several days' worth of drug in the therapeutic range. However, with repeated dosing the half-life becomes shorter, and the dosing needs to increase in amount and frequency.

There are very little data on any of the protease inhibitors in children younger than 3 months of age

Table 7–2
Neonatal Antiretroviral Medication Doses

DRUG	AGE GROUP	DOSING SCHEDULE	COMMENTS
Zidovudine (ZDV)	Premature (<34 weeks)	1.5 mg/kg/q12h for 2 weeks, then 2 mg/kg q8h age 2–8 weeks	Dosing based on preliminary information. Full studies pending.[28]
	Newborn	2 mg/kg q6h or 3 mg/kg q8h	q8h schedule is not proved.
Lamivudine (3TC)	<30 days	2 mg/kg bid	Dose doubles after 30 days old to 4 mg/kg bid.
Abacavir (ABC)	1–3 months	8 mg/kg/dose bid	Dosing preliminary: still under study.
Didanosine (ddI)	<90 days	50 mg/m²/dose q12h	Hard to assess toxicity in newborns.
Stavudine (d4T)	N/A	No information yet	ZDV and d4T interact unfavorably: do not use both simultaneously.
Zalcitabine (ddC)	N/A	No information	No liquid preparation.
Efavirenz (EFZ)	N/A	No information	
Nevirapine (NVP)	<3 months	5 mg/kg qd × 14 days, 120 mg/m² q12 × 114 days, then 200 mg/m² q12h	The latter two steps are standard pediatric dosing. The 5 mg/kg/day dose is unique to infants.
Amprenavir (AMP)	N/A	No information	Formulation not suitable for children <3 years old.
Indinavir (IDV)	N/A	No information	Since IDV can produce hyperbilirubinemia, it is not suitable for infants.
Nelfinavir (NLV)	Uncertain	40 mg/kg/dose bid	Data are only preliminary.
Ritonavir	N/A	No information	ACTG Study 354 will evaluate.
Saquinavir	N/A	No information	No liquid formulation.

Adapted from ATIS Guidelines.[27]

REFERENCES

1. Stiehm ER, Lambert JS, Mofenson LM, et al: Efficacy of zidovudine and human immunodeficiency virus (HIV) hyperimmune immunoglobulin for reducing perinatal HIV transmission from HIV-infected women with advanced disease: Results of Pediatric AIDS Clinical Trials Group protocol 185. J Infect Dis 1999;179:567–575.
2. Von Rompay KK, Marthas ML, Ramos RA, et al: Simian immunodeficiency virus (SIV) infection of infant rhesus macaques as a model to test antiretroviral drug prophylaxis and therapy: Oral 3′-azido-3′-deoxythymidine prevents SIV infection. Antimicrob Agents Chemother 1992;36:2381–2386.
3. Martin LN, Murphey-Corb M, Soike KF, et al: Effects of initiation of 3′-azido,3′-deoxythymidine (zidovudine) treatment at different times after infection of rhesus monkeys with simian immunodeficiency virus. J Infect Dis 1993;168:825–835.
4. Tsai CC, Follis KE, Sabo A, et al: Prevention of SIV infection in macaques by (R)-9-(2-phosphonylmethoxypropyl)adenine. Science 1995;270:1121–1122.
5. Van Rompay KK, Berardi CJ, Aguirre NNL, et al: Two doses of PMPA protect newborn macaques against oral simian immunodeficiency virus infection. AIDS 1998;12:F79–83.
6. Tsai CC, Follis KE, Grant R, et al: Comparison of the efficacy of AZT and PMEA treatment against acute SIVmne infection in macaques. J Med Primatol 1994;23:175–183.
7. Boucher FD, Modlin JA, Ruff A, et al: A phase I evaluation of zidovudine administered to infants exposed at birth to the human immunodeficiency virus. J Pediatr 1993;122:137–144.
8. Sperling RS, Roboz J, Dische R, et al: Zidovudine pharmacokinetics during pregnancy. Am J Perinatol 1992;9:247–249.
9. Watts DH, Brown ZA, Tartaglione T, et al: Pharmacokinetic disposition of zidovudine during pregnancy. J Infect Dis 1991;163:226–232.

10. O'Sullivan MJ, Boyer PJ, Scott GB, et al: The pharmacokinetics and safety of zidovudine in the third trimester of pregnancy for women infected with human immunodeficiency virus and their infants: Phase I Acquired Immunodeficiency Syndrome Clinical Trials Group Study (Protocol 082). Am J Obstet Gynecol 1993;168:1510–1516.

11. Sperling RS, Shapiro DE, Coombs RW, et al for the Pediatric AIDS Clinical Trials Group Protocol 076 Study Group: Maternal viral load, zidovudine treatment, and the risk of transmission of human immunodeficiency virus type 1 from mother to infant. N Engl J Med 1996;335:1621–1629.

12. Perinatal HIV Guidelines Working Group: U.S. Public Health Service Task Force recommendations for the use of antiretroviral drugs in pregnant women infected with HIV-1 for maternal health and for reducing perinatal HIV-1 transmission in the United States. http://hivatis.org/guidelines/perinatal/Perintal Feb2500.pdf

13. Stiehm ER, Lambert JS, Mofenson LM, et al: Pediatric AIDS Clinical Trials Group Protocol 185 Team. J Infect Dis 1999;179:567–575.

14. Lurie P, Wolfe SM: Unethical trials of interventions to reduce perinatal transmission of the human immunodeficiency virus in developing countries. N Engl J Med 1997;337:853–856.

15. Wilfert CM, Fleming T: Perinatal transmission—successful interventions: Where do we go from here? Int J STD AIDS 1998;9(Suppl 1):22–27.

16. Wade NA, Birkhead GS, Warren BL, et al: Abbreviated regimens of zidovudine prophylaxis and perinatal transmission of the human immunodeficiency virus. N Engl J Med 1998;339:1409–1414.

17. Fiscus SA, Adimora AA, Schoenbach VJ, et al: Trends in human immunodeficiency virus (HIV) counseling, testing, and antiretroviral treatment of HIV-infected women and perinatal transmission in North Carolina. J Infect Dis 1999;180:99–105.

18. Shaffer N, Chuachoowong R, Mock PA, et al: Short-course zidovudine for perinatal HIV-1 transmission in Bangkok, Thailand: a randomized controlled trial. Lancet 1999;353:773–780.

19. Kaiser J: Cheap treatment cuts HIV transmission. Science 1999;283:916–917.

20. Saba J, Petra Trial Study Team: Interim analysis of early efficacy of three short ZDV/3TC combination regimens to prevent mother-to-child transmission of HIV-1: The PETRA Trial. Paper presented at the Sixth Conference on Retroviruses and Opportunistic Infections (Abstract S-7), Chicago, Ill, January 1999, p. 212.

21. Guay LA, Musoke P, Fleming T, et al: Intrapartum and neonatal single-dose nevirapine compared with zidovudine for prevention of mother-to-child transmission of HIV-1 in Kampala, Uganda: HIVNET 012 randomised trial. Lancet 1999;354:795–802.

22. Becker-Pergola G, Guay LL, Mmiro F, et al: Selection of the K103N nevirapine resistance mutation in Ugandan women receiving NVP prophylaxis to prevent HIV-1 vertical transmission (HIVNET-006). In Program and Abstracts of the Seventh Conference on Retroviruses and Opportunistic Infections [Abstract 658], San Francisco, January 30–February 2, 2000.

23. Blanche S, Tardieu M, Rustin P, et al: Persistent mitochondrial dysfunction and perinatal exposure to antiretroviral nucleoside analogues. Lancet 1999; 354:1084–1089.

24. Brinkman K, Ter Hofstede HJM, Burger DM, et al: Adverse effects of reverse transcriptase inhibitors: Mitochondrial toxicity as a common pathway. AIDS 1998;12:1734–1744.

25. Johnson VA, Woods C, Hamilton CD, Fiscus SA: Vertical transmission of an HIV-1 variant resistant to multiple reverse transcriptase and protease inhibitors (Abstract 266). In Program and Abstracts of the 6th Conference on Retroviruses and Opportunistic Infections, Chicago, Ill, Jan 31–Feb 4, 1999, p. 118.

26. Colgrove R, Pitt J, Japour A, Welles S: Zidovudine resistance after vertical transmission of HIV-1 (Abstract 265). In Program and Abstracts of the 6th Conference on Retroviruses and Opportunistic Infections, Chicago, Ill, Jan 31–Feb 4, 1999, p. 118.

Treatment and Virologic Monitoring of Primary HIV-1 Infection in Children

Stephen A. Spector

Treatment of infants and children perinatally infected with HIV-1 presents unique opportunities and challenges. Because in nonbreastfeeding populations the timing of primary infection is known to be either in utero or intrapartum, initial therapy for the perinatally infected infant recognized shortly after birth is in many ways similar to the identification and treatment of adults with primary infection. In contrast, the child who is untreated beyond the first year or two of age is past the time of the most rapid disease progression and may not require the same level of intensive therapy as the newly identified infected infant.

GENERAL PRINCIPLES FOR APPROACHING ANTIRETROVIRAL THERAPY

Treatment and management of the HIV-infected child have become increasingly complex. Therefore, whenever possible, the management of the infected child should be by or in consultation with a multidisciplinary team that specializes in the care of HIV-infected children. Issues associated with adherence are important considerations when deciding when and with what drugs treatment should be initiated. Antiretroviral therapy has the highest likelihood for success when given to antiretroviral-naive children. The development of antiretroviral resistance is a common problem and can have a significant impact on future antiretroviral options and treatment success. Treatment should be considered in the context of a continuum of care, of which the antiretrovirals selected must be supported by a multidisciplinary team that can help the patient and family manage daily therapy by providing the necessary medical care, health education, social services, nutrition counseling, and community support.

When to Start Treatment (Table 8–1)

Infant

HIV-1 disease progression is the most rapid within the first year of life. Infants who developed symptomatic disease within the first year without therapy in one study had a mortality rate of about 50% at 3 years.[1, 2] Of 529 HIV-infected children followed in the Italian Register, of which 112 were followed from birth, 82% developed HIV-1–related disease at a median of 5 months, with symptoms being associated with shorter survival.[3] In a more recent study performed in Uganda, HIV-infected infants had a 34% rate of mortality within 12 months, 66% by 3 years, and 75% by 5 years.[4] These findings are quite similar to those of a cohort of infants followed in the United States prior to the availability of antiretrovirals.[5] Numerous other reports strongly support the treatment of any infant identified as HIV-1 infected within the first 12 months of life.

Children Older than 1 Year

The point at which infants are better able to control HIV-1 infection and move from the rapid progression associated with infancy to a rate of progression more consistent with that of adolescents

Table 8-1
Indications for Initiation of Antiretroviral Therapy in Children with HIV Infection*

- Clinical symptoms associated with HIV infection (i.e., clinical categories A, B, or C).
- Evidence of immune suppression, indicated by CD4+ T cell absolute number or percentage (i.e., immune category 2 or 3).
- Age < 12 months, regardless of clinical, immunologic, or virologic status.
- For asymptomatic children aged ≥1 year with normal immune status, two options can be considered[†]:
  Option 1: Initiate therapy, regardless of age or symptom status.
  Option 2: Defer treatment in situations in which the risk for clinical disease progression is low and other factors (i.e., concern for the durability of response, safety, and adherence) favor postponing treatment. In such cases, the healthcare provider should regularly monitor virologic, immunologic, and clinical status. Factors to be considered in deciding to initiate therapy include the following:
   - High or increasing HIV RNA copy number.
   - Rapidly declining CD4+ T cell number or percentage to values approaching those indicative of moderate immune suppression (i.e., immune category 2).
   - Development of clinical symptoms.

*Indications for initiation of antiretroviral therapy need to address issues of adherence. Post-pubertal adolescents should follow the Guidelines for the Use of Antiretroviral Agents in Adults and Adolescents (http://www.hivatis.org).
[†]The exact age of a perinatally infected child as to when it may be safe not to initiate antiretroviral therapy is unknown. Few children <2 years of age have no symptoms associated with their HIV-1 infection. Because of the risk of developmental delays and neurocognitive impairment in young children, this author believes that except in rare circumstances HIV-1–infected children <2 years of age should receive treatment.
From "Guidelines for the Use of Antiretroviral Agents in Pediatric HIV Infection" developed by the Working Group on Antiretroviral Therapy and Medical Management of HIV-Infected Children convened by the national Pediatric and Family HIV Resource Center.

and adults has not been clearly defined. However, children perinatally infected with HIV-1 who are asymptomatic and have maintained normal CD4+ lymphocyte counts are at lower risk of progression and may not require antiretroviral treatment until they show evidence of disease progression, as defined by the criteria of when to start treatment for HIV-infected adolescents and adults (see later).

Some experts continue to believe that all children infected with HIV-1 should be started on therapy regardless of current CD4+ lymphocyte count or viral load. The potential benefits of this approach are as follows: (1) Earlier initiation of therapy offers the best opportunity to prevent or slow disease progression and allow for continued normal development. (2) Normal immune function can be maintained before there is loss of function. (3) With lower virus loads, there will be a greater likelihood of sustained viral suppression with less risk of resistance. The benefits of early intervention must be weighed against potential risks, including the following: (1) drug-related decline in quality of life; (2) greater cumulative drug-related adverse events; (3) earlier development of drug resistance if viral suppression suboptimal; and (4) limitation of antiretroviral options.

A second approach that is gaining favor among experts (particularly for children beyond 2 or 3 years of age) is to defer treatment in asymptomatic children with normal immune status in whom the risk of clinical progression is low. Most HIV-1–infected children who appear to be clinically well will have evidence of immunosuppression based on their CD4+ lymphocyte count. Advantages of delaying therapy include (1) avoiding the negative impact that taking antiretrovirals can have on a child's quality of life, (2) avoiding antiretroviral associated adverse effects, (3) delaying the development of antiretroviral resistance, and (4) preserving the maximal number of antiretroviral options for the future. However, risks are also associated with delaying antiretroviral intervention particularly in younger children, including (1) the risk of irreversible immune system depletion, (2) greater difficulty in suppressing viral replication in the future, and (3) the development of irreversible impairment of development, including neurocognitive capability. The impact of HIV-1 infection on growth, development, and neurocognitive function may initially be subtle and may not be recognized until there has been a significant delay. Although some catch-up growth and improved neurologic function can occur with effective antiretroviral therapy, the full capability of reversing such delays is unknown.

If the decision is made to defer antiretroviral therapy, children should be monitored regularly (every 3 months) for virologic, immunologic, and clinical status. Neurocognitive status must also be evaluated at least every 6 months. Antiretroviral therapy should be initiated if there is a high or significantly increasing plasma HIV-1 RNA level, rapidly declining CD4+ lymphocyte count, or percentage values indicative of moderate suppression (immune category 2; see Table 8–1), the development of clinical symptoms and any evidence of a decline or failure to progress in achieving neurocognitive milestones or school difficulties that could be related to HIV-1 infection. With normal immune function, the plasma HIV-1 RNA load that should trigger initiation of treatment remains controversial. Children with plasma RNA levels above 100,000 copies/mL are at increased risk for progression, and most experts believe should be encouraged to initiate antiretroviral therapy. Current guidelines for adults and adolescents recommend that treatment be initiated for plasma HIV-1 RNA levels above 55,000 copies/mL using the Roche Amplicor assay (Table 8–2). Such a level in an asymptomatic child suggests an increased likelihood that the patient will become symptomatic, and most experts would initiate treatment in these cases. Similarly, for all adults and adolescents with a CD4+ lymphocyte count less than 200/mm^3 experts agree that treatment should be started, and most would initiate treatment in patients with between 200 and 350/mm^3 CD4+ lymphocytes.

Table 8–2
Indications for the Initiation of Antiretroviral Therapy in the Chronically HIV-1–Infected Adult or Adolescent Patients

CLINICAL CATEGORY	CD4+ T CELL COUNT	PLASMA HIV RNA	RECOMMENDATION
Symptomatic (AIDS, severe symptoms)	Any value	Any value	Treat
Asymptomatic, AIDS	CD4+ T cells <200/mm^3	Any value	Treat
Asymptomatic	CD4+ T cells >200/mm^3 but <350/mm^3	Any value	Treatment should generally be offered, although controversy exists.*
Asymptomatic	CD4+ T cells >350/mm^3	>30,000 (bDNA) or >55,000 (RT-PCR)	Some experts would recommend initiating therapy, recognizing that the 3-year risk of developing AIDS in untreated patients is >30%. In the absence of very high levels of plasma HIV RNA, some would defer therapy and monitor the CD4+ T cell count and level of plasma HIV RNA more frequently. Clinical outcomes data after initiating therapy are lacking.
Asymptomatic	CD4+ T cells >350/mm^3	<30,000 (bDNA) or <55,000 (RT-PCR)	Many experts would defer therapy and observe, recognizing that the 3-year risk of developing AIDS in untreated patients is <15%.

bDNA, branched DNA; RT-PCR, reverse transcriptase polymerase chain reaction.
*Clinical benefit has been demonstrated in controlled trials only for patients with CD4+ T cells <200/mm^3. However, most experts would offer therapy at a CD4+ T cell threshold <350/mm^3. All decisions to initiate therapy should be based on prognosis for disease-free survival in the absence of treatment, as determined by the CD4+ T cell count and level of plasma HIV RNA, the potential benefits and risks of therapy, and the willingness of the patient to accept therapy.
From "Guidelines for the Use of Antiretroviral Agents in HIV-Infected Adults and Adolescents" developed by the Panel on Clinical Practices for Treatment of HIV Infection convened by the Department of Health and Human Services and the Henry J. Kaiser Family Foundation (http://www.hivatis.org).

Choice of Antiretrovirals at Initiation of Therapy (Table 8–3)

A full review of specific antiretrovirals is not possible in this chapter. The interested reader is referred to the website http://www.hivatis.org, which has the living document, "Guidelines for the Use of Antiretroviral Agents in Pediatric HIV infection." New antiretrovirals are added to this document as they become available and as recommendations for the treatment of children change.

The goal of antiretroviral therapy is to provide the combination of drugs that most effectively lowers viral load and maintains or restores immunologic function while resulting in the fewest adverse effects. Antiretroviral therapy with at least three drugs is recommended for children when initiating treatment. Table 8–3 summarizes the antiretroviral regimens for initial therapy of HIV-1 infection in children.

Combination therapy with at least three antiretrovirals, usually from at least two different classes of drugs, is considered necessary when initiating treatment of the HIV-1–infected child. Mono- or dual-therapy is no longer acceptable treatment. A single agent, zidovudine, is effective when given to an infant born to an HIV-1–infected mother combined with a treatment regimen given to the mother to prevent mother-to-infant transmission. If a newborn is identified as HIV-1 infected while receiving zidovudine prophylaxis, the infant should be switched to a treatment regimen containing at least three drugs from at least two classes of drugs.

When initiating therapy for the HIV-1–infected infant whose mother received antiretrovirals during pregnancy, it is usually not necessary to select drugs based on maternal antiretroviral usage. Most data suggest that almost all infected infants born to mothers receiving antiretrovirals have virus sensitive to the drugs to which the mother has been exposed.[6–8] However, this is an evolving area that may require more careful consideration as the number of HIV-1–infected women who are highly antiretroviral experienced giving birth to second and third children increases.

Importance of Viral Load Monitoring

Viral load monitoring has become an integral part of the care for the HIV-1–infected child. Abundant data support the use of plasma HIV-1 RNA determinations for the assessment of the risk for disease progression and to monitor the successful suppression of virus by antiretrovirals. Combined with CD4+ lymphocyte counts, the current HIV-1–related disease status and future risk for disease progression can be predicted.

Plasma HIV-1 RNA

The use of plasma HIV-1 RNA to monitor infected children receiving antiretrovirals has become standard of care in the United States and other resource-rich countries. Whereas plasma HIV-1 RNA is predictive for future disease progression, the CD4+ lymphocyte count best identifies the current risk that a child will experience an HIV-1–related complication. Using the Multi-Center AIDS Cohort Study (MACS) cohort, Mellors and coworkers and Gange and coworkers[9–12] demonstrated that as the plasma HIV-1 RNA load increases, the risk that an infected adult will develop AIDS increases (Table 8–4). Refining these data, at viral loads (plasma HIV-1 RNA as determined by reverse-transcriptase polymerase chain reaction) greater than 55,000 copies/mL with a CD4+ lymphocyte count of 200/µL or less, the risk for developing AIDS-defining complications for the MACS cohort was 85.5% by 3 years. In contrast, persons with plasma viral loads of less than 1500 and greater than 350 CD4+ lymphocytes/µL have a less than 2% risk of developing AIDS-defining complications; this risk increases to 15% if the viral load is between 20,000 and 55,000 copies/mL and to 40% with a plasma viral load more than 55,000 copies/mL.

Similar studies of plasma HIV-1 RNA have been performed in children. Of note, the mean HIV-1 RNA load for young children is approximately 10-fold higher than that for the HIV-1–infected adult. In data from PACTG 152, a study in which children received zidovudine, didanosine, or both drugs, children younger than 30 months of age with plasma HIV-1 RNA loads of less than 150,000 copies/mL had an 11% risk of disease progression or death at 2 years, which rose to a 42% risk for viral loads above 1.7 million copies/mL (Table 8–5). For children older than 30 months of age, plasma HIV-1 RNA loads were considerably lower than observed in younger children. Among the children 30 months of age or older, children with plasma HIV-1 RNA loads less than 15,000 copies/mL had no disease progression or death within 2 years, whereas children with plasma HIV-1 RNA levels greater than 150,000 copies/mL had a 34% rate of disease progression or death. In another study by Mofenson and colleagues, children with 100,000 or fewer copies/mL of HIV-1 RNA with 15% or greater CD4+ lymphocytes had a 15% risk

Table 8-3
Recommended Antiretroviral Regimens for Initial Therapy for HIV Infection In Children

Strongly Recommended
Clinical trial evidence of clinical benefit and/or sustained suppression of HIV replication in adults and/or children.
- One highly active protease inhibitors (nelfinavir or ritonavir) plus two nucleoside analogue reverse transcriptase inhibitors.
- Recommended dual NRTI combinations: the most data on use in children are available for the combinations of *ZDV* and *ddI ZDV and 3TC, and d4T and ddI*. More limited data are available for the combinations of *d4T* and *3TC** and *ZDV* and *ddC*.†
- For children who can swallow capsules: the NNRTI efavirenz‡ plus two NRTIs, or efavirenz plus nelfinavir and one NRTI.

Recommended as an Alternative
Clinical trial evidence of suppression of HIV replication, but (1) durability may be less in adults and/or children than with strongly recommended regimens or may not yet be defined; or (2) evidence of efficacy may not outweigh potential adverse consequences (e.g., toxicity, drug interactions, cost); (3) experience in infants and children is limited.
- Nevirapine and two NRTIs
- Abacavir in combination with ZDV and 3TC
- Lopinavir/ritonavir with two NRTIs or one NRTI and NNRTI§
- Indinavir or saquinavir soft gel capsule with two NRTIs for children who can swallow capsules

Offered Only in Special Circumstances
Clinical trial evidence of either (1) virologic suppression that is less durable than for the Strongly Recommended or Alternative regimens or (2) data are preliminary or inconclusive for use as initial therapy but may be reasonably offered in special circumstances.
- Two NRTIs
- Amprenavir in combination with two NRTIs or abacavir

Not Recommended
Evidence against use because (1) overlapping toxicity may occur and/or (2) use may be virologically undesirable.
- Any monotherapy¶
- d4T and ZDV
- ddC† and ddI
- ddC† and d4T
- ddC† and 3TC

ddC, zalcitabine; ddI, didanosine; d4T, stavudine; NNRTI, non-nucleoside reverse transcriptase inhibitor; NRTI, nucleoside reverse transcriptase inhibitor; 3TC, lamivudine; ZDV zidovudine.
*The author has had considerable experience with the combination of d4T and 3TC and has found this to be a highly effective and well tolerated combination when combined with a protease inhibitor with or without an NNRTI.
†ddC is not available commercially in a liquid preparation, although a liquid formulation is available through a compassionate use program of the manufacturer (Hoffman-La Roche Inc., (http://www.rocheusa.com), Nutley, NJ). ZDV and ddC are a less preferred choice for use in combination with a protease inhibitor.
‡Efavirenz is currently available only in capsule form, although a liquid formulation is available through an expanded access program of the manufacturer (Dupont Pharmaceutical Company (http://www.dupontpharma.com), Wilmington, Del). There are currently no data on appropriate dosage of efavirenz in children younger than 3 years of age.
§The data presented to the Food and Drug Administration for review during the drug approval process provided significant data on the pharmacokinetics and safety in children receiving lopinavir/ritonavir (Kaletra) for 24 weeks. The combination of lopinavir/ritonavir with either two NRTIs or one NRTI and an NNRTI may be moved up to the Strongly Recommended category as experience with this drug is gained by US investigators.
¶Except for ZDV chemoprophylaxis administered to HIV-exposed infants during the first 6 weeks of life to prevent perinatal HIV transmission; if an infant is confirmed as HIV-infected while receiving ZDV prophylaxis, therapy should be changed to a combination antiretroviral drug regimen.
From "Guidelines for the Use of Antiretroviral Agents in Pediatric HIV Infection" developed by the Working Group on Antiretroviral Therapy and Medical Management of HIV-Infected Children convened by the national Pediatric and Family HIV Resource Center. (http://www.hivatis.org).

for death after a mean follow-up of 5.1 years, as compared with a 63% risk of death if the CD4+ lymphocyte percentage was less than 15% (Table 8–6). For plasma HIV-1 RNA levels greater than 100,000 copies/mL, children with 15% or greater CD4+ lymphocytes had a 36% risk of death compared with 81% for those who began with less than 15% CD4+ lymphocytes.

Table 8–4
Risk of Progression to AIDS-Defining Illness in a Cohort of Homosexual Men Predicted by Baseline CD4+ T Cell Count and Viral Load*

CD4+ ≤200 PLASMA VIRAL LOAD (COPIES/ML)†		% AIDS (AIDS-DEFINING COMPLICATION)‡			
bDNA	RT-PCR	n	3 Years	6 Years	9 Years
≤500	≤1500	0§	–	–	–
501–3000	1501–7000	3§	–	–	–
3001–10,000	7001–20,000	7	14.3	28.6	64.3
10,001–30,000	20,001–55,000	20	50.0	75.0	90.0
>30,000	>55,000	70	85.5	97.9	100.00
CD4+ 201–350 PLASMA VIRAL LOAD (COPIES/ML)		**% AIDS (AIDS-DEFINING COMPLICATION)**			
bDNA	RT-PCR	n	3 Years	6 Years	9 Years
≤500	≤1500	3§	–	–	–
501–3000	1501–7000	27	0	20.0	32.2
3001–10,000	7001–20,000	44	6.9	44.4	66.2
10,001–30,000	20,001–55,000	53	36.4	72.2	84.5
>30,000	>55,000	104	64.4	89.3	92.9
CD4+ > 350 PLASMA VIRAL LOAD (COPIES/ML)		**% AIDS (AIDS-DEFINING COMPLICATION)**			
bDNA	RT-PCR	n	3 Years	6 Years	9 Years
≤500	≤1500	119	1.7	5.5	12.7
501–3000	1501–7000	227	2.2	16.4	30.0
3001–10,000	7001–20,000	342	6.8	30.1	53.5
10,001–30,000	20,001–55,000	323	14.8	51.2	73.5
>30,000	>55,000	262	39.6	71.8	85.0

bDNA, branched DNA; RT-PCR, reverse-transcriptase polymerase chain reaction.
*Data from the Multi-Center AIDS Cohort Study. These data are likely applicable to adolescents.
†MACS numbers reflect plasma HIV RNA values obtained by bDNA testing. RT-PCR values are consistently 2 to 2.5-fold higher than bDNA values, as indicated.
‡In this study, AIDS was defined according to the 1987 Centers for Disease Control and Prevention definition and does not include asymptomatic individuals with CD4+ T cells <200 mm³.
From "Guidelines for the Use of Antiretroviral Agents in HIV-Infected Adults and Adolescents" developed by the Panel on Clinical Practices for Treatment of HIV Infection convened by the Department of Health and Human Services and the Henry J. Kaiser Family Foundation. (http://www.hivatis.org).

Plasma HIV-1 RNA Kinetics in Children Receiving Antiretrovirals

Luzuriaga and associates[13] examined HIV-1 turnover and kinetics in children aged 15 days to 2 years following initiation of antiretroviral therapy including zidovudine, lamivudine, and nevirapine. Viral decay rates used to estimate viral turnover suggested that during the first phase of virus decay, half of the plasma virus turned over approximately every 30 hours during infancy and approximately every 14 hours in older children. Their findings further suggested that HIV-1 production in children is at least as rapid as for adults[14–16] and that older infants and children have more rapid production and turnover of HIV-1 in plasma than adults.

Spector and colleagues[17] examined the plasma HIV-1 RNA response of children receiving potent antiretroviral therapy including one or two nucleoside reverse transcriptase inhibitors, efavirenz and nelfinavir. Their data demonstrate a rapid decline in plasma HIV-1 RNA with the median times to achieving a plasma HIV-1 RNA level of less than 400 and less than 50 copies/mL of 4 and 20 weeks, respectively. Thus, half of the children with detectable plasma HIV-1 RNA between 50 and 400 copies/mL continued to have a decline in RNA levels for more than 5 months after the initiation of a new course of antiretroviral therapy. The median time from less than 400 copies/mL to less than 50 copies/mL was 6 weeks. Although the time to reaching either less than 400 copies/mL or less than 50 copies/mL did not affect the durability of suppression, those children who failed to achieve a level of less than 50 copies/mL had a less sustained

Table 8-5
Association of Baseline HIV RNA Quartile by Age at Entry with Risk for Disease Progression or Death During Study Follow-up among HIV-Infected Children Receiving Antiretroviral Treatment*

AGE AT ENTRY	BASELINE HIV RNA QUARTILES, COPIES/ML[†]	PATIENTS, N	DISEASE PROGRESSION OR DEATH, N(%)
<30 months[§]	<1000–150,000	79	9 (11)
	150,001–500,000	66	13 (20)
	500,001–1,700,000	76	29 (38)
	>1,700,000	81	42 (52)
≥30 months[¶]	<1000–15,000	66	0 (0)
	15,001–50,000	54	7 (13)
	50,001–150,000	80	13 (16)
	>150,000	64	22 (34)

*Data from the Pediatric AIDS Clinical Trip Group protocol 152.
[†]Tested by NASBA assay (manufactured by Organon Teknika, Durham, North Carolina) on frozen stored serum.
[§]Mean age, 1.1 years.
[¶]Mean age, 7.3 years.
From "Guidelines for the Use of Antiretroviral Agents in Pediatric HIV Infection" developed by the Working Group on Antiretroviral Therapy and Medical Management of HIV-Infected Children convened by the national Pediatric and Family HIV Resource Center (http://www.hivatis.org). Reprinted with modifications from Palumbo PE, Raskino C, Fiscus S, et al: Disease progression in HIV-infected infants and children: Predictive value of quantitative plasma HIV RNA and CD4 lymphocyte count. *JAMA* 1998; 279:756–761.

Table 8-6
Association of Baseline HIV RNA Copy Number and CD4+ T Cell Percentage with Long-Term Risk for Death in HIV-Infected Children*

BASELINE HIV RNA[†] (COPIES/ML)	BASELINE CD4+ T CELL PERCENTAGE	PATIENTS, N[‡]	DEATHS, N (%)[§]
≤ 100,000			
	≥15	103	15 (15)
	<15	24	15 (63)
> 100,000			
	≥15	89	32 (36)
	<15	36	29 (81)

*Data from the National Institute of Child Health and Human Development Intravenous Immunoglobulin Clinical Trial.
[†]Tested by NASBA assay (manufactured by Organon Teknika, Durham, North Carolina) on frozen stored serum.
[‡]Mean age, 3.4 years.
[§]Mean follow-up, 5.1 years.
From "Guidelines for the Use of Antiretroviral Agents in Pediatric HIV Infection" developed by the Working Group on Antiretroviral Therapy and Medical Management of HIV-Infected Children convened by the national Pediatric and Family HIV Resource Center. (http://www.hivatis.org). Reprinted with modifications from Mofenson LM, Korelitz J, Meyer WA, et al: The relationship between serum human immunodeficiency virus type 1 (HIV-1) RNA level, CD4 lymphocyte percent, and long-term mortality risk in HIV-1 infected children. J Infect Dis 1997; 175:1029–1038.

reduction in viral load than those who did reach a level of less than 50 copies/mL.

The monitoring of plasma HIV-1 RNA has become an essential component of providing safe and effective antiretroviral treatment for children as well as adults. A child who fails to achieve virologic suppression of fewer than 400 copies/mL should have the reasons for virologic failure evaluated. Although resistance must be considered and has become increasingly common among antiretroviral-experienced children, issues of adherence must also be reviewed with the child and family. Frequently, adherence is found to be a major factor in repeated virologic failures and requires the efforts of social workers, health educators, case managers, and other health care professionals to work with the child and family to develop a treatment regimen and plan that can result in sustained virologic suppression for that child.

Cerebrospinal Fluid HIV-1 RNA

Limited research has been performed to evaluate the association between cerebrospinal fluid (CSF) levels of HIV-1 RNA and the presence or development of neurocognitive impairment. Pratt and associates[18] found that CSF HIV-1 RNA levels greater than 10,000 copies/mL were highly associated with neurocognitive impairment of children. Higher RNA levels were associated with abnormal brain imaging scans and with increased risk of neurocognitive deficits. Similar studies performed by Sei and associates[19] also found an association between higher HIV-1 load in CSF and the presence of neurologic deficits. Thus, in children with neurologic disease associated with HIV-1 infection, monitoring of HIV-1 within CSF may provide an additional marker of antiretroviral efficacy with the objective of reducing viral load within the CSF to undetectable. Although no study in children has systematically evaluated the direct effect of decreasing HIV-1 RNA within CSF and improved neurocognitive function in children, significant central nervous system benefit has been observed in children treated with effective antiretroviral therapy. Therefore, children who are suspected of HIV-1–related neurologic impairment should have their CSF evaluated for possible persistent HIV-1 within the central nervous system. If HIV-1 RNA is detected within CSF, an antiretroviral regimen that will reduce the viral load to undetectable is desirable.

Intracellular HIV-1 DNA

Until recently, assays evaluating the presence of intracellular HIV-1 DNA were used solely for the identification of the HIV-1–infected infant or to determine the infection status of an at-risk adult who might not yet have developed HIV-1 antibody. Recently, however, with the use of highly active antiretroviral therapy, there has been an interest in the identification and monitoring of HIV-1 reservoirs of latently infected or low replicating virus. Increasing data in adults have demonstrated that HIV-1 DNA can be detected in peripheral blood mononuclear cells of patients with sustained viral loads below 50 copies/mL as measured by the Roche Amplicor ultrasensitive assay. Standard cultures of these patients are usually negative for infectious virus, but several groups have demonstrated that cultures that select for CD4+ cells can often be positive, indicating that, despite sustained virologic suppression as determined by plasma RNA assay, infectious virus is still present within circulating peripheral cells.[20–25] Moreover, virus has been demonstrated to remain in lymph nodes of patients with undetectable HIV-1 RNA in plasma.[20,21,26,27] Additional research in adults has demonstrated that viral DNA with 2-LTR (long terminal repeat) circles can be found in peripheral blood mononuclear cells despite undetectable levels of HIV-1 RNA, suggesting that a low level of viral replication exists despite there being no detectable viral RNA in the plasma.[28–30]

Recently, Saitoh and colleagues examined intracellular DNA levels of children with sustained suppression of plasma HIV-1 RNA for more than 2 years. Their findings demonstrated that HIV-1 DNA remains detectable in the peripheral blood mononuclear cells (PBMC) of infected children despite sustained plasma HIV-1 RNA levels lower than 50 copies/mL. The HIV-1 DNA levels gradually declined from baseline through week 48, reaching a plateau from week 80 through week 104. The mean quantity of intracellular HIV-1 DNA decreased from baseline by 73% at week 8, 61% at week 20, and 63% at week 48. The estimated half-life of HIV-1 DNA for this patient population by regression coefficient analysis was 60 weeks (about 14 months), which is longer than the previously reported viral half-lives for infected adults receiving effective antiretroviral therapy that were estimated to be between 5 and 10 months.[15,31,32] Thus, despite the failure to detect viral RNA in plasma, PBMC continued to harbor HIV-1 DNA that could be quantified for at least 2 years and can be used as a maker of continued virologic suppression.

Intracellular levels of HIV-1 DNA at baseline were predictive of future quantities of DNA in the children evaluated in this study. Children with high HIV-1 DNA values at baseline continued to have higher quantities of DNA throughout the 104 weeks of follow-up. Similar findings have been reported for HIV-1–infected adults receiving highly active antiretroviral therapy, independent of CD4+ lymphocyte counts at baseline.[31,32] At baseline and while there continued to be active HIV-1 replication (during the first 8 weeks of therapy), quantities of intracellular HIV-1 DNA correlated with quantities of plasma HIV-1 RNA. By week 20, correlations between HIV-1 DNA and RNA were no longer meaningful, as RNA became undetectable (<50 copies/mL) in almost all members of the subgroup studied here.

HIV-1 p24 Antigen

The first marker identified as useful for the monitoring of potential efficacy of antiretrovirals, the determination of plasma/serum p24 antigen, has fallen from favor and has been almost universally supplanted by HIV-1 RNA assays. This is unfortunate, because p24 antigen determinations could be of considerable use as antiretrovirals are introduced in the developing world. The initial studies of HIV-1 p24 antigen demonstrated that an antiretroviral active against HIV-1 such as zidovudine decreased serum levels of p24 antigen while an inactive drug such as ribavirin failed to have an impact on p24 antigen.[33] These findings were supported in children. A concern with the initially used p24 antigen assays was that the tests failed to identify serum p24 antigen in 25% to 50% of persons known to be infected with HIV-1. Although this proportion is considerably lower in children than in adults, the standard assay was felt to have considerable limitations. Immune complex dissociation of p24 antigen-antibody complexes (ICD-p24 antigen) increased the sensitivity of these assays, particularly in children who routinely have higher circulating levels of HIV-1 in blood than adults. Mofenson and associates[34] found that the level of ICD-p24 antigen levels in children correlated with an increased risk of mortality. In an additional study, Spector and coworkers (unpublished data) also found that as the quantity of p24 antigen increased, the risk of children experiencing disease progression or death in PACTG 152 also increased. Thus, assays for p24 antigen may prove useful in certain settings.

The p24 antigen assay presents several advantages over assays determining plasma levels of HIV-1 RNA. First, the antigen detection assays are considerably less complicated and can be performed by technicians with limited laboratory experience. Secondly, the assays are considerably less expensive and are more affordable in developing countries where resources are urgently needed for the purchase of antiretrovirals. Thirdly, as noted earlier, most children will be p24 antigen positive. Thus, p24 antigen assays could provide a simple and inexpensive method for monitoring the course of antiretroviral therapies. Additionally, the plasma HIV-1 RNA level might be of interest if only the p24 antigen assay were determined to be negative, because persons who are p24 antigen positive can be safely assumed to have circulating HIV-1 RNA in their plasma as well.

IMPORTANCE OF RESISTANCE TESTING

(Table 8–7)

For children failing antiretroviral therapy, most experts believe that resistance testing to determine antiretroviral susceptibility should be used to increase the likelihood that a child will respond to the new therapeutic regimen selected. The use of resistance testing, whether genotypic or phenotypic testing, in antiretroviral-naive or zidovudine-exposed children is more controversial. Most experts believe that resistance testing is unnecessary in such cases. As noted previously, very few children identified as perinatally infected with HIV-1 have been infected with resistant virus. However, as the number of women who are highly antiretroviral-experienced give birth, the risk for the transmission of resistant virus from mother to infant will likely increase. For this reason, although most experts do not recommend resistance testing for children when initiating therapy, if a child fails to respond to initial treatment and adherence to treatment regimens is thought to be good, the possibility of primary resistance should be considered. In such cases, resistance testing is critical prior to the initiation of a new regimen. If plasma from pretreatment is available, this specimen should also be tested to assess for the presence of primary resistance.

CONCLUSION

Remarkable progress has been made in improving treatments for children infected with HIV-1. Despite this progress, many challenges remain, including the development of more effective agents that can be given infrequently and with minimal risk to children. To accomplish these improved treatments, much research will be required to enable the evaluation of new drugs for children. Additionally, the advances made for children living in resource-rich countries must be extended to all children infected with HIV-1 regardless of the wealth of the nation where they live. This challenge can be met only through a concerted international effort involving governments, pharmaceutical companies, international charities and institutions, and health care providers. Research will be necessary to determine the optimal approaches to the most efficient use of antiretrovirals that will lead to the most benefit with the least toxicity at the lowest

Table 8-7
Recommendations for the Use of Drug Resistance Assays

CLINICAL SETTING/RECOMMENDATION	RATIONALE
Recommended	
Virologic failure during highly active antiretroviral therapy	Determine the role of resistance in drug failure and maximize the number of active drugs in the new regimen if indicated.
Suboptimal suppression of viral load after initiation of antiretroviral therapy	Determine the role of resistance and maximize the number of active drugs in the new regimen if indicated.
Consider	
Acute HIV infection	Determine if drug-resistant virus was transmitted and change regimen accordingly.
Not Generally Recommended	
Chronic HIV infection prior to initiation of therapy	Uncertain prevalence of resistance virus. Current assays may not detect minor drug-resistant species.
After discontinuation of drugs	Drug resistance mutations may become minor species in the absence of selective drug pressure. Current assays may not detect minor drug-resistant species.
Plasma viral load <1000 HIV RNA copies/mL	Resistance assays cannot be reliably performed because of low copy number of HIV RNA.

From "Guidelines for the Use of Antiretroviral Agents in HIV-Infected Adults and Adolescents" developed by the Panel on Clinical Practices for Treatment of HIV Infection convened by the Department of Health and Human Services and the Henry J. Kaiser Family Foundation. (http://www.hivatis.org).

cost. Recent research within the PACTG has demonstrated in the United States that successful treatment of children can be achieved; the challenge for the future will be to sustain current treatment successes and extend these advances to children throughout the world.

Acknowledgments

Dr. Spector's research is supported by the Pediatric AIDS Clinical Trials Group (AI-52254) and by Grants from the National Institute of Allergy and Infectious Diseases (AI-39004, AI-27563, AI-33835, AI-41110, and AI-36214; University of California, San Diego Center for AIDS Research) and the National Institute of Children Health and Development (HD-40464).

Much of the information for this chapter has been gleaned from the "Guidelines for the Use of Antiretroviral Agents in Pediatric HIV Infection" developed by the Working Group on Antiretroviral Therapy and Medical Management of HIV-Infected Children convened by the national Pediatric and Family HIV Resource Center and "Guidelines for the Use of Antiretroviral Agents in HIV-Infected Adults and Adolescents" developed by the Panel on Clinical Practices for Treatment of HIV Infection convened by the Department of Health and Human Services and the Henry J. Kaiser Family Foundation. These living documents can be accessed on the HIV/AIDS Treatment Information Service Website (http://www.hivatis.org).

References

1. Blanche RC, Moscato M: A prospective study of infants born to women seropositive for human immunodeficiency virus type 1. N Engl J Med 1989; 320:1643-1648.
2. Blanche S, Newell ML, Mayaux MJ, et al: Morbidity and mortality in European children vertically infected by HIV-1. The French Pediatric HIV Infection Study Group and European Collaborative Study. J Acquir Immune Defic Syndr Hum Retrovirol 1997;14:442-450.
3. Tovo PA, de Martino M, Gabiano C, et al: Prognostic factors and survival in children with perinatal HIV-1 infection. The Italian Register for HIV Infections in Children. Lancet 1992;339:1249-1253.
4. Marum LH, Tindyebwa D, Gibb D: Care of children with HIV infection and AIDS in Africa. AIDS 1997;11(Suppl B):S125-134.

5. Spencer LT, Ogino MT, Dankner WM, Spector SA: Clinical significance of human immunodeficiency virus type 1 phenotypes in infected children. J Infect Dis 1994;169:491–495.
6. Eastman PS, Shapiro DE, Coombs RW, et al: Maternal viral genotypic zidovudine resistance and infrequent failure of zidovudine therapy to prevent perinatal transmission of human immunodeficiency virus type 1 in pediatric AIDS Clinical Trials Group Protocol 076. J Infect Dis 1998;177:557–564.
7. McSherry GD, Shapiro DE, Coombs RW, et al: The effects of zidovudine in the subset of infants infected with human immunodeficiency virus type-1 (Pediatric AIDS Clinical Trials Group Protocol 076). J Pediatr 1999;134:717–724.
8. Stiehm ER, Lambert JS, Mofenson LM, et al: Efficacy of zidovudine and human immunodeficiency virus (HIV) hyperimmune immunoglobulin for reducing perinatal HIV transmission from HIV-infected women with advanced disease: Results of Pediatric AIDS Clinical Trials Group protocol 185. J Infect Dis 1999;179:567–575.
9. Mellors JW, Kingsley LA, Rinaldo CR Jr, et al: Quantitation of HIV-1 RNA in plasma predicts outcome after seroconversion. Ann Intern Med 1995;122:573–579.
10. Mellors JW, Rinaldo CR Jr, Gupta P, et al: Prognosis in HIV-1 infection predicted by the quantity of virus in plasma (see comments) (published erratum appears in Science 1997;275:14). Science 1996;272:1167–1170.
11. Mellors JW, Munoz A, Giorgi JV, et al: Plasma viral load and CD4+ lymphocytes as prognostic markers of HIV-1 infection (see comments). Ann Intern Med 1997;126:946–954.
12. Gange SJ, Mellors JW, Lau B, et al: Longitudinal patterns of HIV type 1 RNA among individuals with late disease progression. AIDS Res Hum Retroviruses 2001;17:1223–1229.
13. Luzuriaga K, Wu H, McManus M, et al: Dynamics of human immunodeficiency virus type 1 replication in vertically infected infants. J Virol 1999;73:362–367.
14. Ho DD, Neumann AU, Perelson AS, et al: Rapid turnover of plasma virions and CD4 lymphocytes in HIV-1 infection. Nature 1995;373:123–126.
15. Perelson AS, Essunger P, Cao Y, et al: Decay characteristics of HIV-1-infected compartments during combination therapy (see comments). Nature 1997;387:188–191.
16. Perelson AS, Neumann AU, Markowitz M, et al: HIV-1 dynamics in vivo: Virion clearance rate, infected cell life-span, and viral generation time. Science 1996;271:1582–1586.
17. Spector SA, Hsia K, Yong FH, et al: Patterns of plasma human immunodeficiency virus type 1 RNA response to highly active antiretroviral therapy in infected children. J Infect Dis 2000;182:1769–1773.
18. Pratt RD, Nichols S, McKinney N, et al: Virologic markers of human immunodeficiency virus type 1 in cerebrospinal fluid of infected children. J Infect Dis 1996;174:288–293.
19. Sei S, Stewart SK, Farley M, et al: Evaluation of human immunodeficiency virus (HIV) type 1 RNA levels in cerebrospinal fluid and viral resistance to zidovudine in children with HIV encephalopathy. J Infect Dis 1996;174:1200–1206.
20. Wong JK, Hezareh M, Günthard HF, et al: Recovery of replication-competent HIV despite prolonged suppression of plasma viremia (see comments). Science 1997;278:1291–1295.
21. Wong JK, Günthard HF, Havlir DV, et al: Reduction of HIV-1 in blood and lymph nodes following potent antiretroviral therapy and the virologic correlates of treatment failure. Proc Natl Acad Sci U S A 1997;94:12574–12579.
22. Finzi D, Blankson J, Siliciano JD, et al: Latent infection of CD4+ T cells provides a mechanism for lifelong persistence of HIV-1, even in patients on effective combination therapy (see comments). Nat Med 1999;5:512–517.
23. Finzi D, Hermankova M, Pierson T, et al: Identification of a reservoir for HIV-1 in patients on highly active antiretroviral therapy (see comments). Science 1997;278:1295–1300.
24. Persaud D, Pierson T, Ruff C, et al: A stable latent reservoir for HIV-1 in resting CD4(+) T lymphocytes in infected children. J Clin Invest 2000;105:995–1003.
25. Cavert W, Notermans DW, Staskus K, et al: Kinetics of response in lymphoid tissues to antiretroviral therapy of HIV-1 infection (see comments) (published erratum appears in Science 1997 May 30;276[5317]:1321). Science 1997;276:960–964.
26. Gray CM, Lawrence J, Ranheim EA, et al: Highly active antiretroviral therapy results in HIV type 1 suppression in lymph nodes, increased pools of naive T cells, decreased pools of activated T cells, and diminished frequencies of peripheral activated HIV type 1-specific CD8+ T cells. AIDS Res Hum Retroviruses 2000;16:1357–1369.
27. Gunthard HF, Havlir DV, Fiscus S, et al: Residual human immunodeficiency virus (HIV) Type 1 RNA and DNA in lymph nodes and HIV RNA in genital secretions and in cerebrospinal fluid after suppression of viremia for 2 years. J Infect Dis 2001;183:1318–1327.
28. Ibanez A, Puig T, Elias J, et al: Quantification of integrated and total HIV-1 DNA after long-term highly active antiretroviral therapy in HIV-1-infected patients. AIDS 1999;13:1045–1049.
29. Sharkey ME, Teo I, Greenough T, et al: Persistence of episomal HIV-1 infection intermediates in patients on highly active anti-retroviral therapy. Nat Med 2000;6:76–81.
30. Zazzi M, Romano L, Catucci M, et al: Evaluation of the presence of 2-LTR HIV-1 unintegrated DNA as a simple molecular predictor of disease progression. J Med Virol 1997;52:20–25.

31. Andreoni M, Parisi SG, Sarmati L, et al: Cellular proviral HIV-DNA decline and viral isolation in naive subjects with ≤5000 copies/ml of HIV-RNA and ≥500 × 10(6)/l CD4 cells treated with highly active antiretroviral therapy. AIDS 2000;14:23–29.
32. Izopet J, Salama G, Pasquier C, et al: Decay of HIV-1 DNA in patients receiving suppressive antiretroviral therapy. J Acquir Immune Defic Syndr Hum Retrovirol 1998;19:478–483.
33. Spector SA, Kennedy C, McCutchan JA, et al: The antiviral effect of zidovudine and ribavirin in clinical trials and the use of p24 antigen levels as a virologic marker. J Infect Dis 1989;159:822–828.
34. Mofenson LM, Lambert JS, Stiehm ER, et al: Risk factors for perinatal transmission of human immunodeficiency virus type 1 in women treated with zidovudine. Pediatric AIDS Clinical Trials Group Study 185 Team. N Engl J Med 1999;341:385–393.

Immune-Based Therapies for HIV Infection

*Javier Chinen and
William T. Shearer*

Control of HIV infection is currently one of the most challenging problems in medicine. HIV targets the immune system, specifically CD4+ T cells and monocytes, cells that play a significant role directing the specific immune response against pathogens. The immune dysfunction induced by HIV infection is associated with an increased frequency and severity of opportunistic and regular infections, as well as autoimmune phenomena and neoplasia. Several approaches have been taken to control HIV infection, resulting primarily in the development of drugs that inhibit one of two key viral enzymes: reverse transcriptase and viral protease. These drugs are currently used in multiple combination regimens, also known as highly active antiretroviral therapy (HAART) because of their efficacy on reducing the viral load, restoring CD4+ T cell counts, and decreasing the incidence of opportunistic infections and the rate of mortality from HIV disease.[1] However, significant limitations of antiretroviral therapeutic regimens have become evident in the last few years. Although suppression of plasma viral load to undetectable levels is achieved, HIV is not eradicated; several reports have shown that when these drugs are stopped, a rebound in viral replication is observed.[2,3] In addition, severe drug adverse effects, incomplete immune reconstitution, problems with patient adherence to therapy, and the emergence of viral strains resistant to HAART justify the search for alternative antiretroviral strategies.

Anti-HIV immune-based therapy could be defined as any strategy designed to treat HIV infection, working with elements of the immune response. These elements include T cells, active and passive immunization, and soluble factors such as cytokines and chemokines (Table 9–1). Understanding how the immune system interacts with HIV infection is essential (Figure 9–1; see Chapter 3). In animal models using nonhuman primates infected with simian immunodeficiency virus (SIV), the presence of SIV-specific cytolytic CD8+ T cells is associated with better control of infection. When these cells are depleted, viral load increases. Similarly, in HIV-infected individuals, the development of strong HIV-specific CD4+ T cells and cytolytic responses is associated with slow progression of disease and viremia control.[4,5] Pregnant women with high CD4+ T cell counts are less likely to transmit HIV to their babies. Conversely, low CD4+ T cell counts and low neutralizing antibody titers are associated with increased risk

Table 9–1
Immune-Based Strategies for Creating HIV Infection

Cytokines: interleukin-2, interleukin-12
Growth factors: granulocyte colony-stimulating factor; granulocyte-macrophage colony-stimulating factor
Chemokine analogues and chemokine receptor inhibitors
Immunoglobulins: IVIG, anti-HIV monoclonal antibodies, and CD4-IgG2
Therapeutic vaccines
Adoptive cellular immunotherapy
Immunosuppressant agents: cyclosporine A, thalidomide

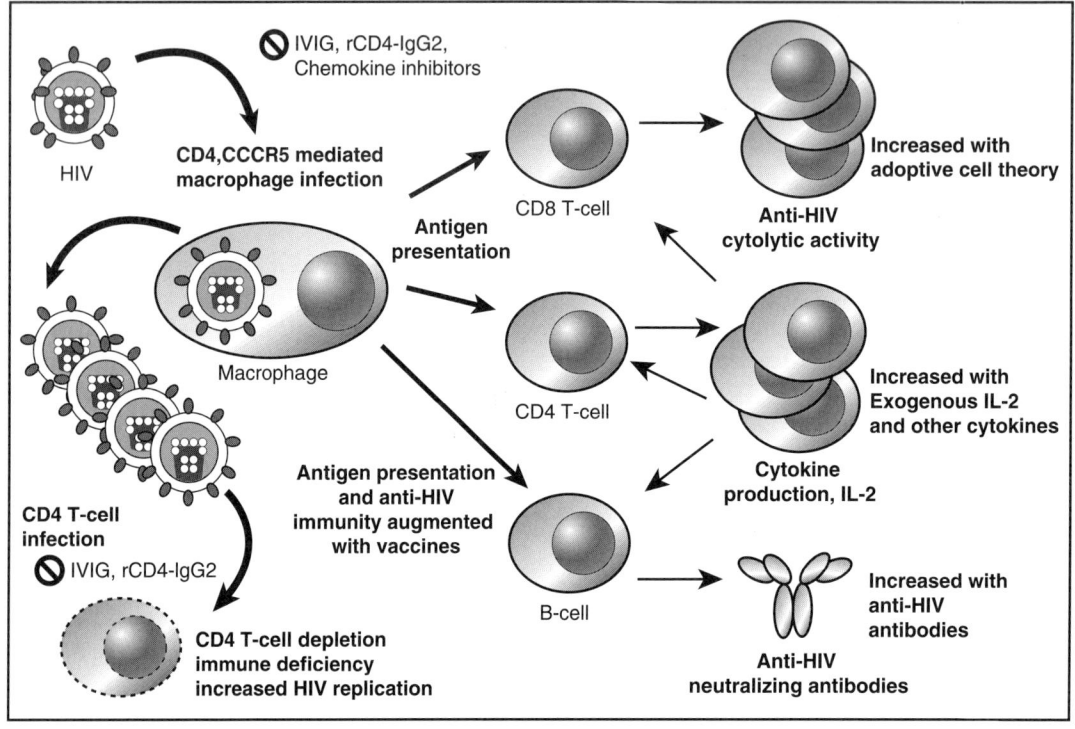

Figure 9–1. Simplified scheme of the development of specific anti-HIV immunity and immune-based strategies for therapeutic intervention (in red).

of viral transmission.[6–8] Based on this evidence, most immune-based efforts are designed to enhance HIV-specific cellular immunity. Other strategies focus on the interactions between HIV and the target cell surface receptor. Soon after it was known that the CD4+ molecule was the T cell receptor for the virus entry, some of the initial studies used soluble recombinant CD4+ molecule (srCD4) infusions in an attempt to neutralize the virus attachment to T cells. In vitro tests were encouraging, but very high doses of srCD4 were needed to demonstrate a reduction in plasma virus titers in HIV-infected subjects, making this approach impractical.[9] A third-generation CD4+ blocker fusion protein, exhibiting a longer serum half-life and multiple HIV gp120 binding sites, has renewed the interest in this approach (see later discussion).

In this review, we present some of the most promising immune-based approaches to controlling HIV infection, with emphasis on those that have been tested in clinical trials.

CYTOKINES AND CHEMOKINES

Cytokines and chemokines are glycoproteins secreted by different types of cells that activate immune system cells, enhancing their function. For example, interleukin-2 and interleukin-7 expand the T cell pool by activating T cells and inducing their replication. Other cytokines, granulocyte colony stimulating factor (GCSF) and granulocyte-macrophage colony stimulating factor (GMCSF), increase the number of neutrophils. Interferon-α inhibits viral replication in macrophages. Several cytokines have been tested for therapeutic effect in HIV infection, as measured by a decrease in viral load or an increase in CD4+ T cell count. To date, interleukin-2 has proven to be the most successful, and it may be used in combination with antiretroviral drugs. Not all cytokines tested have been demonstrated to produce a beneficial effect. Interleukin-10 inhibits HIV replication in macrophages in vitro[10] but has not produced any significant changes in HIV RNA levels or CD4+ T cell counts, when tested in a 4-week, placebo-controlled, double-blind trial with 39 HIV-infected subjects.[11] Similarly, based on the upregulation of HIV expression that is observed when interleukin-1 is added to HIV-infected T cell cultures, a clinical trial testing soluble interleukin-1 receptor (sIL-1R) at doses of 125 to 1250 μg/m^2 was conducted with 12 HIV-infected patients. After 3 months, there were no significant changes of peripheral blood

CD4+ T cell counts nor plasma HIV viral load. Seven patients reported improvement of general systemic symptoms, most likely because of the anti-inflammatory effect of sIL-1R.[12]

Interleukin-2 (Table 9–2)

Interleukin-2 is produced by activated CD4+ T cells and plays a significant role on the activation and replication of T cells, preferentially naive cells, and natural killer (NK) cells. Early clinical trials were encouraged by the in vitro evidence of cellular immunity defects in HIV-infected patients that were reversible with interleukin-2.[13] The results of these trials failed to show clear evidence of therapeutic advantage, and the adverse effects (malaise, fever) were significant.[14] However, some of the patients receiving continuous intravenous interleukin-2 had moderate increases in their CD4+ T cell counts, prompting subsequent studies using alternative methods of administration of interleukin-2. Recent reports using interleukin-2 for 5-day cycles every 6 to 8 weeks, in addition to antiretrovirals, have shown that these increases in CD4+ T cells counts can be sustained.[15] The success of these approaches may be related to the availability of new antiretroviral drugs, or differences in doses and mode of administration of interleukin-2. Because activation of T cells may also trigger HIV replication in infected cells, protocols using interleukin-2 in HIV-infected patients should be administered with antiretroviral drug therapy.[16] Compared with patients using antiretrovirals alone, HIV-infected patients with CD4+ T cell counts greater than 200 cells/mm^3 and receiving interleukin-2 benefit with an increase of CD4+ T cell numbers; their viral load appears not to be affected.[15–17]

Most recent studies have used a regimen of daily subcutaneous injections of 1.5 to 7.5 million international units (IU). A randomized placebo-controlled trial of interleukin-2 (in addition to antiretroviral therapy) in 83 patients showed a 113% increase of CD4+ T cell counts after 1 year, compared with 18% in subjects receiving antiretroviral drugs alone. There was also a significant viral load decrease of 0.28 log^{10} compared with 0.09 log^{10}, respectively. Kovacs and collaborators have shown an increase in CD4+ T cell counts (428 cells/mm^3 to 916 cells/mm^3, after 12 months) in HIV-infected patients using subcutaneous interleukin-2 therapy at doses of 18 million IU daily, in contrast to a decrease (406 cells/mm^3 to 349 cells/mm^3) in the group receiving only conventional antiretroviral treatment. The adverse effects were analyzed, showing that most patients had flu-like symptoms only during the infusion days.[15,18] A similar study with 64 HIV-infected patients subcutaneous receiving interleukin-2 (9 million IU/day) reported fewer incidents of Kaposi sarcoma and opportunistic infections, a mean CD4+ T cell count increase of 100 cells/mm^3, and improvement of the delayed hypersensitivity response skin test to HIV antigens after 1 year of treatment.[19] When subcutaneous interleukin-2 was used three times a week, patients showed an increase of CD4+ T cell counts, but progressively higher doses were required to maintain the effect, and the viral RNA levels were not reduced.[20]

Because of the significant adverse effects with doses of interleukin-2 greater than 1.5 million IU/m^2, studies using interleukin-2 at low-doses from 250,000 to 1.2 million IU/m^2 daily for 6 months have been performed in HIV-infected patients with CD4+ T cell counts between 200 and 500 cells/mm^3. No significant side effects were reported. A small significant increase of CD4+ T cell counts (3.5%) was demonstrated, with a marked improvement of delayed hypersensitivity skin test to common recall antigens. NK cell numbers increased as compared with those of control patients (156 cells/mm^3 versus 20 cells/mm^3).[21,22] Intermediate doses of interleukin-2 (3 million IU/m^2) have also shown a significant increase of CD4+ T cell counts, after 24 weeks, as compared with antiretroviral drugs alone (105 cells/mm^3 and 30 cells/mm^3, respectively).[23] A direct comparison between low-dose (1.5 million IU twice a day) and high-dose (7.5 million IU twice a day) subcutaneous interleukin-2 given during 5-day cycles every 8 weeks resulted in a 95% increase in mean CD4+ T cell counts over baseline, compared with 19% in the low-dose recipients, after 6 months. Although high-dose recipients had more constitutional side effects, they were not dose-limiting.[24]

The route of administration of interleukin-2 was compared in a trial involving 94 asymptomatic HIV-infected patients who had not received antiretroviral treatment. Interleukin-2 was given as 12 million IU/day intravenously, 3 million IU/m^2 twice a day subcutaneously, or 2 million IU/m^2 every 2 months in intravenous bolus with polyethyleneglycol. Equivalent increases in CD4+ T cell counts were observed with both intravenous and subcutaneous routes, and they were significantly better than interleukin-2 with polyethylene glycol. No

Table 9-2
Selected Interleukin-2 Clinical Trials for HIV Infection

AUTHOR STUDY	YEAR	PATIENTS, N	ROUTE	DAILY DOSE OF INTERLEUKIN-2	DURATION	COMMENTS
Volberding et al[14]	1987	87	IV	1-2 million IU/m^2 (daily)	8 wks	No benefits; side effects: fever, myalgia, fatigue, arthralgia
Kovacs et al[15]	1996	60	IV	18 million IU (5d q8wk)	48 wks	CD4 increase
Davey et al[18]	2000	82	SC	7.5 million IU bid (5d q8wk)	48 wks	CD4 increase, viral load decrease
Hengge et al[19]	1998	64	SC	9 million IU qd (5d q6wk)	48 wks	CD4 increase; reduced HIV disease progress
Jacobson et al[21]	1996	16	SC	250,000 IU/m^2 (daily)	24 wks	Small CD4+ increase, NK cells increase; Less toxicity
Lalezari et al[22]	2000	115	SC	1.2 million IU/m^2 (daily)	24 wks	NK cells increase
Arno et al[23]	1999	25	SC	3 million IU (5d q8wk)	24 wks	Moderate CD4+ increase
Levy et al[25]	1999	94	IV, SC	12 million, 3 million IU (q8wk)	50 wks	Equal CD4+ increases
Miller et al[27]	2001	22	SC	7.5 million IU bid	32 wks	Optimal cycle: 5d q8wk

NK, natural killer.

differences were found in viral load.[25] A similar study evaluated 20 HIV patients receiving 9 million IU/day of interleukin-2, either intravenously or subcutaneously, in addition to HAART. Both groups had a more than 200% increase in CD4+ T cell counts, and an over 100% increase in CD8+ T cell counts. There were no viral load changes in either group, but there were fewer side effects in the subcutaneous group.[26] To optimize the frequency of interleukin-2 cycles and the cycle duration, Miller and collaborators studied 22 HIV-infected patients with CD4+ T-cell counts between 200 and 500 cells/mm^3.[27] Patients were randomized into three groups: the first group received the standard interleukin-2 cycle of 5 days every 8 weeks; the second group received interleukin-2 every 2 weeks for a number of days determined by the peak cell cycle; and the third group received 5 days of interleukin-2 every time CD4+ T cell counts fell from a predetermined value. There were no immunologic differences between the three groups, although more frequent or longer cycles led to an increased frequency of side effects. Interleukin-2 has also been successfully used in HIV-1–related lymphoma[28] and in combination with interferon-α to treat Kaposi sarcoma.[29]

The use of interleukin-2 in the treatment of HIV infection is still investigational. It has been shown to be safe and most useful for those patients with good CD4+ T cell counts (>200 cells/mm^3) and low viremia, as an adjunct to HAART. Clinical trials in HIV-infected children are currently being conducted.

Interferon-γ, Interferon-α, Interleukin-12, and Interleukin-16

Other T_H1 cytokines are being tested in clinical trials with the objective of enhancing cellular immunity and controlling viral replication. Interferon-γ is a glycoprotein secreted by T cells and NK cells. Its function is to activate macrophages, enhancing its phagocytic activity and the oxidative burst reaction. Initial studies showed good tolerability, with activity against Kaposi sarcoma.[30] Because of its importance in antimycobacterial immunity, interferon-γ protocols have been used to reduce the incidence of mycobacterial and other opportunistic infections in HIV patients with CD4+ T cell counts lower than 100 cells/mm^3, at doses of 50 μg/m^2 three times a week for 48 weeks. One placebo-controlled study showed a decrease from 3.45 opportunistic infections per month in the placebo group to 1.71 in the patient group receiving interferon-γ; and a 3-year survival rate of 28% as compared with 18% in patients receiving placebo.[31] There was a greater effect on the reduction of infections caused by *Candida* spp, cytomegalovirus, and herpes simplex, and side effects (headache, myalgia, fatigue, depression, and granulocytopenia) were reversible.[31] Shearer and collaborators studied the use of interferon-γ at doses of 50 to 100 μg/m^2 subcutaneously three times per week, for 24 weeks, in HIV-infected children who were receiving antiretroviral monotherapy. There were no significant changes in viral load or CD4+ T cell counts, and the therapy was well tolerated. The incidence of infections was not evaluated in this short-term trial.[32]

Interferon-α is a polypeptide produced by mononuclear cells in response to infections by double-stranded RNA or DNA viruses. It induces synthesis of enzymes that interfere with viral transcription and MHC class I expression. Clinical benefit was documented in early trials using interferon-α in addition to zidovudine, resulting on more patients becoming HIV culture negative and not progressing to AIDS,[33] and demonstrating increased CD4+ T cell counts and a decrease of serum HIV p24 antigen.[34] However, larger trials did not confirm these results, reporting transient small decreases in viral load and severe general adverse effects, including hematologic and neurologic toxicities.[35–37] Studies of the antiretroviral effect of interferon-α in addition to HAART have not been reported.

Interleukin-12 enhances the activity of NK cells and cytolytic CD8+ T cells as well as increasing the in vitro lymphoproliferative responses to mitogens. Interleukin-12 given to monkeys chronically infected with SIVmac, an SIV strain, has been shown to induce T_H1 responses and NK cell activity, although no change in viral load was observed.[38] Interleukin-12 given subcutaneously at a dose up to 300 ng/kg was well tolerated in 47 HIV-infected patients with CD4+ T cell counts of 100 to 500 cells/mm^3.[39] No significant effects on plasma HIV RNA levels and moderate increases of CD8+ T cells, NK cells, and serum interferon-γ levels were observed.[39] The use of interleukin-12 in the treatment of HIV infection is still experimental.

Interleukin-16 is a T_H1 cytokine secreted preferentially by CD8+ T cells and monocytes. It induces the secretion of other proinflammatory cytokines, such as interleukin-6, interleukin-15, and tumor necrosis factor (TNF)-α. It also works as a chemokine for CD4+ T cells. Interleukin-16 has also shown in vitro anti-HIV activity in CD4+ T cells and dendritic cells. When added at the time of infection, it induces a block of viral entry and reducing proviral DNA levels. The mechanisms of these effects are not known but do not involve induction of suppressive chemokines or cytokines.[40] Interleukin-16 has not been tested in HIV-infected patients.

Growth Factors

Granulocyte colony stimulation factor (GCSF) is a hematopoietic growth factor that maintains the circulating number of neutrophils by stimulating their production in bone marrow. Neutropenia is frequently found in HIV-infected patients; it increases the incidence of severe infections and contributes to the activation of HIV replication. GCSF is elevated in HIV-infected patients with bacterial infections, but not in patients with neutropenia alone. Treatment with GCSF reverses HIV-induced neutropenia and reduces the number of infection-related hospitalizations.[41] Therapy with GCSF does not increase HIV viral load. Thirty HIV-infected patients on HAART with CD4+ T cell counts less than 350 cells/mm^3 were given GCSF three times a week for 12 weeks in a placebo-controlled trial. Small increases of CD4+ (20 cells/mm^3) and CD8+ (100 cells/mm^3) T cell counts were demonstrated as well as increased expression of the cell surface activation marker CD38. HIV viral load remained stable throughout the trial. These parameters returned to baseline at the 24-week follow-up examination.[42] GCSF is currently indicated for HIV-induced neutropenia.

Granulocyte-monocyte colony stimulating factor (GMCSF) is produced by T cells, fibroblasts, and endothelial cells. It induces growth and activates neutrophils and macrophages. GMCSF was shown to be safe and well tolerated in HIV patients, with no effect on viral load, when given with HAART.[43] GMCSF may increase viral load in patients not receiving therapy.[44] In a phase III clinical trial in AIDS patients designed to assess its effect on mortality and opportunistic infections, GMCSF was used in combination with antiretroviral treatment at a dose of 250 µg subcutaneously three times a week. It reduced the incidence of infections but not the overall mortality rate. No changes in HIV viral load and only a small increase in CD4+ T cell counts were found.[45] In 105 HIV-infected patients, with CD4+ T cell counts less than 300 cells/mm^3, GMCSF was given at 50, 125, and 250 µg/m^2 daily producing a significant decrease of HIV-RNA levels of more than 0.5 log^{10}. There were no differences in CD4+ T cell counts. After 6 months of GMCSF therapy, no differences in mortality rate or in the incidence of opportunistic infections were demonstrated.[46,47]

Chemokines

Chemokines are molecules that were initially characterized by their ability to induce leukocyte chemotaxis. Recently it was discovered that several chemokine receptors, particularly CCR5 and CXCR4 (monocyte/macrophages and CD4+ T cells, respectively), were the long-sought coreceptors needed for HIV entry to host cells. Chemokine receptor expression determines the tropism of different HIV strains for either T cells or monocytes. Individuals who are homozygous for a 32-base pair deletion in the *CCR5* gene are protected against HIV infection, and HIV-infected subjects heterozygous for this deletion have slower progression of the disease. Subjects who do not express the normal CCR5 receptor have a normal immune response to other pathogens, with no detected abnormalities, likely because of the redundancy of the different chemokine receptor family members.[48] The therapeutic use of chemokines or chemokine analogues to inhibit HIV entry is currently being tested, although it seems that large concentrations are needed to produce a significant inhibitory effect.[49] Inhibitors based on chemokine structure have been designed to interfere with HIV entry, and human trials are in progress.[50–52] An indirect strategy proposed to use a cytokine, TNF-α, to induce production of the chemokine RANTES (regulated on activation of normal T cells expressed and secreted) by monocytes exposed to viral infection. This in vitro study showed that RANTES suppressed HIV replication in a dose-dependent manner.[53]

Genetic engineering has been applied to design an intracellular molecule based on chemokines and antibodies, named *intrakines*. The intrakine gene is introduced into T cell with a viral vector. Intrakines block CXCR-4 cell surface expression by binding to this receptor molecule in the endoplasmic reticulum, and this complex is degraded before it reaches the cell membrane. Modified T cells become immune to T-tropic HIV virus infection, because of the need of CXCR4 as a coreceptor for viral entry.[54] A similar strategy has been developed with ribozymes designed to inhibit the expression of CC chemokine receptor genes, although this inhibition occurs at the nuclear level.[55]

THERAPEUTIC VACCINES
(Table 9–3)

Immunization with vaccines is one of the most successful strategies in medicine. With vaccines, it has been possible to eradicate smallpox infection worldwide; and other diseases, including polio and measles, are no longer occurring in areas of the world with appropriate immunization coverage. Efforts to develop a vaccine for HIV infection have been underway since the early 1980s. Unfortunately, an efficient vaccine has not been achieved yet. A therapeutic or a prophylactic anti-HIV vaccine remains a priority because the HIV epidemic is most prevalent in economically depressed regions of the world, where the cost of antiretroviral drugs is prohibitive. Therapeutic vaccines could be used to decrease the rate of HIV disease progression in HIV-infected patients. Thus, an ideal therapeutic vaccine would be able to induce sterilizing immunity that would lead to virus eradication.[56] The development of a successful anti-HIV vaccine has found many hurdles, mainly related to the extremely high mutation rate of the viral transcriptase that leads promptly to variant escape mutants, in addition to the poor protective effect of the elicited neutralizing antibodies with present-day vaccines. Several different HIV protein vaccines and immunization strategies have been proposed, with more than 20 candidate vaccines tried in humans, including: Env, Gag, Pol, and Nef peptides, gp120, gp160, multimeric gp120, and gp120 V3 loop peptides.

Viral vectors and nonviral approaches are used to induce immune responses to HIV antigens. The most favored delivery viral vectors currently being tested are derived from the vaccinia virus and the canarypox virus. Alphaviruses (e.g., Venezuelan equine encephalitis virus), poliovirus, adenovirus, adeno-associated virus, herpes virus, rabies virus, and vesicular stomatitis virus, are also being investigated as potential vaccine vectors.[56] Venezualan equine encephalitis vectors target dendritic cells, which are efficient antigen-presenting cells. A Venezuelan equine encephalitis vector carrying SIV Env has provided protection against viral challenge in macaques and has elicited strong humoral and cellular response.[57] Adenoviral and poliovirus vectors have been tested to stimulate the mucosal immune system of macaques through nasal and oral immunization, respectively, with

Table 9–3
Selected Anti-HIV Vaccine Strategies

AUTHOR	YEAR	STRATEGY, ANTIGEN	COMMENTS
Davis et al[57]	2000	VEE vector, SIV Env	Targets dendritic cells, elicits strong humoral and cellular response
Crotty et al[59]	1999	Poliovirus vector, SIV Env	Oral route, induces systemic mucosal immune response
Seth et al[63]	2000	Vaccinia vector, SIV Gag-Pol	Protective Gag-specific CTLs in a macaque model
Team TAVEGP[67]	2001	Canarypox vector, HIV Env, Gag, Pol	30% of vaccinees developed CTLs, weak neutralizing antibodies
Shiver et al[76]	2002	Adenoviral vector and protein booster	Most efficient strategy to develop anti-HIV cellular immunity
Lambert et al[70]	1998	Recombinant HIV gp120, gp160	30–60% of vaccinees with lymphoproliferative responses
Borkowsky et al[72]	2000	Recombinant HIV gp120 in infants	56% of vaccinees developed lymphoproliferative responses
Boyer et al[73]	2000	DNA vaccine, HIV env/rev	Induction of strong cellular response
Lisziewicz et al[75]	2001	Transduced dendritic cells, HIV env/gag	Strong cytotoxic response in a macaque model
Goebel et al[80]	1999	Recombinant HIV gp160	No significant benefit in HIV disease progression
Tsoukas et al[81]	1998	Recombinant HIV gp160	No significant disease in HIV disease progression
Kahn et al[84]	2000	HIV immunogen, inactivated virion	No significant benefit in HIV disease progression

moderate protection against viral vaginal challenge in macaques and induction of systemic mucosal response in humans.[58,59]

The need for inducing specific anti-HIV CD8+ T cell response has been suggested by several studies on populations exposed to HIV infection. Sex workers resistant to HIV infection do not have HIV-specific antibodies but make a strong specific CD8+ T cell response.[60] In macaques, induction of SIV-specific CD8+ T cells protects them from SIV infection, despite the absence of neutralizing antibodies.[61] The choice of an HIV viral epitope for an immunization strategy should be one that is shared by most HIV strains, as demonstrated by a successful immunization protocol in the macaque animal model, using SIVmn gp160, which protected only for homologous viral challenges but failed to offer protection to a different viral strain challenge.[62] Seth and coworkers showed that a vaccination protocol using *Gag-pol* genes, in a modified vaccinia virus, induces protective cytotoxic T-cells specific for Gag epitopes that correlate with SIV viremia reduction, similar to the association between development of specific CD8+ T cells and slow disease progression found in humans.[63,64] Currently, several phase I safety trials are being conducted in HIV-infected and noninfected humans, with the major concern being the possibility of viral recombination with reconstitution of wild-type HIV. To date, tested vaccines have been demonstrated to be safe, although most of them elicit only modest levels of HIV-specific CD4+ and CD8+ T cell responses. A canarypox vaccine carrying Env, Gag, and Pol epitopes has been shown to induce a response that lasts up to 9 months in uninfected subjects. One third of persons who received the vaccine develop specific cytotoxic T cells and have weak neutralizing antibodies, although the antibodies can be boosted with a dose of recombinant viral proteins.[65–68] Recombinant HIV envelope proteins offer a protection that is limited to the strain used and induce poor neutralizing antibodies.[69] Studies in HIV-infected children and neonates have demonstrated the safety of HIV recombinant proteins with adjuvant vaccines. HIV envelope vaccines induced lymphoproliferative responses in up to 56% of HIV-infected volunteers without altering CD4+ T cell counts or viral load[70] and induced antibody responses in 63% of HIV-exposed neonates by age 12 weeks.[71] Borkowsky and collaborators tested the immunogenicity of two recombinant HIV gp120 vaccines that are carried with different adjuvants, given to 109 neonates born to HIV-infected mothers and given at birth and at 1 month, 3 months, and 5 months of age. HIV-specific lymphoproliferative responses developed in more than 56% of the patients and lasted up to 104 weeks.[72]

DNA vaccines offer the advantages of lower cost, simplicity, and fewer storage requirements. A few anti-HIV DNA vaccine candidates are in phase I trials. Using DNA plasmid-carrying HIV *env* and *rev* genes, Boyer and collaborators have shown induction of a strong T-cell response in non-HIV-infected volunteers, in addition to an increase of β-chemokine secretion.[73] Research to improve the immunogenicity of DNA vaccines is very active, with several adjuvants being tested, including the coadministration of cytokine-encoding plasmids and immunostimulatory DNA sequences. In mice, these strategies elicit good mucosa-specific antibodies and cytotoxic activities, highly desirable for an anti-HIV vaccine.[74] Lisziewicz and coworkers transduced dendritic cells with DNA plasmids encoding for HIV Env and Gag proteins and infused them back into nonhuman primates. This strategy takes advantage of the well-known property of dendritic cells to efficiently present antigens and to induce a strong cellular response. The animals produced a strong cytotoxic response and a high cytokine production in response to viral challenge. This unique approach may increase the efficacy of specific immunity induction.[75]

Most recently, a comparison between different modalities, including a plasmid DNA vector, a modified vaccinia vector, and a replication-incompetent adenovirus vector, was published, showing that the adenovirus vector was most efficient in eliciting protective cellular immunity.[76] Simultaneously, it was reported that a single amino-acid change resulted in a viral escape mutant from cytotoxic T cells in an infected macaque believed to have developed protective cellular immunity, with no clinical progression and decreased viremia. This finding points out the extreme variability of the virus and the need for continued viral screening.[77]

Vaccination studies are also performed in HIV-infected patients to test for a therapeutic effect. It has been shown that patients who develop lymphoproliferative responses are those who have high CD4+ T cell counts and are at an early stage of disease.[78] Two large trials were conducted in Europe (200 and 835 HIV-infected patients) to test recombinant HIV gp160 given every 3 months to HIV-infected patients in addition to antiretroviral therapy. Both studies showed induction of specific lymphoproliferative responses but no significant benefit in the natural history of disease at 2 and 3 years, as compared with results in subjects receiving placebo.[79,80] Similarly, an active immunization protocol of 278 HIV patients with a recombinant HIV envelope protein showed no effect on progression of disease.[81] A smaller protocol evaluated a DNA-based vaccine carrying the *env* and *rev* genes in 15 HIV-infected adults and demonstrated safety and the induction of specific cellular immunity.[82] Another randomized, placebo-controlled trial using HIV gp120 in 570 HIV-infected patients did not demonstrate differences in disease progression after a 15-month trial.[83] The largest study, including more than 2500 HIV-infected patients, tested the HIV-1 immunogen (an inactivated gp120-depleted HIV virion) that had previously shown no side effects or viral recombination events. The results were disappointing, with no differences observed in rate of disease progression or viral load, although specific lymphoproliferative responses were generated.[84] In summary, several efforts to develop a therapeutic vaccine have already been conducted, with demonstration of adequate safety and newly induced HIV-specific cellular and humoral responses. However, no clinical impact or decrease of viral load has been achieved. New vaccines delivering multiple immunogenic peptides, the use of new adjuvants, and schedules of immunization are currently being researched.

IMMUNOGLOBULINS

Intravenous Immunoglobulins

The therapeutic effects of intravenous immunoglobulins (IVIG) in HIV-infected children were reported by Mofenson and collaborators in 1992, who conducted a multicenter, randomized, placebo-controlled trial using monthly doses of IVIG at 400 mg/kg on children with CD4+ T cell counts greater than 200 cells/mm^3. There was a significant reduction in the incidence of viral and bacterial infections but not in the occurrence of opportunistic infections.[85] Spector and collaborators studied the effect of IVIG in 255 children who had AIDS or AIDS-related complex in reducing the incidence of severe bacterial infections over 2 years, as compared with placebo. There was a decreased risk of infections (16.9% versus 24.3%; $P = .07$); however, the benefit was significant only for the children who were not on cotrimoxazole prophylaxis (11.3% versus 26.8%; $P = .03$). The 2-year survival rate was similar in both groups.[86]

Although IVIG is still an alternative to reduce the number of infections in HIV-infected pediatric patients, its high cost and the effectiveness of HAART regimens have reduced the usefulness of immunoglobulin infusions.

Intravenous Immunoglobulins Containing High Anti-HIV Antibody Titers

Early trials had shown the clinical benefit of using heat-inactivated plasma from HIV-seropositive individuals, reporting less mortality and fewer patients entering the AIDS stage in randomized, placebo-controlled trials over 12-month periods. For example, in one of these studies, 86 symptomatic HIV-infected patients received 300 mL of either plasma rich in anti-HIV p24 antibody or seronegative plasma every 14 days, in addition to zidovudine and standard prophylactic therapy. Seven AIDS-related deaths occurred in the treatment group, versus 11 in the control group.[87,88] The practice of using plasma from HIV-infected patients has been abandoned because of concerns related to the possibility of remaining non-inactivated viruses or the presence of other unknown blood-borne pathogens.

Hyperimmune immunoglobulin infusions that include HIV-specific antibodies have been administered during pregnancy but have not been shown to significantly decrease perinatal HIV transmission (4.1%), compared with the group that received standard IVIG (6.0%; $P = .36$); both regimens were given in addition to zidovudine in women with CD4+ T cell counts lower than 500 cells/mm^3.[89] It was decided that follow-up studies to determine whether this difference was real would not be conducted because they would have required a large number of study subjects, when the declining perinatal HIV transmission rate was taken into account (Pediatrics AIDS Clinical Trial Group 185).

Monoclonal Anti-HIV Antibodies

Several attempts have been made to develop a neutralizing anti-HIV monoclonal antibody that would confer passive immunity. In a trial to reduce viral load, specific mouse anti-HIV antibodies with neutralizing properties were infused to 11 HIV-infected patients. Anti-mouse and anti-idiotypic antibodies appeared in 8 cases. Plasma gp120 protein decreased, but viral load was not consistently reduced.[90]

Mascola and collaborators used a SIV/HIV chimeric virus (SHIV) macaque model to evaluate two humanized anti-HIV monoclonal antibodies (2F5 and 2G12) and to test protection against SHIV viral vaginal challenge. These antibodies are specific for amino acid sequences from the HIV envelope glycoprotein gp41 and have been shown to neutralize different primary HIV-1 isolates in vitro. High viremia developed in all control monkeys and in 6 of 14 monkeys pretreated with the monoclonal antibodies, although they became undetectable at week 12. The control monkeys had persistent viremia up to week 22. None of the monkeys infused with the monoclonal antibodies had CD4+ T cell depletion, which was seen in all five control animals. Furthermore, the anti-HIV antibodies were detected in all mucosal compartments.[91] These antibodies have already been examined in a phase I trial with seven HIV-infected adults. After a follow-up period of 22 weeks, safety and tolerability were demonstrated but no significant changes in HIV viral load or CD4+ T cells were detected.[92] Studies in HIV-infected humans are being proposed.

CD4-IgG2

Shearer and collaborators have developed a recombinant dimeric molecule that uses the virus-binding domains of CD4 coupled with IgG, as a soluble competitor for HIV gp120 binding to CD4, on the T cell membrane. CD4-IgG was demonstrated to be safe for both mother and infant and crossed the placenta barrier.[93] Based on this previous study, a new CD4+ blocker (PRO542; Fig. 9–2) has been developed by Progenics Pharmaceuticals (Tarrytown, NJ). This new drug has four copies of the human CD4+ molecule fused with conserved domains of the constant region of human IgG2. It has an extended half-life (>2 days) and multiple binding sites for gp120. It neutralizes primary HIV-1 regardless of genotype or phenotype.[94] In a recent study, 18 children received 10 mg/kg of rCD4-IgG2. It was well tolerated and appeared to produce sustained decreases in serum HIV-1 RNA concentrations, up to 2 $\log_{10}$ at 2 weeks after the infusion (Pediatric Clinical Trial Group Protocol 351).[95] In HIV-infected adults, CD4-IgG2 has been shown to be safe and well tolerated, with a significant reduction of plasma HIV-RNA up to 2 $\log_{10}$, after a single intravenous infusion.[96]

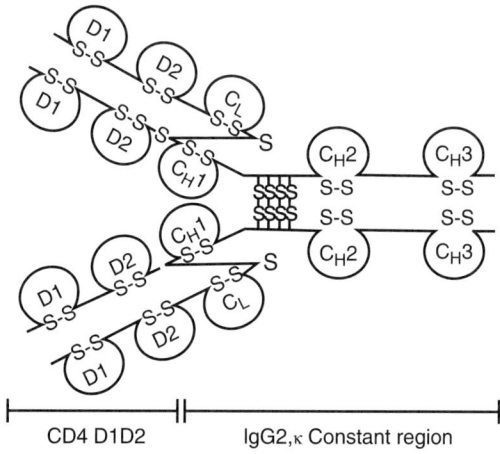

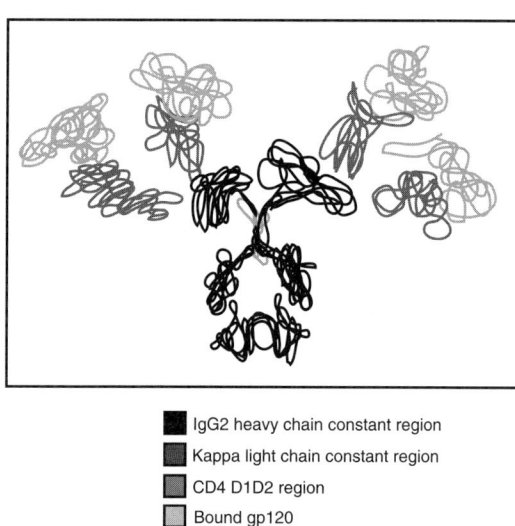

Figure 9–2. Diagram and tridimensional image of rCD4-IgG2 structure. (Reproduced from Zhu et al: J Virol 2001; 75: 6682, with permission).

ADOPTIVE LYMPHOCYTE TRANSFER

HIV-infected patients who receive adequate antiretroviral treatment have a slower progression of disease and a lower rate of mortality. This improvement is mainly attributed to the recovery of CD4+ T cell counts. However, restoration of the immune system is usually incomplete, with not all specific clones represented uniformly. This nonhomogeneous immune reconstitution of HIV-infected patients probably depends on how early therapy was started.[97] Several attempts to improve reconstitution of the immune system rely on the transfer of donor or stimulated lymphocytes to HIV-infected patients. The goals of these efforts have been to increase the number of circulating CD4+ T cells or CD8+ T cells and to restore immune responses to pathogens. Some protocols modified these cells to enhance their specificity against certain viruses, that is, cytomegalovirus and HIV.[98] It has been shown, however, that specific cytolytic T cells transferred to HIV-infected patients have a short half-life and undergo apoptosis when they encounter the HIV antigen.[99] In a different strategy, HIV-infected volunteers received engineered autologous T cells, expressing a modified CD4-ζ chain, to induce activation upon contact with HIV. One to 3% of modified cells persisted up to 8 weeks, and 0.1% after 1 year, with detectable presence of these cells in rectal tissue. No decrease in serum viral load occurred, but a demonstrable decrease in HIV present in rectal tissue was reported.[100] Tsoukas and coworkers[101] described a direct strategy consisting of the infusion of lymphocytes obtained from seronegative identical twin siblings and stimulated 5 days in vitro with interleukin-2. The HIV-infected patients who received these infusions demonstrated dramatic increases of CD4+ T cell numbers and new and increased specific anti-HIV cellular immune responses. Lieberman and coworkers[102] expanded clones of HIV-epitope–specific T cells in vitro and reinfused these cells into patients, showing a transient increase in specific cellular responses. Unfortunately, although these infusions were well tolerated, these cells and the increased cellular responses were short lived.

More recently, it has been shown that reinfusion of 3 to 30 × 10^9 autologous CD4+ T cells stimulated in vitro with CD3 and CD28 produced significant and sustained increments of peripheral blood CD4+ T cell count up to 1 year after the infusion, with corresponding threefold decreases of viral load.[103] The effect was not obtained if the cells were stimulated with the mitogen concanavalin A and interleukin-2. These results are likely explained by the downregulation of CCR5 receptor and enhanced secretion of β chemokines, effects that were observed when CD3 and CD28 were used for T cell activation in vitro. This approach may induce resistance to HIV infection because of the need for the chemokine receptor for viral entry to the cells. The possible side effects of inducing autoimmune phenomena or increasing viral replication did not occur in this trial. Furthermore, lymphoproliferative responses to several mitogens and antigens were improved, and production of interleukin-2, GMCSF, and interferon-γ were increased.[103]

IMMUNOSUPPRESSIVE DRUGS

Thalidomide

Thalidomide inhibits the effects of TNF-α and has been used to treat wasting syndrome and oral aphthous ulcers in HIV-infected patients. TNF-α activates HIV replication; therefore, thalidomide should have the potential of reducing HIV viral load. In vitro studies have shown that thalidomide inhibits the lipopolysaccharide-induced upregulation of chemokine receptors in CD4+ T cells[104] and stimulates delayed hypersensitivity responses and interleukin-12 production in HIV-infected patients not taking antiretroviral therapy.[105] Although these changes were associated with a moderate increase of viral load, they returned to baseline when the drug was stopped.[105] Recently, the immunologic effects of thalidomide (at the low dose of 3 mg/kg/day for 28 days) were studied in eight HIV-infected children who were not receiving antiretroviral therapy. The viral load did not change significantly, and the activation markers of CD8+ T cells increased, as did the activity of HIV *Gag*-specific CD8+ T cells.[106]

Cyclosporine A

Cyclosporine A inhibits T cell proliferation and cytokine expression by binding to cyclophilin, a protein needed for T cell activation. Cyclosporine A is commonly used in the prevention of transplant rejection and in selected autoimmune disorders. When it was found that cyclophilin was necessary for HIV particle maturation, investigators conducted protocols that tested cyclosporine A as an anti-HIV agent, unfortunately without effect on viral load or disease progression.[107] More recently, Martin and coworkers[108] administered cyclosporine A to seven SIVmac-infected monkeys, demonstrating a decrease of viral load and plasma HIV p27 level. Protocols that test cyclosporine A in addition to HAART in humans have not been published.

CONCLUSIONS

The management of HIV has improved considerably with the introduction of drug combination regimens that include reverse transcriptase inhibitors and protease inhibitors. However, multidrug treatments have several limitations, including difficult compliance and the emergence of resistant HIV strains. These clinical studies have shown the need of developing novel approaches for the control of HIV infection. Immune-based therapies are attractive because they are designed to intervene in the pathogenesis of the disease. They are novel and still experimental, but they promise to be adjuvant to current antiretroviral regimens, to achieve a better and sustained control of viral replication. Priority is placed on the development of vaccines that have the potential double role of preventing and treating HIV infection by eliciting protective immunity. Several variables that complicate the evaluation of these immune-based approaches need to be defined and include doses and schedules of treatment, end points, disease severity, and the use of concomitant antiretroviral therapy. In addition, because most clinical trials have been performed in adult populations, clinical studies including HIV-infected children are critically needed.

ACKNOWLEDGMENT

This work was supported in part by NIH grants AI-27551, AI-39131, AD-41983, HL-61184, AI-07456, AI-36211, and RR-0188 and by the Pediatric AIDS Fund and Immunology Research Fund of Texas Children's Hospital.

REFERENCES

1. Autran B, Carcelain G, Li TS, et al: Positive effects of combined antiretroviral therapy on CD4 T-cell homeostasis and function in advanced HIV disease. Science 1997;277:112–116.
2. Natarajan V, Bosche M, Metcalf JA, et al: HIV-1 replication in patients with undetectable plasma virus receiving highly active antiretroviral therapy. Lancet 1999;353:119–120.
3. Wong JK, Hezareh M, Gunthard HF, et al: Recovery of replication-competent HIV despite prolonged suppression of plasma viremia. Science 1997;278:1291–1295.
4. Bucy RP, Kilby JM: Perspectives on inducing efficient immune control of HIV-1 replication: A new goal for HIV therapeutics. AIDS 2001;15:S36–S42.
5. Rosenberg ES, Billingsley JM, Caliendo AM, et al: Vigorous specific CD4 T-cell responses are associated with control of viremia. Science 1997;278:1447–1450.
6. Scarlatti G, Albert J, Rossi P, et al: Mother to child transmission of HIV-1: Correlation with neutralizing antibodies against primary isolates. J Infect Dis 1993;168:207–210.
7. Mofenson LM, Lambert JS, Stiehm ER, et al: Risk factors for perinatal transmission of human immunodeficiency virus type 1 in women treated with zidovudine. N Engl J Med 1999;341:385–393.
8. Sperling RS, Shapiro DE, Coombs RW, et al: Maternal viral load, zidovudine treatment, and the risk of transmission of human immunodeficiency type 1 from mother to infant. N Engl J Med 1996;335:1621–1629.
9. Schacker T, Collier AC, Coombs R, et al: Phase I study of high-dose intravenous rsCD4 in subjects with advanced HIV-1 infection. J Acquir Immune Defic Syndr Hum Retrovirol 1995;9:145–152.
10. Chang J, Naif HM, Li S, et al: The inhibition of HIV replication in monocytes by interleukin 10 is linked to inhibition of cell differentiation. AIDS Res Hum Retroviruses 1996;12:1227–1235.
11. Angel JB, Jacobson MA, Skolnik PR, et al: A multicenter, randomized, double-blind, placebo-controlled trial of recombinant human interleukin-10 in HIV-infected subjects. AIDS 2000;14: 2503–2508.
12. Takebe N, Paredes J, Pino MC, et al: Phase I/II trial of the type I soluble recombinant human interleukin-1 receptor in HIV-1 infected patients. J Interferon Cytokine Res 1998;18:321–326.
13. Lifson JD, Benike CJ, Mark DF, et al: Human recombinant interleukin-2 partly reconstitutes deficient in-vitro immune responses of lymphocytes from patients with AIDS. Lancet 1984;1:698–702.
14. Volberding P, Moody DJ, Beardslee D, et al: Therapy of acquired immune deficiency syndrome with recombinant interleukin-2. AIDS Res Hum Retroviruses 1987;3:115–124.
15. Kovacs JA, Vogel S, Albert JM, et al: Controlled trial of interleukin-2 infusions in patients infected with the human immunodeficiency virus. N Engl J Med 1996;335:1350–1356.
16. Kovacs JA, Baseler M, Dewar R, et al: Increases in CD4 T lymphocytes with intermittent courses of interleukin-2 in patients with human immunodeficiency virus infection: A preliminary study. N Engl J Med 1995;332:567–575.
17. Emery S, Capra WB, Cooper DA, et al: Pooled analysis of three randomized controlled trials of interleukin-2 therapy in adult human immunodeficiency virus type 1 disease. J Infect Dis 2000;182:428–434.
18. Davey RT, Murphy RL, Graziano FM, et al: Immunologic and virologic effects of subcutaneous interleukin 2 in combination with antiretroviral therapy: A randomized controlled trial. JAMA 2000;284:183–189.
19. Hengge UR, Goos M, Esser S, et al: Randomized, controlled phase II trial of subcutaneous interleukin-2 in combination with highly active antiretroviral therapy (HAART) in HIV patients. AIDS 1998;12:F225–233.

20. Larsen CS, Ostergard L, Moller BK, Buhl MR: Subcutaneous interleukin-2 combination with antiretroviral therapy for treatment of HIV-1-infected subjects. Scan J Infect Dis 2000;32:153–160.
21. Jacobson EL, Pilaro F, Smith KA: Rational interleukin 2 therapy for HIV-positive individuals: Daily low doses enhance immune function without toxicity. Proc Natl Acad Sci U S A 1996;93:10405–10410.
22. Lalezari JP, Beal JA, Ruane PJ, et al: Low-dose daily subcutaneous interleukin-2 in combination with highly active antiretroviral therapy in HIV+ patients: A randomized controlled trial. HIV Clin Trials 2000;1:1–15.
23. Arno A, Ruiz L, Juan M, et al: Efficacy of low-dose subcutaneous interleukin-2 to treat advanced human immunodeficiency virus type 1 in persons with microL CD4 T cells and undetectable plasma virus load. J Infect Dis 1999;180:56–60.
24. Davey RT, Chaitt DG, Albert JM, et al: A randomized trial of high versus low dose subcutaneous interleukin-2 outpatient therapy for early human immunodeficiency virus type 1 infection. J Infect Dis 1999;179:849–858.
25. Levy Y, Capitant C, Houhou S, et al: Comparison of subcutaneous and intravenous interleukin-2 in asymptomatic HIV-1 infection: A randomized controlled trial ANRS 048 study group. Lancet 1999;353:1923–1929.
26. Witzke O, Winterhagen T, Reinhardt W, et al: Comparison between subcutaneous and intravenous interleukin-2 treatment in HIV disease. J Intern Med 1998;244:235–240.
27. Miller KD, Spooner K, Herpin BR, et al: Immunotherapy of HIV-infected patients with intermittent interleukin-2: Effects of cycle frequency and cycle duration on degree of CD4 T-lymphocyte expansion. Clin Immunol 2001;99:30–42.
28. Shah MH, Baiocchi RA, Fehniger TA, et al: Cytokine replacement in patients with HIV-1 non-Hodgkin's lymphoma: The rationale for low-dose interleukin-2 therapy. Cancer J Sci Am 2000;6:S45–S51.
29. Schnittman SM, Vogel S, Baseler M, et al: A phase I study of interferon-alpha 2b in combination with interleukin-2 in patients with human immunodeficiency virus infection. J Infect Dis 1994;169:981–989.
30. Heagy W, Groopman J, Schindler J, Finberg R: Use of IFN-gamma in patients with AIDS. J Acquir Immune Defic Syndr 1990;3:584–590.
31. Riddell LA, Pinching AJ, Hill S, et al: A phase III study of recombinant human interferon gamma to prevent opportunistic infections in advance HIV disease. AIDS Res Hum Retroviruses 2001;17:789–797.
32. Shearer WT, Kline MW, Abramson SL, et al: Recombinant human gamma interferon in human immunodeficiency virus-infected children: Safety, CD4+ lymphocyte count, viral load, and neutrophil function (AIDS Clinical Trial Group Protocol 211). Clin Diagn Lab Immunol 1999;6:311–315.
33. Lane HC, Davey V, Kovacs JA, et al: Interferon-alpha in patients with asymptomatic human immunodeficiency virus (HIV) infection: A randomized, placebo-controlled trial. Ann Intern Med 1990;112:805–811.
34. Frissen PH, van der Ende ME, ten Napel CH, et al: Zidovudine and interferon-alpha combination therapy versus zidovudine monotherapy in subjects with symptomatic human immunodeficiency virus type 1 infection. J Infect Dis 1994;169:1351–1355.
35. Fernandez-Cruz E, Lang JM, Frissen J, et al: Zidovudine plus interferon-alpha versus zidovudine alone in HIV-infected symptomatic or asymptomatic persons with CD4+ cell counts >150 × 10 (6)/L: Results of the Zidon trial. AIDS 1995;9:1025–1035.
36. Fischl MA, Richman DD, Saag M, et al: Safety and antiviral activity of combination therapy with zidovudine, zalcitabine, and two doses of interferon-alpha2a in patients with HIV. AIDS Clinical trials group Study 197. J Acquir Immune Defic Syndr Hum Retrovirol 1997;16:247–253.
37. Haas DW, Lavelle J, Nadler JP, et al: A randomized trial of interferon alpha therapy for HIV type 1 infection. AIDS Res Hum Retroviruses 2000;16:183–190.
38. Watanabe N, Sypek JP, Mitter S, et al: Administration of recombinant human interleukin 12 to chronically SIVmac-infected rhesus monkeys. AIDS Res Hum Retroviruses 1998;14:393–399.
39. Jacobson MA, Hardy D, Connick E, et al: Phase 1 trial of a single dose of recombinant human interleukin-12 in human immunodeficiency virus-infected patients with 100–500 CD4 cells/microliter. J Infect Dis 2000;182:1070–1076.
40. Truong MJ, Darcissac EC, Hermann E, et al: Interleukin-16 inhibits human immunodeficiency virus type 1 entry and replication in macrophages and dendritic cells. J Virol 1999;73:7008–7013.
41. Kuritzkes DR, Parenti D, Ward DJ, et al: Filgrastim prevents severe neutropenia and reduces infective morbidity in patients with advanced HIV infection: Results of a randomized, multicenter, controlled trial. AIDS 1998;12:65–74.
42. Aladdin H, Ullum H, Dam Nielsen S, et al: Granulocyte colony stimulating factor increases CD4+ T-cell counts of human immunodeficiency virus-infected patients receiving stable, highly active antiretroviral therapy: Results from a randomized, placebo-controlled trial. J Infect Dis 2000;181: 1148–1152.
43. Skowron G, Stein D, Drusano G, et al: The safety and efficacy of granulocyte-macrophage colony-stimulating factor (Sargramostim) added to indinavir- or ritonavir-based antiretroviral therapy: A randomized double-blind, placebo-controlled trial. J Infect Dis 1999;180:1064–1071.
44. Pluda JM, Yarchoan R, Smith PD, et al: Subcutaneous recombinant granulocyte-macrophage colony stimulating factor used as single agent and in an alternating regimen with azidothymidine in leukopenic patients with severe human immunodeficient virus infection. Blood 1990;76:463–472.

45. Angel JB, High K, Rhame F, et al: Phase III study of granulocyte macrophage colony-stimulating factor in advanced HIV disease: Effect on infections, CD4 cell counts and HIV suppression. Leukine/HIV Study Group. AIDS 2000;14:387–395.
46. Brites C, Badaro R, Pedral-Sampaio D, et al: A randomized placebo-controlled trial of granulocyte-macrophage colony-stimulating factor and nucleoside analogue therapy in AIDS. J Infect Dis 2000;182: 1531–1535.
47. Scadden DT, Pickus O, Hammer SM, et al: Lack of in vivo effect of granulocyte-macrophage colony stimulating factor on human immunodeficiency virus type 1. AIDS Res Hum Retroviruses 1996;12:1151–1159.
48. Paxton WA, Martin SR, Tse D, et al: Relative resistance to HIV-1 infection of CD4 lymphocytes despite multiple high-risk exposures. Nat Med 1996;2:412–417.
49. Cocchi F, DeVico AL, Garzino-Demo A, et al: Identification of RANTES, MIP-1alpha, MIP-1beta as the major HIV-1 suppressive factors produced by CD8 T-cells. Science 1996;270:1811–1814.
50. Doranz BJ, Filion LG, Diaz-Mitoma F, et al: Safe use of the CXCR4 inhibitor ALX40-4C in humans. AIDS Res Hum Retroviruses 2001;17:475–486.
51. Ghezzi S, Menzo S, Brambilla A, et al: Inhibition of R5X4 dual tropic HIV-1 primary isolates by single chemokine co-receptor ligands. Virology 2001;15: 253–261.
52. Howard OM, Oppenheim JJ, Hollingshead MG, et al: Inhibition and in vitro and in vivo HIV replication by a distamycin analogue that interferes with chemokine receptor function: A candidate for chemotherapeutic and microbicidal application. J Med Chem 1998;41:2184–2193.
53. Lane BR, Markovitz DM, Woodfor NL, et al: TNF-alpha inhibits HIV-1 replication in peripheral blood monocytes and alveolar macrophages by inducing the production of RANTES and decreasing C-C chemokine receptor 5 (CCR5) expression. J Immunol 1999;163:3653–3661.
54. Chen JD, Bai X, Yang AG, et al: Inactivation of HIV-1 chemokine co-receptor CXCR-4 by a novel intrakine strategy. Nat Med 1997;3:1110–1116.
55. Bai J, Rossi J, Akkina R: Multivalent anti-CCR ribozymes for stem cell based HIV type 1 gene therapy. AIDS Res Hum Retroviruses 2001;17:385–399.
56. Mascola JR, Nabel GJ: Vaccines for prevention of HIV disease. Curr Opinion Immunol 2001;13:489–495.
57. Davis NL, Caley IJ, Brown KW, et al: Vaccination of macaques against pathogenic simian immunodeficiency virus with Venezuelan equine encephalitis virus replication particles. J Virol 2000;74:371–378.
58. Buge SL, Murty L, Arora K, et al: Factors associated with slow disease progression in macaques immunized with an adenovirus-simian immunodeficiency virus (SIV) envelope priming-gp120 boosting regimen and challenged vaginally with SIVmac251. J Virol 1999;73:7430–7440.
59. Crotty S, Lohman BL, Lu FX, et al: Mucosal immunization of cynomolgus macaques with two serotypes of live poliovirus vectors expressing simian immunodeficiency virus antigens: Stimulation of humoral, mucosal and cellular immunity. J Virol 1999;73:9485–9495.
60. Rowland-Jones SL, et al: Cytotoxic T-cell responses to multiple conserved HIV epitopes in HIV resistant prostitutes in Nairobi. J Clin Invest 1998;102:1758–1765.
61. Lifson JD, Rossio JL, Piatak MJ, et al: Containment of simian immunodeficiency virus infection: Cellular immune responses and protection from rechallenge following transient post-inoculation antiretroviral treatment. J Virol 2000;74:2584–2593.
62. Polacino P, Stallard V, Klaniecki JE, et al: Limited breadth of the protective immunity elicited by simian immunodeficiency virus SIVmne gp160 vaccines in a combination immunization regimen. J Virol 1999;73:618–630.
63. Seth A, Ourmanov I, Schmitz JE, et al: Immunization with a modified vaccinia virus expressing simian immunodeficiency virus (SIV) Gag-Pol primes for an anamnestic Gag-specific cytotoxic T-lymphocyte response and is associated with reduction of viremia after SIV challenge. J Virol 2000;74:2502–2509.
64. Koup RA, Safrit JT, Cao Y, et al: Temporal association of cellular immune responses with the initial control of viremia in primary immunodeficiency virus type 1 infection syndrome. J Virol 1994;68:4650–4655.
65. Gorse GJ, Patel GB, Belshe RB: HIV type 1 vaccine-induced T cell memory and cytotoxic T lymphocyte responses in HIV type-1 uninfected volunteers. AIDS Res Hum Retroviruses 2001;17:1175–1179.
66. McElrath MJ, Corey L, Montefiori D, et al: A phase II study of two HIV type 1 envelope vaccines, comparing their immunogenicity in populations at risk of acquiring HIV type 1 infection. AIDS Res Hum Retroviruses 2000;16:907–919.
67. Team TAVEGP: Cellular and humoral responses to a canarypox vaccine containing immunodeficiency virus type 1 Env, Gag and Pro in combination with rpg120. J Infect Dis 2001;183:563–570.
68. Verrier F, Burda S, Belshe R, et al: A human immunodeficiency virus prime-boost immunization regimen in humans induces antibodies that show interclade cross-reactivity and neutralize several X4, R5 and dual tropic clade B and C primary isolates. J Virol 2000;74:10025–10033.
69. Cho MW, Kim YB, Lee MK, et al: Polyvalent envelope glycoprotein vaccine elicits a broader neutralizing antibody response but is unable to provide sterilizing protection against heterologous simian/human immunodeficiency virus infection in pigtailed macaques. J Virol 2001;75:2224–2234.
70. Lambert JS, McNamara J, Katz SL, et al: Safety and immunogenicity of HIV recombinant envelope in HIV-infected infants and children. NIH-sponsored Pediatrics AIDS Clinical Trials Group (ACTG-218).

J Acquir Immune Defic Syndr Hum Retrovirol 1998;19:451–461.
71. McFarland EJ, Borkowsky W, Fenton T, et al: Human immunodeficiency virus type 1 (HIV-1) gp-120-specific antibodies in neonates receiving an HIV-1 recombinant gp120 vaccine. J Infect Dis 2001;184:1331–1335.
72. Borkowsky W, Wara D, Fenton T, et al: Lymphoproliferative responses to recombinant HIV-1 envelope antigens in neonates and infants receiving gp120 vaccines. J Infect Dis 2000;181:890–896.
73. Boyer JD, Cohen AD, Vogt S, et al: Vaccination of seronegative volunteers with a human immunodeficiency virus type 1 env/rev DNA vaccine induces antigen-specific proliferation and lymphocyte production of beta chemokines. J Infect Dis 2000;181:476–483.
74. Chattergoon M, Boyer J, Weiner DB: Genetic immunization: A new era of vaccines and immune therapeutics. FASEB J 1997;11:753–763.
75. Lisziewicz J, Gabrilovich DI, Varga G, et al: Induction of potent human immunodeficiency virus type-1 specific T-cell restricted immunity by genetically modified dendritic cells. J Virol 2001;75:7621–7628.
76. Shiver JW, Fu TM, Chen K, et al: Replication-incompetent adenoviral vaccine vector elicits effective anti-immunodeficiency-virus immunity. Nature 2002;415:331–335.
77. Barouch DH, Kunstman J, Kuroda MJ, et al: Eventual AIDS vaccine failure in a rhesus monkey by viral escape from cytotoxic T lymphocytes. Nature 2002;415:335–339.
78. Schooley RT, Spino C, Kuritzkes D, et al: Double-blinded, randomized, comparative trials of 4 human immunodeficiency virus type 1 (HIV-1) envelope vaccines in HIV-1-infected individuals across a spectrum of disease severity: AIDS clinical trial groups 209 and 214. J Infect Dis 2000;182:1357–1364.
79. Sandstrom E, Wahren B: Therapeutic immunisation with recombinant gp160 in HIV-1 infection: A randomised double-blind placebo-controlled trial. Nordic VAC-04 Study Group. Lancet 1999;353:1735–1742.
80. Goebel FD, Mannhalter JW, Belshe RB, et al: Recombinant gp160 as a therapeutic vaccine for HIV-infection: Results of a large randomized, controlled trial. European Multinational IMMUNO AIDS Vaccine study group. AIDS 1999;13:1461–1468.
81. Tsoukas CM, Raboud J, Bernard NF, et al: Active immunization of patients with HIV infection: A study of the effect of VaxSyn, a recombinant HIV envelope subunit vaccine, on progression of immunodeficiency. AIDS 1998;12:175–182.
82. MacGregor RR, Boyer JD, Ugen KE, et al: First human trial of DNA-based vaccine for treatment of human immunodeficiency virus type-1 infection: Safety and host response. J Infect Dis 1998;178:92–100.
83. Eron JJ, Ashby MA, Giordano MF, et al: Randomized trial of MNrgp120 HIV-1 vaccine in symptomless HIV-1 infection. Lancet 1996;15:105–113.
84. Kahn JO, Cherng DW, Mayer K, et al: Evaluation of HIV-1 immunogen, an immunologic modifier, administered to patients infected with HIV having 300 to 549 × 10(6) CD4 cell counts: A randomized controlled trial. JAMA 2000;284:2193–2202.
85. Mofenson LM, Moye JJ, Bethel J, et al: Prophylactic intravenous immunoglobulin in HIV-infected children with CD4+ counts of 0.20 × 10(9)/L or more: Effect on viral, opportunistic, and bacterial infections. The National Institute of Child Health and Human Development Intravenous Immunoglobulin Clinical Trial Study Group. JAMA 1992;268:483–488.
86. Spector SA, Gelber RD, McGrath N, et al: A controlled trial of intravenous immunoglobulin for the prevention of serious bacterial infections in children receiving zidovudine for advanced human immunodeficiency virus infection. Pediatrics AIDS Clinical Trials Group. N Engl J Med 1994;331:1181–1187.
87. Levy J, Youvan T, Lee ML: Passive hyperimmune plasma therapy in the treatment of acquired immunodeficiency syndrome: Results of a 12-month multicenter double-blind controlled trial. The Passive Hyperimmune Therapy Study Group. Blood 1994;84:2130–2135.
88. Vittecoq D, Chevert S, Morand-Joubert L, et al: Passive immunotherapy in AIDS: A double-blind randomized study based on transfusions of plasma rich in anti-human immunodeficiency virus 1antibodies vs. transfusions of seronegative plasma. Proc Nat Acad Sci U S A 1995;92:1195–1199.
89. Stiehm ER, Lambert JS, Mofenson LM, et al: Efficacy of zidovudine and human immunodeficiency virus (HIV) hyperimmune immunoglobulin for reducing perinatal transmission from HIV-infected women with advanced disease: Results of Pediatric AIDS Trial Group Protocol 185. J Infect Dis 1999;179:567–575.
90. Hinkula J, Bratt G, Gilljam G, et al: Immunological and virological interactions in patients receiving passive immunotherapy with HIV-1 neutralizing monoclonal antibodies. J Acquir Immune Defic Syndr 1994;7:940–951.
91. Mascola JR, Stiegler G, VanCott TC, et al: Protection of macaques against vaginal transmission of a pathogenic HIV-1/SIV chimeric virus by passive infusion of neutralizing antibodies. Nat Med 2002;6:207–210.
92. Armbruster C, Stiegler GM, Vcelar BA, et al: A phase I trial with two human monoclonal antibodies (hMAb 2F5, 2G12) against HIV-1. AIDS 2002;16:227–233.
93. Shearer WT, Duliege AM, Kline MW, et al: Transport of recombinant CD4-IgG across the human placenta: Pharmacokinetics and safety in six mother-infant pairs in AIDS clinical trial protocol group 146. Clin Diag Lab Immunol 1995;2:281–285.
94. Trkola A, Ketas T, KewalRamani VN, et al: Neutralization sensitivity of human immunodeficiency virus type 1 primary isolates to antibodies

94. and CD4-based reagents is independent of coreceptor usage. J Virol 1998;72:1876–1885.
95. Shearer WT, Israel RJ, Starr S, et al: Recombinant CD4-IgG2 in human immunodeficiency virus type1-infected children: Phase 1/2 study. J Infect Dis 2000;182:1774–1779.
96. Jacobson JM, Lowy I, Fletcher CV, et al: Single-dose safety, pharmacology and antiviral activity of the human immunodeficiency virus (HIV) type I entry inhibitor to PRO 542 in HIV-infected adults. J Infect Dis 2000;182:326–329.
97. Carcelain G, Debre P, Autran B: Reconstitution of CD4+ T-lymphocytes in HIV-infected individuals following antiretroviral therapy. Curr Opin Immunol 2001;13:483–488.
98. Riddell SR, Greenberg PD: T-cell therapy of cytomegalovirus and human immunodeficiency virus infection. J Antimicrob Chemother 2000;45(Suppl T3):35–43.
99. McKinney DM, Lewinsihn DA, Riddell SR, et al: The antiviral activity of HIV-specific CD8 CTL clones is limited by elimination due to encounter with HIV-infected targets. J Immunol 1999;163:861–867.
100. Mitsuyasu RT, Anton PA, Deeks SG, et al: Prolonged survival and tissue trafficking following adoptive transfer of CD4zeta gene modified autologous CD4 and CD8 T cells in human immunodeficiency virus-infected subjects. Blood 2000;96:785–793.
101. Tsoukas CM, Turner HM, Hatzakis GE, et al: Improvement of HIV-specific immunity in HIV-infected twins treated with highly active antiretroviral therapy, interleukin-2, and syngeneic adoptively transferred cells. AIDS Res Hum Retroviruses 2001;17:887–900.
102. Lieberman J, Fabry JA, Shankar P, et al: Expansion of HIV type 1-specific cytolytic T-cells from HIV type 1-seropositive subjects. AIDS Res Hum Retroviruses 1995;11:257–271.
103. Levine BL, Bernstein WB, Aronson NE, et al: Adoptive transfer of costimulated CD4+ T cells and decreased CCR5 expression in HIV infection. Nat Med 2002;8:47–53.
104. Juffermans NP, Verbon A, Olszyna DP, et al: Thalidomide suppresses up-regulation of human immunodeficiency virus co-receptors CXCR4 and CCR5 on CD4+ T cells in humans. J Infect Dis 2000;181:1813–1816.
105. Haslett PA, Klausner JD, Makonkawkeyoon S, et al: Thalidomide stimulates T cell responses and interleukin 12 production in HIV-infected patients. AIDS Res Hum Retroviruses 1999;15:1169–1179.
106. Hanekom WA, Hughes J, Haslett PA, et al: The immunomodulatory effects of thalidomide on human immunodeficiency virus-infected children. J Infect Dis 2001;184:1192–1196.
107. Levy R, Jais JP, Tourani JM, et al: Long-term follow up of HIV positive asymptomatic patients having received cyclosporin A. Adv Exp Med Biol 1995;374:229–234.
108. Martin LN, Murphey-Corb M, Mack P, et al: Cyclosporin A modulation of early virologic and immunologic events during primary simian immunodeficiency virus infection in rhesus monkeys. J Infect Dis 1997;176:374–383.

10
Infectious Complications of Pediatric HIV Infection

Wayne M. Dankner,
Toni Frederick, and
Jeanne Bertolli

At the onset of the HIV epidemic, the hallmark of the disease was an unusual susceptibility to opportunistic pathogens. Although most of these opportunistic infections (OIs) had been observed previously in other immunocompromised hosts, their prevalence in HIV-infected individuals far exceeded that observed in other immunologically impaired patients, and they quickly became the major defining events for the clinical diagnosis of AIDS.[1,2] Since the initial epidemic in the United States was expressed predominantly in adults, the criteria for AIDS-defining illnesses were weighted toward the diseases recognized in this population. The list of opportunistic pathogens that make up the category C AIDS diagnoses has changed little since the early years of the epidemic.[3] As perinatal transmission of HIV became more widely prevalent, however, we began to appreciate both similarities and important differences in the OIs experienced by the pediatric age group.

Our understanding of the expression of OIs in AIDS has been greatly enhanced by the identification of the etiologic agent for HIV disease, the role of CD4+ lymphocytes in defining the susceptibility to opportunistic pathogens encountered by this population of children and adults, and, more recently, the interaction between HIV viral replication (as measured by HIV viral RNA load) and CD4+ counts in the determination of this increased susceptibility.[4–7] The CD4+ count has been the best predictor of the risk of OIs and has therefore become the major determinant in guidelines for the treatment and prevention of OIs.[8] The importance of the CD4+ count as a predictor of HIV-related morbidity (especially for events related to opportunistic infection) was recognized by the inclusion of a threshold of 200 cells/mm^3 for adolescents and adults as an AIDS-defining event in the 1993 revised AIDS classification system and by the use of CD4+ counts to define levels of immunosuppression in the revised pediatric classification system in 1994.[3,4,9] The importance of CD4+ counts made the description of age-related differences critical to understanding both the risks of and the expression of opportunistic pathogens and other infectious agents in the pediatric age group. This step has been difficult, however, because of the lower rates of OIs in children, except for bacterial infections, and the smaller numbers of HIV-infected children identified since the start of the epidemic. As a result, pediatricians have relied heavily on the understanding of OIs in HIV-infected adults and adopted a more empirical approach in the determination of immunologic thresholds for the initiation of prophylaxis in children. In this chapter, we focus on the increasing body of pediatric specific data, supplemented as necessary with adult data, to provide a better understanding of the pathogenesis, treatment, and prevention of specific opportunistic pathogens in the HIV-infected pediatric patient.

TRENDS IN THE OCCURRENCE OF OPPORTUNISTIC PATHOGENS

The HIV epidemic has changed dramatically since the first descriptions of this disease. The most pronounced changes have been in significant reductions in both the HIV-related mortality rate and the incidence of OI events.[10–14] These improvements have been directly related to several factors, especially the careful epidemiologic and clinical investigations that have led to linking levels of immunosuppression with the occurrence of specific infections. Once these diseases were identified and immunologic thresholds described for their occurrence, it was possible to institute clinical trials to determine optimal treatment and prophylactic regimens to decrease their actual incidence. From these trials and related clinical experience of HIV experts, guidelines for the prevention and treatment of OIs have been developed and updated on a regular basis.[8,15,16]

The combination of antiretroviral therapy, even prior to the availability of highly active combination therapy, and effective prophylactic regimens contributed to the gradual decline in OIs.[11,17–21] It is important to note that these studies not only demonstrated the importance of OIs as causes of significant morbidity but also showed that many of these infections (cytomegalovirus, disseminated *Mycobacterium avium* complex [DMAC], *Pneumocystis carinii* pneumonia [PCP], toxoplasmosis, cryptosporidiosis, progressive multifocal leukoencephalopathy, and *Candida* esophagitis) were significantly associated with mortality, independent of the effect of CD4+ cell counts. The greatest impact on mortality and the occurrence of OIs, however, has been the development and subsequent availability of highly active antiretroviral therapy (HAART) regimens. These regimens, which may include protease inhibitors, non-nucleoside reverse transcriptase inhibitors, or triple nucleoside reverse transcriptase inhibitors, all have one element in common: dramatic reductions in HIV replication leading to improvement in immune function and restoration of CD4+ cell counts. Despite debates about the nature and degree of immune function restored by these regimens, the overall effect appears to be related to elevation of CD4+ cell counts to levels above the relatively well-established thresholds associated with significant risks for the occurrence of OI events. Although there are some important caveats regarding the rise in CD4+ counts and the risk of OI events, which are covered later in the chapter, the overall impact on the incidence of OI diseases has been dramatic. Rates for essentially every OI have been reduced several-fold. These effects have been seen across geographic regions, gender, race, and HIV risk behavior groups. Not only has there been a striking decrease in the incidence of OIs, but there has also been an impressive effect on the outcomes of these diseases in individuals actively or chronically infected with these pathogens. As we will discuss later, the prospects of discontinuing prophylactic medicines, withdrawing maintenance therapy for chronic infections with DMAC, cytomegalovirus retinitis, systemic fungal infections, and toxoplasmosis, and even improving the outcome of progressive multifocal leukoencephalopathy, cryptosporidiosis, and microsporidiosis, for which previous therapeutic interventions held little promise, has changed the way we think about and approach these diseases.[22–33]

Although most of these dramatic changes have been best illustrated in the adult population, there is now a growing body of information about surveillance of OIs, the impact of antiretroviral therapy, and the determination of immunologic thresholds for the prevention of these pathogens in HIV-infected children. Early pediatric series contributed to our knowledge about many of these pathogens and highlighted some of the differences from adult disease, but the data from three particular sources are particularly useful in defining the impact of these diseases on the pediatric HIV population.[34–48] These include Centers for Disease Control and Prevention (CDC) surveillance, which receives data from all 50 states in the United States and Puerto Rico on AIDS-defining illnesses; the Pediatric Spectrum of Disease (PSD) database, which encompasses a prospective cohort of HIV-exposed and -infected children from Los Angles County in California, Washington DC, Texas, New York City, Puerto Rico, and Massachusetts and, for purposes of the analyses presented here, also included the San Francisco Bay Area and North Carolina; and the Pediatric AIDS Clinical Trials Groups (PACTGs), which have been conducting HIV treatment trials in the United States and Puerto Rico (and were recently expanded to include international sites from Europe, South America, Southern Africa, and Thailand) since 1989. Although there is definite overlap between the data accumulated by each group, the information provided by each dataset complements the others.

Data from the CDC AIDS surveillance branch are presented in Table 10–1. For comparison, we have presented the AIDS-defining OI events in

Table 10–1
AIDS-Defining Conditions for HIV-Infected Children for 1992–1998 with Comparison to Adults with Similar Diagnoses for 1997*

FIRST AIDS-DEFINING CONDITION[†]	1992, N (%)	1993, N (%)	1994, N (%)	1995, N (%)	1996, N (%)	1997, N (%)	1998, N (%)	1997 ADULT AIDS DATA, N (%)
Pneumocystis carinii pneumonia	233 (26.2)	236 (27.0)	195 (24.9)	141 (21.4)	112 (22.6)	74 (24.2)	47 (20.9)	5763 (24)
Lymphoid interstitial pneumonia	181 (20.3)	158 (18.1)	133 (17.0)	113 (17.1)	88 (17.7)	36 (11.8)	27 (11.8)	NA
Recurrent bacterial infections	118 (13.3)	126 (14.4)	107 (13.6)	94 (14.3)	82 (16.5)	51 (16.6)	41 (18.0)	NA
Encephalopathy	118 (13.3)	111 (12.7)	110 (14.0)	112 (17.0)	81 (16.3)	58 (18.9)	28 (12.2)	1196 (5)
wasting	121 (13.6)	111 (12.7)	109 (13.9)	85 (12.9)	68 (13.6)	40 (13.0)	45 (19.7)	4212 (18)
Esophageal candidiasis	103 (11.6)	92 (10.5)	96 (12.2)	79 (11.9)	53 (10.7)	27 (8.8)	17 (7.5)	2057 (9)
Cytomegalovirus disease	47 (5.3)	58 (6.6)	58 (7.4)	26 (4.0)	25 (4.9)	11 (3.4)	10 (4.6)	1638 (7)
Mycobacterium avium complex	34 (3.8)	46 (5.3)	35 (4.5)	26 (4.0)	19 (3.8)	14 (4.6)	9 (3.8)	941 (4)
Chronic herpes simplex	40 (4.5)	30 (3.4)	24 (3.1)	32 (4.9)	14 (2.9)	13 (4.2)	9 (4.0)	1250 (5)

*Pediatric cases reported through December 1999, adjusted for reporting delay, unweighted for age, include definitive and presumptive diagnoses. Adult cases include definitive diagnoses only.
[†]Children may be diagnosed with more than one AIDS-defining condition.
Unpublished data provided courtesy of Dr. MaryLou Lindegren, Division of HIV AIDS Prevention, Centers for Disease Control and Prevention.
Data partially derived from Centers for Disease Control and Prevention: HIV/AIDS Surveillance Report, Vol. 9. Atlanta, GA, CDC, 1998, pp 1–41.

adults from the last year these data were published in the HIV Surveillance Report (1997).[49] Once again, this comparison demonstrates the magnitude of the difference in the number of events between children and adults and explains why the vast majority of information regarding pathogenesis, treatment, and prevention has been derived from adult cohorts. It is important to note that the pediatric data have not been weighted for age, an important consideration with the recent decline in perinatal HIV transmission rates. Despite this reduction in the HIV perinatal transmission rate, the dramatic decline of AIDS-defining events in 1997 and 1998 is still more likely a reflection of the improved immune status of those children currently living with HIV infection.

The PSD database has been particularly important because of its prospective cohort design and its similarity to the design of the Adult Spectrum of Disease (ASD) database, which has provided important information on the trends of HIV disease in adolescents and adults.[10,17,18,50] The PSD data, presented in Table 10–2, illustrate the incidence of the most common AIDS-defining conditions (ADCs), including OIs, among HIV-infected children from 1992 through 1998. Noninfectious ADCs are included in this table to provide perspective on the ADCs of interest in this chapter. All ADCs examined, except candidiasis of the lung, declined during this time period. For *M. avium*, the decline was observed only during the period of 1996 through 1998. In 1992, incidence rates were 3% for the high-incidence ADCs (PCP, lymphoid interstitial pneumonia, and HIV encephalopathy) and declined to less than 1% in 1998. For ADCs with the more moderate incidence (wasting syndrome, bacterial infections, esophageal candidiasis, and *M. avium* infection), rates ranged from 1% to 2% in 1992 and declined to less than 1% in 1998. Ratios comparing 1992 rates with 1998 rates showed at least a sixfold decline for lymphoid interstitial pneumonia (RR, 11.4), cryptosporidiosis (RR, 6.6), wasting (RR, 6.5), and *M. avium* infection (RR, 6.5). A comparison of the 1995/1998 ADC rate ratios and 1992/1995 ratios demonstrated that for each ADC, the decline in the period from 1995 through 1998 was greater than the decline in period from 1992 through 1998.

Although not shown in the table, the incidence of any ADC (whether the primary or subsequent ADC) has declined from 14% in 1992 to 4% in 1998, with most of the decline occurring after 1996. Similarly, the incidence of a primary ADC declined from 1992 to 1998, with the greatest decline after 1996, culminating in a low of only 39 primary ADCs in 1998. Rates of a subsequent ADC showed the greatest decline from 20% in 1992 to 4% in 1998, with a consistently steep decline after 1995.

During the study period, the mean age of the cohort of HIV-infected children increased from 4.9 years in 1992 to 8.7 in 1998 (Table 10–3). The proportion of children younger than 6 years of age decreased from 67% in 1992 to 29% in 1998, whereas the proportion children 6 years of age or older increased from 33% in 1992 to 71% in 1998. At the same time, the mean age at first ADC increased from 3.5 years in 1992 to 6.3 in 1998. The proportion of first ADCs among children younger than 1 year of age decreased from 32% in 1992 to 18% in 1998, whereas the proportion of children 10 years or older increased from 10% to 31%. Controlling for the potentially confounding effect of the changing age distribution, the 1992 to 1998 decline was significant at $P < .05$ for the high and moderate incidence of ADCs, with the exception of PCP and multiple bacterial infections. The observed decline for PCP noted in Table 10–1 was due to the dramatic reduction in newly infected infants between 1992 and 1998, who were at the highest risk for PCP. The proportion of cases of PCP among children younger than 1 year of age decreased from 63% in 1992 to 31% in 1998, whereas the proportion children 10 years of age or older increased from 4% in 1992 to 38% in 1998. Numbers for the low-incidence ADCs were too small to evaluate the potentially confounding effect of age.

Complementary data have also been derived from the Pediatric AIDS Clinical Trials Group (PACTG) datasets. Recently, an analysis of 13 PACTG studies, conducted prior to the widespread use of HAART regimens, was performed to determine rates of OIs and to better define the CD4+ count thresholds that posed a significant risk for these OIs.[51] Although this dataset is not from a truly prospective cohort (patients were chosen by inclusion/exclusion criteria for each study and often data were collected only for the duration of each study), there is still value to this determination because of the large number of children followed. The analysis shows similar event rates for specific OIs, as depicted in Table 10–4, to the rate observed in the PSD prospective cohort, confirms the importance of bacterial infections as a significant cause of morbidity in HIV-infected children, and demonstrates low rates for most of the other classic OIs. Once again, however, when compared with rates derived from the ASD study and also

Table 10–2
Percentage of HIV-Infected Children with Selected AIDS-Defining Conditions, 1992–1998

AIDS-DEFINING CONDITION	YEAR							RATE RATIO		
	1992	1993	1994	1995	1996	1997	1998	'92/'98	'92/'95	'95/'98
High Incidence										
Pneumocystis carinii pneumonia	2.88 (79/2743)	2.77 (77/2781)	2.69 (74/2752)	2.44 (64/2627)	1.87 (45/2406)	1.15 (24/2089)	0.8 (14/1798)	3.6	1.2	3.1
Lymphoid Interstitial pneumonia	3.43 (91/2654)	2.74 (73/2662)	2.66 (70/2631)	2.46 (61/2478)	2.05 (45/2245)	0.73 (14/1927)	0.3 (5/1647)	11.4	1.4	11.4
HIV encephalopathy	2.93 (82/2797)	3.81 (108/2834)	2.93 (82/2801)	3.24 (86/2657)	2.67 (65/2435)	1.42 (30/2111)	0.6 (10/1817)	4.9	.9	5.4
Moderate Incidence										
Wasting syndrome	1.96 (56/2861)	2.20 (64/2905)	1.83 (53/2899)	1.80 (50/2772)	1.74 (43/2553)	0.76 (17/2223)	0.3 (6/1916)	6.5	1.1	6.0
Bacterial infections	.97 (27/2797)	1.57 (45/2860)	1.09 (31/2851)	1.40 (38/2716)	1.04 (26/2489)	0.55 (12/2165)	0.2 (4/1855)	4.9	1.4	7.0
Esophageal candidiasis	1.51 (43/2854)	1.58 (46/2915)	1.38 (40/2898)	1.52 (42/2768)	0.99 (25/2538)	0.81 (18/2216)	0.7 (13/1901)	2.2	1.0	2.2
Disseminated Mycobacterium avium complex	1.80 (52/2883)	1.75 (51/2922)	1.65 (48/2910)	1.73 (48/2773)	1.88 (48/2550)	1.13 (25/2219)	0.3 (6/1901)	6.0	1.0	5.8
Low Incidence										
Cytomegalovirus—other	0.76 (22/2881)	0.82 (24/2928)	0.48 (14/2922)	0.72 (20/2797)	0.39 (10/2585)	0.27 (6/2251)	0.4 (7/1935)	1.9	1.1	1.8
Cryptosporidiosis	0.66 (19/2889)	0.20 (6/2941)	0.54 (16/2943)	0.46 (13/2803)	0.31 (8/2575)	0.22 (5/2248)	0.1 (2/1937)	6.6	1.4	4.6
Cytomegalovirus retinitis	0.41 (12/2897)	0.37 (11/2955)	0.27 (8/2951)	0.46 (13/2819)	0.38 (10/2599)	0.18 (4/2263)	0.1 (2/1949)	4.1	1.1	4.6
Candidiasis of the lung	0.1 (3/2895)	0.17 (5/2960)	0.27 (8/2955)	0.07 (2/2822)	0.08 (2/2600)	0.18 (4/2267)	0.05 (1/1952)	2.0	1.4	1.4

*Includes HIV-infected at risk of first Aids-defining condition (ADC).
†Includes only HIV-infected with their first ADC in prior years.
Unpublished data courtesy of Dr. Toni Frederick for the Pediatric Spectrum of Disease project.

Table 10-3
Age Characteristics of HIV-Infected Children by Year of Study

AGE CHARACTERISTICS	YEAR		
	1992 (2905)*	1995 (2834)	1998 (1963)
Mean Age, Y	4.9	6.2	8.7
% <1 Year of Age	13	8	1
% >10 Years of Age	12	19	34
Mean age at primary AIDS-defining condition	3.5 (248)†	4.3 (197)	6.3 (39)

*Number of HIV-infected children followed in database for each year listed, respectively.
†Number of HIV-infected children with primary AIDS-defining condition for each year listed, respectively.
Data courtesy of Dr. Toni Frederick on behalf of the Pediatric Spectrum of Disease group.

Table 10-4
Comparison of Pediatric and Adult Opportunistic Infection Event Rates Before Highly Active Antiretroviral Therapy* Using Pediatric ACTG Cumulative Data and ASD 1994 Surveillance Data

DIAGNOSIS	EVENT RATE	
	Pediatric†	Adult†
Serious bacterial infection	15.1	2.6‡
Herpes zoster	2.9	NR§
Disseminated *Mycobacterium avium* complex	1.8	7.9
Pneumocystis carinii pneumonia	1.3	8.8
Candidiasis	1.2	6.2
Cryptosporidiosis	0.6	1.8
Cytomegalovirus retinitis	0.5	5.4
Tuberculosis	0.4	1.8
Cytomegalovirus—other	0.2	3.4
Fungal infection¶	0.1	2.1
Toxoplasmosis	0.06	1.5
Progressive multifocal lenkoencephalopathy	0.06	0.9

†Rates per 100 person-years.
‡Not directly reported in ASD. Event rate is for recurrent pneumonia (recurrent pneumonia rate from PACTG dataset: 3.0 events/100 person-year).
§Not reported by ASD.
¶Fungal includes the systemic mycoses: cryptococcosis/coccididiomycosis/histoplasmosis.
Data partially derived from Dankner et al[51] and CDC.[17]

determined prior to widespread use of HAART regimens, it is apparent that adults experience greater numbers and increased frequency of OIs except for presumed bacterial pneumonia.[17]

Despite not being a truly prospective cohort, the intensive nature of follow-up incorporated into the PACTG studies allowed the investigators to collect CD4+ cell counts near the time of an OI event and thus to determine the CD4+ cell count thresholds related to these events. These determinations, categorized by age group and CD4 counts, are depicted in Table 10-5. Several points are evident from this analysis. The low number of events for most of the OIs (with the exception of PCP) in children younger than 2 years of age severely limits the ability to determine with any precision what the CD4+ thresholds should be for consideration of initiating prophylactic regimens. For patients 2 to 6 years of age, the published thresholds seem reasonable, based on the PACTG analysis. For children older than 6 years of age, the thresholds used for adults are quite appropriate and lend support to the dynamic age-related changes in CD4+ cell counts, which plateau by the sixth year of life.

The importance of these trend data cannot be overstated. Continued surveillance of OI events in both pediatric and adult populations will be critical to assessment of the continued impact of HAART on the expression of these diseases, to determine the impact of treatment failures on these rates, and to address existing and potentially new prevention strategies. However, the kind of data derived from these sources may not be applicable to all HIV-infected pediatric populations. The current data have been derived from HIV-infected patients residing in the United States and should be quite applicable to children residing in other developed nations, such as those in Europe, where there are equivalent levels of care, access to antiretroviral drugs, and general sanitation. Comparable data from mid-developing and developing nations are scant or altogether lacking. The acquisition of such data should be made a priority because the burden of pediatric HIV disease, even more so than in the past, is increasingly concentrated in these countries, which have not shared in the success of

Table 10-5
Oppunistic Infection Event Rates by CD4+ Counts

DIAGNOSIS	CD4 COUNT, CELLS/MM³	EVENTS, N	EVENT RATE PER 100 PERSON-YEARS
Serious bacterial infection	≤50	205	23.8
	51–100	54	20.4
	101–200	60	16.4
	201–600	231	14.1
	601–1000	157	12.8
	>1000	171	11.8
Herpes zoster	≤50	54	5.0
	51–100	18	6.0
	101–200	23	5.3
	201–600	64	3.4
	601–1000	16	1.1
	>1000	24	1.5
Disseminated *Mycobacterium avium* complex*	≤50	96	8.4
	51–100	9	2.7
	101–200	10	2.2
	201–600	7	0.4
	601–1000	3	0.2
Pneumocystis carinii pneumonia	≤50	51	4.4
	51–100	8	2.4
	101–200	9	2.0
	201–600	13	0.7
	601–1000	5	0.3
	>1000	6	0.4
Candidiasis	≤50	52	4.5
	51–100	6	1.8
	101–200	11	2.4
	201–600	14	0.7
	601–1000	2	0.1
	>1000	2	0.1
Cryptosporidiosis	≤50	21	1.8
	51–100	3	0.9
	101–200	7	1.5
	201–600	6	0.3
	601–1000	0	0.0
	>1000	4	0.2
Cytomegalovirus retinitis	≤50	20	1.7
	51–100	1	0.3
	101–200	4	0.9
	201–600	5	0.3
	601–1000	1	0.1
	>1000	2	0.1
Tuberculosis	≤50	9	0.8
	51–100	1	0.3
	101–200	5	1.1
	201–600	5	0.3
	601–1000	5	0.3
	>1000	2	0.1
Cytomegalovirus—other	≤50	8	0.7
	51–100	0	0.0
	101–200	3	0.7
	201–600	1	0.1
	601–1000	1	0.1

Continued

Table 10–5
Oppunistic Infection Event Rates by CD4+ Counts Continued

DIAGNOSIS	CD4 COUNT, CELLS/MM^3	EVENTS, N	EVENT RATE PER 100 PERSON-YEARS
	>1000	2	0.1
Fungal infection	≤50	5	0.4
	51–100	0	0.0
	101–200	0	0.0
	201–600	3	0.2
Toxoplasmosis†	≤50	4	0.3
Progressive multifocal leukoencephalopathy†	≤50	4	0.3

*No events at >1000 CD4+ cell count level
†No events above 50 CD4+ count level

perinatal treatment regimens at reducing HIV transmission rates as seen in the developed nations nor in the dramatic impact that HAART has had upon the morbidity and mortality of those children who are HIV-infected.[52–54] Where appropriate, we refer to pathogens identified in developing nations that have been, or may be, affected by concurrent HIV infection in the pediatric population.

SERIOUS BACTERIAL INFECTIONS

Although unusual and exotic infections have drawn attention during the HIV era, common bacteria have accounted for many of the infections experienced by HIV-infected children. Serious bacterial infections were deemed such an important indicator of immunologic dysfunction in the pediatric HIV-infected population that repeated infections were recognized as an AIDS-defining illness early in the description of this syndrome.[55]

Susceptibility to these infections is best understood as derangements in both cellular immunity and humoral immunity, which is especially important in the defense against encapsulated bacteria. T-cell defects are primarily responsible for susceptibility to many opportunistic pathogens and also contribute to the B cell dysfunctions that lead to this impaired humoral response. Although these humoral defects were first identified in adults, they have been best demonstrated in HIV-infected children.[56–58]

Polymorphonuclear neutrophils may also be dysfunctional. Studies of the polymorphonuclear neutrophil function of 25 (12 symptomatic and 13 asymptomatic) HIV-infected children against *Staphylococcus aureus* revealed depression of chemotaxis and defective bactericidal activity, in spite of intact superoxide generation.[59] Similar findings have been reported for HIV-infected adults.[60, 61] These abnormalities may be accentuated by the administration of medications to treat HIV or its related complications, which can cause or aggravate neutropenia.

Epidemiology

Early in the description of pediatric HIV disease, the most common manifestations of recurrent bacterial infections included bacteremia and sinopulmonary infections, but infection at other sites, such as the urinary tract, meninges, skin, and soft tissue, were also observed.[62,63] The most common offenders were *Streptococcus pneumoniae*, *Salmonella* species, and *H. influenzae* type b. These infections were equally common before children acquired an AIDS-defining illness, indicating that severe immunosuppression was not a prerequisite for the susceptibility to these infections, as is true with many other opportunistic pathogens.[62,63] These case series were supported by larger cohort studies, including those from Europe, demonstrating that serious bacterial infections were not often fatal but still contributed heavily to morbidity.[34,64–68] Rates of serious recurrent infections among these cohorts ranged from 13% to 20%, and disease manifestations were identical to those described previously. Pneumonia and sepsis were the most common presentations. Although the risk of bacterial infection was highest in children with advanced HIV infection and AIDS, bacterial infections were also common among children with less advanced disease. Two early treatment trials, NICHD IVIG study and ACTG 051, which explored the role of intravenous immunoglobulin (IVIG) in the prevention of recurrent bacterial infections, were also instrumental in defining the incidence of bacterial infections in children during the monotherapy era and were performed in the setting of a controlled clinical trial.[69–71] Both showed once again that pneumonia and bacteremia were the most common presentations. Both studies revealed fairly significant infection rates for children with low CD4+ counts (~40 events/100 patient years of follow-up), and the NICHD, which enrolled children across a broader spectrum of immunologic dysfunction, corroborated the earlier series demonstrating that bacterial infections could occur across the entire CD4+ count spectrum, as did the meta-analysis of multiple ACTG studies performed prior to the HAART era.[51,70] All of these studies continued to demonstrate that *Pneumococcus* was the most common pathogen. Analysis of studies from mid-developing and developing countries are complicated by the cofactor of malnutrition, but *Pneumococcus*, *Salmonella*, and other gram-negative rods appear to predominate.[72–76]

Investigators from the National Cancer Institute (NCI) have noted that *Pseudomonas* spp. caused a significant number of bacteremic (13) and nonbacteremic (25) infections in a cohort of 236 patients.[77] Interestingly, neutropenia was not a common risk factor for these infections, although the presence of a central venous catheter was. Common nonbacteremic sites of infection included central venous catheter exit sites, lungs (pneumonia), and ear canals (otitis externa).[77,78] Other pediatric investigations have identified *Pseudomonas aeruginosa* as a significant cause of end-stage bacteremia.[37,79] This experience has also been reported by several different investigators caring for adults with HIV infection.[80,81] Unlike pneumococcal infections, both adults and children with *Pseudomonas* infections have relatively advanced HIV disease. The incidence of pseudomonal infections has decreased in the HAART era.[82]

Because adolescents account for an increasing proportion of the pediatric HIV population in developed nations, it will be important to identify differences in the patterns and frequency of bacterial infections in this age group as compared with younger cohorts. Currently, the closest experience that can be drawn upon is from reports in HIV-infected adults. These reports emphasize the importance of pneumococcal disease and recurrent current pneumonia as the leading causes of bacterial infections in adults. But they have also demonstrated that prophylactic regimens for PCP or *M. avium* complex have had a concomitant impact on bacterial infections.[83–86] It will be especially important to follow these trends in the incidence and types of bacterial infections affecting HIV-infected adolescents, regardless of their initial route of HIV infection, especially with the unknown duration of HAART-induced immune restoration and the availability of new interventions such as conjugated pneumococcal vaccine. In this regard, two studies are best situated to observe and follow adolescents as they become young adults, the PSD surveillance study and the Long-Term Outcomes Study (ACTG 219) within the PACTG.

The NICHD study also looked at nonserious infections and showed that these were relatively common in HIV-infected children.[70] Otitis media and recurrent and chronic sinusitis are frequent complications of HIV disease, as might be expected in patients with altered humoral immune responses.[87,88] Although these less serious infections may not lead to hospitalization or place the child at risk for significant morbidity or mortality, they increase the children's need for medical intervention, affect aspects of daily living for patients and their families, and contribute to speech delays if conditions such as otitis media are frequent or chronic in nature.

Treatment and Prevention

The clinical importance and high incidence of both minor and serious bacterial infections has made the development of strategies to prevent these infections a high priority in the management of pediatric HIV infection. These strategies have taken three different but complementary approaches: the use of passive immune therapy, antibiotic prophylaxis, and active immunization. The initial clinical trials used IVIG with or without trimethoprim-sulfamethoxazole (TMP-SMX) prophylaxis.[69–71] The NICHD trial, which accrued 376 HIV-infected children between the ages of 1 month and 12 years and stratified patients on the basis of a CD4+ count threshold of 200 cells/mm^3, demonstrated that the use of IVIG prolonged the infection-free time for serious bacterial infections, including pneumococcal disease, minor bacterial infections, and viral infections. It was also associated with a reduced rate of hospitalization for acute care. These statistically significant results were noted only in the subjects with CD4+ cells counts greater than 200/mm^3, whereas the small number of patients with CD4 cell counts less than 200/mm^3 reduced the power to detect such a difference.[70, 71] Although the recommendations for PCP prophylaxis with TMP-SMX and the availability of zidovudine therapy for children were not established at the initiation of the protocol, a post hoc analysis of the data, taking into account the use of these agents by patients later in the series, showed that IVIG still accounted for the favorable outcomes.[71]

The ACTG 051 IVIG study was also randomized, blinded, and placebo-controlled, but it included the universal use of zidovudine at entry for all subjects and increased use of TMP-SMX as standard prophylaxis for PCP (30–40% were receiving prophylaxis before entry).[69] Once again, IVIG was associated with lower rates of bacterial infections and decreased hospital use but did not bestow any advantage to patients with CD4+ cell counts less than 200/mm^3. The major difference as compared with the NICHD trial was that the statistical advantage of IVIG over placebo was evident only in patients who were not receiving prophylactic TMP-SMX concomitantly. Thus, in the presence of TMP-SMX, IVIG did not appear to provide any distinct benefit.[69]

A more recent study, PACTG 254, was designed to compare standard TMP-SMX prophylaxis with a combination of two newer agents, atovaquone and azithromycin. This study demonstrated the equivalence of the combination of the newer agents to TMP-SMX for prevention of infection with multiple opportunistic pathogens, most specifically bacterial infections, and also provided some insight into the natural history of these complications in HIV-infected children who met the criteria for PCP prophylaxis. In this study, the rate of bacterial infections (including pneumonia, bacteremia, sinusitis, and deep abscesses) was only half of that observed in the NICHD and the PACTG 051 studies.[89] The two ACTG studies (051 and 254) highlight the effectiveness of TMP-SMX and azithromycin as prophylactic agents against recurrent bacterial infections in addition to their already established roles against PCP and DMAC. However, as pointed out in the USPHS guidelines, indiscriminate use (when not indicated for PCP, toxoplasmosis, or DMAC prophylaxis) could jeopardize the benefits of these agents by promoting resistant bacterial pathogens.[8]

Although IVIG was found to be of clinical value, its use has been limited by risks of transmission of hepatitis C, shortages of the product related to the previous problems with hepatitis C contamination, the perceived and observed benefits of antibiotic prophylaxis, and the inconvenience of parenteral administration. Many centers reserved the use of IVIG for patients with recurrent serious bacterial infections. As with many therapeutic interventions, its use has become even less frequent with the introduction and success of HAART.

Because of concerns about the development of bacterial resistance to the commonly used prophylactic agents and the problems associated with IVIG use, it is logical to turn to solutions such as active immunization, which might provide long-term immunity to bacterial pathogens. The development of effective protein-conjugate vaccines against *H. influenzae* type b, specifically for the age groups most susceptible to this invasive bacterial agent, has already had significant impact on the incidence of this infection.[90] The immunologic response to these vaccines has been reported for both children and adults.[91–94] Overall, infants younger than 9 months of age responded best to the conjugate vaccines regardless of immunologic disease category or viral load, whereas older toddlers demonstrated less robust responses. In HIV-infected adults, patients with low CD4+ counts responded better to the unconjugated vaccines than to the conjugated vaccines (which depends on more intact T cell function) but overall was still less than optimal. None of the studies have addressed the duration of the immune response or the effect of boosters on either relatively immunocompetent or more immunocompromised children. Thus, it is likely that the earlier these vaccines are administered, the better the response, especially since T cell–dependent mechanisms are engaged by the conjugate vaccines.

The predominance of *Pneumococcus* in serious bacterial infections in both developed and developing nations provides the opportunity to demonstrate the advantages of these conjugate vaccines over polysaccharide vaccines, or at least to demonstrate significant reductions in the incidence of pneumococcal disease over historical controls. The efficacy of these vaccines has already been demonstrated in large cohorts of immunocompetent children.[95] Although prior studies in HIV-infected patients given the 23-valent polysaccharide vaccine revealed suboptimal immunologic responses, studies of HIV-infected adults have demonstrated effectiveness for patients with CD4+ cell counts greater than 200/mm^3.[85, 91, 96] Thus 23-valent polysaccharide vaccine is recommended for children older than 2 years of age. This intervention should be provided early in their medical evaluation.

The potential advantages of the conjugate pneumococcal vaccines for both young infants and older children are being addressed. A study by King and associates[97] using an earlier five-valent pneumococcal conjugate vaccine in a convenience sample of children younger than 2 years of age demonstrated that three doses of this vaccine were both safe and immunogenic across CDC HIV disease categories. Two studies within the ACTG have evaluated or are in the process of evaluating the immunogenicity and safety of these vaccines in HIV-infected infants and older children. PACTG 292 found the currently licensed seven-valent pneumococcal conjugate vaccine to be both safe and immunogenic in infants enrolled prior to 6 months of age when given as a primary series, even those with symptomatic HIV infection.[98] PACTG P1024 is studying the safety and immunogenicity of this vaccine in children older than 2 years of age. Large-scale efficacy trials will not be possible in developed nations, and such trials in developing nations will first require thoughtful discourse over the best use of precious human and financial resources and the benefits these vaccines might bestow if access to antiretroviral therapy remains limited. It is apparent that prevention of deterioration or restoration of the immune system of HIV-infected children provides the best insurance that these strategies will be relatively successful. Thus, simultaneous development of more effective and longer-sustaining antiretroviral drugs or immunomodulators is imperative.

FUNGAL PATHOGENS

Pneumocystis carinii

Pneumocystis carinii pneumonia is classically associated with the HIV epidemic and is the most frequent life-threatening opportunistic infection in children with HIV. *P. carinii* was originally thought to be a protozoan based on its morphology and response to antiprotozoal drugs, but it is now considered to be a fungus related to ascomycetous yeasts.[99, 100] An important question is whether PCP is actively acquired, or reacquired, in susceptible patients or is a reactivated latent infection. Although a reasonable amount of firm evidence supports actively acquired infection, especially in HIV-infected infants, newer molecular techniques have shown that reactivation of PCP can also occur.[101–104] Airborne transmission and exposure to environmental sources may be the most likely routes, but this remains an area of continued investigation. Person-to-person transmission has also been suggested but did not account for the majority of cases in a study of case clusters.[103–106]

Although PCP was the first disease for which CD4 cell counts were shown to have significant predictive value for the development of disease, this measure of immune function has not been as reliable a marker of high risk for PCP in younger children, especially those younger than 1 year of age. One study found that approximately 20% of infants younger than 1 year of age had CD4+ cell counts greater than 1500/mm^3 at the time of PCP diagnosis.[21] This is an important observation, as age is a strong risk factor for PCP. Most of the PCP cases among HIV-infected children occur before the age of 2 years; the remainder represent mainly prophylaxis failures in older, severely immunocompromised children. The risk of PCP among children with perinatally acquired HIV peaks between 3 and 6 months of age. The incidence of PCP among perinatally infected infants during the first year of life has been estimated at 12% in Europe and 13% to 25% in the United States before guidelines for prophylaxis were published.[20, 67, 107] In HIV-infected adults in developing countries, *P. carinii* may not cause severe pneumonia as commonly as tuberculosis and other bacteria.[108, 109] The true incidence of PCP in HIV-infected children in much of the developing world is unknown, owing to the frequent nonavailability of diagnostic tests that can clearly establish this diagnosis in symptomatic children. A few studies in developing countries, however, indicate that PCP is common among HIV-infected children, with rates of 10% to 30% observed in children with severe pneumonia or from autopsy studies.[73, 110–112]

Clinical Manifestations

Children with PCP commonly present with dyspnea at rest, tachypnea, cough, and fever. Partial pressure of oxygen (PaO$_2$) is often decreased below 70 mm Hg, with an increase in the alveolar-arterial oxygen gradient of over 30 mm Hg. In infants, extensive pulmonary exudates often lead to massive acute respiratory failure. The course of illness tends to progress more slowly in older children. PCP is frequently fatal, with an associated mortality rate of approximately 30%.[107] In an early report, the median survival of children diagnosed with PCP as their first AIDS-defining condition was 1 month.[68] A study of older children has estimated the median survival time at 19 months.[107]

Prophylaxis with TMP-SMX is highly effective in the prevention of PCP, but breakthrough infections do occur. Studies of adults have shown that breakthrough rates increase with decreasing CD4+

counts.[113] Chest radiographs can be useful but are not specific. The chest radiograph typically shows bilateral diffuse perihilar alveolointerstitial infiltrates, but findings can range from normal to focal or patchy infiltrates and cavities to "white lungs." Pleural effusions and various air leaks (pneumothoraces, pneumomediastinum, pneumopericardium) occur. Lactate dehydrogenase activity is increased, although this is not specific for PCP. Infections with other pathogens, such as cytomegalovirus, *Mycobacterium avium-intracellulare*, and respiratory viruses can manifest similarly and should be considered in the differential diagnosis of PCP in HIV-infected children.

Because *P. carinii* cannot be cultured, a definitive diagnosis has traditionally relied on microscopic identification on conventional histologic stains or immunofluorescence of respiratory material, although polymerase chain reaction (PCR) technology has shown promise as a diagnostic tool and may be more sensitive in detecting low burdens of this organism.[114, 115] Classically, respiratory sources for diagnostic testing have included induced sputum, bronchoalveolar lavage, or transbronchial biopsy obtained from bronchoscopic procedures, tracheal aspirate, or open lung biopsy.[116-118] However, except in pediatric tertiary care settings, these specimens are not easily obtained from small infants. The use of PCR as described, with its increased sensitivity, may allow the use of more easily obtained specimens such as throat swabs, nasal lavage fluids, or gastric aspirates.

Untreated, the outcome of PCP is fatal for nearly all patients. Even with the use of effective antimicrobial therapy and improved management of HIV infection, the risk of death for children diagnosed with PCP remains high, especially in those with respiratory failure. Immediate treatment is critical because the disease progresses rapidly. For these reasons, prevention of PCP should be the paramount objective.

Treatment and Prevention

Several drugs are effective against PCP. TMP-SMX is the standard treatment for HIV-infected children with PCP. A three-week course of treatment is recommended for severe infections, but milder ones may be treated for a minimum of 2 weeks. Intravenous administration in four daily doses is preferred, but this can be changed to an oral formulation after sustained clinical improvement. Other agents used in the treatment of PCP, primarily in patients intolerant to TMP-SMX, have been intravenous pentamidine, dapsone-trimethoprim, clindamycin-primaquine, atovaquone, and trimethatrexate-leucovorin.[119] Intravenous pentamidine is considered the second choice for treating children with PCP and is reserved for children who do not improve clinically. If no improvement is noted in 5 to 7 days, TMP-SMX treatment should be changed to pentamidine. Adverse reactions may be more frequent with the use of pentamidine and include hematologic, cardiac, hepatic, renal, and metabolic (hypo- or hyperglycemia) along with rash and injection site reaction toxicities.[120-122]

Adjunctive corticosteroid therapy has been associated with reduced morbidity in HIV-infected adults and children with PCP, although no randomized clinical trials involving the use of this adjunctive therapy have been performed in the pediatric HIV-infected population.[123-126] Prednisone, 2 to 4 mg/kg/day divided every 6 hours, or equivalent doses of other corticosteroids can be administered for 4 or 5 days and then tapered off for an additional week. Before administering corticosteroid therapy, the clinician should rule out infection with cytomegalovirus, *Mycobacterium tuberculosis*, or invasive fungal pathogens such as aspergillus, *Histoplasma*, or coccidioidomycosis.

The efficacy of PCP prophylaxis for HIV-infected children has been well documented.[127] Primary PCP prophylaxis among HIV-infected infants reduces the risk for PCP and early death by more than fourfold, even after adjustment for the CD4+ level.[20] TMP-SMX is recommended as the first-line drug for PCP prevention because its failure rate is only 3% in HIV-infected children and adults. Interestingly, one study found that when standard TMP-SMX prophylaxis was given concomitantly with azithromycin, at doses used to prevent DMAC, these two agents combined provided additional protection against PCP over that of standard PCP prophylaxis.[128] Dapsone, atovaquone, and aerosolized or intravenous pentamidine are alternatives to TMP-SMX for prophylaxis against PCP, although these drugs have demonstrated considerably higher failure rates than TMP-SMX.[113,119,127, 129-131] Dapsone and atovaquone are preferred to aerosolized pentamidine because they are more effective when CD4+ cell counts are lower than 100, they are easier to administer, and their use eliminates the risk of transmission of other respiratory pathogens during administration. Based on pharmacokinetic data, a dose of 2 mg/kg/day is the recommended dose for children, up to a maximum of 100 mg.[132]

Given that PCP can manifest early in the course of HIV disease in infants, early identification of HIV-infected infants is one key to prevention of this OI. Early guidelines recommended initiation of PCP prophylaxis based on CD4+ cell counts or percentages.[133] However, monitoring CD4+ cell count proved to be of limited value for early identification of children at high risk for PCP.[107,134] Current guidelines recommend prophylaxis for all infants born to women infected with HIV, starting at 4 to 6 weeks of age, regardless of their CD4+ count. The guidelines recommend continuing prophylaxis until HIV infection can be reasonably excluded on the basis of two or more negative viral diagnostic tests (HIV culture or PCR), both of which are performed after 1 month of life and one of which is performed after 4 months of life. HIV-infected children should continue prophylaxis until 12 months of age. After the first year of life, PCP prophylaxis should be continued or restarted for children whose CD4+ cell count or percentage indicates severe immunosuppression (Table 10-6).

Invasive Yeasts

As shown in the Tables, *Candida albicans* and the other *Candida* species are the most common causes of yeast infection in the pediatric HIV population. *Candida* esophagitis and tracheobronchial mucositis are associated with a higher rate of mortality than other *Candida* infections, in both adult and pediatric populations, independent of the CD4+ count.[46, 50, 135, 136] Although oropharyngeal and post-pubertal vaginal candidiasis are much more common complications in this group of immunocompromised hosts, they rarely lead to death, and we do not cover them in this chapter.[137] Nevertheless, any *Candida* infection may be a warning of major immunologic dysfunction or higher viral loads that could contribute directly to increased risk of mortality.

Esophageal and tracheobronchial candidiasis are often preceded by involvement of the oral cavity. The symptoms associated with these more severe forms of mucosal involvement include hoarseness and possible airway problems in patients with tracheobronchial disease or substernal pain, dysphagia, odynophagia, and failure to thrive in patients with esophageal involvement. Although the diagnosis of tracheobronchial disease and esophageal disease is often based on clinical signs and symptoms and confirmed by response to appropriate antifungal treatment, it is important to remember that some affected patients are asymptomatic and that cytomegalovirus and herpes simplex virus can cause clinically indistinguishable disease. Thus, it is wise to establish the definitive diagnosis by culture of endoscopic brushings or biopsies, or both, of the affected areas. Refractory or recurrent disease must be evaluated endoscopically with biopsies and cultures. Fungal cultures provide the added benefits of determining the specific species of *Candida* and sensitivity testing, primarily to the azoles (fluconazole or itraconazole). The risk of resistance has risen, especially in those patients who have been on antifungal prophylaxis or have had repeated courses of these drugs.

Although oropharyngeal or vaginal candidiasis can often be treated with topical agents, more serious mucosal involvement of the esophagus and tracheobronchial tree require systemic antifungal therapy. Oral fluconazole or itraconazole (preferably the solution formulation) are the first choices because of the ease of administration and advantage of outpatient management. Intravenous amphotericin may be indicated for patients unresponsive to these agents or those with severe enough symptoms to impair oral intake. Fluconazole and itraconazole are now available in intravenous formulations and could be used in patients who have not yet failed oral azole therapy but are too ill to take the azoles by mouth. Although primary and secondary prophylaxis against oropharyngeal candidiasis is discouraged because of concerns for the potential for development of drug-resistant strains, the possibility of drug interactions, side effects, and cost, patients with recurrent tracheobronchial or esophageal disease should be considered candidates for oral prophylaxis with azoles, taking into account the concerns listed above. Drug and dose recommendations for acute disease management and prophylaxis are included in Tables 10-6 and 10-7.

Although extrapulmonary cryptococcosis is the most common life-threatening fungal infection in HIV-infected adults, it is distinctly uncommon in the pediatric age group (see Table 10-4). It is seen primarily in older children and adolescents with advanced HIV disease.[43, 138] The impact of antiretroviral therapy on the expression of this pathogen in the adult population suggests that it will remain uncommon in the pediatric population who are similarly treated with more active antiretroviral regimens. The portal of entry for *Cryptococcus neoformans* is the respiratory tract. Although the pulmonary component of this

Table 10-6
Recommendations for Opportunistic Infection Prophylaxis

OPPORTUNIST PATHOGEN	INDICATIONS	RECOMMENDED DRUGS*
Strongly Recommended		
Pneumocystis carinii pneumonia	<1 year of age: all infected or indeterminate infants 1–6 years of age: CD4+ count <500 cells/mm³ or CD4+ % <15% >6 years of age: CD4+ count <200 cells/mm³ or CD4+ % <15% or <250 cells/mm³ and symptomatic HIV disease	✓ TMP-SMX 150/750 mg/m² daily divided bid three times weekly (max, one double-strength tab) on consecutive or alternate days ▶ Dapsone 2 mg/kg daily (max, 100 mg) ▶ Atovaquone 30 mg/kg daily (max, 1500 mg) ▶ Pentamidine aerosol 300 mg inhaled monthly via Respigard II nebulizer†
Mycobacterium avium complex	CD4+ count <50 cells/mm³	✓ Azithromycin 20 mg/kg weekly (max, 1200 mg) ✓ Clarithromycin 7.5 mg/kg bid (max, 500 mg) ▶ Rifabutin 300 mg daily‡
Toxoplasmosis	CD4+ count <100 cells/mm³ and IgG antibody to toxoplasma	✓ TMP-SMX, 150/750 mg/m²/daily divided bid (max one single-strength tablet/dose) ▶ Dapsone 2 mg/kg (max, 50 mg) *plus* Pyrimethamine 1 mg/kg daily *plus* Leucovorin 5 mg/kg every 3 days
Tuberculosis	PPD ≥5 mm and negative chest radiograph or close contact of infectious patient	✓ Isoniazid 10–15 mg/kg daily (max, 300 mg) or 20–30 mg/kg (max, 900 mg) twice weekly ▶ Rifampin 10–15 mg/kg daily (max, 600 mg) or Rifabutin 300 mg daily *plus* Pyrazinamide 25 mg/kg daily (max, 2 g) for 2 months
	For exposure to multidrug-resistant strains	▶ Consult a tuberculosis specialist
Streptococcus pneumoniae infection	<2 years of age ≥2 years	✓ Pneumococcal conjugate vaccine ✓ Pneumococcal conjugate vaccine followed by 23-valent polysaccharide vaccine
Generally Recommended		
Hepatitis B	Susceptible subjects (HepB$_s$Ag and HepB$_c$Ab negative)	✓ Hepatitis B vaccine, three doses
Influenza virus	All patients	✓ Influenza vaccine, yearly prior to influenza season
Varicella virus	Susceptible (varicella Ab negative) >12 months of age with CD4+ ≥2.25%	✓ Varicella vaccine
Generally Not Recommended		
Cytomegalovirus	CD4+ count <50 cells/mm³ and Cytomegalovirus IgG Ab+	Oral ganciclovir 30–40 mg/kg/dose tid (max, 1 g)
Fungal Infections	CD4+ counts <100 cells/mm³	

Table 10–6
Recommendations for Opportunistic Infection Prophylaxis *Continued*

OPPORTUNIST PATHOGEN	INDICATIONS	RECOMMENDED DRUGS*
Cryptococcus neoformans		Fluconazole 3–6 mg/kg daily (max, 200 mg)
Histoplasma capsulatum		Itraconazole 2–5 mg/kg daily (max, 200 mg)

✓, First-line regimens; ▶, alternative regimens; TMP-SMX, trimethoprim-sulfamethoxazole.
*All drugs except for vaccinations are orally dosed.
†For children >5 years.
‡For children > 6 years (safety and tolerance not well established in children).
Data adapted from 1999 USPHS/IDSA Guidelines.[8]

disease is often clinically unapparent, it may harbor live cryptococci and seed the central nervous system (CNS), especially in cases of immunodeficiency, and cause the most common manifestation of this disease, meningoencephalitis. The clinical presentation consists predominantly of headache, with or without fever, and altered mental status. The diagnostic test of choice is a cryptococcal antigen test on the serum and cerebrospinal fluid (CSF) (if a lumbar puncture is not clinically contraindicated). Cultures of CSF and blood are the diagnostic gold standards, but the clinical impact on management is delayed compared with the more rapid antigen test. Where antigen testing is unavailable, both Gram stain and India ink stains can be of value but require some skill in evaluating the CSF stains to avoid false-positive results. Low CSF cell counts have been observed commonly in adult patients with CNS disease.

The mainstay of treatment is the administration of amphotericin B and 5FC for 2 weeks followed, in stable patients, by high-dose fluconazole (Table 10–7) for another 8 weeks.[139] As with adult patients, unless there is improvement in the child's immunologic function, lifelong suppressive therapy with lower dose fluconazole is indicated to prevent relapsing meningoencephalitis.[140, 141] Because the use of intravenous formulations may not be possible in developing nations, effective oral regimens would be of value in these countries. Initial treatment with fluconazole alone has not been recommended, but the combination of fluconazole and 5FC has shown promise as an effective alternative to 5FC and intravenous amphotericin and may be a suitable regimen in regions of the world where access to administration of intravenous therapy is limited.[142, 143] Cryptococcal antigen titers should be followed during the acute treatment phase to monitor the response to therapy and during the maintenance phase to identify potential relapse. If CSF antigen titers do not fall or rise during acute therapy, early relapse or microbiologic failure must be considered, whereas a rise in titer during maintenance therapy could indicate relapse.[144] In contrast to the utility of CSF antigen testing, monitoring of serum titers has not been found to be useful in the management of HIV patients on treatment.[145]

Despite the serious morbidity and potential mortality of this disease, primary prophylaxis has not been endorsed. Although both fluconazole and itraconazole prophylaxis have been found to be effective by reducing the occurrence of this disease in randomized trials, the lack of impact on overall mortality, the relative infrequency of cryptococcal disease (even in the adult population), and the same cautions stated previously about primary prophylaxis for candidal infections have prevented recommendations for prophylaxis.[146, 147] It is important to note, however, that although itraconazole has been shown to be effective in preventing cryptococcal disease and disseminated histoplasmosis (as will be discussed later), it was not as effective as fluconazole for maintenance therapy of previously established cryptococcal disease and, therefore, should not be used for that purpose.[147, 148]

Dimorphic Fungi

The dimorphic fungi that are important causes of infection in HIV patients include *Histoplasma capsulatum*, *Coccidioides immitis*, and *Penicillium marneffei*.[135, 149–154] Infections caused by these fungi must be considered by clinicians living in geographic regions where these organisms are prevalent, and a thorough history regarding previous residence in, and travel to, endemic areas is indicated even in areas of low incidence because these infections can reactivate when the immune system becomes markedly impaired. Coccidioidomycosis has been an uncommon OI in the adult

Table 10–7
Recommendations for Treatment of Opportunistic Infections

OPPORTUNIST PATHOGEN	TREATMENT OF PRIMARY DISEASE	MAINTENANCE REGIMENS
Fungal Pathogens		
Pneumocystis carinii pneumonia	TMP-SMX 15/75 mg/kg IV or PO divided qid × 21 days ▶ Pentamidine 4 mg/kg IV qd × 21 days ▶ Clindamycin 600 mg IV q8h or 300–450 mg PO q6h plus primaquine 30 mg base PO qd × 21 days* ▶ Atovaquone 750 mg PO bid × 21 days*	▶ No maintenance regimen but secondary prophylaxis strongly recommended (see Table 10–6)
Esophageal candidiasis	✓ Fluconazole 3–6 mg/kg qd (max 200–400 mg) ▶ Itraconazole 2–5 mg/kg qd (max 100–200 mg) × 2–3 wk ▶ Amphotericin B 0.3–0.5 mg/kg qd × 5–7d	▶ Fluconazole 3 mg/kg qd (max, 100 mg)†
Cryptococcosis	✓ Amphotericin B 0.7 mg/kg IV ± Flucytosine 100 mg/kg PO divided qid × 10–14 d then Fluconazole 6 mg/kg (max, 400 mg) × 8–10 wks ▶ Fluconazole 6 mg/kg qd (max, 400 mg) plus Flucytosine 100 PO divided mg/kg qd × 6–10 wks	✓ Fluconazole 3–6 mg/kg qd (max, 200 mg) ▶ Itraconazole 2–5 mg/kg every 12-24 hrs (max, 200 mg) ▶ Amphotericin B 0.5–1.0 mg/kg IV 1–3x/week
Histoplasmosis	✓ Amphotericin B 0.5–1.0 mg/kg IV × 7–14d ▶ Itraconazole 300 mg mg bid × 3d, then 100 mg bid (oral suspension)	✓ Itraconazole 2–5 mg/kg every 12-24 hours ▶ Amphotericin B 1.0 mg/kg IV weekly
Coccidioidomycosis	✓ Amphotericin B 0.5 mg/kg IV qd × ≥8 wks ✓ Fluconazole 6–12 mg/kg (max, 400–800 mg) IV or PO qd (can be divided bid)	Fluconazole 6 mg/kg qd ▶ Amphotericin B 1.0 mg/kg IV weekly
Penicilliosis	✓ Amphotericin B 0.7–1.0 mg/kg IV qd ▶ Itraconazole 400 mg PO qd	✓ Itraconazole 200 mg PO qd
Mycobacterial Pathogens		
Disseminated Mycobacterium avium complex	Clarithromycin 7.5 mg/kg (max, 500 mg) PO qd plus Ethambutol 15 mg/kg (max, 900 mg) PO qd ± Rifabutin 5 mg/kg (max, 300 mg) PO qd‡	✓ Clarithromycin 7.5 mg/kg, (max 500 mg) qd plus Ethambutol 15 mg/kg (max, 900 mg) qd ± Rifabutin 5 mg/kg qd (max, 300 mg)‡ ▶ Azithromycin 10 mg/kg (max, 500 mg) PO plus Ethambutol ± Rifabutin
Mycobacterium tuberculosis infection	For regimens not using a PI or NNRTI: ✓ Isoniazid 10–15 mg/kg (max, 300 mg) PO qd plus Rifampin 10–15 mg/kg (max, 600 mg) plus Pyrazinamide 25 mg/kg (max, 2 g) PO plus Ethambutol 15–20 mg/kg (max, 2.5 g) PO × 8 wks	No maintenance regimen recommended after completion of primary treatment

Table 10–7
Recommendations for Treatment of Opportunistic Infections *Continued*

OPPORTUNIST PATHOGEN	TREATMENT OF PRIMARY DISEASE	MAINTENANCE REGIMENS
	✓ Then INH *plus* Rifampin × an additional 18 wks (minimum)§ *For regimens using a PI or NNRTI:* ✓ Substitute Ribabutin 5 mg/kg PO (max 300 mg) for Rifampin‡	
Parasitic Pathogens		
Toxoplasmosis	Sulfadiazine 85–120 mg/kg PO in 2–4 divided doses *plus* Pyramethamine 2 mg/kg loading dose then 1 mg/kg PO daily *plus* Leucovorin 5 mg/kg PO every 3 days × at least 6 wks ✓ Clindamycin 600 mg IV or PO three or four times day *plus* Pyramethamine 2 mg/kg loading dose then 1 mg/kg daily *plus* Leucovorin 5 mg/kg every 3 days × at least 6 weeks*	▶ Sulfadiazine 85–120 mg/kg in two to four divided doses *plus* Pyramethamine 1 mg/kg daily *plus* Leucovorin 5 mg/kg every 3 days
Cryptosporidiosis	▶ Paromomycin 25–35 mg/kg PO divided bid or qid ✓ Successful response to HAART likely to provide best opportunity for remission	No recommendations
Isosporosis	✓ TMP-SMX one double-strength tablet PO qid ×10d, then bid × 3 wks*	No recommendations
Microsporidiosis	✓ Albendazole 400–800 mg PO bid × > 3 weeks*¶	No recommendations
Viral Pathogens		
Cytomegalovirus retinitis	✓ Ganciclovir 5mg/kg IV bid × 2–3 wks	Ganciclovir 5 mg/kg IV qd or 30–40 mg/kg PO tid (max, 1–2 g)
	▶ Foscarnet 60 mg/kg IV q8h or 90 mg/kg IV q12h × 2–3 wks	▶ Foscarnet 90–120 mg/kg IV qd ▶ Cidofovir 5 mg/kg IV every other wk* ▶ Intraocular Ganciclovir q6 mo ± oral Ganciclovir 1 g tid*
Cytomegalovirus—end-organ disease other than retinitis	Same as above	Ganciclovir regimen as above ▶ Foscarnet regimen as above
Progressive multifocal leukoencephalopathy	No JC virus-specific antiviral regimen found to be effective ✓ Successful response to HAART likely to provide best opportunity for remission	No recommendations

✓, First-line regimens; ▶, alternative regimens; HAART, highly active antiretroviral therapy; NNRTI, non-nucleoside reverse transcriptase inhibitor; PI, protease inhibitor; TMP-SMX, trimethoprim-sulfamethoxazole.
*Minimal or no clinical experience or published data on efficacy or safety of these regimens in pediatric patients (<13 years of age).
†Maintenance therapy not generally recommended.
‡Rifabutin dosing not established for children younger than 6 years of age. No approved pediatric formulation available.
§For recommendations on choosing regimens for suspected or confirmed drug resistant strains of *M. tuberculosis*, contact tuberculosis expert.
¶Efficacy of albendazole is established only for infections involving *Septata intestinalis*.

HIV population and rarely described in the pediatric age group. In the largest adult series reported, the most commonly reported symptoms were fever, chills, weight loss, and night sweats.[152] The lung was the most commonly involved organ and the CNS the second (similar to that described for other immunocompromised hosts). The nature of the pulmonary involvement was unusual, however. Diffuse reticulonodular infiltrates were common and mortality was very high (60% overall and rising to 68% for those with reticulonodular findings on chest radiograph). Traditional serologic tests for detecting disseminated coccidioidomycosis were negative in a quarter of the patients. Treatment with amphotericin followed by lifelong treatment with fluconazole was recommended.[149, 152, 153, 155] Because the disease is infrequent, antifungal prophylaxis is not recommended.

Although disseminated histoplasmosis has also been reported uncommonly in HIV-infected children, it has garnered more attention because it is endemic in a wider region of the United States and in other temperate zones around the world, including Third World nations.[135] In adults, the most common presentation is the disseminated form, which often manifests with fever, weight loss, pulmonary symptoms, cutaneous lesions, hepatosplenomegaly, and lymphadenopathy. A hyperacute syndrome resembles septic shock. Laboratory abnormalities include pancytopenia and elevated liver function tests. The organism can be best identified by microscopic examination of Giemsa-stained bone marrow biopsy or aspirate and peripheral blood smears. Urine antigen detection is a rapid, reliable diagnostic tool. Examination of a bone marrow aspirate or biopsy may also help to establish the diagnosis of disseminated disease. Cultures of blood and bone marrow are reliable but can require 1 to 6 weeks for growth of this fastidious organism.[156] The yield from sputum cultures is much lower. Treatment is usually initiated with amphotericin B, followed by itraconazole, which should be continued indefinitely.[154] The use of a colloidal suspension of amphotericin B was studied recently in adult patients, and, although preliminary in nature, the findings of more rapid clearance and lower adverse event rates as compared with itraconazole are encouraging.[157]

Disseminated disease due to *Penicillium marneffei* is important in areas of high endemicity, such as Southeast Asia.[150, 151, 158] The most common presenting signs and symptoms include fever, generalized adenopathy, hepatosplenomegaly, pulmonary infiltrates, weight loss, anemia, and a generalized papular skin rash. The fungus can be easily grown from blood, bone marrow, and skin lesions. The diagnosis can sometimes be established even more rapidly by microscopic review of smears of skin lesions, bone marrow aspirates, or biopsies. Although an oral regimen would be ideal for treatment, especially in poorer nations, initiation of therapy with oral itraconazole led to an unacceptable delay in the time to sterilization of fungal blood cultures. Thus, treatment should be begun with intravenous amphotericin, but a recent study revealed that the course of amphotericin B could be shortened from the previously recommended 6 to 8 weeks to 2 weeks, followed by itraconazole for another 10 weeks.[150] Lifelong suppressive therapy with itraconazole is indicated to prevent relapses.[151] As with the other fungal pathogens, although primary prophylaxis with itraconazole was found to be effective in reducing the incidence of this opportunistic pathogen, no survival advantage was observed for patients with advanced HIV disease.[159]

Aspergillus

Monomorphic or filamentous fungi have also been noted to cause disease in HIV-infected individuals. The most commonly reported organisms are *Aspergillus* species, which may cause invasive aspergillosis, especially in patients with advanced disease and marked immunosuppression.[135, 160] Additional risk factors coincide with those previously described for other immunocompromised patients and include previous pulmonary or sinus infections, corticosteroid use, neutropenia, and tissue trauma. Pulmonary disease is the most common manifestation and, as observed in other compromised patients, the diagnosis is often made late in the disease course or at autopsy. A thorough discussion of diagnostic assays and treatment options is beyond the scope of this chapter; the reader is referred to more complete discussions on these topics. However, the mainstay of treatment consists of amphotericin B or one of the liposomal products (for those failing or intolerant of standard therapy). Itraconazole has a role in the long-term treatment of invasive disease, and a new azole, voriconazole, may hold promise for patients who fail other treatment regimens.

MYCOBACTERIAL PATHOGENS

Except for PCP, nowhere have the effects of HIV infection had more impact than on the expression of mycobacterial disease, both with the rise of disseminated *Mycobacterium avium* complex (DMAC) as a major pathogen and the resurgence of *Mycobacterium tuberculosis*, especially as it has affected worldwide efforts to gain control of this age old disease.

Mycobacterium avium

Epidemiology and Clinical Features

The ubiquitous organism *Mycobacterium avium*, which can be found in water, soil, dairy products, and domesticated farm and household animals, had previously been infrequently encountered in human disease. Although the environmental sources for the actual acquisition of this organism still remain unclear, both the respiratory and gastrointestinal tract have been identified as portals of entry, with the gastrointestinal tract thought to be the most common site for colonization and subsequent dissemination of this opportunistic pathogen.[161] As with most other agents addressed in this chapter, the incidence of the disease associated with this agent in the pediatric population is much lower than that in the adult HIV-infected population.[36–38, 162, 163] This difference may be due to a higher degree and length of environmental exposure of adults. This hypothesis supports the notion that the pathogenesis of this disease is dissemination from persistently colonized sites and emphasizes the importance of long-term exposure versus recent acquisition. Nonetheless, DMAC is a late-stage disease in both children and adults and is associated with a severely compromised immune system (CD4+ counts below 50 cells/mm^3). It is also associated with reduced survival time in children and adults independent of other risk factors.[50, 164, 165] Since it may be a marker for increased viral load, there is no reason to believe that it would not be associated with decreased survival in similarly affected children and adolescents.

Localized manifestations of *M. avium* complex include cervical adenitis, pneumonitis, liver function abnormalities, skin lesions, and abscesses. However, the hallmark of this opportunistic infection in HIV-infected individuals is disseminated disease, and it may present with such nonspecific features as recurrent fevers, weight loss, night sweats, diarrhea, and abdominal pain. Prominent laboratory abnormalities include anemia and elevated alkaline phosphatase. Elevated alkaline phosphatase is less specific in children, since they have naturally higher levels. Diagnosis is best established by isolation from the blood, although bone marrow aspirates or core biopsies and tissue from other sterile body sites are also indicative of disseminated disease. Because of the availability and efficacy of current antimycobacterial regimens, bone marrow aspirates and core biopsies should be pursued in patients at significant risk when the Bactec (Becton Dickinson, Sparks, MD) blood culture is sterile. Bone marrow core biopsies should be obtained in conjunction with marrow aspirates because they have greater *M. avium* loads than marrow aspirates.[166] The Bactec culture system for unprocessed blood or bone marrow aspirates often leads to the detection of acid-fast bacilli in 7 to 14 days. Liquid media should not be relied upon as the sole method for detection of mycobacteria, including *M. avium*. The concomitant use of solid media ensures the highest yield. DNA probe technology permits rapid speciation of tuberculous and nontuberculous bacteria directly from culture media. The first-line drugs that should be included in susceptibility testing are the macrolides (with clarithromycin as the class drug), rifabutin, and ethambutol. Additional useful information may be obtained by testing both amikacin and ciprofloxacin, but there is no consensus on breakpoints, and only sensitivity results to clarithromycin correlate clearly with clinical results.

Treatment and Prevention

A major advance in the treatment and prophylaxis of DMAC has been the development of the newer macrolides, clarithromycin and azithromycin. The value of treating these infections to improve survival and quality of life is no longer in doubt. Previous regimens without macrolides had some impact on short-term clinical, bacteriologic, and survival outcomes, but results were not sustained.[167] Subsequent trials including macrolides revealed the lack of definitive clinical benefit from the addition of clofazimine and also demonstrated increased mortality when clarithromycin was used in doses greater than 500 mg twice a day.[168, 169] More recent results suggest that the addition of rifabutin to a combination of clarithromycin and ethambutol may help prevent the emergence of resistance to clarithromycin but did not improve the bacteriologic response rate or survival when compared with the two-drug combination.[170] Prophylaxis trials with rifabutin demonstrated its efficacy and activity in the prevention of DMAC, although toxicity and drug interactions have resulted in rifabutin being supplanted by either clarithromycin or azithromycin as the prophylactic agents of choice.[83, 167, 171] The combination of azithromycin and rifabutin, but not clarithromycin and rifabutin, is more effective than azithromycin alone.[83, 172] Owing to the problems associated with rifabutin, however, and the absence of overall survival benefit, this combination is not routinely recommended. Despite the efficacy of azithromycin prophylaxis, clarithromycin is considered to be the first-line agent when devising treatment regimens. In children, the availability of pediatric formulations for both clarithromycin and azithromycin make them the prophylactic drugs of choice. There is no licensed pediatric formulation for rifabutin and little pharmacokinetic data to support its use for M. avium prophylaxis. Because there have not been any treatment or prophylaxis trials in the pediatric population, the dosing recommendations provided in Tables 10–6 and 10–7 are based on best estimates.

Mycobacterium tuberculosis

Epidemiology and Clinical Features

Owing to the worldwide burden of both HIV and tuberculosis, tuberculosis is now the most common opportunistic infection in developing nations.[42, 53, 173, 174] Some investigators have debated whether the actual rates of tuberculosis in HIV-infected children are significantly higher than those in uninfected children, but the impact of HIV on the progression of tuberculosis in HIV-infected children is dramatic.[111, 175–177] This disease has also received considerable attention in industrialized nations because of the significant reversal in the decline of tuberculosis associated with the spread of HIV. Among the reasons for this resurgence are increased rates of reactivation tuberculosis in HIV-infected individuals, rapid progression to active disease in severely immunocompromised patients, associated risks of nosocomial transmission in both traditional and nontraditional settings, and increased rates of drug-resistant M. tuberculosis.[178,179] Although the trend data presented earlier indicate that tuberculosis is uncommon in HIV-infected children in the United States, this important worldwide pathogen deserves particular attention.

HIV-infected individuals are at markedly increased risk for progressive primary or reactivation tuberculous disease and for exogenous reinfection. The level of immunosuppression in adults also has a significant impact on the expression of tuberculous disease; more immunosuppressed patients (CD4+ cell counts below 200–300/mm^3) exhibit greater rates of mycobacteremia, extrapulmonary manifestations, and, when presenting with pulmonary disease, mediastinal adenopathy, a radiologic finding more classically observed in non–HIV-infected children. Abdominal disease is more likely to manifest with visceral lesions and intra-abdominal lymphadenopathy with necrosis. Meningitis presentations may be similar to immunocompetent patients, but intracranial lesions are more common. Children, especially those younger than 5 years of age, are already at increased risk for extrapulmonary disease, although the degree of increase when coinfected with HIV remains to be determined.

Owing to the protean nature of tuberculosis expression in HIV-infected individuals, acid-fast bacillus smears and mycobacterial cultures should be routinely included in the evaluation of bodily fluids or tissues obtained from patients with acute or chronic illnesses. Although mycobacterial cultures remain the gold standard of diagnosis, two new rapid techniques that detect either ribosomal RNA (MTD, Gen-Probe, San Diego, CA) or DNA (Amplicor, Roche Molecular Systems, Branchburg, NJ) are approved for detection of M. tuberculosis in acid-fast bacillus smear–positive sputum specimens.[179] These tests may prove quite useful in HIV-infected children in developed countries, where the risk for tuberculosis is lower and where a positive rapid test would allow for timely institution of therapy and potentially obviate further invasive diagnostic procedures. A negative result, although not ruling out active tuberculosis, may permit the clinician to withhold antituberculous therapy with its potential for drug interactions and toxicity while further evaluation is pursued. The same may not be true in developing nations, where the risk of tuberculosis is higher, the test itself would likely be unaffordable, and acid-fast bacillus smear positivity would warrant institution of therapy.

Treatment and Prevention

Treatment and prevention of tuberculosis in HIV-infected individuals during the protease treatment era has caused difficult clinical and policy decisions.[179, 180] Unfortunately, the effective drugs for the treatment of HIV and tuberculosis have deleterious interactions. The major problem has been the drug-drug interactions between rifamycins, especially rifampin, and the protease inhibitors and the non-nucleoside reverse transcriptase inhibitors. Rifampin induces the activity of cytochrome p450 CY3A that, in turn, reduces the levels of protease inhibitors and non-nucleoside reverse transcriptase inhibitors to subtherapeutic levels. The substitution of rifabutin, a less potent inducer of CYP3A, for rifampin appears to allow the use of either concurrent indinavir or nelfinavir as part of an antiretroviral regimen. Caution should be exercised when using rifabutin in conjunction with the non-nucleoside reverse transcriptase inhibitors as the drug interactions can go in either direction, making it difficult to predict therapeutic or toxic levels for either. More recently, the use of low-dose ritonavir, a potent inhibitor of CYP3A, in conjunction with a variety of the potent protease inhibitors has been touted as a means to allow the concomitant use of rifampin, an important component of effective tuberculosis therapy.[181]

Another area of uncertainty involves the length of treatment. Although 6-month short-course treatment has become the mainstay for drug-susceptible tuberculosis in HIV-negative individuals, this regimen may not be adequate for HIV-infected individuals, especially when rifampin has been substituted with rifabutin. Although some investigators have recommended longer treatment regimens, the most recent CDC guidelines state that the minimal duration of therapy is 6 months.[180] A slow clinical or bacteriologic response, however, warrants either a 9-month course or continuation of therapy for 4 months after cultures are sterile. Nonetheless, the choice of antiretroviral drugs and antituberculous drugs for coinfected patients is complicated enough that it warrants consultation with experienced pharmacologists or pharmacists and HIV clinicians before final decisions are made and, where possible, the concomitant use of directly observed therapy to facilitate successful completion of antituberculous therapy.

The routine use of bacillus Calmette-Guérin vaccine in countries with a high prevalence of tuberculosis to decrease the risk of extrapulmonary disease in young children has been debated. Although this strategy has been relatively successful in reducing the incidence of serious tuberculosis in young children, the targeted countries are those that also have or are at risk of having the highest rates of pediatric HIV disease. Early concerns regarding the risks for disseminated bacillus Calmette-Guérin infections have not been borne out, likely due to the early age (before 1 month of age) at which these infants receive the vaccine.[182] However, continued surveillance for any increase in bacillus Calmette-Guérin infections would be prudent.

Recent reviews have confirmed the efficacy of chemoprophylaxis in HIV-infected patients with either positive tuberculin skin tests, a previous positive skin test without prior chemoprophylaxis, or recent close contact with a potentially infectious source.[183,184] The currently recommended regimens are described in Table 10–6. Nevertheless, there is no convincing evidence for the utility of chemoprophylaxis for anergic HIV-infected patients, nor has anergy testing itself been reproducible.[180,185] Therefore, anergy testing is no longer recommended in conjunction with specific tuberculosis testing to assess the risk of tuberculosis. HIV patients not on chemoprophylaxis must be observed carefully for evidence of reactivation tuberculosis.

VIRAL PATHOGENS

Although viral infections, especially herpesviruses, JC virus and, more recently, hepatitis C virus, have also classically been a hallmark of the AIDS epidemic, once again their incidence and prevalence in the pediatric population is dwarfed by that encountered in the adult population. Exposure rates are one significant contributing factor to the lower incidence rates, and these lower incidence rates, combined with the smaller number of HIV-infected children than adults, account for the much smaller prevalence numbers. These factors make it difficult to accurately describe the epidemiology of these diseases in the pediatric population and even more difficult to design interventional studies that can test the safety and efficacy of therapies that have shown some promise or benefit in adults. Nevertheless, as with other areas of treatment for opportunistic infections, extrapolation of adult data provides the basis for much of the therapeutic decisions made in pediatric patients. Thus it remains important to understand the pharmacodynamic rationale of drug therapy in adults with viral OIs, so that small-scale pharmacokinetic studies can be designed to ensure that children receive equivalent drug exposure to regimens with demonstrated efficacy in adults.

Cytomegalovirus

Epidemiology and Clinical Features

Clearly, the herpesviruses, most importantly cytomegalovirus, have figured predominately in causes of morbidity and mortality in adults. Cytomegalovirus disease is manifested by end-organ involvement, most commonly in the form of retinitis, but it also involves the gastrointestinal tract, central nervous system, liver, and lungs. As in adult disease, it would appear that the cytomegalovirus disease entities mentioned earlier also occur in children with very low CD4+ counts, except in children younger than 2 years of age in whom there are too few data to determine at what CD4+ threshold the risk of cytomegalovirus disease is at its greatest.[39,41,45,186] In some respects, this comparable CD4+ threshold risk allows for the implementation of prevention strategies found to be helpful in adults. It has been clearly demonstrated that cytomegalovirus viremia either precedes or is coincident with end organ disease.[47,187–189] This factor provides for a mechanism for surveillance in the highest risk patients (those who are cytomegalovirus-seropositive with low CD4+ counts) to determine who may need more careful clinical evaluation (retinal examinations, review of signs and symptoms that may warrant referral for invasive tests such as endoscopy, lumbar puncture, biopsies, or CNS imaging) or even preemptive therapy. Surveillance may be particularly important in the youngest children who may not be able to describe referable symptoms, especially visual symptoms, that could lead to a diagnosis of retinitis.[186] The surveillance tests used include PCR for detection of cytomegalovirus DNA in plasma or detection of cytomegalovirus early antigens in white blood cell smears.[187]

A particular area of interest for pediatricians in regard to cytomegalovirus is perinatal transmission from HIV/cytomegalovirus-coinfected women and the risks this places on their offspring. Data from several sources suggest that congenital disease may not be increased in either HIV-infected or uninfected infants when born to coinfected mothers, but the risk for acquired cytomegalovirus infection by 6 months of age in the HIV-infected offspring appears to be higher as compared with their HIV-uninfected counterparts.[190–192] However, the occurrence of coinfection with cytomegalovirus early in life in HIV-infected infants may be a risk factor for more rapid HIV disease progression.[190,192]

Treatment and Prevention

Once cytomegalovirus disease is diagnosed, treatment is warranted; otherwise, disease will progress, potentially involving other organ systems, and could be fatal. The treatment of retinitis has received the most attention and has evolved from primarily parenteral therapy to options for oral therapy or local intravitreal drug delivery. Although parenteral agents such as ganciclovir, foscarnet, and cidofovir have been used in the adult population, only ganciclovir has been used enough in the pediatric population to determine its safety and efficacy.[193,194] The other two agents may be used in cases of ganciclovir-resistant infections, but recommendations on dosing are primarily empiric. The use of intravitreal drug delivery systems has seen very little use in pediatric patients and no specific recommendations can be provided regarding its use other than to consider its potential benefits on a case-by-case basis. Should intravitreal therapy be utilized, it may be best to combine its use with a systemic agent to prevent viremic spread to other organ systems or to an uninvolved eye.[193] The role of oral therapy has taken a significant step forward with the availability of valganciclovir, an oral prodrug of ganciclovir, which achieves ganciclovir levels nearly equivalent to what previously could be only achieved by the parenteral route. Although oral ganciclovir pharmacokinetics have been established for HIV-infected children with quiescent cytomegalovirus disease or those at risk for cytomegalovirus disease, the difficulties of identifying a suitable liquid formulation for valganciclovir have not allowed similar pharmacokinetic studies to be performed in children.[194,195]

Prior to the availability of the currently more potent antiretroviral combinations, treatment for cytomegalovirus retinitis was indefinite. Even with maintenance therapy, the course of this infection was marked by the need for reinduction therapy due to clinical and virologic relapses, serious risk of progression to blindness due to episodes of relapse or lack of response to antiviral therapy, and retinal detachment. Additionally, the risk of viral resistance associated with the need for long-term therapy has been clearly observed in this disease and is a one of the definitive causes for evidence of either clinical or virologic failure.[193,196] Given the overall severity of cytomegalovirus disease, it is clearly desirable to develop interventions to prevent the manifestations of this viral pathogen in those patients at greatest risk for the disease. Even though oral ganciclovir has been shown to be effective in reducing the risk of cytomegalovirus disease in high-risk individuals, like antifungal prophylaxis it has not been officially recommended within the Public Health Service OI guidelines, owing to issues of adverse events, debate over demonstrating a clear survival benefit, risk of viral resistance, and cost of therapy.[197] Potentially targeting preemptive therapy in those at greatest risk, specifically low CD4+ counts and with evidence of cytomegalovirus antigenemia/DNAemia, could prove more productive and more cost-effective.[198]

Treatment of the other forms of cytomegalovirus-related disease reveal discordant results.

Gastrointestinal disease usually responds well to cytomegalovirus-specific antiviral therapy, whereas there are debates regarding the need for maintenance therapy. In contrast is the treatment of CNS disease, in which therapeutic interventions, including combination therapy, have produced disappointing results.[193]

Varicella Zoster

Although the varicella-zoster virus does not produce any AIDS-defining illnesses, it still must be reckoned with as a cause of morbidity and, much less frequently, as a cause of mortality for HIV-infected children and adolescents.[199, 200] The recurrent episodes of herpes zoster, shingles, were all too familiar to those who treated HIV-infected children, given the ubiquitous nature of prior exposure to varicella in early childhood. Although often not life-threatening, these episodes diminished the quality of life for these afflicted patients and, unlike other opportunistic infections, could occur at less advanced stages of immunosuppression. Recurrent episodes occur more frequently in those children who acquired their primary varicella in the setting of low CD4+ counts.[199] Varicella is also a risk to those who were still susceptible (usually the youngest children) and although the risk of serious disease increases with increasing severity of immunosuppression, despite earlier reports to the contrary, in most children, even those with low CD4+ counts, the disease course is often not severe.[199] Acyclovir therapy has been the mainstay of treatment for patients with these infections, with oral therapy (20 mg/kg/dose given four to five times/day) often the initial choice and parenteral therapy used for those with evidence of severe disease. The advantages of valacyclovir, the oral prodrug of acyclovir, with its ability to produce acyclovir levels nearing those associated with parenteral therapy, have not been extended to the pediatric population due to lack of a suitable oral formulation for younger children and the absence of pharmacokinetic CPK studies in older children. A similar lack of experience with famciclovir, another oral drug with good activity against varicella-zoster virus, also limits recommendations regarding its use for this disease indication. However, the key to prevention of complications associated with the varicella-zoster virus lies in active immunization. The effect would be twofold: first, prevention of primary varicella, and second, through the use of this live attenuated virus, the strong likelihood of preventing episodes of shingles. There is already movement with this mode of intervention with the favorable safety and immunologic results of a phase II study (ACTG 265) involving the use of the live varicella virus vaccine in HIV-infected children with CD4+ counts above 25% (CDC Immunologic Category 1), leading to the Advisory Committee on Immunization Practices (ACIP) recommendation to vaccinate this group of children.[201, 202] This study has been extended to children in CDC Immunologic Category 2 (15–24% CD4+ count) and to those children who were previously in Immunologic Category 3 (<15% CD4+ count) but had recovered to greater than 15% with treatment by potent antiretroviral therapy. The results of this study are pending but should provide further opportunities to offer vaccination against varicella across a wider spectrum of those children infected with HIV.

Human Herpesvirus 8

Although human herpesvirus 8, believed to be responsible for Kaposi sarcoma and other associated syndromes, has been rarely reported as an opportunistic pathogen in the pediatric population, the chapter would be remiss if it did not mention this herpesvirus.[203] Despite the rarity of this condition in developed nations, the potential for this virus to cause disease in HIV-infected children in the developing world is supported by the vertical and horizontal transmission (presumably among young children via saliva) in human herpesvirus-8–endemic regions and thus should be looked for as efforts to increase survival of HIV-infected children in these regions is pursued.[204–206] As noted earlier, the role of this virus in pediatric HIV disease has been quite limited, but with increasing numbers of adolescents being infected with HIV, the potential for this virus to manifest itself in this older population needs to be considered. Surveillance efforts should be directed toward this age group to monitor for serologic and virologic evidence of this virus, along with other sexually transmitted pathogens. Currently, although chemotherapeutic agents have shown varying success in treating Kaposi sarcoma, the best treatment remains HAART and restoration of immune function.

Polyomavirus

JC virus, the agent responsible for progressive multifocal leukoencephalopathy, has been known for some time to cause disease in immunosuppressed individuals. However, before the AIDS epidemic, progressive multifocal leukoencephalopathy was quite uncommon. Believed to be primarily a reactivation phenomenon, this disease, like cytomegalovirus and DMAC, is only seen in patients with very severe immunosuppression. It is because of the need for prior exposure to this pathogen (which would appear to be less ubiquitous than cytomegalovirus and DMAC) and severe immunosuppression that the incidence and prevalence of this disease in the pediatric population have thankfully been very low. However, given the relatively older age of the pediatric patients who have been reportedly afflicted by this disease, the manifestations and disease course are essentially the same as described in adults. The disease usually causes progressive neurologic deterioration leading to death. Its disease course must be distinguished from that of HIV encephalopathy, CNS lymphoma, and CNS toxoplasmosis. The magnetic resonance imaging appearance is quite useful to provide a presumptive diagnosis, but prior to the development of PCR tests for detection of the virus in CSF, the only definitive means of diagnosis was by brain biopsy.[207,208]

Even with definitive diagnosis, however, the therapeutic options have been limited and, except for some preliminary uncontrolled data regarding the use of cidofovir, have been almost uniformly unsuccessful in preventing the eventual fatal outcome of this disease.[207,209] As already seen with other OIs, the best intervention appears to be a positive response to HAART, although this intervention cannot always be counted on to reverse the course of this disease.[25,32,33,209]

Hepatitis C

Hepatitis C, the virus most commonly associated with blood transfusions and intravenous drug abuse, now threatens to reverse some of the gains made in extending life expectancy in HIV-infected adults with the advent of improved antiretroviral regimens.[210,211] Although many questions regarding the pathogenesis of the phenomenon remain unanswered in the adult population, it appears that the progression of hepatitis C disease is accelerated in HIV-infected individuals, leading sometimes to progressive cirrhosis and hepatic failure.[210–212] The underlying hepatic involvement associated with hepatitis C can also complicate the antiretroviral management of the patients' HIV disease, putting them at risk for HIV disease progression. Therapeutic interventions such as interferon therapy alone, combination interferon and ribavirin, and pegylated interferon (with or without ribavirin) are being studied in coinfected adults, but early studies suggest that these treatments are likely to be less successful than observed in non–HIV-infected individuals and potentially have an increased adverse event rate profile.

With these sobering thoughts in mind, some issues specific to pediatric HIV disease should be covered. Except for adolescents with adult risk behaviors, the primary mode of transmission of hepatitis C in the pediatric HIV population has been through mother-to-infant transmission, likely during the birth process. The data on transmission rates are somewhat limited, but epidemiologic evidence suggests that the rates of vertical transmission can be two- to threefold higher (14–19%) than in HIV-uninfected mothers (4–8%).[213–217] It does not appear that this rate is affected by the HIV status of the child, although data are limited by the small size of the cohorts studied to date. The factors affecting vertical transmission rates have not been clearly delineated, but both HIV and hepatitis C viral loads are likely to be among the factors. What has yet to be determined is the overall prevalence of this disease in HIV-infected children, but clearly it will be linked with the epidemiology of HCV disease in HIV-infected women and could be of significant importance in populations of women with a history of intravenous drug abuse. The PACTG has initiated a study to determine the current burden of hepatitis C disease in a random sample of perinatally HIV-infected children (1–21 years of age) in an attempt to understand the scope of this copathogen in the pediatric HIV population and to identify the capacity for future clinical trials. Although no interventional strategies are currently available to prevent maternal-child transmission, it is still imperative for both the mother's and the infant's health to screen all HIV-infected mothers for the presence of hepatitis C virus. If the mother is determined to be positive, follow-up testing of the infant is warranted through at least the first year of life (longer if found to be infected). At least for HIV-infected infants, it is recommended that hepatitis C PCR tests be used when hepatitis C antibody test results are negative, as it is currently uncertain what percentage (if any) of coinfected infants may not manifest their hepatitis C infection through production of hepatitis C antibodies.

PARASITIC PATHOGENS

Toxoplasma gondii

Toxoplasmosis is a disease highly associated with severe immunosuppression and evidence of prior infection as determined by IgG serology. Thus, the vast majority of cases of disease are believed to represent reactivation as opposed to new acute infection. As with other diseases discussed in this chapter, toxoplasmosis is quite uncommon in the pediatric HIV-infected population; the low incidence is likely related directly to lack of exposure to this pathogen. The disease is much more common in Europe than in the United States, owing the higher seroprevalence in both the HIV-infected populations and the general populations in these regions.[218] Because the seroprevalence is also believed to be higher in many developing nations, surveillance in these populations is warranted. The most prominent manifestation of disease is the cerebral form, with pulmonary, ocular, and disseminated disease much less common. It is important to note that the clinical presentation of pulmonary toxoplasmosis is relatively indistinguishable from that of PCP. The clinical manifestations of CNS toxoplasmosis include headache, fevers, confusion, and lethargy. Seizures may occur in up to 30% of patients and are the most common cause of seizures secondary to OIs in HIV-infected individuals. The diagnosis of cerebral toxoplasmosis should be considered in those individuals with lesions, usually ring-enhancing, noted on computed tomography or magnetic resonance imaging scan of the head (magnetic resonance imaging scans are more sensitive at detecting cerebral lesions), low CD4+ counts, and previous evidence of seropositivity. Lumbar puncture is indicated (if there is no evidence of increased intracranial pressure on neuroimaging) to eliminate other opportunistic pathogens. The gold standard for definitive diagnosis is brain biopsy, which can demonstrate toxoplasma cysts or trophozoites or provide tissue diagnosis of the other two entities, CNS lymphoma or progressive multifocal leukoencephalopathy, that may present with similar clinical and neuroradiologic findings. However, a presumptive diagnosis of toxoplasmosis can be established by demonstrating a clinical and radiologic response to specific toxoplasma therapy. PCR of both CSF and serum has also been used as a noninvasive alternative to brain biopsy in patients with suspected disease.

A unique situation exists in the pediatric age group and relates to congenital transmission of this organism from previously seroimmune mothers. Although classic teaching has held that congenital transmission of this parasite occurs only during primary maternal infection, there are well-documented cases of vertical transmission occurring during reactivation of toxoplasmosis in previously seroimmune HIV-infected mothers. However, other investigators have found the overall risk for congenital toxoplasmosis to be low in children born to HIV-infected women.[219, 220]

As mentioned earlier, treatment should be instituted in those patients with suspected cerebral lesions and positive toxoplasma serology. The treatment of choice includes pyrimethamine and sulfadiazine, although the combination of pyrimethamine and clindamycin is a very useful alternative regimen for patients who are intolerant of sulfa drugs. Subsequent life-long suppression with daily pyrimethamine, sulfadiazine, and folinic acid is required for those individuals who cannot achieve reconstitution of their CD4+ cell counts above 200. For the uncommon infant who may have congenital toxoplasmosis and HIV infection, treatment recommendations are similar. Primary prophylaxis should be provided to those with CD4+ cell counts less than 200/mm^3 and positive toxoplasma serology. TMP-SMX, as used for PCP prophylaxis, has been shown to be very effective in the prevention of toxoplasmosis in high-risk populations. Alternative regimens for patients intolerant of TMP-SMX are provided in Table 10–6, but either they are less effective or there is less clinical experience currently available.

Cryptosporidium, Microsporidia, Isospora

Epidemiology and Clinical Features

This group of enteric pathogens has been responsible for a significant percentage of cases of diarrhea in case series of AIDS-related enteropathy.[221,222] Although *Cryptosporidium parvum* was the first major pathogen to be described, organisms belonging to the microsporidial group, *Encephalitozoon intestinalis*, *Enterocytozoon bieneusi*, and *Encephalitozoon hellem*, have been shown to cause a comparable amount of disease in the adult HIV-infected population.[223] Cryptosporidiosis is the most common diarrheal pathogen of this group in HIV-infected children.[44,48] There has been little published information regarding microsporidiosis in this age group. This is somewhat surprising given the degree of diarrheal disease caused by microsporidia in the adult HIV population. Whether this represents a real lack of exposure and a resultant reduced risk of subsequent disease or a lack of diagnosis is not known. Since water and food may serve as vehicles for exposure to both enteric parasites, it seems more likely that the lower rates for microsporidiosis are related to missed diagnoses.

The symptoms associated with cryptosporidiosis and microsporidiosis are relatively indistinguishable, and both infections occur in patients with markedly impaired immune systems. Symptoms include large-volume, watery diarrhea, often associated with abdominal pain and cramping and lack of associated fever. Disease is usually progressive, but periods of spontaneous remissions may occur. Spontaneous cures in those who are most immunologically impaired is rare. Management of these diseases in developing countries is even further complicated by underlying malnutrition.[224,225] *Isospora* produces a similar clinical picture but is identified much less commonly than either cryptosporidia or microsporidia.

Diagnosis can now be established for all three pathogens by examination of stool specimens. Cryptosporidiosis can be identified by the use of either modified acid-fast stains or with the use of fluorescent antibody staining. *Isospora* can also be identified by modified acid-fast stain, but the cysts are much larger than *Cryptosporidium* (20–30 μm vs. 4–6 μm). Microsporidia are much smaller and more difficult to detect on routine microscopic review of stool samples and routine histologic stains of small bowel biopsies. Definitive diagnosis often required electron microscopy of small bowel biopsies. More recently, modified Giemsa and special trichrome stains read by experienced personnel have provided reasonable diagnostic yields. The development of species-specific PCR probes may add improved diagnostic capability to the detection of these organisms, but this methodology is not commercially available and its application in routine clinical laboratories is currently severely restricted.[226]

Treatment and Prevention

Except for *Isospora*, which responds well to treatment and suppressive therapy with TMP-SMX, the results of treatment and prevention of cryptosporidial and microsporidial disease have been disappointing. In cases of cryptosporidial disease, clinical responses have been reported to paromomycin and azithromycin in uncontrolled trials, but neither drug has shown any proven efficacy in controlled studies.[227,228] A new drug, nitazoxanide, is currently in clinical trials, but results demonstrating its efficacy are still pending. Similarly, no standard treatment exists for microsporidiosis. Drugs such as metronidazole, albendazole, and atovaquone have been used with mixed results and no specific controlled trials have been attempted.[223,229] Currently, there are no specific recommendations for the prevention of these enteric parasites, although the successful treatment and subsequent suppression of *Isospora* by TMP-SMX may suggest that the routine use of this antimicrobial for PCP and toxoplasmosis prophylaxis may also prevent infection with this pathogen. An interesting post hoc analysis of data from a large *M. avium* prophylaxis trial comparing rifabutin to clarithromycin to the combination of these two agents demonstrated a treatment benefit of rifabutin but not clarithromycin in the prevention of cryptosporidiosis in HIV-infected adults with severe immunosuppression.[230] The biologic mechanism of action could not be elucidated, as the prevention of cryptosporidiosis was not one of the original intents of the study. The use of HAART and subsequent improvement in immunologic function and control of HIV replication, as will be discussed later, holds the most promise for both eradication and prevention of these diarrheal pathogens.[31,231] It should be pointed out that all of these infections occur in developing nations, where the impact of HAART on their course and incidence is unlikely to be felt.

Other Parasitic Infections

With regard to tropical diseases, there has been a conspicuous absence of evidence of a biologic interaction between malaria and HIV or an upsurge of disease caused by metazoan parasites, including *Strongyloides* hyperinfestation syndrome, which has been described in other immunosuppressed populations.[111,232] Additionally, in a large prospective study of HIV-infected children in central Africa, investigators were unable to demonstrate any evidence that HIV infection led to an increased susceptibility to malaria or worsened the course of falciparum malaria or that malarial infection led a progression of HIV disease.[233]

Although currently uncommonly reported in HIV-infected children, leishmaniasis, specifically visceral leishmaniasis, is another tropical disease that occurs in many regions where HIV disease is prevalent. Interestingly, in southwestern Europe, there has been a reversal of age distribution of visceral leishmaniasis cases, with greater prevalence among young HIV-infected adults over what was traditionally a pediatric disease. Additionally, the clinical features of visceral leishmaniasis, which include fever, weight loss, hepatosplenomegaly, and pancytopenia, are difficult to distinguish from those caused by HIV disease. As with other opportunistic infections, HIV-infected individuals with severely compromised immune function are at increased risk to develop visceral leishmaniasis once infected, and infections relapse rates are high after initial treatment with traditional and newer agents, such as pentavalent antimony, amphotericin B, and its liposomal derivatives. Optimal regimens for secondary prophylaxis have not been determined.[232, 234]

WITHDRAWAL OF OPPORTUNISTIC INFECTION THERAPY AND PROPHYLAXIS

Although advances have been made in the treatment and prevention of OIs during the last two decades, the most dramatic impact on these infections has been the restoration of immune function associated with the introduction of the more potent antiretroviral regimens. Several important observations from the current literature and from ongoing studies now make it possible to determine the feasibility and safety of withdrawing either the primary or secondary prophylactic regimens that we have described previously. Even more radical efforts to discontinue maintenance treatment of chronic infections such as DMAC, cytomegalovirus, and cryptococcal meningitis now seem possible when indefinite treatment or suppressive therapy appeared to be a foregone conclusion.[22,28,235–239] Finally, the ability to induce resolution of diseases such as progressive multifocal leukoencephalopathy, cryptosporidiosis, and microsporidiosis, where effective therapy had previously eluded clinicians, has also been reported recently.[31–33, 240]

The literature is now replete with evidence that primary PCP prophylaxis can be safely discontinued in adult patients whose CD4+ counts rise above 250 cells/mm^3, and there is accumulating data that this approach is also safe for those receiving secondary prophylaxis for prior episodes of PCP.[27,29,30,241,242] Studies that address the withdrawal of primary prophylaxis for diseases such as DMAC and toxoplasmosis have also been reported.[27,243–246]

In pediatric patients, guidelines for the withdrawal of PCP prophylaxis will have to rely on the results from adult HIV patients, as the incidence of these diseases is too low in older children to make observational studies feasible. For infants of younger than 1 year of age, however, not enough data are available on the impact of immune reconstitution to change the current CDC recommendation to provide PCP prophylaxis to all HIV-infected children in this age group.

Although it may not be possible to study the withdrawal of PCP and DMAC prophylaxis in children as it relates to those specific OIs, the impact of withdrawing these therapies on recurrent bacterial infections can be determined in the pediatric population. PACTG P1008 is exploring this clinical question and a 1-year interim review of infection rates revealed to be clinically comparable to those seen in patients on antimicrobial prophylaxis. This study, which was planned to complete follow-up in late 2002, should provide ongoing risk assessment of the withdrawal of PCP prophylactic regimens on bacterial and PCP infections in children. These continually accumulating data are now being incorporated into the 2001 US Public Health guidelines on the prevention of opportunistic infections to provide clinicians with guidance regarding the discontinuation of primary and secondary prophylaxis.

Despite these exciting advances, some cautionary notes are necessary. Although CD4+ count thresholds provide the simplest method for determining when to withdraw OI prophylaxis, viral loads are still likely to have an impact on the patient's risk of developing an OI while on HAART. It has been observed that patients may still develop OIs in the first few months after initiating HAART.[247–249] This has occurred most frequently during the first 3 months but can occur as late as 6 months into therapy. It would seem prudent to follow the response to HAART and consider discontinuing prophylaxis against pathogens such as *P. carinii*, *M. avium*, and cytomegalovirus after documenting a sustained response (rise in CD4+ counts and decline in viral load) for at least 3 months into HAART therapy. Another important observation has been the occurrence of an inflammatory immune response in patients soon after receiving potent antiretroviral therapy.[250, 251] This has now been described for flares of herpes viruses, mycobacterial diseases, and cytomegalovirus retinitis (in the form of vitritis) soon after evidence of immune reconstitution related to HAART is apparent.[180,252–254] These phenomena represent not a failure of antiretroviral therapy but a restored immunologic response to microbial antigens, and they often do not require specific antimicrobial therapy. This will prove to be an important clinical presentation that will challenge clinicians until more experience is gained regarding prevention or treatment options (such as the use of anti-inflammatory agents). Lastly, failure of antiretroviral therapy may lead to a subsequent decline in previously improved immune function. Close surveillance of these patients is warranted to allow timely reinitiation of prophylaxis or prior maintenance therapy to avoid new or recurrent OI events.[255, 256]

CONCLUSIONS

As presented in this chapter, opportunistic infections continue to cause serious morbidity and mortality in HIV-infected children; however, the last decade has seen a dramatic improvement in the control of viral replication and, with it, a concomitant improvement in immune function. For most developed nations, this has led to a significant decline in OIs and deaths in both children and adults and a positive impact on their quality of life. These positive results contrast sharply with the rising burden of HIV disease in developing countries, where the vast majority of HIV-infected children die before 3 years of age from complications of both common and opportunistic infections and from nutritional deprivation. This dichotomy poses several challenges for the coming decade. Despite the sharp decline in OIs in the last few years, it will still be important to maintain active surveillance for these diseases, as antiretroviral therapy failure may cause patients to return to the previous low levels of immune function that had placed them at risk for OIs originally. In developing nations, improved surveillance systems, which include efficient, sensitive, and inexpensive field tests for diagnosing infectious diseases, are necessary to understand the local epidemiology of these diseases so that experience gained in the treatment and prevention of OIs in developed nations can be applied to these underserved regions. Of equal concern is the possibility that the current decline in OIs in developed nations (where many of the drugs used for treatment and prevention are most affordable) may lead to less emphasis on research and development of alternative agents with potentially improved efficacy, decreased toxicity, and fewer drug-drug interactions. This could have a serious impact on the efforts to control OIs in developing nations and even in developed nations should the current failure rate of new antiretroviral drugs lead to a resurgence of severe immune dysfunction and a new rise in OI incidence. With the advances of the last few years, vigilance, and a strong focus on new research and development, we can continue to reduce the burden of OIs that had so dominated the management of HIV disease.

REFERENCES

1. Chan I, Neaton J, Saravolatz L, et al: Frequencies of opportunistic diseases prior to death among HIV-infected persons. AIDS 1995;9:1145–1151.
2. Selik R, Karon J, Ward J: Effect of the human immunodeficiency virus epidemic on mortality from opportunistic infections in the United States in 1993. J Infect Dis 1997;176:632–636.
3. Castro K, Ward J, Slutsker L, et al: 1993 Revised classification system for HIV infection and expanded surveillance case definition for AIDS among adolescents and adults. MMWR 1993;41(RR–17):1–18.
4. Kovacs J, Masur H: Prophylaxis against opportunistic infections in patients with human immunodeficiency virus infection. N Engl J Med 2000;342:1416–1429.
5. Williams P, Currier J, Swindels S: Joint effects of HIV-1 RNA levels and CD4 lymphocyte cells on the risk of specific opportunistic infections. AIDS 1999;13:1035–1044.
6. Lyles R, Chu C, Mellors J, et al: Prognostic value of plasma HIV RNA in the natural history of *Pneumocystis carinii* pneumonia, cytomegalovirus and *Mycobacterium avium* complex. AIDS 1999;13:341–349.
7. Kaplan J, Hanson D, Jones J, et al: Viral load as an independent risk factor for opportunistic infections in HIV-infected adults and adolescents. AIDS 2001;15:1831–1836.
8. USPHS/IDSA: 1999 USPHS/IDSA guidelines for the prevention of opportunistic infections in persons infected with human immunodeficiency virus. MMWR 1999;48(RR–10):1–59, 61–66.
9. Centers for Disease Control and Prevention: 1994 revised classification system of human immunodeficiency virus infection in children less than 13 years of age. MMWR 1994;43(RR–12):1–10.
10. Kaplan J, Hanson D, Dworkin M, et al: Epidemiology of human immunodeficiency virus–associated opportunistic infections in the United States in the era of highly active antiretroviral therapy. Clin Infect Dis 2000;30(Suppl 1):S5–S14.
11. Brodt H, Kamps B, Gute P, et al: Changing incidence of AIDS-defining illnesses in the era of antiretroviral combination therapy. AIDS 1997;11:1731–1738.
12. Palella F, Delaney K, Moorman A, et al: Declining morbidity and mortality among patients with

advanced human immunodeficiency virus infection. N Engl J Med 1998;338:853–860.
13. Moore R, Chaisson R: Natural history of HIV infection in the era of combination antiretroviral therapy. AIDS 1999;13:1933–1942.
14. Paul S, Gilbert H, Ziecheck W, et al: The impact of potent antiretroviral therapy on the characteristics of hospitalized patients with HIV infection. AIDS 1999;13:415–418.
15. USPHS/IDSA: USPHS/IDSA guidelines for the prevention of opportunistic infections in persons infected with human immunodeficiency virus: A summary. MMWR 1995;44(RR–8):1–34.
16. USPHS/IDSA: 1997 USPHS/IDSA guidelines for the prevention of opportunistic infections in persons infected with human immunodeficiency virus: Disease-specific recommendations. Clin Infect Dis 1997;25(Suppl 3):S313–S335.
17. Centers for Disease Control and Prevention: Surveillance for AIDS-defining opportunistic illnesses, 1992–1997. MMWR 1999;48(SS–2):1–22.
18. Frederick T, Bertolli J, Mascola L: Trends in the incidence of AIDS-defining conditions among children infected with HIV: 1992–1997. Paper presented at the Seventh Conference on Retroviruses and Opportunistic Infections, San Francisco, CA, January/February 2000.
19. McNaghten A, Hanson D, Jones J, et al: Effects of antiretroviral therapy and opportunistic illness primary chemoprophylaxis on survival after AIDS diagnosis. AIDS 1999;13:1687–1695.
20. Thea D, Lambert G, Weedon J, et al: Benefit of primary prophylaxis before 18 months of age in reducing the incidence of *Pneumocystis carinii* pneumonia and early death in a cohort of 112 human immunodeficiency virus-infected infants. Pediatrics 1996;97:59–64.
21. Simonds R, Lindegren M, Thomas P, et al: Prophylaxis against *Pneumocystis carinii* pneumonia among children with perinatally acquired human immunodeficiency virus infection in the United States. N Engl J Med 1995;332:786–790.
22. Macdonald J, Torriani F, Morse L, et al: Lack of reactivation of cytomegalovirus (CMV) retinitis after stopping CMV maintenance therapy in AIDS patients with sustained elevations in CD4 T cells in response to highly active antiretroviral therapy. J Infect Dis 1998;177:1182–1187.
23. Powderly W: Impact of protease inhibitors on resolution of opportunistic infections. HIV Treatment Update 1999;July:12–16.
24. Schneider M, Borleffs J, Stolk R, et al: Discontinuation of prophylaxis for *Pneumocystis carinii* pneumonia in HIV-1–infected patients treated with hightly active antiretroviral therapy. Lancet 1999;353:201–203.
25. Tantisiriwat W, Tebas P, Clifford D, et al: Progressive multifocal leukoencephalopathy in patients with AIDS receiving highly active antiretroviral therapy. Clin Infect Dis 1999;28:1152–1154.
26. Tural C, Romeu J, Sirera G, et al: Long lasting remission of cytomegalovirus retinitis without maintenance therapy in human immunodeficiency virus-infected patients. J Infect Dis 1998;177:1080–1083.
27. Kirk O, Lundgren J, Pedersen C, et al: Can chemoprophylaxis against opportunistic infections be discontiued after an increase in CD4 cells induced by highly active antiretroviral therapy. AIDS 1999;13:1647–1651.
28. Aberg JA, Yajko DM, Jacobson MA: Eradication of disseminated *Mycobacterium avium* complex after twelve months anti-mycobacterial therapy and response to highly active antiretroviral therapy. J Infect Dis 1998;178:1446–1449.
29. Furrer H, Egger M, Opravil M, et al: Discontinuation of primary prophylaxis against *Pneumocystis Carinii* pneumonia in HIV-1–infected adults treated with combination antiretroviral therapy. N Engl J Med 1999;340:1301–1306.
30. Weverling G, Mocroft A, Ledergerber B, et al: Discontinuation of *Pneumocystis carinii* pneumonia prophylaxis after start of highly active antiretroviral therapy in HIV-1 infection. Lancet 1999;353:1293–1287.
31. Maggi P, Larocca A, Quarto M, et al: Effect of antiretroviral therapy on cryptosporidiosis and microsporidiosis in patients infected with human immunodeficiency virus type 1. Eur J Clin Microbiol Infect Dis 2000;19:213–217.
32. Clifford D, Yiannoutsos C, Glicksman M, et al: HAART improves prognosis in HIV associated progressive multifocal leukoencephalopathy. Neurology 1999;52:623–625.
33. Dworkin M, Wan P, Hanson D, et al: Progressive multifocal leukoencephalopathy: Improved survival of human immunodeficiency virus-infected patients in the protease inhibitor era. J Infect Dis 1999;180:621–625.
34. Thomas P, Singh T, Williams R, et al: Trends in survival for children reported with maternally transmitted acquired immunodeficiency syndrome in New York City, 1982 to 1989. Pediatr Infect Dis J 1992;11:34–39.
35. Horsburgh CR Jr, Caldwell MB, Simonds RJ: Epidemiology of disseminated nontuberculous mycobacterial disease in children with acquired immunodeficiency syndrome. Pediatr Infect Dis J 1993;12:219–222.
36. Hoyt L, Oleske J, Holland B, et al: Nontuberculous mycobacteria in children with acquired immunodeficiency syndrome. Pediatr Infect Dis J 1992;11:354–360.
37. Johann-Liang R, Cervia J, Noel G: Characteristics of human immunodeficiency virus-infected children at the time of death: An experience in the 1990s. Pediatr Infect Dis J 1997;16:1145–1150.
38. Lewis L, Butler K, Husson R, et al: Defining the population of human immunodeficiency virus-

infected children at risk for *Mycobacterium avium-intracellular* infection. J Pediatr 1992;121: 677–683.
39. Reik R, Rodríguez M, Hensley G: Infections in children with human immunodeficiency virus/acquired immunodeficiency syndrome: An autopsy study of 30 cases in south Florida, 1990–1993. Pediatr Pathol Lab Med 1995;15:269–281.
40. Drut R, Anderson V, Greco M, et al: Opportunistic infections in pediatric HIV infection: A study of 74 autopsy cases from Latin America. The Latin American AIDS Pathology Study Group. Pediatr Pathol Lab Med 1997;17:569–576.
41. Chandwani S, Kaul A, Bebenroth D, et al: Cytomegalovirus infection in human immunodeficiency virus type 1-infected children. Pediatr Infect Dis J 1996;15:310–314.
42. Chintu C, Zumla A: Childhood tuberculosis and infection with the human immunodeficiency virus. J R Coll Physicians Lond 1995;29:92–95.
43. Gonzalez C, Shetty D, Lewis L, et al: Cyptococcosis in human immunodeficiency virus-infected children. Pediatr Infect Dis J 1996;15:796–800.
44. Guarino A, Castaldo A, Russo S, et al: Enteric cryptosporidiosis in pediatric HIV infection. J Pediatr Gastroenterol Nutr 1997;25:182–187.
45. Kitchen B, Engler H, Gill V, et al: Cytomegalovirus infection in children with human immunodeficiecyvirus infection. Pediatr Infect Dis J 1997;16: 358–363.
46. Morris C, Araba-Owoyele L, Spector S, et al: Disease patterns and survival after acquired immunodeficiency syndrome diagnosis in human immunodeficiency virus-infected children. Pediatr Infect Dis J 1996;15:321–328.
47. Nigro G, Krzysztofiak A, Gattinara G, et al: Rapid progression of HIV disease in children with cytomegalovirus DNAemia. AIDS 1996;10:1127–1133.
48. Saredi N, Bava J: Cryptosporidiosis in pediatric patients. Rev Inst Med Trop Sao Paulo 1998;40:197–200.
49. Centers for Disease Control and Prevention: HIV/AIDS Surveillance Report, Vol. 9. Atlanta, GA, CDC, 1998, pp 1–41.
50. Hsu H, Pelton S, Williamson J, et al: Survival in children with perinatal HIV infection and very low CD4 lymphoctye counts. J Acquir Immune Defic Syndr 2000;25:269–275.
51. Dankner W, Lindsey J, Levin M, et al: Correlates of opportunistic infections in children with human immunodeficiency virus managed before highly active antiretroviral therapy. Pediatr Infect Dis J 2001;20:40–48.
52. Tudor-Williams G: HIV infections in children in developing countries. Trans R Soc Trop Med Hyg 2000;94:3–4.
53. Graham SC, Coulter JB, Gilks CF: Pulmonary disease in HIV-infected African children. Int J Tuberc Lung Dis 2001;5:12–23.
54. Dray-Spira R, Lepage P, Dabis F: Prevention of infectious complications of paediatric HIV infection in Africa. AIDS 2000;14:1091–1099.
55. Centers for Disease Control and Prevention: Classification system for human immunodeficiency virus (HIV) infection in children under 13 years of age. MMWR 1987;36:225–236.
56. Ammann A, Schiffman G, Abrams D, et al: B-cell immunodeficiency in acquired immune deficiency snydrome. JAMA 1984;251:1447–1449.
57. Bernstein L, Ochs H, Wedgwood R, et al: Defective humoral immunity in pediatric acquired immune deficiency syndrome. J Pediatr 1985;107:352–357.
58. Pahwa S, Fikrig S, Menez R, et al: Pediatric acquired immunodeficiency syndrome: Demonstration of B lymphocyte defects in vitro. Diag Immunol 1986;4: 24–30.
59. Rollides E, Mertins S, Eddy J, et al: Impairment of neutrophil chemotactic and bactericidal function in children infected with human immunodeficiency virus type 1 and partial reversal after in vitro exposure to granulocyte-macrophage colony-stimulating factor. J Pediatr 1990;117:531–540.
60. Murphy P, Lane H, Fauci A, et al: Impairment of neutrophil bactericidal capacity in patients with AIDS. J Infect Dis 1988;158:627–630.
61. Ellis M, Gupta S, Galant S, et al: Impaired neutrophil function in patients with AIDS or AIDS-Related Complex: A comprehensive evaluation. J Infect Dis 1988;158:1268–1276.
62. Krasinski K, Borkowsky W, Bonk S, et al: Bacterial infection in human immunodeficiency virus infected children. Pediatr Infect Dis J 1988;7:323–328.
63. Bernstein L, Krieger B, Novick B, et al: Bacterial infection in the acquired immunodeficiency syndrome of children. Pediatr Infect Dis J 1985;4: 472–475.
64. Ruiz-Contreras J, Ramos J, Hernández-Sampelayo T, et al: Sepsis in children with human immunodeficiency virus infection. The Madrid HIV Pediatric Infection Collaborative Study Group. Pediatr Infect Dis J 1995;14:522–526.
65. Tovo P, DeMartino M, Gaviano C, et al: Prognostic factors and survival in children with perinatal HIV-1 infection. Lancet 1992;339:1249–1253.
66. Principi N, Marchisio P, Tornaghi R, et al: Occurrence of infections in children infected with human immunodeficiency virus. Pediatr Infect Dis J 1991;10:190–193.
67. European Collaborative Study: Natural history of vertically acquired human immunodeficiency virus-1 infection. Pediatrics 1994;94:815–819.
68. Scott G, Hutto C, Makuch R, et al: Survival in children with perinatally acquired human immunodeficiency virus type 1 infection. N Engl J Med 1989;321:1791–1796.
69. Spector S, Gelber R, McGrath N, et al: A controlled trial of intravenous immune globulin for the prevention of

serious bacterial infections in children receiving zidovudine for advanced human immunodeficiency virus infection. New Engl J Med 1994;331:1181–1187.
70. The National Institute of Child Health and Human Development Intravenous Immunoglobulin Study Group: Intravenous immune globulin for the prevention of bacterial infections in children with symptomatic human immunodeficiency virus infection. N Engl J Med 1991;325:73–80.
71. Mofenson L, Moye J: Intravenous immune globulin for the prevention of infections in children with symptomatic human immunodeficiency virus infection. Pediatr Res 1993;33(Suppl):S80–S89.
72. Nathoo K, Chigonde S, Nhembe M, et al: Community-acquired bacteremia in human immunodeficiency virus-infected children in Harare, Zimbabwe. Pediatr Infect Dis J 1996;15:1092–1097.
73. Ikeogu M, Wolf B, Mathe S: Pulmonary manifestations in HIV seropositivity and malnutrition in Zimbabwe. Arch Dis Child 1997;76:124–128.
74. Jones N, Huebner R, Khoosal M, et al: The impact of HIV on *Streptococcus pneumoniae* bacteraemia in a South African population. AIDS 1998;12:2177–2184.
75. Jean S, Pape J, Verdier R, et al: The natural history of human immunodeficiency virus 1 infection in Haitian infants. Pediatr Infect Dis J 1999;18:58–63.
76. Madhi S, Madhi A, Petersen K, et al: Impact of human immunodeficiency virus type 1 infections on the epidemiology and outcome of bacterial meningitis in South African children. Int J Infect Dis 2001;5: 119–125.
77. Rollides E, Marshall D, Venzon D, et al: Bacterial infections in human immunodeficiency virus type 1 infected children: The impact of central venous catheters and antiretroviral agents. Pediatr Infect Dis J 1991;10:813–819.
78. Rollides E, Butler K, Husson R, et al: *Pseudomonas* infections in children with human immunodeficiency virus infection. Pediatr Infect Dis J 1992;11:547–553.
79. Flores G, Stavola J, Noel G: Bacteremia Due to *Pseudomonas aeruginosa* in children with AIDS. Clin Infect Dis 1993;16:706–708.
80. Shepp D, Lang I, Ramundo M, et al: Serious *Pseudomonas aeruginosa* infections in patients with AIDS. J Acquir Immune Defic Syndr 1994;7:823–831.
81. Nelson M, Shanson D, Barter G, et al: *Pseudomonas* septicaemia assoicated with HIV. AIDS 1991;5:761–763.
82. Golden M, Goldie S: Changing epidemiology of *Pseudomonas aeruginosa* in HIV-infected patients. Infect Med 2000;17:109–111, 115–116.
83. Havlir D, Dube P, Sattler F, et al: Prophylaxis against disseminated *Mycobacterium avium* complex with weekly azithromycin, daily rifabutin or both. N Engl J Med 1996;335:392–398.
84. El-Sadr W, Luskin-Hawk R, Yurik T, et al: A randomized trial of daily and thrice-weekly trimethoprim-sulfamethoxazole for the prevention of *Pneumocystis carinii* pneumonia in human immunodeficiency virus-infected persons. Clin Infect Dis 1999;29:775–783.
85. Dworkin M, Ward J, Hanson D, et al: Pneumococcal disease among HIV-infected persons: Incidence, risk factors, and impact of vaccination. Clin Infect Dis 2001;32:794–800.
86. Osmond D, Chin D, Glassroth J, et al: Impact of bacterial pneumonia and *Pneumocystis carinii* pneumonia on human immunodeficiency virus disease progression. Clin Infect Dis 1999;29:536–543.
87. Barnett E, Klein J, Pelton S, et al: Otitis media in children born to human immunodeficiency virus infected mothers. Pediatr Infect Dis J 1992;11:360–364.
88. Principi N, Marchisio P, Tornaghi R, et al: Acute otitis media in human immunodeficiency virus infected mothers. Pediatr 1991;88:566–571.
89. Dankner W, Yogev R, Hughes W, et al: Phase II/III, randomized, double-blind trial to compare atovaquone plus azithromycin to trimethoprim-sulfamethoxazole in the prevention of multiple opportunistic pathogen infections in HIV-infected children. Paper presented at the Pediatric Academic Societies and American Academy of Pediatrics Joint Meeting, Boston, Mass, May, 2000.
90. Adams W, Deaver K, Cochi S, et al: Decline of childhood *Haemophilus influenzae* type B (Hib) disease in the Hib vaccine era. JAMA 1993;269:221–226.
91. Gibb D, Spoülou V, Giacomelli A, et al: Antibody responses to *Haemophilus influenzae* type b and *Streptococcus pneumoniae* vaccines in children with human immunodeficiency virus infection. Pediatr Infect Dis J 1995;14:129–135.
92. Peters V, Sood S: Immunity to *Haemophilus influenza* type b polysaccharide capsule in children with human immunodeficiency virus infection immunized with a single dose of *Haemophilus* vaccine. J Pediatr 1994;125:74–77.
93. Read J, Frasch C, Rich K, et al: The immunogenicity of *Haemophilus influenzae* type b conjugate vaccines in children born to human immunodeficiency virus-infected women. Women and Infants Transmission Study Group. Pediatr Infect Dis J 1998;17:391–397.
94. Steinhoff M, Auerbach B, Nelson K, et al: Antibody responses to *Haemophilus influenzae* type b vaccines in men with human immunodeficiency virus infection. N Engl J Med 1991;325:1837–1841.
95. Shinefield H, Black S: Efficacy of pneumococcal conjugate vaccines in large scale field trials. Pediatr Infect Dis J 2000;19:394–397.
96. Breiman R, Keller D, Phelan M: Evaluation of the effectiveness of 23-valent pneumococcal capsular polysaccharide vaccine for HIV-infected patients. Arch Intern Med 2000;160:2633–2638.
97. King J, Vink P, Farley J, et al: Safety and immunogenicity of three doses of a five-valent pneumococcal conjugate vaccine in children younger than two years with and without human immunodeficiency virus infection. Pediatrics 1997;99:575–580.
98. Nachman S, Kim S, King J: A double blind, placebo-controlled trial of the safety and immunogenicity of

a seven valent conjugate pneumococcal vaccine in HIV-infected infants. Paper presented at the meeting of the European Society for Pediatric Infectious Diseases, Istanbul, Turkey, March 2001.
99. Wakefield A, Peters S, Banerji S, et al: *Pneumocystis carinii* shows DNA homology with the ustomycetous red yeast fungi. Mol Microbiol 1992;6:1903–1911.
100. Stringer J, Edman J, Cushion M, et al: The fungal nature of *Pneumocystis carinii*. J Med Vet Mycol 1992;30(Suppl 1):271–278.
101. Tsolaki A, Miler R, Underwood A, et al: Genetic diversity at the internal transcribed spacer regions of the rRNA operon among isolates of *Pneumocystis carinii* from AIDS patients with recurrent pneumonia. J Infect Dis 1996;174:1141–1156.
102. Vargas S, Hughes W, Wakefield A, et al: Limited persistence in and subsequent elimation of *Pneumocystis carinii* from the lungs after *P. carinii* pneumonia. J Infect Dis 1995;172:506–510.
103. Hughes W: Current issues in the epidemiology, transmission, and reactivation of *Pneumocystis carinii* pneumonia. Semin Respir Infect 1998;13:282–288.
104. Beard C, Carter J, Keely S, et al: Genetic variation in *Pneumocystis carinii* isolates from different geographic regions: Implications for transmission. Emerg Infect Dis 2000;6:265–272.
105. Chave J, David S, Wauters J, et al: Transmission of *Pneumocystis carinii* from AIDS patients to other immunosuppressed patients: A cluster of *Pneumocystis carinii* pneumonia in renal transplant recipients. AIDS 1991;5:927–932.
106. Walzer P: *Pneumocystis carinii* pneumonia: New clinical spectrum? N Engl J Med 1991;324:263–265.
107. Simonds R, Oxtoby M, Caldwell M, et al: *Pneumocystis carinii* pneumonia among US children with perinatally acquired HIV infection. JAMA 1993;270:470–473.
108. Abouya Y, Beaumel A, Lucas S, et al: *Pneumocystis carinii* pneumonia: An uncommon cause of death in African patients with acquired immune deficiency syndrome. Am Rev Respir Dis 1992;145:617–620.
109. Batungwanayo J, Taelman H, Lucas S, et al: Pulmonary disease associate with the human immunodeficiency virus in Kigali, Rwanda: A fiberoptic bronchoscopic study of 111 cases of undetermined etiology. Am J Respir Crit Care Med 1994;149:1591–1596.
110. Jeena P, Coovadia H, Chrystal V: *Pneumocystis carinii* and cytomegalovirus infections in severely ill, HIV-infected African infants. Ann Trop Paediatr 1996;16:361–368.
111. Lucas S, Peacock C, Hounnou A, et al: Disease in children infected with HIV in Abidjan, Côte d'Ivoire. BMJ 1996;312:335–338.
112. Graham S, Mtitimila E, Kamanga H, et al: Clinical presentation and outcome of *Pneumocystis carinii* pneumonia in Malawian children. Lancet 2000;355:369–373.
113. Bozzette S, Finkelstein D, Spector S, et al: A randomized trial of three antipneumocystis agents in patients with advanced human immunodeficiency virus infection. N Engl J Med 1995;332:693–699.
114. Baughman R, Liming J: Diagnostic strategies in *Pneumocystis carinii* pneumonia. Front Biosci 1998;3:E1–E12.
115. Martino A, Visconti E, Zolfo M, et al: Noninvasive diagnosis of *Pneumocystis carinii* pneumonia on oral washes in an HIV-infected child. Pediatric Pulmonol 1999;28:352–355.
116. Abadco D, Amaro-Gonzalez R, Rao M, et al: Experience with flexible fiberoptic bronchoscopy with bronchoalveolar lavage as a diagnostic tool in children with AIDS. Am J Dis Child 1992;146:1056–1059.
117. Amaro-Galves R, Rao M, Abadco D, et al: Nonbrochoscopic bronchoalveolar lavage in ventilated children with acquired immune deficiency syndrome: A simple and effective diagnostic method for *Pneumocystis carinii* infection. Pediatr Infect Dis J 1991;10:473–475.
118. Ognibene F, Gill V, Pizzo P, et al: Induced sputum to diagnose *Pneumocystis carinii* pneumonia in immunosuppressed pediatric patients. J Pediatr 1989;115:430–433.
119. Castro M: Treatment and prophylaxis of *Pneumocystis carinii* pneumonia. Semin Respir Infect 1998;13:296–303.
120. Harel Y, Scott W, Szeinberg A, et al: Pentamidine-induced torsades de pointes. Pediatr Infect Dis J 1993;12:692–694.
121. McSherry G, Wright M, Oleske J, et al: Frequency of serious adverse reactions to trimethoprim-sulfamethoxzaole and pentamidine among children with human immunodeficiency virus 1 infection. Paper presented at the 38th Interscience Conference on Antimicrobial Agents and Chemotherapy, San Diego, CA, 1998.
122. Miller R, Noury J, Corbett E, et al: *Pneumocystis carinii* infection: Current treatment and prevention. J Antimicrob Chemother 1996;37(Suppl B):33–53.
123. Bye M, Cairns-Bazarian A, Ewig J: Markedly reduced mortality associated with corticosteroid therapy of *Pneumocystis carinii* pneumonia in children with acquired immunodeficiency syndrome. Arch Pediatr 1994;148:638–641.
124. McLaughlin G, Satranjan S, Schleien C, et al: Effect of corticosteroids on survival of children with acquired immunodeficiency syndrome and *Pneumocystis carinii*-related respiratory failure. J Pediatr 1995;126:821–824.
125. Sleasman J, Hemenway C, Klein A, et al: Corticosteroids improve survival of children with AIDS and *Pneumocystis carinii* pneumonia. Am J Dis Child 1993;147:30–34.
126. Bozzette S, Sattler F, Chiu J, et al: A controlled trail of early adjunctive treatment with corticosteroids

for *Pneumocystis carinii* in the acquired immunodeficiency syndrome. N Engl J Med 1990;323:1451–1457.
127. Rigaud M, Pollack H, Leibovitz B, et al: Efficacy of primary chemoprophylaxis against *Pneumocystis carinii* pneumonia during the first year of life in infants infected with human immunodeficiency virus type 1. J Pediatr 1994;125:476–480.
128. Dunne M, Bozzette S, McCutchan J, et al: Efficacy of azithromycin in prevention of *Pneumocystis carinii* pneumonia: A randomised trial. Lancet 1999;354:891–895.
129. Chan C, Montaner J, Lefebvre E, et al: Atovaquone suspension compared with aerosolized pentamidine for prevention of *Pneumocystis carinii* pneumonia in human immunodeficiency virus-infected subjects intolerant of trimethoprim or sulfonamides. J Infect Dis 1999;180:369–376.
130. El-Sadr W, Murphy R, Yurik T, et al: Atovaquone compared with dapsone for the prevention of *Pneumocystis carinii* pneumonia in patients with HIV infection who cannot tolerate trimethoprim, sulfonamides, or both. N Engl J Med 1998;339:1889–1895.
131. Mueller B, Pizzo P: Failure of intravenous pentamidine prophylaxis for *Pneumocystis carinii* pneumonia. J Pediatr 1993;121:163–164.
132. Mirochnick M, Cooper E, McIntosh K, et al: Pharmacokinetics of dapsone administered daily and weekly in human immunodeficiency virus-infected children. Antimicrob Agents Chemother 1999;43:2586–2591.
133. CDC: Guidelines of prophylaxis against *Pneumocystis carinii* pneumonia for children infected with human immunodeficiency virus. MMWR 1991;40(RR–2):1–13.
134. Group ECS: CD4 T cell count as predictor of *Pneumocystis carinii* pneumonia in children born to mothers infected with HIV. BMJ 1994;308:437–440.
135. Müller F, Groll A, Walsh T: Current approaches to diagnosis and treatment of fungal infections in children infected with human immunodeficiency virus. Eur J Pediatr 1999;158:187–199.
136. Chiou C, Groll A, Gonzalez C, et al: Esophageal candidiasis in pediatric acquired immunodeficiency syndrome: Clinical manifestations and risk factors. Pediatr Infect Dis J 2000;19:729–734.
137. Schuman P, Capps L, Peng G, et al: Weekly fluconazole for the prevention of mucosal candidiasis in women with HIV infection: A randomized, double-blind, placebo-controlled trial. Ann Intern Med 1997;126:689–696.
138. Abadi J, Nachman S, Kressel A, et al: Cryptococcosis in children with AIDS. Clin Infect Dis 1999;28:309–313.
139. Saag M, Graybill R, Larsen R, et al: Practice guidelines for the management of cryptococcal disease. Clin Infect Dis 2000;30:710–718.
140. Powderly W, Saag M, Cloud G, et al: A controlled trial of fluconazole or amphotericin B to prevent relapse of cryptococcal meningitis in the acquired immunodeficiency syndrome. N Engl J Med 1992;326:793–798.
141. Bozzette S, Larsen R, Chiu J, et al: A controlled trial of maintenance therapy with fluconazole after treatment of cryptococcal meningitis in the acquired immunodeficiency syndrome. N Engl J Med 1991;324:580.
142. Mayanja-Kizza H, Oishi K, Mitarai S, et al: Combination therapy with fluconazole and flucytosine for cryptococcal meningitis in Ugandan patients with AIDS. Clin Infect Dis 1998;26:1362–1366.
143. Larsen R, Bozzette S, Jones B, et al: Fluconazole combined wih flucytosine for treatment of cryptococcal meningitis in patients wih AIDS. Clin Infect Dis 1994;19:741–745.
144. Powderly W, Cloud G, Dismukes W, et al: Measurement of cryptococcal antigen in serum and cerebrospinal fluid: Value in the management of AIDS-associated cryptococcal meningitis. Clin Infect Dis 1994;18:789–792.
145. Aberg J, Watson J, Segal M, et al: Clinical utility of monitoring serum cryptococcal antigen (sCRAG) titers in patients with AIDS-related cryptococcal disease. HIV Clin Trials 2000;1:1–6.
146. Havlir DV, Dubé MP, McCutchan JA, et al: Prophylaxis with weekly versus daily fluconazole for fungal infections in patients with AIDS. Clin Infect Dis 1998;27:1369–1375.
147. McKinsey D, Wheat L, Cloud G, et al: Itraconazole prophylaxis for fungal infections in patients with advanced human immunodeficiency virus infection: Randomized, placebo-controlled, double-blind study. Clin Infect Dis 1999;28:1049–1056.
148. Saag M, Cloud G, Graybill J, et al: A comparison of intraconazole versus fluconazole as maintenance therapy for AIDS-associated cryptococcal meningitis. Clin Infect Dis 1998;28:291–296.
149. Wheat J: Endemic mycoses in AIDS: A clinical review. Clin Microbiol Rev 1995;8:146–159.
150. Sirisanthana T, Supparatpinyo K, Perriens J, et al: Amphotericin B and intraconazole for treatment of disseminated *Penicillium marneffei* infection in human immunodeficency virus-infected patients. Clin Infect Dis 1998;26:1107–1110.
151. Supparatpinyo K, Perriens J, Nelson K, et al: A controlled trial of itraconazole to prevent relapse of *Penicillium marneffei* infection in patients infected with the human immunodeficiency virus. N Engl J Med 1998;339:1739–1744.
152. Singh V, Smith D, Lawrence J, et al: Coccidioidomycosis in patients infected with human immunodeficiency virus: A review of 91 cases at a single institution. Clin Infect Dis 1996;23:563–568.
153. McNeil M, Ampel N: Opportunistic coccidioidomycosis in patients infected with human

immunodeficiency virus: Prevention issues and priorities. Clin Infect Dis 1995;21(Suppl 1):S111–S113.
154. McKinsey D, Spiegel R, Hutwagner L, et al: Prospective study of histoplasmosis in patients infected with human immunodeficiency virus: Incidence, risk factors, and pathophysiology. Clin Infect Dis 1999;24:1195–1203.
155. Galgiani J, Catanzaro A, Cloud G, et al: Comparison of oral fluconazole and itraconazole for progressive, nonmeningeal coccidioidomycosis: A randomized, double-blind trial. Ann Intern Med 2000;133:676–686.
156. Wheat L: Laboratory diagnosis of histoplasmosis. Semin Respir Infect 2001;16:131–140.
157. Wheat L, Cloud G, Johnson P, et al: Clearance of fungal burder during treatment of disseminated histoplasmosis with liposomal amphotericin B versus itraconazole. Antimicrob Agents Chemother 2001;45:2354–2357.
158. Sirisanthana T, Supparatpinyo K: Epidemiology and management of pencilliosis in human immunodeficiency virus-infected patients. Int J Infect Dis 1998;3:48–53.
159. Chariyalertsak S, Supparatpinyo K, Sirisanthana T, et al: A controlled trial of itraconazole as primary prophylaxis for systemic fungal infections in patients with advanced human immunodeficiency virus infection in Thailand. Clin Infect Dis 2002;34:277–284.
160. Khoo S, Denning D: Invasive aspergillosis in patients with AIDS. Clin Infect Dis 1994;19(Suppl 1):S41–S48.
161. Chin D, Hopewell P, Yajko D, et al: *Mycobacterium avium* complex in the respiratory or gastrointestinal tract and the risk of *M. avium* complex bacteremia in patients with human immunodeficiency virus infection. J Infect Dis 1994;169:289–295.
162. Horsburgh C Jr: *Mycobacterium avium* complex infection in the acquired immunodeficiency syndrome. N Engl J Med 1991;324:1332–1338.
163. Rutstein R, Cobb P, McGowan K, et al: *Mycobacterium avium intracellulare* complex infection in HIV-infected children. AIDS 1993;7:507–512.
164. Chin D, Reingold A, Stone E, et al: The impact of *Mycobacterium avium* complex bacteremia and its treatment on survival of AIDS patients: A prospective study. J Infect Dis 1994;170:578–584.
165. Horsburgh C, Metchock B, Gordon S, et al: Predictors of survival in patients with AIDS and disseminated *Mycobacterium avium* complex disease. J Infect Dis 1994;170:573–577.
166. Hafner R, Inderlied C, Peterson D, et al: Correlation of quantitative bone marrow and blood cultures in AIDS patients with disseminated *Mycobacterium avium* complex infection. J Infect Dis 1999;180:438–447.
167. Masur H: Recommendations on prophylaxis and therapy for disseminated *Mycobacterium avium* complex disease in patients infected with the human immunodeficiency virus. N Engl J Med 1993;329:898–904.
168. Chaisson R, Keiser P, Pierce M, et al: Clarithromycin and ethambutol with or without clofazimine for the treatment of bacteremic *Mycobacterium avium* complex disease in patients with HIV infection. AIDS 1997;11:311–317.
169. Ward T, Rimland D, Kauffman C, et al: Randomized, open-label trial of azithromycin plus ethambutol vs. clarithromycin plus ethambutol as therapy for *Mycobacterium avium* complex bacteremia in patients with human immunodeficiency virus infection. Clin Infect Dis 1998;27:1278–1285.
170. Gordin F, Sullam P, Shafran S, et al: A randomized, placebo-controlled study of rifabutin added to a regimen of clarithromycin and ethambutol for treatment of disseminated infection with *Mycobacterium avium* complex. Clin Infect Dis 1999;28:1080–1085.
171. Pierce M, Crampton S, Henry D, et al: A randomized trial of clarithromycin as prophylaxis against disseminated *Mycobacterium avium* complex infections in patients with advanced acquired immunodeficiency syndrome. N Engl J Med 1996;335: 384–391.
172. Benson C, Williams P, Cohn D, et al: Clarithromycin or rifabutin alone or in combination for primary prophylaxis of *Mycobacterium avium* complex disease in patients with AIDS: A randomized, double-blinded, placebo-controlled trial. J Infect Dis 2000;181:1289–1297.
173. Schaaf H, Geldenduys A, Gie R, et al: Culture-positive tuberculosis in human immunodeficiency virus type 1-infected children. Pediatr Infect Dis J 1998;17:599–604.
174. Dhurat R, Manglani M, Sharma R, et al: Clinical spectrum of HIV infection. Ind Pediatr 2000;37:831–836.
175. Coovadia H, Jeena P, Wilkinson D: Childhood human immunodeficiency virus and tuberculosis co-infections: Reconciling conflicting data. Int J Tuberc Lung Dis 1998;2:844–851.
176. Jeena PM, Mitha T, Bamber S, et al: Effects of the human immunodeficiency virus on tuberculosis in children. Tuber Lung Dis 1996;77:437–443.
177. Kiwanuka J, Graham S, Coulter J, et al: Diagnosis of pulmonary tuberculosis in children in an HIV-endemic area, Malawi. Ann Trop Paediatr 2001;21: 5–14.
178. Huebner R, Castro K: The changing face of tuberculosis. Annu Rev Med 1995;46:47–55.
179. Havlir D, Barnes P: Tuberculosis in patients with human immunodeficiency virus infection. N Engl J Med 1999;340:367–373.
180. Centers for Disease Control and Prevention: Prevention and treatment of tuberculosis among patients infected with human immunodeficiency virus: Principles of therapy and revised recommendations. MMWR 1998;47(RR–20):1–58.
181. Centers for Disease Control and Prevention: Updated guidelines of the use of rifabutin or rifampin for the treatment and prevention of tuberculosis among

HIV-infected patients taking protease inhibitors or non-nucleoside reverse transcriptase inhibitors. MMWR 2000;49:185–189.
182. O'Brien K, Ruff A, Louis M, et al: Bacillus Calmette-Guérin complications in children born to HIV-1–infected women with a review of the literature. Pediatrics 1995;95:414–418.
183. Wilkinson D, Squire S, Garner P: Effect of preventive treatment for tuberculosis in adults infected with HIV: Systematic review of randomised placebo controlled trials. BMJ 1998;317:625–629.
184. Bucher H, Griffith L, Guyatt G, et al: Isoniazid prophylaxis for tuberculosis in HIV infection: A meta-analysis of randomized controlled trials. AIDS 1999;13:501–507.
185. Gordin F, Matts J, Miller C, et al: A controlled trial of isoniazid in persons with anergy and human immunodeficiency virus infection who are at high risk for tuberculosis. N Engl J Med 1997;337:315–320.
186. Du L, Coats D, Kline M, et al: Incidence of presumed cytomegalovirus retinitis in HIV-infected pediatric patients. J AAPOS Am Assoc Pediatr Opthalmol Strabismus 1999;3:245–249.
187. Spector S: Detection and quantification of human cytomegalovirus (CMV) as a marker for the development of CMV disease and survival in patients with AIDS. Antiviral Ther 1997;2:200–205.
188. Spector S, Wong R, Hsia K, et al: Plasma cytomegalovirus (CMV) DNA load predicts CMV disease and survival in AIDS patients. J Clin Invest 1998;101:497–502.
189. Boriskin Y, Sharland M, Dalton R, et al: Viral loads in dual infection with HIV-1 and cytomegalovirus. Arch Dis Child 1999;80:132–136.
190. Kovacs A, Schluchter M, Easly K, et al: Cytomegalovirus infection and HIV-1 disease progression in infants born to HIV-1 infected women. N Engl J Med 1999;341:77–84.
191. Mussi-Pinhata M, Yamamoto A, Figueiredo L, et al: Congenital and perinatal cytomegalovirus infection in infants born to mothers infected with human immunodeficiency virus. J Pediatr 1998;132:285–290.
192. Mentzer D, Kreuz W: CMV coinfection and disease progression in vertically acquired HIV infection. Arch Dis Child 1999;81:189.
193. Whitley R, Jacobson M, Friedberg D, et al: Guidelines for the treatment of cytomegalovirus diseases in patients with AIDS in the era of potent antiretroviral therapy. Arch Intern Med 1998;158:957–969.
194. Frenkel L, Capparelli E, Dankner W, et al: Oral ganciclovir in children: Pharmacokinetics, safety, tolerance and antiviral effects. J Infect Dis 2000;182:1616–1624.
195. Curran M, Noble S: Valganciclovir. Drugs 2001;61:1145–1150.
196. Jabs D, Enger C, Dunn J, et al: Cytomegalovirus retinitis and viral resistance: Ganciclovir resistance. J Infect Dis 1998;177:770–773.
197. Spector S, McKinley G, Lalezari J, et al: Oral ganciclovir for the prevention of cytomegalovirus disease in persons with AIDS. N Engl J Med 1996;334:1491–1497.
198. Paltiel A, Goldie S, Losina E, et al: Preevaluation of clinical trial data: The case of preemptive cytomegalovirus therapy in patients with human immunodeficiency virus. Clin Infect Dis 2001;32:783–793.
199. Derryck A, LaRussa P, Steinberg S, et al: Varicella and zoster in children with human immunodeficiency virus infection. Pediatr Infect Dis J 1998;17:931–933.
200. Rongkavilit C, Mitchell C, Nachman S: Varicella zoster infection in HIV-infected children. Paediatric Drugs 2000;2:291–297.
201. Centers for Disease Control and Prevention: Prevention of varicella-updated recommendations of the Advisory Committee on Immunizations Practices (ACIP). MMWR 1999;48(RR–6):1–5.
202. Levin M, Gershon A, Weinberg A, et al: Immunization of HIV-infected children with varicella vaccine. J Pediatr 2001;139:305–310.
203. Gnann J, Pellett P, Jaffe H: Human herpesvirus 8 and Kaposi's sarcoma in persons infected with human immunodeficiency virus. Clin Infect Dis 2000;30(Suppl 1):S72–S76.
204. Sitas F, Newton R, Boshoff C: Increasing probability of mother to child transmission of HHV-8 with increasing maternal antibody titer for HHV-8. N Engl J Med 1999;340:1923.
205. Plancoulaine S, Abel L, van Beveren M, et al: Human herpesvirus 8 transmission from mother to child and between siblings in an endemic population. Lancet 2000;356:1062–1065.
206. He J, Bhat G, Kankasa C, et al: Seroprevalence of human herpesvirus 8 among Zambian women of childbearing age without Kaposi's sarcoma (KS) and mother-child bears with KS. J Infect Dis 1998;178:787–790.
207. De Luca A, Giancola M, Cingolani A, et al: Clinical and virological monitoring during treatment with intrathecal cytarabine in patients with AIDS-associated progressive multifocal leukoencephalopathy. Clin Infect Dis 1999;28:624–628.
208. Bogdanovic G, Priftakis P, Hammarin A, et al: Detection of JC virus in cerebrospinal fluid (CSF) samples from patients with progressive multifocal leukoencephalopathy but not in CSF samples from patients with herpes simplex encephalitis, enteroviral meningitis or multiple sclerosis. J Clin Microbiol 1998;36:1137–1138.
209. Berenguer J, Miralles P, Arrizabalaga J, et al: Clinical course and prognostic factors of AIDS-associated progressive multifocal leukoencephalopathy (PML) in patients treated with HAART (GESIDA 11/99). Paper presented at the Eight Conference on Retroviruses and Opportunistic Infections, Chicago, Ill, February, 2001.
210. Dodig M, Tavill A: Hepatitis C and human immunodeficiency virus coinfections. J Clin Gastroenterol 2001;33:367–374.

211. Indilman R, Colantoni A, De Maria N, et al: Effect of human immunodeficiency virus on the outcome of hepatitis C virus infection. Scand J Gastroenterol 2001;36:225–234.
212. Staples C, Rimland D, Dudas D: Hepatitis C in the HIV (human immunodeficiency virus) Atlanta V.A. (Veterans Affairs Medical Center) Cohort Study (HAVACS): The effect of coinfection on survival. Clin Infect Dis 1999;29:150–154.
213. Nigro G, D'Orio F, Catania S, et al: Mother to infant transmission of coinfection by human immunodeficiency virus and hepatitis C virus: Prevalence and clinical manifestations. Arch Virol 1997;142:453–457.
214. Papaevangelou C, Pollack H, Rochford G, et al: Increased transmission of vertical hepatitis C virus (HCV) infection to human immunodeficiency virus (HIV)-infected infants of HIV- and HCV-coinfected women. J Infect Dis 1998;178:1047–1052.
215. Resti M: Mother-to-infant transmission of hepatitis C virus. Ital J Gastroenterol Hepatol 1999;31:489–493.
216. Thomas S, Newell M, Peckham C, et al: A review of hepatitis C vertical transmission: Risks of transmission to infants born to mothers with and without HCV viraemia or human immunodeficiency virus infection. Int J Epidermiol 1998;27:108–117.
217. Mast E, Alter M: Hepatitis C. Semin Pediatr Infect Dis 1997;8:17–22.
218. Belanger F, Derouin F, Grangeot-Keros L, et al: Incidence and risk factors of toxoplasmosis in a cohort of human immunodeficiency virus-infected patients: 1988–1995. Clin Infect Dis 1999;28:575–581.
219. European Collaborative Study and Research Network on Congenital Toxoplasmosis: Low incidence of congenital toxoplasmosis in children born to women infected with human immunodeficiency virus. Eur J Obstet Gynecol Reprod Biol 1996;68:93–96.
220. Dunn D, Newell M, Gilbert R: Low risk of congenital toxoplasmosis in children born to women infected with human immunodeficiency virus. Pediatr Infect Dis J 1997;16:84.
221. Manabe Y, Clark D, Moore R, et al: Cryptosporidiosis in patients with AIDS: Correlates of disease and survival. Clin Infect Dis 1998;27:536–542.
222. Moore R, Chaisson R: Natural history of opportunistic disease in an HIV-infected urban clinical cohort. Ann Intern Med 1996;124:633–642.
223. Dascomb K, Clark R, Aberg J, et al: Natural history of intestinal microsporidiosis among patients Infected with human immunodeficiency virus. J Clin Microbiol 1999;37:3421–3422.
224. Johnson S, Hendson W, Crewe-Brown H, et al: Effect of human immunodeficiency virus infection on episodes of diarrhea among children in South Africa. Pediatr Infect Dis J 2000;19:972–979.
225. Amadi B, Kelly P, Mwiya M, et al: Intestinal and systemic infection, HIV, and mortality in Zambian children with persistent diarrhea and malnutrition. J Pediatr Gastroenterol Nutr 2001;32: 550–554.
226. Liguory O, David F, Sarfati C, et al: Diagnosis of infections caused by *Enterocytozoon bieneusi* and *Encephalitozoon intestinalis* using polymerase chain reaction in stool specimens. AIDS 1997;11:723–726.
227. Hicks P, Zweiner R, Squires J, et al: Azithromycin therapy for *Cryptosporidium parvum* infection in four children infected with human immunodeficiency virus. J Pediatr 1996;129:297–300.
228. Griffiths J: Human cryptosporidiosis: Epidemiology, transmission, clinical disease, treatment, and diagnosis. Adv Parasitol 1998;40:37–85.
229. Molina J, Chastang C, Goguel J, et al: Albendazole for treatment and prophylaxis of microsporidiosis due to *Encephalitozoon intestinalis* in patients with AIDS: A randomized double-blind controlled trial. J Infect Dis 1998;177:1373–1377.
230. Fichtenbaum C, Zackin R, Feinberg J, et al: Rifabutin but not clarithromycin prevents cryptosporidiosis in persons with advanced HIV infection. AIDS 2000;14:2889–2893.
231. Kartalija M, Sande M: Diarrhea and AIDS in the era of highly active antiretroviral therapy. Clin Infect Dis 1999;28:701–707.
232. Karp C, Neva F: Tropical infectious diseases in human immunodeficiency virus-infected patients. Clin Infect Dis 1999;28:947–963.
233. Greenberg A, Nsa W, Ryder R, et al: *Plasmodium falciparum* malaria and perinatally acquired human immunodeficiency virus type 1 infection in Kinshasa, Zaire. N Engl J Med 1991;325:105–109.
234. Pintado V, Martin-Rabadan P, Rivera M, et al: Visceral leishmaniasis in human immunodeficiency virus (HIV)-infected and non-HIV-infected patients: A comparative study. Medicine 2001;80:54–73.
235. Jabs D, Bolton S, Dunn J, et al: Discontinuing anticytomegalovirus therapy in patients with immune reconstitution after combination antiretroviral therapy. Ann J Ophthalmol 1998;126:817–822.
236. Jouan M, Saves H, Tubiana R, et al: Discontinuation of maintenance therapy for cytomegalovirus retinitis in HIV infected patients receiving highly active antiretroviral therapy. AIDS 2001;15:23–31.
237. Nwokolo N, Fisher M, Gazzard B, et al: Cessation of secondary prophylaxis in patients with cryptococcosis. AIDS 2001;15:1438–1439.
238. Aberg J, Price R, Heeren D, et al: Discontinuation of antifungal therapy for cryptococcosis after immunologic response to antiretroviral therapy (Abstract 250). Paper presented at the Seventh Conference on Retroviruses and Opportunistic Infections, San Francisco, Calif, January 30–February 2, 2000.
239. Mussini C, Cossarizza A, Pezzotti P, et al: Discontinuation or continuation of maintenance therapy for cryptococcal meningitis in patients with AIDS treated with HAART (Abstract 546). Paper presented at the Eighth Conference on Retroviruses

and Opportunistic Infections, Chicago, Ill, February, 2001.
240. Foudraine N, Weverling G, van Gool T, et al: Improvement of chronic diarrhoea in patients with advanced HIV-1 infection during potent antiretroviral therapy. AIDS 1998;12:35–41.
241. Ledergerber B, Mocroft A, Reiss P, et al: Discontinuation of secondary prophylaxis against *Pneumocystis carinii* pneumonia in patients with HIV infection who have a response to antiretroviral therapy. N Engl J Med 2001;344:168–174.
242. Lopez J, Miro J, Pena J, et al: A randomized trial of the discontinuation of primary and secondary prophylaxis against *Pneumocystis carinii* pneumonia after HAART in patients with HIV infection. N Engl J Med 2001;344:159–167.
243. El-Sadr W, Burman W, Grant L, et al: Discontinuation of prophylaxis against *Mycobacterium avium* complex disease in HIV-infected patients who have a response to antiretroviral therapy. N Engl J Med 2000;342:1085–1087.
244. Currier J, Williams P, Koletar S, et al: Discontinuation of *Mycobacterium avium* complex prophylaxis in patients with antiretroviral therapy-induced increases in CD4+ cell count. A randomized, double-blind, placebo-controlled trial. Ann Intern Med 2000;133:493–503.
245. Furrer H, Oparavil M, Bernasconi E, et al: Stopping primary prophylaxis in HIV-1 infected patients at high risk of toxoplasma encephalitis. Lancet 2000; 355:2217–2218.
246. Furrer H, Rossi M, Telenti A, et al: Discontinuing or withholding primary prophylaxis against *Mycobacterium avium* in patients on successful antiretroviral combination therapy. AIDS 2000;14: 1409–1412.
247. Michelet C, Arvieux C, Francois C, et al: Opportunistic infections occurring during highly active antiretroviral treatment. AIDS 1998;12:1815–1822.
248. Rodriguez-Rosado R, Soriano V, Cona C, et al: Opportunistic infections shortly after beginning highly active antiretroviral therapy. Antiviral Therapy 1998;3:229–231.
249. Ledergerber B, Egger M, Erard V, et al: AIDS-related opportunistic illnesses occurring after initiation of potent antiretroviral therapy: The Swiss HIV Cohort Study. JAMA 1999;23:2220–2226.
250. DeSimone J, Pomerantz R, Babinchak T: Inflammatory reactions in HIV-1–infected persons after initiation of highly active antiretroviral therapy. Ann Intern Med 2000;133:447–454.
251. Foudraine N, Hovenkamp E, Notermans D, et al: Immunopathology as a result of highly active antiretroviral therapy in HIV-1–infected patients. AIDS 1999;13:177–184.
252. Narita M, Ashkin D, Hollender E, et al: Paradoxical worsening of tuberculosis following antiretroviral therapy in patients with AIDS. Am J Respir Crit Care Med 1998;158:157–161.
253. Karavellas M, Plummer D, Macdonald J, et al: Incidence of immune recovery vitritis in cytomegalovirus retinitis patients following institution of successful highly active antiretroviral therapy. J Infect Dis 1999;179:697–700.
254. Miralles P, Berenguer J, Lacruz C, et al: Inflammatory reactions in progressive multifocal leukoencephalopathy after highly active antiretroviral therapy. AIDS 2001;15:1900–1902.
255. Torriani F, Freeman W, MacDonald J, et al: CMV retinitis recurs after stopping treatment in virological and immunological failures of potent antiretroviral therapy. AIDS 2000;14:173–180.
256. Cinti S, Kaul D, Sax P, et al: Recurrence of *Mycobacterium avium* infection in patients receiving highly active antiretroviral therapy and antimycobacterial agents. Clin Infect Dis 2000;30: 511–514.

Respiratory Compromise in Children Infected with HIV

Meyer Kattan

HISTORICAL PERSPECTIVE

At the onset of the AIDS epidemic almost two decades ago, children were identified in the first few years of life when they presented with advanced symptoms of the disease. The presenting symptoms of the illness were most commonly pulmonary in origin. Opportunistic pulmonary infections, particularly *Pneumocystis carinii* pneumonia (PCP) became markers of the infection.[1] Acute pulmonary infections were a major cause of morbidity and mortality throughout the world.[2] Lymphocytic interstitial pneumonia (LIP) was a common pulmonary diagnosis in those children with subacute disease.[3] LIP was believed to be so characteristic of HIV infection that chronic reticulonodular radiographic findings in children younger than 13 years of age became one of the specifically identified conditions in the Centers for Disease Control and Prevention (CDC) classification.[4]

The identification of HIV infection within the first few months of life, even in asymptomatic infants, resulted in earlier diagnosis, prophylaxis, and treatment of pulmonary infections and improved survival. Subsequently, the use of intensive antiretroviral therapy in infected infants has lowered the rates of acute pulmonary disease. Children with HIV infection now live longer and chronic pulmonary conditions are more evident, but the nature, incidence, and prognosis of these conditions need to be more precisely determined.

The emerging countries in Africa and Asia have the majority of HIV-infected patients worldwide.[5] In these areas, early identification and treatment of HIV infection and its complications is not standard, and the pulmonary manifestations of HIV infection are a problem of epidemic proportions. What may be a historical description of the pulmonary manifestations in parts of North America and Western Europe is a tragic reality in other regions of the world.

EFFECTS OF HIV IN THE LUNG

The profound immunologic alterations caused by HIV result in a spectrum of infectious and noninfectious lung diseases. In the lung, as in peripheral blood, HIV infects pulmonary lymphocytes, and infection can be identified in lymphocytes obtained from bronchoalveolar lavage fluid.[6] The virus decreases numbers of lung CD4+ cells as it does in all tissues. It also causes infiltration of CD8+ cells in the interstitial and alveolar spaces. This is mediated by cytokines, including interleukin-15, from alveolar macrophages that induce T cell proliferation and stimulate T cell migration.[7] Alveolar macrophages obtained by bronchoalveolar lavage can also be infected with HIV.[8] Although some components of macrophage defense are preserved during HIV infection, lack of activation signals from T lymphocytes impairs effective defense by macrophages. The T lymphocytes from HIV-infected individuals do not produce interferon-γ normally in response to antigens, which is necessary for macrophage activation. The inability to elaborate this predicts progression of disease.[9]

HIV is also associated with alterations in humoral (B cell) immunity, despite elevated immunoglobulin levels.[10] There is an impaired ability of HIV-infected T cells to activate B cells.[11] This results in increased susceptibility to bacterial pneumonia in HIV-infected persons.

Infants who are infected by vertical transmission have no recognizable pulmonary disease at birth attributable to the infection.[12] The incidence of respiratory distress syndrome and bronchopulmonary dysplasia is similar in infected and uninfected children born to HIV-infected mothers.[13] A pulmonary problem has been the first manifestation of HIV infection in more than half of the cases.[14,15] Between 1981 and 1993, of 1261 pediatric AIDS cases reported in New York City, pulmonary problems were the diseases most frequently diagnosed.[14]

With the successful prevention of mother-to-infant transmission because of antiretroviral regimens, there is a growth population of uninfected infants born to HIV-infected mothers. Prospective studies indicate that the uninfected children born to HIV-infected mothers are not more susceptible to pulmonary disease than those born to uninfected mothers.[16,17] In areas where there is a high rate of pneumonia, the rates and types of pneumonia are similar in uninfected children born to infected and uninfected mothers.[17]

PNEUMONIA

Respiratory infections are predominant causes of morbidity and mortality in HIV-infected children younger than 12 years of age.[18,19] In a prospective cohort followed from birth in the United States, the rate of lower respiratory tract infections in HIV-infected children in the first year of life was approximately 2.8 times greater than the rate in uninfected children born to HIV-infected mothers.[16] In a prospective study from Rwanda, the risk of developing severe pneumonia among infected children was three times greater than among uninfected children.[17] The highest incidence of pneumonia occurs in the first 12 months of life. The incidence rate for pneumonia (excluding PCP) is between 20 and 25 per 100 child-years during the first 12 months.[16,20] In a prospective cohort enrolled at a mean age of 40 months, 25% of the children developed an acute pneumonia over 3 years, and multiple episodes occurred in 34% of children.[20]

In one report, risk factors for the development of acute pneumonia were a prior history of an AIDS-defining recurrent bacterial infection and a lower CD4+ count.[20] In a subgroup of these patients, higher levels of baseline HIV-1 RNA titers (especially when RNA was greater than 1,000,000 copies/mL) were associated with a higher rate of acute pneumonia. In children younger than 12 months of age, a low CD4+ cell count in the infant and low maternal CD4+ cell count but not viral load appear to be risk factors for pneumonia.[16] The rate of decline of CD4+ cells during the first year of life is also associated with development of lower respiratory tract infections (Table 11–1).

The origin of the pulmonary infections is varied. Bacterial pneumonias with both gram-negative and gram-positive organisms and viral pneumonias occur more frequently in HIV-infected children. Mixed infections with multiple bacterial isolates or bacterial and viral isolates are sometimes found. In many cases, no organisms are isolated. This is, in part, a result of the difficulty in obtaining diagnostic specimens in children. The incidence of PCP has declined with highly active antiretroviral therapy, but the effect of antiretroviral therapy on the rates of bacterial and viral pneumonia is not known.[21] The rates of PCP and tuberculosis remain high in regions with poor medical infrastructure and limited availability of drugs.

Bacterial Pneumonia

Bacterial and viral pneumonia occur more frequently in HIV-infected children. The bacterial

Table 11–1
Mean Rate of Decline of CD4+ Lymphocyte Count in First Year of Life Prior to Developing LRI or PCP

PATIENT STATUS	CELLS/MM³/MO
HIV-uninfected	55 ± 9
HIV-infected No LRI	134 ± 20
HIV-infected With LRI	266 ± 61
HIV-infected With PCP	375 ± 112

LRI, lower respiratory tract infection; PCP, *Pneumocystis carinii* pneumonia.
Data from Kattan M, Platzker A, Mellins RB, et al: Respiratory diseases in the first year of life in children born to HIV-1 infected women. Pediatr Pulmonol 2001;31:267–276.

isolates reported in Western countries and Africa are remarkably similar.[22,23] *Streptococcus pneumoniae* and *Staphylococcus aureus* are the most commonly documented gram-positive organisms. Using postmortem percutaneous lung aspirates from children in Zimbabwe, Ikeogu[23] found *Klebsiella* and *Pseudomonas* species to be the most common gram-negative organisms. *Bordetella pertussis* has been recovered in children with respiratory distress and cough.[24]

Isolation of bacterial organisms in cases of pneumonia is problematic in young children because invasive procedures are often required. Children often do not have a productive cough, and induced sputum for bacterial pneumonia is not reliable. A positive blood culture finding with a new radiographic infiltrate may establish the cause of pneumonia. An organism other than common oral flora accompanied by neutrophils obtained from bronchial lavage fluid strongly suggests a bacterial cause of pneumonia.

Intravenous immunoglobulin (IVIG) may be effective in reducing some bacterial infections in patients with symptomatic HIV infection and peripheral CD4+ cell counts of 200/mm^3 or greater. Data from the National Institute of Child Health and Human Development IVIG Clinical Trial, which was performed in an era with no antiretroviral therapy and limited PCP prophylaxis, indicated that IVIG was associated with a 48% reduction in the rate of acute laboratory-proven bacterial or clinically diagnosed pneumonia episodes per 100 patient-years in patients with CD4+ cell counts of 200/mm^3 or higher.[25] The AIDS Clinical Trials Group Protocol 051 reported that the beneficial effect of IVIG was limited to those children not receiving trimethoprim-sulfamethoxazole (TMP-SMX) prophylaxis.[26] IVIG is currently recommended in HIV-infected children in combination with antiretroviral agents only for hypogammaglobulinemia (IgG <250 mg/dL), in children with two or more serious bacterial infections, and in children who fail to form antibodies to common antigens.[27]

Pneumococcal vaccination is indicated for children 2 months and older with asymptomatic or symptomatic HIV infection in view of the high incidence of invasive pneumococcal infection.[27] Reimmunization after 3 to 5 years is recommended. HIV-infected children should be immunized with *Haemophilus influenzae* type b vaccine according to the routine childhood immunization schedule.

Tuberculosis

Tuberculosis remains a major public health problem throughout the world. An increase in the incidence of tuberculosis has paralleled the AIDS epidemic, and the two diseases are strongly related.[28] In one report from Zambia, the HIV seroprevalence rate in children with tuberculosis disease was 55.8%, compared with 9.6% in a control population.[29] Birth cohorts of perinatally HIV-infected infants and children followed prospectively in the United States have found only a small number of cases of tuberculosis, but there are reports of tuberculosis and HIV infection in the United States.[30,31] Because of the association of tuberculosis and HIV infection, children with tuberculosis disease should be tested for HIV disease.[27]

It is not clear whether HIV infection increases susceptibility to tuberculosis. Children with HIV infection are more likely to be in contact with HIV-infected adults with tuberculosis and therefore are increasingly susceptible to tuberculous infection and disease. Control of tuberculosis in children with HIV infection rests predominantly with adequate public health measures to control tuberculosis in the community by contact and source tracing and ensuring adherence to medication regimens.

Fever, cough, lobar pneumonia, and lymphadenopathy may indicate infection with *Mycobacterium tuberculosis*. Pulmonary tuberculosis is the predominant clinical manifestation, although extrapulmonary disease can occur.[31]

Annual screening of HIV-infected children for tuberculosis infection or disease is recommended with the Mantoux tuberculin skin test. A reaction greater than 5 mm is considered to be positive.[32] Many children with HIV infection have negative skin test reactions to control antigens; therefore, a negative tuberculin skin test finding may not rule out infection. If there is a high index of suspicion for pulmonary tuberculosis (e.g., contact with a person with tuberculosis) in an HIV-infected child with a pulmonary infiltrate who is anergic, attempts to isolate the organism may be warranted to rule out *M. tuberculosis* infection.

Bacteriologic confirmation of pulmonary tuberculosis in infants and children remains difficult. Examination of expectorated sputum is the initial test performed to diagnose tuberculosis in the older child with a productive cough. In the younger child, gastric lavage is a common procedure to obtain specimens for staining and culture. The organism can be isolated from bronchial lavage fluid or from lung tissue obtained from biopsy. Some studies suggest that the yield for *M. tuberculosis* is higher with gastric lavage compared with bronchoalveolar lavage.[33,34] Sputum induction for isolation of the organism has been reported to be successful in infants and children with HIV infection.[35] In that study, induced sputum had a better yield for pulmonary tuberculosis than gastric lavage.

A study in HIV-infected adults has demonstrated the efficacy of a 1-year course of isoniazid prophylaxis in decreasing the frequency of active tuberculosis in symptom-free HIV-seropositive adults with a positive tuberculin skin test.[36] There are limited data on the efficacy of prophylaxis for *M. tuberculosis* in the context of HIV infection. Preventive therapy for HIV-infected children with a positive tuberculin skin test result but no evidence of active disease is 9 months of isoniazid. In patients for whom the source case is likely to have an isoniazid-resistant strain, rifampin should be used. If the child is anergic but has a history of exposure, isoniazid should be given. If the contact is known to have a multidrug-resistant strain, the child should be treated with two drugs to which the strain is susceptible.[37]

Recommended treatment of pulmonary infections in children with a sensitive strain is isoniazid, rifampin, and pyrazinamide for 2 months followed by isoniazid and rifampin for a total of 12 months of therapy. In areas where there is a high prevalence of multidrug-resistant strains, infection should be treated with four drugs if the susceptibility pattern is unknown: isoniazid, rifampin, pyrazinamide, and ethambutol for 2 months followed by isoniazid and rifampin if the patient has responded well to the initial treatment. Streptomycin, cycloserine, or ethionamide may be substituted for ethambutol. If the isolate is known to be isoniazid and rifampin resistant, two or three drugs to which the organism is sensitive should be given for 18 to 24 months after culture conversion. Some second-line drugs may be necessary, such as clarithromycin, azithromycin, and ciprofloxacin. Daily or twice-weekly regimens are acceptable. Directly observed therapy should be used whenever possible to ensure administration of the medication. Contact-tracing is an essential part of the management.

The rate of mortality with this disease is high, either from the tuberculosis infection itself or by acceleration of the natural history of HIV disease. In a comparison of children with tuberculosis with and without HIV infection, those with coinfection had a poorer clinical and radiologic response to treatment at 6 months. The mortality rate was higher in the HIV-infected group (6 of 40 HIV-infected versus 0 of 40 uninfected).[38]

In the United States and other areas of low tuberculosis prevalence, bacillus Calmette-Guérin vaccine is not recommended.[27] However, in areas where the prevalence is high, the World Health Organization recommends that bacillus Calmette-Guérin be given to all infants at birth if they are asymptomatic.

Mycobacterium avium complex

Mycobacterium avium complex (MAC) causes disease predominantly in immunocompromised patients. The organism can be found in the blood, lung tissue, liver, and bone marrow. In HIV-infected patients, respiratory symptoms are not a prominent feature, and the clinical manifestations are usually due to extrapulmonary disease. In one series of 196 children with HIV infection, of 22 children with MAC, none had respiratory symptoms.[39] The significance of the organism in the bronchial secretions is unclear but most likely reflects disseminated disease rather than pulmonary infection. Disseminated disease has been reported in 8% to 11% of cases of HIV-infected children.[14,39]

Symptoms are often nonspecific, with intermittent fever, weight loss, night sweats, cachexia, and diarrhea. Children with MAC are older and have lower CD4+ cell counts without MAC. Patients with disseminated MAC have a poor prognosis.[40] In one report, of children who died, 42% had disseminated MAC and in 24% it was the underlying cause of death.[41]

With any regimen, a minimum of two agents is recommended to minimize the risk of proliferation of resistant strains. Recommendations for prophylaxis and therapy for disseminated MAC disease in patients with HIV infection have been published.[37,42] Every treatment regimen should include either azithromycin or clarithromycin. Ethambutol is recommended as a second drug. The addition of a third or fourth drug from one of the following is suggested: clofazimine, rifabutin, rifampin, ciprofloxacin, and amikacin. Prophylaxis with clarithromycin or azithromycin to prevent a first episode is recommended for children aged 6 years and older with CD4+ cell counts less than 50/µL, 2 to 6 years with CD4+ cell counts less than 75/µL, and 1 to 2 years with CD4+ counts less than 500/µL.

Viral Pneumonia

Viral pneumonia with common pathogens, such as respiratory syncytial virus, parainfluenza, herpes simplex virus, and adenovirus occurs in HIV-infected children.[2,43] Prolonged duration of respiratory syncytial virus antigen shedding for up to 90 days has been observed in HIV-infected children.[44] Concomitant bacterial or opportunistic infection must be ruled out in those patients with persistent symptoms or clinical deterioration with respiratory syncytial virus. In a report from Côte d'Ivoire, Africa, measles giant cell pneumonia was more common in children older than 15 months who were HIV positive than in children who were HIV negative.[19]

Cytomegalovirus is a herpesvirus that can cause retinitis, encephalitis, and colitis in HIV-infected patients. Its role in causing pneumonitis is less clear. Cytomegalovirus pneumonia was found in 7% of HIV-seropositive infants from Zimbabwe on autopsy.[23] The virus has been isolated in bronchial lavage fluid in 35% to 78% of HIV-infected adults with respiratory illness and has also been found in bronchial lavage fluid in children.[45,46] However, isolation of cytomegalovirus from lavage fluid sometimes occurs without tissue evidence of cytomegalovirus pneumonia. Confirmation of pneumonia requires lung tissue. Histologically, alveolar macrophages, type II pneumocytes, bronchial and bronchiolar epithelial cells, and capillary endothelial cells may manifest cytomegaly and nuclear and cytoplasmic inclusions. The degree of interstitial pneumonitis varies because of the presence of concomitant infections. Cytomegalovirus is often found with other pathogens in the lung. The presence or absence of cytomegalovirus with PCP made no difference in the short-term outcome or long-term survival in adults and children.[47,48] Ganciclovir is the most effective drug in the treatment of cytomegalovirus infection.

When feasible, prevention of viral infection is warranted. Yearly influenza vaccine should be considered for children 6 months of age or older. HIV-infected children mount antibody responses to influenza vaccinations, but the titers are lower than in HIV-negative control subjects.[49] Routine immunization with measles vaccine is recommended.

FUNGAL INFECTION

Opportunistic fungal infections can cause severe pulmonary disease in children with HIV infection, but the number of reported cases is small. The most common infections are with *Cryptococcus neoformans*, *Histoplasma capsulatum*, and *Coccidioides immitis*. Dissemination of infection is common and treatment is difficult. Constitutional symptoms such as weight loss and fever may reflect extrapulmonary involvement.

Cryptococcus infection usually manifests as meningitis but can involve the lungs, causing an interstitial pneumonia.[50] *Histoplasma capsulatum* most commonly affects the lungs but is likely to become disseminated in HIV-infected patients.[51] Standard serologic tests can be positive for both coccidioidomycosis and histoplasmosis, but false-negative test results occur in the most profoundly immunocompromised patients.[52] Skin testing is not useful because of problems with anergy and lack of standardization of most fungal skin test preparations. Cultures of bone marrow, cerebrospinal fluid, and lymph node or lung biopsy can make the diagnosis.

Candida species are often found in the oropharynx and esophagus in HIV-infected children. Isolation of *Candida* from bronchoalveolar lavage fluid most likely represents an oropharyngeal contaminant, because pulmonary infection is rarely confirmed on lung biopsy. *Candida* supraglottitis has been described with a slowly progressive course and lesions on the epiglottis, arytenoids, cartilages, and aryepiglottic folds.[53]

Aspergillus infection has been reported in patients with HIV infection. It occurs late in the course of HIV infection and usually follows corticosteroid use or neutropenia.[54] Aspergilloma and invasive cavitary aspergillosis have been described.[55,56] *Aspergillus* infection can cause necrosis of the tracheobronchial tree with formation of a fungal pseudomembrane, resulting in severe airway obstruction.[57] Transmural and peribronchial extension of the infection occurs.

Amphotericin-B is the drug of choice for most life-threatening fungal infections. However, even with treatment, rates of relapse and mortality are high. Some form of chronic suppressive therapy is often given following amphotericin.

Pneumocystis Carinii Pneumonia

Children with HIV infection have a high propensity to develop PCP. *Pneumocystis carinii* was originally classified as a protozoan. Analysis of ribosomal RNA sequences suggest a homology between fungi and *Pneumocystis carinii*.[58,59] The organism is now classified as a fungus. Two morphologic forms of the organism are found in infected lungs: thin-walled single-nucleated trophozoites adherent to type I pneumocytes and thick-walled cysts containing four to eight single-nucleated sporozoites. The organism attaches to the alveolar epithelium, resulting in desquamation of alveolar cells. As the infection progresses, a diffuse desquamative alveolitis ensues and the alveoli become filled with a foamy exudate consisting of alveolar macrophages and cysts containing sporozoites. Interstitial inflammation becomes evident.[60]

Reports from the early stages of the HIV pandemic found that PCP occurred in more than one third of children with AIDS. PCP is now uncommon in parts of the world where there is early treatment with highly active antiretroviral therapy and PCP prophylaxis. PCP can be the initial manifestation of HIV infection. The median age of presentation is 5 months.[2,3] Children with PCP most commonly present with acute onset of cough, fever, tachypnea, retractions, and marked hypoxemia.

An important risk factor for the development of PCP in adults is a CD4+ cell count less than 1000 cells/mm^3 or a rapid rate of decline in CD4+ count. However, 18% to 26% of children younger than 12 months of age have CD4+ counts greater than 1500 cells/mm^3 at the time of PCP diagnosis.[61, 62] Additional laboratory findings include a normal white blood cell count, an elevated lactate dehydrogenase level and a normal IgG level. Lactate dehydrogenase levels greater than 1000 IU/L are frequently associated with PCP.[2] The chest radiograph most commonly shows a diffuse reticulonodular infiltrate most prominent in the perihilar region and extending peripherally. Air bronchograms, focal infiltrates, and pneumatoceles can also be present on the radiograph.

The diagnosis of PCP relies on the identification of the organism from bronchial washings or lung tissue. Bronchoalveolar lavage with fiberoptic bronchoscopy is a reliable method for establishing the diagnosis.[43] In intubated patients, instillation of two or three aliquots of 5 to 10 mL of saline into the endotracheal tube followed by suctioning also provides a high yield in isolating *P. carinii*.[63] False-negative results rarely occur with lavage using the bronchoscope or via the endotracheal tube. Sputum induction has been used to diagnose PCP in children. Sputum is induced with the use of nebulized hypertonic saline (3% or 5%) for 10 to 30 minutes.[64,65] The diagnostic yield using this technique is variable and is dependent on the experience of the individuals collecting and interpreting the specimen. Nasopharyngeal aspirates have been used to identify *P. carinii*, but results with this technique are also variable.[65, 66]

Methenamine silver, toluidine blue O, and fluorescein-conjugated monoclonal antibody are stains that identify the thick-walled cysts of *P. carinii*. Trophozoite forms are identified with Giemsa stain, modified Wright-Giemsa stain, or fluorescein-conjugated monoclonal antibody.

Most children with PCP have respiratory failure and require mechanical ventilation. Reported experiences in the early years of the pandemic indicate a mortality rate exceeding 40% with the initial episode and the majority of patients surviving less than 1 year subsequent to the episode.[67,68] In reports from Africa, where malnutrition is a complicating factor for the expression of pulmonary disease, the prevalence is high and the mortality rate is approximately 50%.[65] With earlier recognition of PCP, the survival rate from an episode of PCP may increase. Nevertheless, survival of HIV-infected children after PCP is less than with other disease manifestations.[3] A possible explanation for decreased survival after PCP is that the presence of *Pneumocystis carinii* can increase HIV replication. It has been demonstrated that HIV production by alveolar lymphocytes obtained from bronchoalveolar lavage fluid is increased during PCP.[69] Alternatively, acquiring PCP may simply be a marker for a lower CD4+ cell count and progression of disease.

The first-line treatment for PCP is high-dose TMP-SMX intravenously for approximately 3 weeks. Deterioration in the pulmonary status may occur in the first few days of treatment, but improvement is generally apparent by the fifth day of treatment. The earlier treatment is initiated, the greater the chance for survival. Side effects to TMP-SMX include rashes and thrombocytopenia. Intravenous pentamidine can be used in those children with more severe adverse reactions to TMP-SMX or in those in whom there does not appear to be a response after 1 week of treatment with TMP-SMX. The intramuscular route is painful and can cause sterile abscesses and should be avoided if possible. Side effects from pentamidine include pancreatitis, renal dysfunction, and both hyperglycemia and hypoglycemia.

A National Institutes of Health Consensus panel has recommended that corticosteroids be used as an adjunct to therapy in adults with severe PCP based on studies showing improved survival and decreased incidence of respiratory failure.[70] Moderate to severe infection has been defined for this purpose as an arterial oxygen tension less than 70 mm Hg or an alveolar-arterial oxygen gradient more than 35 mm Hg. Controlled clinical trials using corticosteroids in children with PCP have not been conducted, but data from uncontrolled studies suggest that corticosteroids may be beneficial.[71] Reports of increased survival with corticosteroids using historical controls must be interpreted with caution because, with earlier recognition of PCP, the survival rate appears to be improving. Although corticosteroids are often used in the treatment of PCP, the optimal dose in children remains uncertain. The suggested dose of prednisone or its equivalent is 2 mg/kg per day for 7 to 10 days, followed by a tapering dose over 2 weeks.

Pneumocystis carinii pneumonia prophylaxis has had a dramatic effect on reducing the incidence of the disease. Prophylaxis is so effective that lack of adherence to the prophylactic regimen is considered to be the most likely cause of PCP in an HIV-infected child. In recent prospective studies of HIV-infected children who have access to antiretroviral therapy and prophylaxis, the incidence of PCP is less than 10%. Prophylaxis for PCP is recommended in all infants born to HIV-infected mothers beginning at 4 to 6 weeks of age.[72] Once HIV infection in the infant has been excluded, the prophylaxis can be stopped. For HIV-infected children, prophylaxis should be continued throughout the first year of life. From 1 to 5 years, prophylaxis is indicated if the CD4+ count is less than 500/µL or the CD4+/CD8+ ratio is less than 15%. In children 5 years of age or older, prophylaxis is recommended if the CD4+ cell count is less than 200/µL or the CD4+/CD8+ ratio is less than 15%. Prophylaxis is also recommended in patients with severely symptomatic (category C) disease. Lifelong prophylaxis is warranted in those who have had PCP.

Trimethoprim/sulfamethoxazole substantially reduces the risk for PCP among HIV-infected children. If TMP-SMX is not tolerated, alternative prophylactic regimens include dapsone administered orally once daily or, in children 5 years of age and older, aerosolized pentamidine administered via inhaler once monthly. If neither dapsone nor aerosolized pentamidine is tolerated, intravenous pentamidine administered every 2 to 4 weeks may be administered. The current U.S. Public Health Service and Infectious Disease Society of America recommendations state that, in adults, PCP prophylaxis may be discontinued in those with CD4+ cell count greater than 200 cells/µL for at least 3 to 6 months and a sustained reduction in viral load for 3 to 6 months.[43] The safety of discontinuing PCP prophylaxis in HIV-infected children receiving highly active antiretroviral therapy has not been studied.

CHRONIC LUNG DISEASE

The introduction of antiretroviral drugs and combination therapy has resulted in a reduction of the viral load and a better prognosis. In children receiving antiretroviral treatment, the spectrum of lung disease has changed, with fewer opportunistic pulmonary infections and more chronic lung disease. The identification of chronic lung disease usually relies on interpretation of the chest radiograph. In a prospective birth cohort of HIV-infected children, the cumulative incidence of chronic radiographic lung changes was 33% by 4 years of age.[73] Parenchymal consolidation persisting for 6 or more months was present in 8% of HIV-infected children, nodular changes persisting for 6 or more months in 8%, and reticular changes or increased bronchovascular markings persisting for 6 or more months in 14%. These radiographic changes were associated with an increased frequency of clubbing, crackles, tachypnea, and decreased oxygen saturation. Resolution of these chronic changes occurred in 50% to 60% of the cases over the period of the study. This resolution was associated with a declining CD4+ cell count but not with lower rates of clinical abnormalities or viral load and thus may be an indication of progression of the HIV infection. The rate of mortality among the HIV-infected children with chronic radiographic changes was not different from the rate of mortality among HIV-infected children without these changes.

The origin of chronic lung disease in HIV-infected children is varied. Lymphocytic interstitial pneumonia/pulmonary lymphoid hyperplasia (LIP/PLH), nonspecific interstitial pneumonitis, bronchiectasis, and diffuse alveolar damage are reported causes. Pulmonary infections can also be a cause of chronic lung disease. In reports from Africa, tuberculosis is one of the most common causes of chronic lung disease.[74] Chronic PCP infection can result in chronic interstitial disease and cysts.[75,76]

LIP/PLH

The most commonly reported chronic lung disease is LIP/PLH complex. The presence of this condition in an HIV-infected child places a child in the moderately symptomatic category (Category B) of the CDC classification. In retrospective reports, this manifestation of pediatric HIV infection occurred in 20% to 40% of infected children.[2,14] In contrast, a report from a prospective birth cohort indicates that chronic nodular densities are observed in 8% of patients by 5 years of age.[73] In HIV-infected children 5 years of age or younger who died at home in Zimbabwe, 9% had LIP on autopsy.[23] The higher incidence from retrospective reports likely represents selection bias and the inclusion of older children.

The pathology consists of a diffuse infiltration of lymphocytes in the interstitium and scattered nodules of mononuclear cells 0.5 mm in diameter. The mononuclear cells consist of lymphocytes, plasma cells, immunoblasts, and histiocytes. In LIP, the infiltration is diffuse throughout the parenchyma. In PLH, the infiltration is primarily adjacent to the bronchial and bronchiolar walls and consists of bronchial-associated lymphoid tissue hyperplasia. The cause of the abnormal lymphoproliferative response is unclear. The principal hypotheses are that lymphoproliferation is a response to the HIV alone or superinfection with another virus. Epstein-Barr viral DNA has been found in lung biopsy samples of children with LIP, and HIV RNA has been identified in the lungs of infants with LIP.[77–79] However, a causal relationship between Epstein-Barr virus and LIP/PLH has not been confirmed.

The onset of LIP/PLH is insidious and the course is slowly progressive. It usually becomes evident after the first year of life, with a median age of onset of 2.5 to 3.0 years.[2,3] However, reticulonodular changes on chest radiographs may be observed before 12 months of age.[73] Cough or tachypnea may be present. Generalized lymphadenopathy, hepatosplenomegaly, clubbing, and parotid gland enlargement are commonly associated physical findings. Admission rates for lower respiratory tract illness are higher for children with LIP/PLH compared with HIV-infected children without LIP/PLH.[80] The occurrence of LIP/PLH is associated with longer survival.[3,17]

Elevated serum immunoglobulin levels are associated with LIP/PLH.[2] Serum IgG levels greater than 2500 mg/dL are strongly associated with LIP/PLH. The radiograph typically shows a bilateral diffuse interstitial reticulonodular pattern with or without hilar adenopathy. Lung biopsy establishes the diagnosis. However, a presumptive diagnosis of LIP/PLH can be made based on the clinical findings and the typical reticulonodular radiographic pattern lasting more than 2 months without another documented cause. In a longitudinal study, resolution of the chronic nodular radiographic findings occurred in 61% of children.[73]

Treatment of LIP/PLH is nonspecific. Oxygen is administered for hypoxemia as required. Although treatment of LIP/PLH with corticosteroids has been reported to improve hypoxemia in a small number of patients, controlled clinical trials have not been carried out.[81]

Some cases of LIP/PLH progress to a lymphoproliferative disorder characterized by polyclonal, polymorphic B-cell content without evidence of cellular atypia, necrosis, or prominent mitotic activity but with extranodal systemic and prominent pulmonary involvement.[82] Some cases have progressed to malignant lymphoma.

Bronchiectasis

An important cause of chronic infiltrates and atelectasis on chest radiographs is bronchiectasis. This should be suspected when radiographs show persistent abnormalities in the same lobe for more than 6 months. The diagnosis can be confirmed with a computed tomography scan demonstrating dilated tubular structures. Bronchiectasis with HIV infection has been associated with LIP.[83] It is possible that the lymphocytic infiltration into the mucosa and submucosa of the bronchiole leads to destruction, fibrosis, atelectasis, and, subsequently, bronchiectasis. Other mechanisms of development of bronchiectasis include acute or chronic infection, a direct effect of HIV on the lung, or persistent atelectasis. Some children who develop recurrent pneumonia despite the standard medical regimen of cyclic antibiotics and aggressive pulmonary therapy might benefit from adjunctive IVIG therapy at 600 mg/kg per dose, given monthly.

Diffuse Alveolar Damage

Diffuse alveolar damage describes a sequence of events following severe acute lung injury and represents another manifestation of chronic lung disease. The early exudative stage of diffuse alveolar damage occurs over 2 or 3 days and is characterized by alveolar and interstitial edema and hyaline membrane formation. This progresses to a proliferative stage after 1 week in which there is hyperplasia of type II pneumocytes and desquamation of alveolar lining cells and thickening of the interstitium with fibroblast proliferation.[60] Possible causes include viral or opportunistic infections such as *Pneumocystis carinii* infection, adult respiratory distress syndrome, and oxygen toxicity. Clinically, this is characterized by respiratory distress and diffuse pulmonary infiltrates. This entity should be suspected when there is persistent hypoxia following acute respiratory failure from PCP or other opportunistic infections. Recurrent episodes of respiratory failure may represent viral infections superimposed on a lung with diffuse alveolar damage.

PULMONARY TUMORS

Kaposi sarcoma has been associated with HIV infection. It occurs predominantly in homosexual men and is uncommon in children. Although cases have been reported in infants, most cases of Kaposi sarcoma in the pediatric age group have occurred in adolescents.[84] The clinical presentation varies from indolent skin disease to disseminated visceral involvement. The most common manifestation is violaceous plaques of the skin. Pulmonary involvement causes dyspnea, cough, and fever. Examination of the lungs reveals multiple hemorrhagic nodules or violaceous endobronchial lesions, or both. The chest radiograph can show an interstitial pattern, which is usually homogeneous or nodular infiltrates. Pleural effusions are common. The diagnosis is made by biopsy.

Pulmonary tumors of smooth muscle origin in children have been reported. The airways, lungs, and pulmonary veins have been found to have nodular masses that on biopsy have been leiomyoma and leiomyosarcoma.[85] Pseudolymphomas and lymphomas have also been reported.

UPPER AIRWAY DISEASE

The lymphoid proliferation that occurs with HIV infection can be present in tonsillar and adenoidal tissue. The hypertrophy and pharyngeal infiltration of these tissues have resulted in upper airway obstruction in children with HIV infection. It has not been determined whether upper airway obstruction occurs with greater frequency in HIV-infected children than in those not infected.

Noninfectious infiltration of the epiglottis has also been described, with gradual onset of drooling and dysphagia. Biopsy shows acute and chronic inflammation, with granulation tissue and lymphoid follicles in the submucosa.[86]

PULMONARY DISEASE AND MORTALITY

Pulmonary disease is an important cause of HIV-related deaths. Infection is the most prevalent underlying cause (the single cause that initiated the events resulting in death) of death for children younger than 6 years of age. Two thirds of these infections are caused by pulmonary infections. The frequency of pulmonary disease as the underlying cause of death decreases with increasing age. In the prospective Pediatric Pulmonary and Cardiovascular Complications of Vertically Transmitted HIV Study chronic lung disease (diagnosed by case-by-case mortality review) was present in 58% of children who died but was rarely an underlying cause of death.[41]

CONCLUSION

Respiratory diseases play a major role in morbidity and mortality in HIV-infected children, particularly in countries with a poor medical infrastructure. The spectrum of pulmonary diseases in industrialized and emerging countries is similar, but preventable complications such as PCP, tuberculosis, and measles pneumonia are more common in the latter. In the emerging countries, underlying malnutrition complicates the clinical outcome.

REFERENCES

1. Centers for Disease Control: Unexplained immunodeficiency and opportunistic infections in infants: New York, New Jersey, California. MMWR 1982;31:665–667.
2. Marolda J, Pace B, Bonforte RJ, et al: Pulmonary manifestations of HIV infection in children. Pediatr Pulmonol 1991;10:231–235.
3. Scott GB, Hutto C, Makuch RW, et al: Survival in children with prenatally acquired human immunodeficiency virus type 1 infection. N Engl J Med 1989;321:1791–1796.
4. Centers for Disease Control: 1994 Revised classification system for human immunodeficiency virus infection in children less than 13 years of age. MMWR 1994;43:1–10.
5. UNAIDS: Report of the global HIV/AIDS epidemic. Joint United Nations Programme on HIV/Aids 2000. Available at *www.unaids.org/epidemic_update/report/index.html#full.* Accessed September 18, 2000.
6. Landay AL, Schade SZ, Takefman DM, et al: Detection of HIV provirus in bronchoalveolar lavage cells by polymerase chain reaction. J Acquir Immun Defic Syndrome 1993;6:171–175.

7. Agostini C, Zambello R, Facco M, et al: CD8 T-cell infiltration in extravascular tissues of patients with human immunodeficiency virus infection. Interleukin-15 upmodulates costimulatory pathways involved in the antigen-presenting cells-T-cell interaction. Blood 1999; 93:1277–1286.
8. Sierra-Madero JG, Toossi Z, Hom DL, et al: Relationship between load of virus in alveolar macrophages from human immunodeficiency virus type 1-infected person, production of cytokines, and clinical status. J Infect Dis 1994;169:18–27.
9. Murray HW, Hillman JK, Rubin BY, et al: Patients at risk for AIDS-related opportunistic infections: Clinical manifestation and impaired interferon production. N Engl J Med 1985;313:1504–1510.
10. Bernstein LJ, Ochs HG, Wedgwood RD, et al: Defective humoral immunity in pediatric acquired immunodeficiency syndrome. J Pediatr 1985;107: 352–357.
11. Twigg HL 3rd, Spain BA, Soliman DM, et al: Impaired IgG production in the lungs of HIV-infected individuals. Cell Immunol 1996;170:127–133.
12. Blanche S, Mayaux MJ, Rouzioux C, et al: Relation of the course of HIV infection in children to the severity of the disease in their mothers at delivery. N Engl J Med 1994;330:308–312.
13. Martin R, Boyer P, Hammill H, et al: Incidence of premature birth and neonatal respiratory disease in infants of HIV positive mothers. J Pediatr 1997;131: 851–856.
14. AIDS Surveillance Update. Albany, NY, New York State Department of Health, 1993.
15. Oxtoby MJ: Perinatally acquired human immunodeficiency virus infection. Ped Infect Dis J 1990;9: 609–619.
16. Kattan M, Platzker A, Mellins RB, et al: Respiratory diseases in the first year of life in children born to HIV-1 infected women. Pediatr Pulmonol 2001;31:267–276.
17. Spira R, Lepage P, Msellati P, et al: Natural history of human immunodeficiency virus type 1 infection in children: A five-year prospective study in Rwanda. Pediatrics 1999;104:e56. URL:http://www.pediatrics.org/cgi/content/full/104/5/e56.
18. Marolda J, Pace B, Bonforte RJ, et al: Pulmonary manifestations of HIV infection in children. Pediatr Pulmonol 1991;10:231–235.
19. Lucas SB, Peacock CS, Hounnou A, et al: Disease in children infected with HIV in Abidjan, Cote d'Ivoire. BMJ 1996;312:335–338.
20. Diaz C, Hanson C, Cooper ER, et al: Disease progression in a cohort of infants with vertically acquired HIV infection from birth: The Woman and Infants Transmission Study (WITS). J Acquired Immune Defic Hum Retrovirol 1998;18:221–228.
21. Girard P-M: Discontinuing *Pneumocystis carinii* prophylaxis. N Engl J Med 2001;344:222–223.
22. Mofenson LM, Yogev R, Korelitz J, et al: Characteristics of acute pneumonia in human immunodeficiency virus-infected children and association with long term mortality risk. Pediatr Infect Dis J 1998;17:872–880.
23. Ikeogu MO, Wolf B, Mathe S: Pulmonary manifestations in HIV seropositivity and malnutrition in Zimbabwe. Arch Dis Child 1997;76:124–128.
24. Adamson PC, Wu TC, Meade BD, et al: Pertussis in a previously immunized child with human immunodeficiency virus infection. J Pediatr 1989;115:589–591.
25. Mofenson LM, Moye J Jr, Bethel J, et al: Prophylactic intravenous immunoglobulin in HIV-infected children with CD4+ counts of 0.20×10^9/L or more: Effect on viral, opportunistic, and bacterial infections. JAMA 1992;268:483–488.
26. Spector SA, Gelber RD, McGrath N, et al: A controlled trial of intravenous immune globulin for the prevention of serious bacterial infections in children receiving zidovudine for advanced human immunodeficiency virus infection. N Engl J Med 1994;331: 1181–1187.
27. American Academy of Pediatrics: Report of the Committee on Infectious Diseases. Elk Grove Village, Ill, American Academy of Pediatrics, 2000.
28. Murray JF: Cursed duet: HIV-infection and tuberculosis. Respiration 1990;57:210–220.
29. Luo C, Chintu L, Bhat G, et al: Human immunodeficiency virus type-1 infection in Zambian children with tuberculosis: Changing seroprevalence and evaluation of a thiacetzone-free regimen. Tubercle Lung Dis 1994;75:110–115.
30. Moss WJ, Deydo T, Suarez M, et al: Tuberculosis in children infected with human immunodeficiency virus: A report of five cases. Pediatr Infect Dis J 1992;11:114–120.
31. Khouri YF, Mastrucci MT, Hutto C, et al: *Mycobacterium tuberculosis* in children with human immunodeficiency virus type 1 infection. Pediatr Infect Dis J 1992;11:950–955.
32. American Thoracic Society: Diagnostic standards and classification of tuberculosis. Am Rev Respir Dis 1990;142:725–735.
33. Abadco DL, Steiner P: Gastric lavage is better than bronchoalveolar lavage for isolation of *Mycobacterium tuberculosis* in childhood pulmonary tuberculosis. Pediatr Infect Dis J 1992;11:735–738.
34. Somu N, Swaminathan S, Paramasivan CN, et al: Value of bronchoalveolar lavage and gastric lavage in the diagnosis of pulmonary tuberculosis in children. Tuber Lung Dis 1995;76:295–299.
35. Zar HJ, Tannenbaum E, Appoles P, et al: Sputum induction for the diagnosis of pulmonary tuberculosis in infants and children in an urban setting in South Africa. Arch Dis Child 2000;82:305–308.
36. Pape JW, Jean SS, Ho JL, et al: Effect of isoniazid prophylaxis on incidence of active tuberculosis and progression of HIV infection. Lancet 1993;342:268–272.
37. U.S. Public Health Service and Infectious Disease Society of America: 1999 USPHS/IDSA Guidelines for the prevention of opportunistic infections in

persons infected with human immunodeficiency virus. MMWR 1999;48:1–59.
38. Jeena PM, Mitha T, Bamber S, et al: Effect of the human immunodeficiency virus on tuberculosis in children. Tuber Lung Dis 1996;77:437–443.
39. Lewis LL, Butler KM, Husson RN, et al: Defining the population of human immunodeficiency virus-infected children at risk for *Mycobacterium avium intracellulare* infection. J Pediatr 1992;121:677–683.
40. Chaimon RE, Moore RD, Richman DD, et al: Zidovodine Epidemiology Study Group. Incidence and natural history of *Mycobacterium avium* complex infection in patients with advanced human immunodeficiency virus disease treated with zidovudine. Am Rev Respir Dis 1992;146:285–289.
41. Langston C, Cooper ER, Goldfarb J, et al: Human immunodeficiency virus-related mortality in infants and children: Data from the Pediatric Pulmonary and Cardiovascular Complications of Vertically Transmitted HIV (P^2C^2) Study. Pediatrics 2001;107:328–338.
42. Horsburgh CR Jr: *Mycobacterium avium* complete infection in the acquired immunodeficiency syndrome. N Engl J Med 1991;324:1332–1338.
43. Bye MR, Bernstein LJ, Shah K, et al: Diagnostic lavage in children with AIDS. Pediatr Pulmonol 1987;3:425–428.
44. Chadwani S, Borkowsky W, Krasinski K, et al: Respiratory syncytial virus infection in human immunodeficiency virus-infected children. J Pediatr 1990;177:251–254.
45. Murray JF, Felton CP, Garay SM, et al: Pulmonary complications of the acquired immunodeficiency syndrome: Report of a National Heart, Lung and Blood Institute Workshop. N Engl J Med 1984;310:1682–1688.
46. Miles PR, Baughman RP, Linemann CC: Cytomegalovirus in the bronchoalveolar lavage fluid of patients with AIDS. Chest 1990;97:1092–1096.
47. Jacobson MF, Mills J, Rush J, et al: Morbidity and mortality of patients with AIDS and first episode *Pneumocystis carinii* pneumonia unaffected by concomitant pulmonary cytomegalovirus infection. Am Rev Respir Dis 1991;144:6–9.
48. Glaser JH, Schural S, Bernstein O, et al: Cytomegalovirus and *Pneumocystis carinii* pneumonia in children with acquired immunodeficiency syndrome. J Pediatr 1992;120:929–931.
49. Chadwick EG, Chang G, Decker MD, et al: Serologic response to standard inactivated influenza vaccine in human immunodeficiency virus-infected children. Pediatr Infect Dis J 1994;13:206–211.
50. Grant IH, Armstrong D: Fungal infection in AIDS: Cryptococcosis. Infect Dis Clin North Am 1988;2:457–464.
51. Johnson PC, Haml RJ, Sarvosi GA: Clinical review: Progressive disseminated histoplasmosis in the AIDS patient. Semin Respir Infect 1989;4:139–146.
52. Galgiani JN: Coccidioidomycosis in human immunodeficiency virus-infected patients. J Infect Dis 1990;162:165–169.
53. Bye MR, Palomba A, Bernstein L, Shah K: Clinical *Candida* supraglottitis in an infant with AIDS-related complex. Pediatri Pulmonol 1987;3:280–281.
54. Denning DW, Follansbee SE, Scolara M, et al: Pulmonary aspergillosis in the acquired immunodeficiency syndrome. N Engl J Med 1991;324:654–662.
55. Lombardo GT, Anandareo N, Lin CS, et al: Fatal hemoptysis in a patient with AIDS related complex and pulmonary aspergilloma. NY State J Med 1987;87:306–308.
56. Asnis DI, Chitkara RK, Jacobson M, Goldstein JA: Invasive aspergillosis: An unusual manifestation of AIDS. NY State J Med 1988;88:653–655.
57. Pervez NK, Kleinerman J, Kattan M, et al: Pseudomembranous necrotizing bronchial aspergillosis in a patient with hemophilia and acquired immune deficiency syndrome. Am Rev Respir Dis 1985;131:961–963.
58. Edman JC, Kovacs JA, Masur H, et al: Ribosomal RNA sequences show *Pneumocystis carinii* to be a member of the fungi. Nature 1988;334:519–522.
59. Piley FJ, Wakefield NE, Banerji S, et al: Mitochondrial gene sequences show fungal homology for *Pneumocystis carinii*. Molec Microbiol 1991;5:1347–1351.
60. Katzenstein AA, Askin FR: Lung Involvement in the Acquired Immune Deficiency Syndrome (AIDS) in Surgical Pathology of Non-Neoplastic Lung disease. Philadelphia, WB Saunders, 1990.
61. Simonds RJ, Lindegren ML, Thomas P, et al: Prophylaxis against *Pneumocystis carinii* pneumonia among children with perinatally acquired human immunodeficiency virus infection in the United States. N Engl J Med 1995;332:786–790.
62. Leibovitz E, Regaud M, Pollack H, et al: *Pneumocystis carinii* pneumonia in infants infected with the human immunodeficiency virus with more than 450 CD4+ lymphocytes per cubic millimeter. N Engl J Med 1990;323:531–533.
63. Koumbourlis AC, Kurland JA: Nonbronchoscopic bronchoalveolar lavage in mechanically ventilated infants: Technique, efficacy and applications. Pediatr Pulmonol 1993;15:257–263.
64. Ognibene FC, Gill VJ, Pizzo PA, et al: Induced sputum to diagnose *Pneumocystis carinii* pneumonia in immunosuppressed pediatric patients. J Pediatr 1989;115:430–433.
65. Zar HJ, Dechabon A, Hanslo D, et al: *Pneumocystis carinii* pneumonia in South African children infected with human immunodeficiency virus. Pediatr Infect Dis J 2000;19:603–607.
66. Graham SM, Mtitimila EI, Kamanga HS, et al: Clincial presentation and outcome of *Pneumocystis carinii* pneumonia in Malawian children. Lancet 2000;355:369–373.

67. Bernstein LJ, Bye MR, Rubenstein A: Prognostic factors and life expectancy in children with acquired immunodeficiency syndrome and *Pneumocystis carinii* pneumonia. Am J Dis Child 1989;143:775–778.
68. Marolda J, Pace B, Bonforte RJ, et al: Outcome of mechanical ventilation in children with acquired immunodeficiency syndrome. Pediatr Pulmonol 1989;7:230–234.
69. Israel-Biet D, Cadranel J, Even P: Human immunodeficiency virus production by alveolar lymphocytes is increased during *Pneumocystis carinii* pneumonia. Am Rev Respir Dis 1993;148:1308–1312.
70. National Institutes of Health: Consensus statement on the use of corticosteroids as adjunctive therapy for pneumocystis pneumonia in the acquired immunodeficiency syndrome. N Engl J Med 1990; 323:1500–1504.
71. Bye MR, Cairns-Bazarian AM, Ewig JM: Markedly reduced mortality associated with corticosteroid therapy of *Pneumocystis carinii* pneumonia in children with AIDS. Arch Pediatr Adolesc Med 1994;148:638–641.
72. Centers for Disease Control: 1995 Revised guidelines for prophylaxis against *Pneumocystis carinii* pneumonia for children infected with or perinatally exposed to human immunodeficiency virus. MMWR 1995;44:1–10.
73. Norton K, Kattan M, Rao JS, et al: Chronic radiographic lung changes in children with vertically transmitted HIV-1 infection. AJR 2001;176:1553–1558.
74. Jeena PM, Coovadia HM, Thula SA, et al: Persistent and chronic lung disease in HIV-1-infected and uninfected African children. AIDS 1998;12:1185–1193.
75. Wassermann K, Pothoff G, Kirn E, et al: Chronic *Pneumocystis carinii* pneumonia in AIDS. Chest 1993;104:667–672.
76. Evlogias NE, Leonidas JC, Rooney J, et al: Severe cystic pulmonary disease associated with chronic *Pneumocystis carinii* infection in a child with AIDS. Pediatr Radiol 1994;24:606–608.
77. Andiman WA, Eastman R, Martin K, et al: Opportunistic lymphoproliferations associated with Epstein-Barr viral DNA in infants and children with AIDS. Lancet 1985;2:1390–1393.
78. Chayt KJ, Harper ME, Marselle LM, et al: Detection of HTLV-III RNA in lungs of patients with AIDS and pulmonary involvement. JAMA 1986;256:2356–2359.
79. Katz BZ, Berkman AB, Shapiro ED: Serologic evidence of active Epstein-Barr virus associated lymphoproliferative disorders of children with acquired immunodeficiency syndrome. J Pediatr 1992;120:228–232.
80. Sharland M, Gibb DM, Holland F: Respiratory morbidity from lymphocytic interstitial pneumonitis (LIP) in vertically acquired HIV infection. Arch Dis Child 1997;76:334–336.
81. Rubinstein A, Bernstein L, Charytan M, et al: Corticosteroid treatment for pulmonary lymphoid hyperplasia in children with acquired immune deficiency syndrome. Pediatr Pulmonol 1988;4:13–17.
82. Joshi VV, Kauffman S, Oleske J, et al: Polyclonal polymorphic B-cell lymphoproliferative disorder with prominent pulmonary involvement in children with acquired immune deficiency syndrome. Cancer 1987;59:1455–1462.
83. Amorosa JK, Miller RW, Laraya-Cuasay L, et al: Bronchiectasis in children with lymphocytic interstitial pneumonia and acquired immune deficiency syndrome: Plain film and CT observations. Pediatr Radiol 1992;22:603–607.
84. Buck BE, Scott GB, Valdes-Dapena M, Parks WP: Kaposi sarcoma in two infants with acquired immune deficiency syndrome. J Pediatr 1983;103:911.
85. Chadwick EG, Connor EJ, Hanson IC, et al: Tumors of smooth-muscle origin in HIV-infected children. JAMA 1990;263:3182–3184.
86. Diamant EP, Dische RM, Barzilai A, et al: Chronic epiglottitis in a child with acquired immunodeficiency syndrome. Pediatr Infect Dis J 1992;11:770–771.

Infection Control in Hospital, School, and Community: Distinguishing Real Risk from Perceived Danger

Ellen R. Cooper

The last decade has brought dramatic improvements in the chemotherapeutic options for the HIV-infected child. The improvement in life expectancy and sustained periods of well-being has resulted in increased attendance in day care and school as well as expanded involvement in extracurricular activities. In some cases, however, an uneasy interface between the population of HIV-infected children and the general community has developed. Recognition of the severity of disease and a lack of understanding of how HIV is transmitted have led to fear and ostracism of infected children from situations that pose no risk to others.[1] It is important for health care providers to be aware of the many special issues surrounding the daily care of the HIV-infected child, as well as institutional considerations in the prevention of infection. Understanding the modes and relative risks of transmission following different exposures is key to being able to protect the health of the community while still promoting as normal a life as possible for the individual patient.

HIV TRANSMISSION: THE FACTS

The transmission of HIV requires that a sufficient quantity of virus enter the host individual, gain access to the target cell, and be able to establish infection. Large epidemiologic studies have determined that transmission is usually accomplished in one of four settings. These are (1) vertical transmission from mother to infant during pregnancy, delivery, or breastfeeding; (2) direct inoculation of blood or blood-containing tissues through transfusion, transplantation of organs, or penetrating injuries with needles or other sharp objects; (3) sexual activity with resultant transmission through contact with infected semen, vaginal or cervical secretions, or blood through anal or genital mucous membranes; and (4) less commonly, with splattering of blood onto mucous membranes or nonintact skin.[2]

HIV in Body Fluids

HIV has been isolated from a wide variety of body fluids, although transmission has been most often associated with exposure to blood, semen, and breastmilk. HIV preferentially infects and replicates within cells that express the CD4+ antigen. This antigen is expressed on the surface of hematopoietic cell types that circulate throughout the body, although the major cells of this type are a subset of helper T lymphocytes, namely the monocytes and macrophages. The chemokines CCR4 and CCR5 have been shown to function as coreceptors for HIV attachment, thereby contributing to the risk for infection.[3] When the virus has replicated and buds from the cell into the plasma, it is free to infect another cell. HIV can therefore be found both intracellularly and extracellularly. The efficiency with which one can isolate HIV from various body fluids is directly proportional to the number of lymphocytes and monocytes in those fluids, and it stands to reason that exposure to fluids rich in lymphocytes or monocytes poses a greater risk of transmission.

HIV has been isolated from blood, semen, cervical secretions, breastmilk, throat swab samples, saliva, cerebrospinal fluid, and tears.[4–8] It remains difficult to isolate from sweat,[9] stool, vomitus, or urine,[10] when these substances are not contaminated by blood.

The isolation of HIV from saliva and tears has heightened concern over the possibility of HIV transmission with "casual contact." Evidence supports the idea that the efficiency with which HIV is transmitted via exposure to these secretions is very low.[11] Studies of HIV-infected adults have shown that the frequency with which virus can be isolated from saliva varies, ranging from 1.4% to 40%. This probably is related to the variation in total viral load among individuals.[12] Although HIV has been recovered from throat swab samples, it has been theorized that these samples might have been contaminated with lymphocytes from the tonsillar pillars.

One very small study showed that one in seven infected persons had tears with culturable HIV.[4] In spite of this worrisome statistic from a relatively small study, in cases in which exposure has been only to saliva or tears, no transmission has been documented.

Risk of HIV Transmission after True Exposure

As already alluded to, a number of factors may contribute to the efficiency with which HIV is transmitted during an exposure. The route of exposure, the volume of inoculum, the titer of virus present in the secretion, and the antiretroviral therapy being used by the source patient may all play a role. In addition, the replicative integrity of the specific quasispecies of HIV present in the source patient also may contribute to the likelihood of transmission after exposure. Host factors affecting infectivity have been identified through population studies of HIV transmission. The susceptibility of the host may be influenced by factors linked to inflammation or immune activation that alter either the number of susceptible target cells or the receptivity of those cells. These same factors may affect the production of virus within newly infected cells, thereby influencing the infectiousness of the source patient. For example, during immune activation after vaccination with tetanus toxoid, the blood concentration of HIV increases up to 36-fold.[13] Other factors may induce microscopic erosions in the mucous membrane that provide the virus more direct access to the bloodstream, and still others may act by facilitating the survival of HIV in the oral, genital, or rectal mucosa. Vaginal pH may affect the survival of HIV under some conditions.[14]

Epidemiologic data suggest that some individuals show relative resistance to infection with HIV. Some female sex workers and homosexual men have been found to remain uninfected despite repeatedly having unprotected sexual intercourse with HIV-infected partners.[15] A mutation in the chemokine receptor gene has been identified, and this mutation apparently varies greatly according to race. People who are homozygous for the CKR5 mutation appear to be resistant to infection. Heterozygosity for this mutation does not prevent infection altogether but may slow progression of the disease, suggesting that this mutation affects the ability of the virus to replicate once inside the target cell.[16]

The risk of HIV infection after transfusion with contaminated blood is as high as 95% by some reports.[2] The United States instituted strict screening of blood for HIV more than a decade ago.[17] The risk of acquiring HIV after a transfusion that has been screened in the United States is approximately 1 case for every 450,000 to 600,000 donations. The risk of vertical transmission varies with the circumstances surrounding the pregnancy and delivery and is dealt with in detail in another chapter of this book. Transmission through sexual contact now accounts for 75% to 85% of the new infections occurring in the United States in adults and adolescents.[18]

Given the variables discussed, it is difficult to determine the risk of transmission after a single episode of needle sharing or sexual contact.[19–23] Estimates of the rate of transmission of HIV due to unprotected sexual intercourse in adults ranges from 0.8% to 3.2% with a single act of receptive anal intercourse, and from 0.05% to 0.15% for vaginal intercourse.[24] The risk of transmission likely increases when a traumatic injury is present. Most experts agree, however, that barrier protection with condoms during sexual intercourse greatly reduces the risk of transmission of HIV.[25]

Although no large-scale studies investigating percutaneous exposures in children have been published, the average risk for transmission for health care workers exposed to HIV-infected blood is estimated at 0.3% for percutaneous exposures and 0.09% for mucous membrane exposures.[26–28] Kaplan and Heimer, from Yale University School of Medicine, attempted to create a mathematical model to estimate the probability of infection per injection with a contaminated syringe, using data available to them from the New Haven Connecticut legal needle-exchange program.[29] Using the polymerase chain reaction to test for the presence of HIV proviral DNA in a sample of returned needles, they found that 67.5% were positive for HIV. From estimates of shared injection rates and disinfection rates from surveys, they were able to infer that the probability of infection per injection equals 0.0067. This is slightly higher than the estimates from occupational needlestick studies, and higher by a factor of 3 than estimates of the probability of HIV transmission per vaginal sexual act from an infected man to an uninfected woman.[30]

It is difficult to extrapolate these data with confidence to the pediatric population, given the circumstances surrounding their potential exposure to needles and syringes. The risk of HIV transmission after exposure to discarded needles found in parks or alleyways cannot be easily estimated. Variables include the type of injury suffered, the likelihood that the needle or syringe contained infected blood, and environmental factors that can influence the viability of the virus, such as ambient temperature and relative humidity.[31]

Experts agree that the risk of HIV transmission from the type of ordinary contact that occurs among children in households, school, day care, and athletic facilities is vanishingly small.[32–36] Almost 20 studies addressing HIV infection among adult and child household members of infected persons have shown that among 1300 individuals with "casual contact," no individuals were infected except those with independent risk factors for infection. Even studies of household activities that might have involved exposure to blood or other infected body fluid have not identified casual contact as a risk. On the other hand, six cases have been reported that seem to have resulted after exposure to infected body fluid by skin or mucous membrane in a nonhospital environment.[37] In spite of rather complete investigations in all cases, there does remain the possibility of an unidentified blood exposure. In two of the cases, the children had hemophilia, and blood products were being given in the home. There have also been two reports of transmission between an adult and a child in the home.[38] In both cases, there is some question as to whether blood exposure might have been responsible.

Because HIV has been isolated from saliva, biting has been considered an exposure of concern. As early as 1986, there was a report in *The Lancet* of horizontal transmission of HIV infection between two siblings. The only exposure identified was a bite on the forearm remembered by the mother not to have broken the skin. No documentation of the method of transmission could be better identified, and this has been considered a possible mode of transmission since that initial report.[39] HIV transmission by bites, while rare, has been documented, associated with blood-tinged saliva in the wound.[40] In 1996, there was a well-documented seroconversion to HIV following a human bite when there was blood in the mouth of the source patient and a break in the integrity of the skin of a previously uninfected health care worker.[41]

Biting is common among young children, and while most bites do not result in blood contact, it is often difficult to prove, since many are unwitnessed events.[42,43] An estimated 250,000 human bite injuries occur in the United States each year, and the prevalence of bites among children is estimated at one bite per 600 visits to pediatric emergency departments. According to one report, 50% of children at day care centers were bitten at least once in a 1-year period. Given the variables described and the additional variable of direction of bite, it remains impossible even to estimate the magnitude of risk. However, it appears the risk is finite and small.[44,45]

There are two case reports that suggest that blood contamination of saliva as a result of passionate kissing may be a rare method of transmitting HIV.[46] In both cases, there was probably blood exposure from bleeding gums. Nonsexual kissing has not been proven to be a mode of HIV transmission, particularly between children and family members or other loved ones.

In summary, it seems that HIV transmission is unlikely among children and adults from activities common to children's care, education, sports, and play activities. Therefore, restriction from these activities is not recommended, although routine and appropriate precautions should be followed at all times.[33,47–49] In addition, all child care workers should be instructed in the proper response if an exposure occurs in the course of children's activities.

Contact with Infected Health Care Workers

The occurrence of the initial case cluster of dental provider to patient transmission of HIV attracted substantial publicity and public interest. It resulted in tremendous anxiety about the risk of acquiring HIV infection from an infected health care practitioner.[50] A second, more recent cluster of HIV infections was linked to an infected orthopedic surgeon.[51] The epidemiologic investigation of both of these clusters revealed some unusual infection-control practices, although neither case is completely understood. Whatever those circumstances, such instances are rare. In response to unprecedented anxiety, however, the United States Congress passed a statute requiring that states implement the July 1991 Centers for Disease Control and Prevention (CDC) guidelines for managing HIV-infected or hepatitis B–infected providers. The requirement that infected practitioners who plan to perform exposure-prone invasive procedures inform their patients prospectively of the practitioner's infection status was immediately controversial and remains so today. It has been difficult even to find agreement on what constitutes an exposure-prone procedure. The CDC guidelines have not been uniformly adopted by the states. Often, the policy at the hospital level is made by a panel that may include experts in HIV as well as lawyers who weigh the risk of liability. This uneasy environment has decreased the willingness on the part of health care providers to be tested, even in the setting of a potential exposure to them, or to inform the hospital of their infection status should they know it to be positive for infection.

It should be stated, however, that the type of procedures done by the usual pediatrician, either in the office or in the hospital, would not be considered exposure-prone by any accepted criteria. Surgical procedures involving sharp needles, sutures, or scalpels remain controversial, and each state has created its own guidelines.

PREVENTION OF HIV TRANSMISSION

School

In spite of well-publicized instances of discrimination against children with HIV infection at school, no case of transmission occurring in school has to date been reported. The epidemiologic data do not justify excluding children with infection or isolating them to protect other students. Children who are infected with HIV should be encouraged to participate in all school activities as long as their health allows them to do so. Knowledge of a child's HIV status remains unnecessary for public school entry, and disclosure of such status should not be required.[1] Unfortunately, fear of discrimination often prevents parents from disclosing to the school even when the child might benefit. Because of confidentiality issues and the right to privacy of families, it should be recognized that the pediatrician may not notify the school of known infection on the submitted health forms. The decision to disclose infection status should be made in the best interests of the child but remains the responsibility of the parents, who may or may not want to include the pediatrician in the decision. When a decision is made to notify the school that a child is infected, the number of persons aware of the infection can be limited so that information is disclosed only to those who need such knowledge to care for the child. This should include those individuals who would be able to recognize the signs and symptoms that would signal the need for prompt medical attention. These selected individuals also share in the responsibility of maintaining the strict confidentiality of the child's infection status. Children with HIV or other chronic illnesses should be informed of exposure to readily communicable illnesses that could compromise their health.[1,48] Informed personnel should also be able to weigh the risks and benefits to the infected child and to others with respect to specific child-child interactions. Medications may need to be administered at school; this may also influence the choice of whom to inform.

Some scenarios exist that might preclude a child or adolescent from participating in group activities. These include a child or adolescent with weeping wounds that are difficult to cover or a neurologically impaired child with aggressive biting behavior who is unable or unwilling to change the behavior. Because not all families have disclosed infection status, school programs should be uniformly instituted and implemented to inform all families when communicable diseases have been identified in the classroom.

Blood exposures from fights, unintentional injuries, and nosebleeds may occur at school. All schools should be capable of handling blood and potentially infectious materials using standard precautions. Readily available supplies should include gloves, disposable towels, and disinfectants; all staff in the school environment should be educated in the proper use of these precautions within the school setting. Occupational Safety and Health Administration standards require that schools institute an educational program for employees specifically designed to address routine procedures for handling blood or bloody body fluids.[52] The standard precautions used in both hospital and community are listed in Table 12–1.

Important to note as well is that each family makes its own decisions concerning the disclosure of a child's HIV status to the individual child. This decision must be made by the parents or guardians of the child and should take into account the child's age, level of emotional maturity, and cognitive abilities. The timing and location of disclosure should be thought of as a long-term process. It is important for school officials to be cognizant that many children with HIV infection who are attending school do not know of their own diagnosis. The personnel should be careful of their own discussions so that disclosure does not occur in an accidental manner.[53]

The recommended management of exposure to HIV outside of the hospital environment should proceed along the same guidelines established for occupational exposures. This includes prompt reporting to the appropriate authorities, determination of the nature of the exposure, counseling the exposed person and family regarding the use of antiretroviral therapy, and serial testing of the exposed individual. When consent is possible, the testing of the source person is useful in identifying true risk.[54]

Recreational Facilities and School Athletics

In the United States, approximately one third of high-school girls and one half of high-school boys participate in varsity or junior varsity school sports.[55] As children with HIV infection are entering their adolescent years, many are able to fully participate in sports. Therefore, it is expected that the number of children with HIV infection participating in school sports will increase. Although sports-related injuries may involve contact with blood, the risk of HIV transmission is low. Laboratory investigations have revealed that natural sweat does not contain HIV, so exposure to this secretion represents no risk. Blood from an HIV-infected athlete would need to be maintained in sustained contact with a wound or exposed mucous membrane or other portal of entry of the susceptible athlete to threaten an uninfected individual.

The estimation of risk for HIV transmission in contact sports is 1 in 4 million per player per game. The risk of hepatitis B transmission is higher, at 1 in 20,000 per player per game. This is in part because hepatitis B is usually present in higher concentrations in the blood and is more stable in the environment than HIV.[56,57] Only one observational study has investigated the risk of HIV transmission in sports. Eleven teams of the National Football League in the United States were studied. An estimated frequency of less than 1 transmission per 85 million contacts was calculated.[58,59]

In spite of the low risk, guidelines for the prevention of transmission of blood-borne pathogens among athletes should be instituted.[60,61] When a bleeding injury occurs, the game should be temporarily halted. Care to the bleeding athlete should be administered as soon as possible. Injured players should not resume play until the bleeding has stopped and the wound is covered with a dressing. Skin that is exposed to blood, or to other bodily fluids visibly contaminated with blood, should be cleansed with soap and warm water. Skin antiseptics or moist towelettes can be used if soap and water are unavailable. Gloves should be made available to the staff when handling blood.

Table 12–1
Standard Precautions against HIV*

PRECAUTION	COMMENTS
Handwashing	Before and after contact with bodily fluids and after glove removal.
Gloves	When contact with bodily fluid is likely.
Masks/Eye protection	When splattering of bodily fluid is likely.
Nonsterile gown	To protect skin and clothing when splattering of bodily fluid is likely. Dispose of properly for cleaning.
Surface cleaning	Thoroughly clean exposed surfaces with removal of bodily fluids. Disinfect with bleach (1:10 or 1:100 dilution in water).

*Should be practiced in and out of the hospital setting.

Surfaces visibly contaminated with blood should be disinfected with a bleach solution of 1 part bleach to 100 parts water, or 1 tablespoon bleach in a quart of water and allowed to dry before reusing. All young athletes should receive counseling regarding the risk of HIV, especially surrounding sexual behavior and drug use. Should they elect to be tested for HIV, those test results should be maintained with confidentiality. The infected athlete need not be excluded from participation.[60] Special note should be made of the risk of HIV transmission associated with the illicit use of anabolic steroids or other performance-enhancing drugs. Many of these drugs are injected, and athletes may share needles, thereby increasing their risk. Several documented cases of HIV transmission have been attributed to this behavior.[62,63]

Hospital

Health care settings routinely involve the use of needles and other sharp objects. One study investigated the frequency, circumstances, and management of sharp-object injuries in a children's hospital and found that 6 injuries per 100 employees per year were reported. Not surprisingly, these injuries occurred most commonly in the patient room (27%), operating room (25%), and intensive care unit (17%). Most often these accidents involved needles or other procedural devices, and they usually occurred before disposal of the device. However, 20% involved loose sharps found discarded in linen or trash receptacles.[64] As stated previously, injuries from needles contaminated with blood of a patient with HIV are associated with a risk of transmission of approximately 0.3%, although case-controlled studies among health care workers have indicated that there are factors independently associated with increased risk of transmission of HIV. These include deep injury, such as an intramuscular inoculation; large volume of blood, as from a large-bore hollow needle; and high titer of HIV in the inoculum, as would be the case when the source patient has advanced disease with high viral titer.

Children are present in hospitals both as patients and as visitors and are subject to exposures that could place them at risk for HIV infection. The epidemiologic frequency of such exposures has not been well studied, but there are scattered reports of children who were inadvertently exposed to the blood of infected individuals in the health care setting. At our hospital, we were asked to provide consultation regarding postexposure prophylaxis in the case of a poorly supervised young child who climbed on a chair and put his hand into a sharps box while his mother was receiving a gynecologic examination in the same room. The CDC has also received a case report of a child who bit through a glass blood sample tube filled with blood from an adult patient with a history of injection drug use but unknown HIV status. The child suffered lacerations to the oral mucosa.[65] In addition, there have been instances of children receiving needlestick injuries in the hospital from improperly discarded needles in a treatment room. The management of HIV exposure and advisability of postexposure prophylaxis is discussed later in this chapter.

Guidelines to reduce the risk for transmission of all blood-borne and other pathogens in medical facilities have been developed and recently revised. They may also be applied to all settings other than medical facilities. Once referred to as Universal Precautions, they have been renamed Standard Precautions. They are briefly summarized in Table 12–1 and their implementation is expanded upon later in this chapter.[66]

Children with HIV infection and without other potentially contagious illness need not be isolated from other children in the hospital setting, but gloves should be used when contact with bodily fluids is anticipated, including blood, secretions, excretions, mucous membranes, and broken skin. When symptoms are present that may indicate an illness caused by an agent transmitted by the fecal-oral route, or when blood is present in stool, gloves should, of course, be used. Masks and eye protection should be used when splattering of bodily fluid is likely, and nonsterile gowns should be used to protect skin and clothing in this circumstance.

Sharp objects such as needles should be kept out of the reach of small children, and needles and other articles that come into contact with blood should be disposed of in tamper-proof containers out of the reach of children. Infection control material should be made available in all settings in case of the need to handle blood or bodily fluids, and all personnel should be educated as to its use. Exposed surfaces should be thoroughly cleaned. Blood and other bodily fluids should be removed with a disinfectant-containing bleach. Toys that are shared with other children should also be wiped down with disinfectant solution on a regular basis and allowed to dry before being used again. Handwashing remains the key to good infection control. It prevents the spread of all potential pathogens.

Additional considerations are needed for delivery rooms, emergency rooms, and operating rooms, where the potential for exposure to blood and bloody fluids is greatest. Accumulated data from several studies conducted by the CDC show that cutaneous, mucous membrane, and percutaneous blood contact was reported during 30% of vaginal deliveries, 4% of emergency room procedures, and 30% of surgeries.[67–69] In the delivery room, barrier precautions should be used, including eye protection, masks, gloves, and gowns when touching the placenta and when handling the newborn, until blood and amniotic fluid have been washed from the infant's skin. In the nursery, gloves should be worn for umbilical cord care. Infants born to HIV-infected mothers do not need to be isolated.

In the emergency room and intensive care unit, gloves, gowns, and puncture-resistant containers must be easily accessible for emergency situations. There has been no documentation of HIV transmission from mouth to mouth resuscitation, but to minimize the need for this procedure, mouthpieces, resuscitation bags, and other ventilation devices should be easily available for use. To prevent percutaneous injuries during suturing, instruments rather than fingers should be used to manipulate tissue being sutured.

MANAGEMENT OF OCCUPATIONAL HIV EXPOSURES AND THE USE OF POSTEXPOSURE PROPHYLAXIS

Health care workers are no more immune from anxiety than the general public. Few issues have created as much concern in the workplace as did the introduction of HIV and AIDS. Early in the HIV epidemic, the risk of occupational HIV infection of health care workers became apparent. One health care worker who had seroconverted to HIV after a needlestick accident wrote a moving account about the experience and the lack of support he found on the part of hospital administration.[70] This account led to further fear on the part of the general population of health care providers. Some individuals called for a "zero risk" tolerance for occupational HIV infection. Now, 20 years after the onset of the epidemic, our understanding of occupational risks and reasonable strategies to reduce transmission has lessened the number of health care workers who resist caring for infected patients. Accidents do happen, however, and it is important that all institutions have a policy on the management of HIV exposures. A key part of management is postexposure prophylaxis (PEP) with antiretroviral medications.

The premise underlying the use of PEP is that chemoprophylaxis during a window of opportunity may prevent initial cellular infection and local propagation of HIV and thus allow the host's immune defenses to eliminate the inoculum of virus. In the case of needlestick exposures, epidermal Langerhans cells or dermal dendritic cells present virus or viral antigens to T lymphocytes, natural killer cells, and other immune cells.[71] Sexual exposure to HIV through a mucosal surface is not completely analogous but may involve similar host responses.

In the simian model of intravaginal infection, simian immunodeficiency virus (SIV) is taken up by Langerhans cells and macrophages in the lamina propria underlying the epithelium. Within several days, these cells migrate to the regional lymph nodes. Infected T cells and free virus leave the lymph nodes and can be detected in the peripheral blood within 5 days of exposure. As is true for occupational exposures, injection drug exposures usually involve the transcutaneous inoculation of a very small volume of blood, although drug exposure via injection use may also involve direct intravenous injection. Even when the local cutaneous defenses are bypassed, antiretroviral therapy may be able to abort infection by minimizing viral replication.[72]

Other animal studies provide indirect evidence of the efficacy of antiretroviral drugs as agents for postexposure prophylaxis. In most studies, zidovudine (ZDV) was the antiretroviral agent used.[73–77] In more recent animal studies, however, newer agents have also been reported to be effective.[78,79] Data from these remain difficult to interpret, in part because of problems identifying an appropriate model for humans. Most animal studies use a much higher inoculum for exposure than would be expected in cases of human needlestick injury. Choice of viral strain, route of inoculation, timing of prophylaxis initiation, and choice of drug regimen make application of these results to humans of limited utility. Among the animal studies that have showed efficacy of pre-exposure or postexposure prophylaxis, reported outcomes have included suppression of viremia, inhibited viral replication adequate to permit formation of a long-lasting protective cellular immune response, and definitive prevention of infection.[80,81] Studies have demonstrated that early initiation of PEP and small inoculum size are correlates of successful outcome following an experimental exposure. ZDV initiated 1 hour or 24 hours after intravenous exposure to a rapidly lethal variant of SIV in pigtailed macaques prevented infection in one of three animals and modified SIV disease in three of six animals, respectively. PEP initiated at 72 hours had no effect.[82] In another experiment, macaque monkeys were administered either ZDV or another experimental drug called BEA-005 1 to 72 hours after challenge with intravenous SIV. Earlier initiation of PEP was correlated with delayed onset and peak of antigenemia, decreased duration of antigenemia, and reduction in SIV serum titer. The most potent effect was seen when PEP was initiated within 8 hours of exposure.[83] Other studies in primate, murine, and feline animal models have demonstrated that larger inocula decrease prophylactic efficacy.[84] In addition, delaying initiation, shortening the duration, or decreasing the antiretroviral dose of PEP, individually or in combination, decreased prophylactic efficacy.

The first documented human evidence showing that prophylaxis for HIV could prevent infection came from the National Institutes of Health–sponsored AIDS Clinical Trial Group Study ACTG 076, which showed that the use of ZDV was associated with a reduction in perinatal transmission.[85] Efficacy was explained by a prophylactic effect in the fetus or newborn. It was also shown that antiretroviral prophylaxis could prevent SIV infection in macaque monkeys.[86] Not long after, a case-controlled study published in the *New England Journal of Medicine* indicated that health care workers who received ZDV after percutaneous exposure to HIV-infected blood had a reduced risk of seroconversion.[28] In March of 1996, the CDC and National Foundation for Infectious Diseases convened a workshop in Atlanta entitled "HIV Postexposure Management for Healthcare Workers." Participants believed that there was sufficient evidence to recommend PEP after those occupational exposures associated with increased risk.[87] Although it would be optimal to formally study the efficacy of PEP in the occupational setting, this is not likely to be done. A nationwide prospective trial of ZDV administration after percutaneous HIV exposure among health care workers was discontinued because so few had enrolled during the first year.[88] Nevertheless, information from a variety of sources suggests that PEP may be efficacious in aborting the infection, and this is thought to remain biologically plausible. In the retrospective case-controlled study of health care workers, after controlling for other risk factors for HIV infection, the risk for HIV transmission among health care workers who used ZDV as postexposure prophylaxis was reduced by approximately 81% (95% CI, 43–94).[28]

Choice of the best combination of antiretroviral agents for prophylactic treatment also needs to be inferred from the literature available. Several agents from at least three classes of drugs are currently available for the treatment of HIV disease.[89] These include the nucleoside analogue reverse transcriptase inhibitors, non-nucleoside reverse transcriptase inhibitors, and protease inhibitors. Among these drugs, however, ZDV is the best studied agent shown to prevent HIV transmission in humans.[85] Although no data are available for postexposure prophylaxis, clinical data show that even in the presence of genotypic evidence of maternal ZDV resistance, this nucleoside reverse transcriptase inhibitor successfully prevented perinatal transmission.[90] These data have helped ZDV become the first drug of choice for PEP regimens.

There are no data to directly support the addition of other antiretroviral drugs to ZDV to enhance the efficacy of the PEP regimen. In HIV-infected patients, however, combination regimens have proved superior to monotherapy in reducing HIV viral load.[89] Thus, at least theoretically, a combination of drugs whose activity comes at different stages in the viral replication cycle could offer an additive preventive effect in PEP. This is of particular importance with regard to exposures that may pose an increased risk for transmission.

The choice and number of specific agents to use, or when to alter the PEP regimen, remains empiric. Guidelines for the treatment of early HIV infection recommend the use of three drugs (two nucleoside reverse transcriptase inhibitors and a protease inhibitor), although their importance in prophylaxis is unknown.[91] The use of a highly potent regimen can be theoretically justified for exposures that pose increased risk, but it remains unclear whether the potential additional toxicity of a third drug is justified for lower risk circumstances. The United States Public Health Service (USPHS) has issued guidelines that include two- and three-drug PEP regimens that are based on the presumed level of risk for HIV transmission. This estimate of risk is based partly on the type of exposure and the characteristics of the exposure as described earlier in this chapter. These are summarized in Figure 12–1. In addition, in the case of a needlestick when the HIV status of the source patient is unknown, one must estimate the likelihood of transmission. The guidelines adapted from the USPHS also are shown here in Figure 12–2 and Table 12–2. Taken together, recommendations can be made for the individual as to the level of risk and the prophylaxis that should be instituted.

The choice of ZDV and lamivudine has been recommended as a good combination for use in PEP regimens based on greater antiretroviral activity

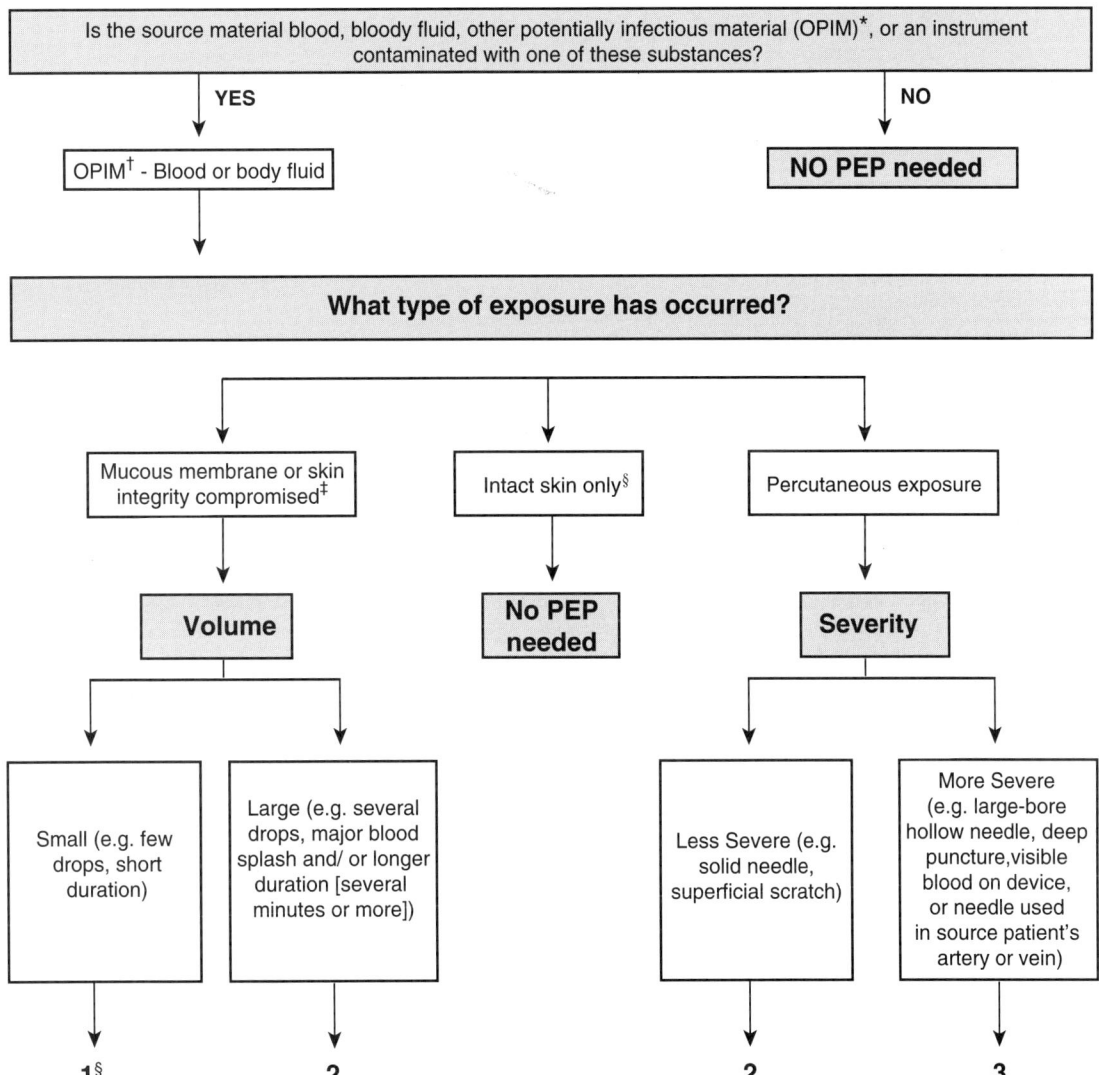

Figure 12–1. Estimation of the risk of an occupatinal exposure to HIV.

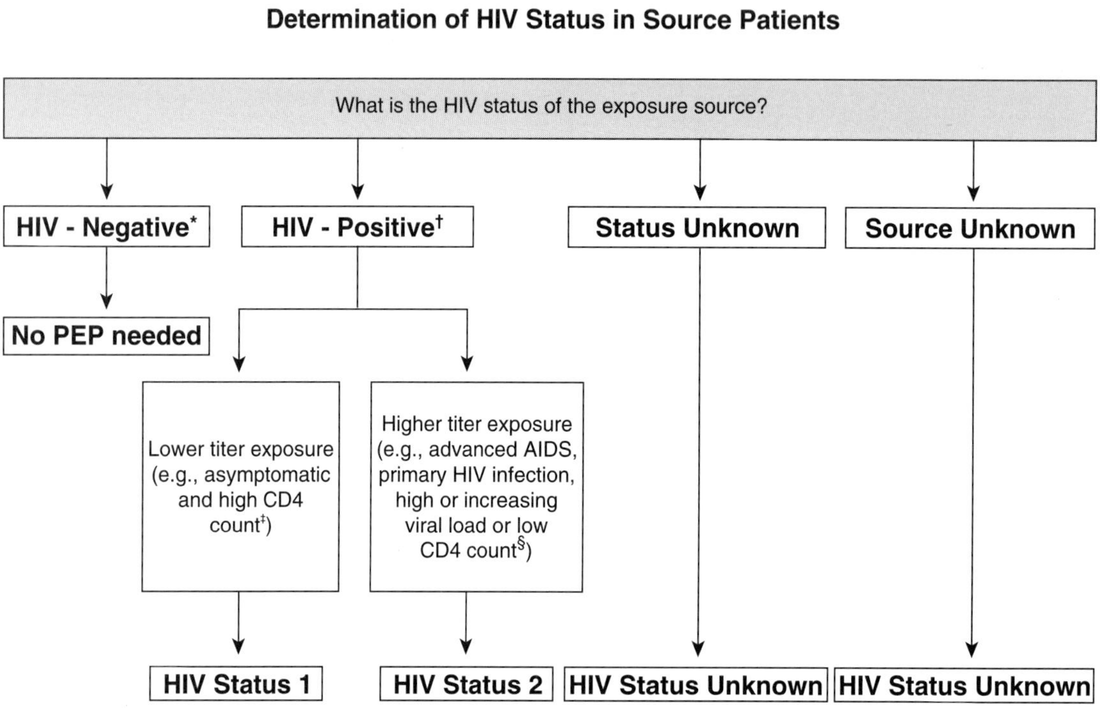

Determination of HIV Status in Source Patients

```
What is the HIV status of the exposure source?
   │            │              │                │
   ▼            ▼              ▼                ▼
HIV-Negative*  HIV-Positive†  Status Unknown   Source Unknown
   │            │
   ▼            │
No PEP needed   │
                ├──────────────┐
                ▼              ▼
          Lower titer     Higher titer exposure
          exposure        (e.g., advanced AIDS,
          (e.g., asymptomatic  primary HIV infection,
          and high CD4    high or increasing
          count‡)         viral load or low
                          CD4 count§)
                │              │              │              │
                ▼              ▼              ▼              ▼
          HIV Status 1   HIV Status 2   HIV Status Unknown   HIV Status Unknown
```

*Semen or vaginal secretions; cerebrospinal, synovial, pleural, peritoneal, pericardial, or amniotic fluids; or tissue.
†Exposure to OPIM must be evaluated on a case-by-case basis. In general, these body substances are considered a low risk for transmission in health care settings. Any unprotected contact with concentrated HIV in a research laboratory or production facility is considered an occupational exposure that rquires clinical evaluation to determine the need for postexposure prophylaxis (PEP).
‡Skin integrity is considered compromised if there is evidence of chapped skin, dermatitis, abrasion, or open wound.
§Contact with intact skin is not normally considered a risk for HIV transmission. However, if the exposure was to blood, and the circumstance suggests a higher volume exposure (e.g., an extensive area of skin was exposed or there was prolonged contact with blood), the risk for HIV transmission should be considered.
¶The combination of these severity factors (eg, large-bore hollow needle *and* deep puncture) contribute to an elevated risk for transmission if the source person is HIV-positive.
(*Adapted from* Centers for Disease Control and Prevention: Public health service guidelines for the management of healthcare workers' exposure to HIV and recommendations for postexposure prophylaxis. MMWR 1998;37:14.)

Figure 12-2. Determination of HIV status in source patients.

and activity against many ZDV-resistant strains without the addition of substantial toxicity. Data also suggest that ZDV-resistant mutations develop more slowly in patients receiving the combination. In vitro studies indicate that the mutation associated with lamivudine resistance may be associated with the reversal of ZDV phenotypic resistance. In addition, the two agents are available in a combination formulation (Combivir, Glaxo Wellcome, North Carolina) and so is more convenient for the patient. Individual clinicians may prefer other combinations of antiretroviral agents, based on their local knowledge of the specific viral characteristics of the source individual.

Indinavir was chosen as the recommended protease inhibitor for the PEP regimen by the USPHS, because of its good bioavailability. However, many clinicians have turned to nelfinavir due to the superior tolerability, especially as it refers to the gastrointestinal symptomatology. In spite of the level of understanding and knowledge on the part of the health care provider, several studies have documented poor compliance with the drug regimen on the part of exposed health care workers because of the toxicity experienced.[92] It may be important to choose the simplest and most easily tolerated regimen, except when the risk is perceived to be the greatest.[93] Based on the level of risk, basic and expanded regimens of antiretroviral agents are outlined in Table 12-3.

Hospitals and other health care organizations should have written protocols available to their personnel outlining the importance of prompt reporting, evaluation, counseling, treatment, and

Table 12-2
Determination of HIV Status in Source Patients

RISK	HIV STATUS	POSTEXPOSURE PROPHYLAXIS (PEP) RECOMMENDATION
1	1	PEP may not be warranted. Exposure type does not pose a known risk for HIV transmission. Whether the risk for drug toxicity outweighs the benefit of PEP should be decided by the exposed health care worker and treating clinician.
1	2	Consider basic regimen. Exposure type poses a negligible risk for HIV transmission. A high HIV titer in the source may justify consideration of PEP. Whether the risk for drug toxicity outweighs the benefit of PEP should be decided by the exposed health care worker and treating clinician.
2	1	Recommend basic regimen. Most HIV exposures are in this category: no increased risk for HIV transmission has been observed, but use of PEP is appropriate.
2	2	Recommend expanded regimen. Exposure type represents an increased HIV transmission risk.
3	1 or 2	Recommend expanded regimen. Exposure type represents an increased HIV transmission risk.
Unknown	Unknown	If the source or, in the case of an unknown source, the setting where exposure occurred suggests a possible risk for HIV exposure and the exposure score is 2 or 3, consider PEP basic regimen (See Table 12-1).

Adapted from Centers for Disease Control and Prevention: Public health service guidelines for the management of healthcare workers' exposure to HIV and recommendations for postexposure prophylaxis. MMWR 1998;47:14.

follow-up of occupational exposures that may place the health care worker at risk for acquiring HIV or any blood-borne pathogen. Access to clinicians who can provide postexposure care should be available during all working hours, including nights and weekends. Antiretroviral agents for PEP should be available for timely administration, and persons responsible for providing the counseling should be familiar with evaluation, treatment, and follow-up protocols. The health care worker should report immediately after the exposure occurs, since PEP is most likely to be effective if implemented as soon after the exposure as possible. Most experts believe that prophylaxis should be initiated within several hours of the exposure, and many attempt to administer the first dose within 60 minutes. Information collected should include the date and time of exposure and other details, including the type and amount of the fluid or material and the severity of the exposure. For a percutaneous exposure, important details include depth of injury and whether the fluid was injected. For a skin or mucous membrane exposure, important details include the estimated volume of material, duration of contact, and condition of the skin. If possible, the source patient should be tested for HIV and other blood-borne pathogens if he or she consents, so that PEP can be discontinued or altered to directly address the characteristics of the viral exposure. Situations in which the source patient is

Table 12-3
Basic and Expanded Regimens for Occupational Postexposure Prophylaxis

REGIMEN CATEGORY	APPLICATION	DRUG REGIMEN
Basic	Occupational HIV exposures for which there is a recognized transmission risk	4 weeks (28 days) of both zidovudine 600 mg every day (i.e., 300 mg twice a day, 200 mg 3x a day, or 100 mg q 4hrs), and lamivudine 150 mg twice a day
Expanded	Occupational HIV exposures that pose an increased risk for transmission (e.g., larger volume of blood and/or higher virus titer in blood)	Basic regimen plus either indinavir 800 mg every 8 hours or nelfinavir 750 mg 3x a day*

*Indinavir should be taken on an empty stomach and with increased fluid consumption (six 8 oz. glasses of water throughout the day); nelfinavir should be taken with meals.

either unknown or of unknown HIV serologic status do occur. Institutional policies must address this issue and must take into account the local and state laws regarding HIV serologic testing.[93] All parts of the management program should keep strict employee confidentiality. In addition, counselors should keep in mind at all times that the exposed individual may be exceedingly anxious and that information might have to be presented multiple times. Even medically sophisticated health care providers have been known to panic when they become victim of a serious needlestick injury.[94]

The actual role that "first aid" has in the reduction of HIV transmission remains unclear, but it seems reasonable that basic first aid techniques should be instituted. Wounds and skin sites should be washed with soap and water or an available disinfectant solution such as iodophor or chlorhexidine, and mucous membranes should be flushed with water. There is no evidence that expressing blood or fluid by squeezing the wound reduces the risk for HIV transmission. The application of caustic agents such as bleach or the injection of antiseptics or disinfectants into the wound is not recommended.

MANAGEMENT OF NONOCCUPATIONAL EXPOSURES TO HIV

The probability of HIV infection from puncture by a contaminated needle is similar to that estimated for a single episode of unprotected receptive anal or vaginal intercourse with an infected partner, or for a single episode of injection drug use with HIV-contaminated equipment.[2,29] HIV has been recovered from syringes maintained at room temperature in excess of 4 weeks.[31] Although the prevalence of HIV in perpetrators of sexual assault is unknown, HIV transmission after rape has been documented.[95] The utility for postexposure prophylaxis for exposures through these routes but outside of the occupational setting has not been adequately studied.[95]

Although the CDC have published recommendations for occupational HIV PEP, no such definitive guidelines for PEP in the nonoccupational setting exist, owing to a lack of efficacy and safety data. Such trials may not be feasible, however. The low frequency of HIV infection after a single exposure means that several thousand participants would be needed for a treatment effect to be demonstrated. Since the efficacy of postexposure prophylaxis among health care workers has been documented, it may not be ethical to enroll subjects in a placebo-controlled trial.

Meanwhile, treatment of people exposed through sexual contact has become commonplace, if not routine, in centers around the country.[96] Some practitioners worry that the availability of postexposure prophylaxis may increase high-risk behavior and promote resistance to antiretroviral drugs. These arguments have seemed less persuasive with regard to the pediatric population with needlestick accidents in nonoccupational settings. The effect of antiretroviral prophylaxis on the resistance of virus in the community continues to be a concern, however.

Very limited information is available concerning the use of HIV PEP in children and adolescents, following either sexual abuse or accidental needlestick. One small series was reported by our group at Boston Medical Center and Boston University School of Medicine. In the interest of eliminating the dichotomy between management of occupational and non-occupational HIV exposures, PEP was offered to children and adolescents initially on a case-by-case basis, then based on a formal departmental policy. The use of HIV PEP in this population produced a considerable management challenge. Only 25% of the children finished the entire 4-week course of prophylaxis. Financial concerns over the cost of the medications, drug tolerability, and psychiatric and substance abuse issues as well as the degree of parental involvement in medical decisions influenced whether PEP and clinical follow-up were completed.[54] The use of postexposure prophylaxis in this setting requires a coordinated effort at the initial presentation to the health care system and at each follow-up visit. These difficulties must be considered before prophylaxis is initiated, and the decision as to whether to implement prophylaxis as well as the choice of the drug regimen should be based on the specific circumstances.

Our group at Boston University undertook a survey of hospital pediatric infectious disease and emergency medicine training programs in the United States and Canada and found that fewer than 25% of the groups responding reported institutional policies for nonoccupational HIV PEP. Infectious disease experts were more comfortable recommending PEP for needlestick or sexual assault scenarios than their emergency medicine colleagues, but there was considerable variation in timing, duration of prophylaxis used, and choice of antiretroviral drugs. Approximately 65% of the responders would offer or recommend HIV PEP for children and adolescents within 24 hours after exposure. There is clearly a need for a national consensus for the use of PEP in cases of nonoccupational HIV exposure.[96]

General considerations regarding the level of risk following nonoccupational exposure to HIV are listed in Table 12–4. They include the type of intercourse, use of condom, bleeding or trauma, and the presence of associated ulcers in either victim or assailant.

The potential benefit of preventing HIV infection needs to be balanced against the potential drug toxicities of the therapy and the limited safety and efficacy data available.[97] Additional considerations are the difficulty of maintaining compliance throughout the course of therapy, the need for close follow-up, and the high cost of therapy. If the HIV status of the assailant can be determined or is known, decisions are more easily made. Psychological support in the emergency department should be provided by a medical social worker or psychiatric nurse familiar with crisis intervention. HIV-related community resources as well as transition to follow-up need to be addressed. Follow-up should be with a physician comfortable with the use of antiretroviral drugs in children and adolescents. Other considerations in victims of sexual assault will not be discussed in detail in this chapter but include forensic evidence collection and both testing and prophylaxis for sexually transmitted diseases other than HIV.

Factors leading to increased transmission risk in cases of accidental needlestick injuries have already been mentioned in this chapter. As suggested in the Public Health Service guidelines for occupational exposures, HIV PEP should not be used for persons with low-risk exposures. Care for the child with accidental needlestick should also include wound care, assessment of tetanus and hepatitis B immunization status via testing, if necessary, and hepatitis C serology.

When it has been decided to use prophylactic antiretrovirals, they should be initiated as soon as possible after exposure, ideally within 1 to 2 hours after exposure, since declining efficacy is expected up to 72 hours. In an attempt to reduce the toxicity and thereby increase potential compliance with the complete duration of therapy, many centers have begun to use a dual-drug regimen of ZDV and lamivudine, leaving the addition of a protease inhibitor to the discretion of the emergency physician and the consulting infectious disease expert for especially high-risk situations. Baseline HIV testing should be performed, as many patients at risk for HIV have not been recently tested, and patients found to be already HIV infected will require ongoing therapy rather than a brief course for prophylaxis. In addition, baseline liver function tests and complete blood count will help in management and follow-up. These laboratory evaluations should be performed again in follow-up at 2 and 4 weeks. In the adolescent, a pregnancy test should be considered. Although antiretroviral drugs have been used in infected pregnant women without significant negative effects on the fetus, decisions as to the use of HIV PEP in uninfected pregnant women should be discussed with a physician with special expertise in this area. In addition, the risk of vertical transmission of HIV is significantly increased when seroconversion occurs during gestation, and the choice of a prophylactic regimen may vary given this additional risk. These guidelines are provided in Table 12–5.

Most experts agree that if postexposure prophylaxis is to work, it must be administered as soon as possible after the exposure. Public health campaigns that encourage clients to seek medical care within hours after an exposure could help. This has been hampered by the fear that false reassurance because of available prophylaxis could encourage risky behavior. It is important that public health

Table 12–4
Factors Associated with Increased HIV Exposure Risk

Sexual Assault
Intercourse: anal receptive > vaginal receptive > insertive anal, insertive vaginal > oral receptive
Lack of condom use
Ulcers, bleeding, trauma
Source patient with higher titer virus or advanced disease
Needle stick injury
Deep injury
Large-bore hollow needle
Visible blood on needle
Needle placed directly in vein or artery
Source patient with titer virus or advanced disease

Table 12–5
Suggested Regimens for HIV Postexposure Prophylaxis (PEP) After Nonoccupational Exposure of Children and Adolescents

Drug Regimen for PEP (4 weeks)

Age	Drug	Dose	Major Toxicities
< 12 Years	Zidovudine	160 mg/m^2 (max 300 mg/dose) tid	Hematologic toxicity, headache
	Lamivudine	4 mg/kg (max 150 mg/dose) bid	Headaches, abdominal complaints, rash, pancreatitis (rare)
> 12 Years	Zidovudine	300 mg bid	
	Lamivudine 4 or Combivir tab	150 mg (lamivudine) or 1 tab (Combivir) bid for either	
	Consider addition of nelfinavir for high risk exposures	25–30 mg/kg (750 mg in older children and adults) q8h	Diarrhea, vomiting, headaches

Baseline Laboratory Tests
Testing in emergency department (HIV related)
HIV serology
Liver function test
Complete blood count
Pregnancy testing (if appropriate)

---

messages be placed in the context of overall programs of health promotion and risk reduction.

CONSIDERATIONS FOR INFECTION CONTROL IN HOSPITAL, SCHOOL, AND DAY CARE

The specific immune defects resulting from HIV infection leaves many infected children particularly susceptible to other infectious diseases. These include opportunistic infections as well as more severe cases of infection with common childhood bacterial, viral, and parasitic pathogens. These secondary pathogens may be passed to other children without HIV infection. Although it is impossible to protect a child from all infectious diseases, health care providers should set as a goal the minimization of this risk.

Guidelines to reduce the risk of transmission of all blood-borne and other pathogens in medical facilities have been developed and recently revised. They may be applied to settings other than medical facilities as well. Once referred to as Universal Precautions,[98] they have been renamed Standard Precautions. The development of Standard Precautions[66] was intended to update the recommendations for all patients without regard to their HIV status.

Recommendations for required isolation for an established diagnosis were divided into three categories based on the mode of transmission: droplet, contact, and airborne. In addition, recommendations are offered requiring temporary implementation of precautions until a definitive diagnosis is made. Table 12–6 summarizes the recommendations in addition to the standard precautions for infections based on the mode of transmission.[99] Although these standard precautions have been recommended for hospital-based practice, application of these guidelines can be useful for the care of children outside the hospital as well.

Handwashing

Handwashing has long been known to be one of the most effective means of preventing the transmission of pathogens.[100] Hands should be washed before and after contact with bodily fluids and after removing gloves. In the day care setting, children should wash their hands upon arrival and departure, before and after eating, after using the toilet or having their diapers changed, after playing on the playground or handling pets, pet cages, or other pet objects, and when hands are visibly soiled. Similarly, providers should be expected to wash their hands upon arrival to and departure from work, before and after handling food, after using or assisting a child in using the toilet or changing dia-

Table 12–6
Transmission-Based Precautions for Hospitalized Patients*

CATEGORY OF PRECAUTIONS	SINGLE ROOM	MASKS	GOWNS	GLOVES
AIRBORNE	Yes, with negative air-pressure ventilation	Yes	No	No
DROPLET	Yes†	Yes, for persons close to patient	No	No
CONTACT	Yes†	No	Yes	Yes

*These recommendations are in addition to the Standard Precautions used for all patients.
†Preferred but not required. Cohorting of children infected with the same pathogen is acceptable.

pers. In addition, providers should wash their hands after contacting a child's bodily fluid, including diapers, runny noses, spit, vomit, and so on, as well as before giving any medication to a child. Even when gloves are used, hands should be washed immediately. The use of gloves alone will not prevent contamination of hands and should not be viewed as a substitute for handwashing.

Gloves

Gloves should be used when contact with bodily fluids is anticipated. The use of gloves has been controversial with regard to exposure to breastmilk, although both the CDC and the American Academy of Pediatrics (AAP) suggest that gloves be worn by health care workers in situations in which exposure to breastmilk might be frequent (such as in breastmilk banks).[2,101] The AAP also notes some other exceptions to using gloves. It has stated that gloves are not necessary for diaper changes, wiping tears, or blowing noses of children in the hospital, although it encourages their use to minimize the transmission of other pathogens and emphasizes the extreme importance of handwashing when gloves are not used.[102]

Masks, Eye Protection, and Gowns

Masks, eye protection, and nonsterile gowns should be used to protect skin, clothing, and eyes if splashes of blood or infected bodily fluids are possible.

Surface Cleaning

All exposed surfaces should be thoroughly cleaned. Blood and other bodily fluids should be removed with the use of a disinfectant containing bleach solution. (See previous sections on day care, athletic injuries, and school accidents on making a bleach-containing disinfectant.) Toys that are shared with other children should be wiped down with disinfectant solution on a regular basis and allowed to dry.[103] Sharp objects, of course, should be kept out of the reach of children, and needles and other articles that come into contact with blood should be disposed of in tamper-proof containers out of the reach of children.[104] Disinfectants and other infection control materials should be made easily available in all settings in case of an emergency need to handle blood or other bodily fluids, but they should be kept out of the immediate reach of young children.

PRECAUTIONS FOR EXPOSURE TO COMMUNICABLE DISEASES OTHER THAN HIV

As stated previously, precautions for exposure to communicable diseases other than HIV have been divided into categories based on the transmission mode for each pathogen. In addition to the standard precautions for preventing blood and bodily fluid exposure among patients in hospitals, transmission-based precautions have been developed for "patients with documented, or suspected to be infected with, highly transmissible or epidemiologically important pathogens for which additional precautions" are needed.[98] These precautions have been combined with others specifically developed for HIV-infected patients and children to give guidance to protect children in out-of-hospital settings.[65,99,103] These are summarized in Table 12–7. The more stringent precautions for day care centers in comparison to schools stems from the higher likelihood of person-to-person spread of pathogens causing gastroenteritis and viral respiratory disease among the younger children who attend these programs. The principles behind these precautions also may be applicable in

TABLE 12-7
Exercise of Precautions for Exposure to Common Infections at Different Locations*

ORGANISM/INFECTION	HOSPITAL†	SCHOOL?	DAY CARE?	COMMENTS
Candida	None	No	No	Ubiquitous, cannot avoid
Cytomegalovirus	None	No	No	Ubiquitous, cannot avoid
Coccidioidomycosis	None	No	No	No person-to-person transmission
Cryptococcus	None	No	No	No person-to-person transmission
Cryptosporidia	Contact	No	Yes	Child with diarrhea should be excluded from day care
Epstein-Barr virus	None	No	No	Ubiquitous
Haemophilus influenzae type b	Droplet	No	No	Prophylaxis of contacts‡
Hepatitis B	None	No	Yes	Avoid biting and blood contact‡
Histoplasmosis	None	No	No	No person-to-person transmission
Herpes simplex	Contact	No	Yes	Exclude child with mouth sores and drooling
Influenza	Droplet	No	No	Common in winter
Isospora hominis	Contact	No	Yes	Pathogenicity negligible in immunocompetent children
Mycobacterium avium-intracellulare	None	No	No	No person-to-person transmission
Measles	Airborne	Yes	Yes	Exclude child until resolved‡
Pertussis	Droplet	Yes§	Yes§	Exclude child until treated‡
Pneumococcus	None	No	No	Ubiquitous in normal children
Pneumocystis carinii	None	No	No	Ubiquitous, cannot avoid
Respiratory syncytial virus	Contact	No	No	Common in winter/spring
Rotavirus	Contact	No	Yes	Child with diarrhea should be excluded from day care, wash hands
Salmonella	Contact	No	Yes	Infected child should be excluded until three stools are negative
Staphylococcus	Contact	Yes‡	Yes‡	Exclude child until resolved
Streptococcus	Contact	Yes‡	Yes‡	High rate of carriage among children
Syphilis	Contact	No	No	Should have been treated in infancy
Toxoplasma	None	No	No	No person-to-person transmission
Tuberculosis	Airborne	Yes	Yes	Exercise precautions until treated
Varicella-zoster virus	Airborne and Contact	Yes	Yes	Exclude child until lesions scabbed

*These are general guidelines; other infection control considerations may apply in certain situations.
†Recommendations from Pickering LK (ed): Red Book: Report of the Committee on Infectious Diseases, 25th ed. Elk Grove Village, IL, American Academy of Pediatrics, 2000, pp. 119-136.
‡Immunization recommended for all children.
§Precautions can be discontinued once the patient has been on therapy at least 24 hours.
Adapted from Chanock SJ, Donowitz LG, Simonds RJ: Medical issues related to provision of care for the HIV-infected child in the hospital, home, day care, school, and community. In: Pizzo PA, Wilfert CM (eds). Pediatric AIDS: The Challenge of HIV Infection in Infants, Children, and Adolescents, 3rd ed. Baltimore, Williams & Wilkins, 1998, p. 655.

other settings, such as family gatherings, summer camps, or recreational facilities.

Most opportunistic infections cannot be prevented by protecting against person-to-person exposure because they are carried by the immunocompromised hosts themselves. On the other hand, many of the pathogens that infect children with HIV infection are prevalent among all children in the community. In most cases, because these organisms are ubiquitous and because school, day care, and other social activities provide important advantages to the life of the infected child, children with HIV infection would not greatly benefit by exclusion merely to avoid these exposures. Many infections can be prevented or ameliorated by active or passive immunization. These are discussed in another chapter of this book, but the importance of either pre- or postexposure immunization or prophylaxis cannot be overemphasized.

Infection Control and Specific Conditions

Although standard precautions as described will protect the transmission of those pathogens carried by blood and bodily fluids, some infections require additional precautions based on their mode of transmission and the likelihood of infecting other susceptible individuals.

Gastrointestinal and Respiratory Infections

Acute gastrointestinal illnesses are common in children and often are highly contagious. They may be especially severe in the HIV-infected child and may be harbored in higher titer. Since most enteric pathogens that cause diarrhea are readily transmissible, especially among children in diapers, it is advisable to exclude these children from group day care until the diarrhea has abated, regardless of the HIV status of the ill child. During an outbreak of diarrheal illness in either day care or school, there should be emphasis on handwashing so as to decrease the frequency of transmission. The HIV-infected child may continue to shed the organism for a longer duration than others. This prolonged infectivity should be considered when applying infection control precautions.

Young children in day care are also commonly infected with respiratory viral infections, such as respiratory syncytial virus, parainfluenza, influenza, or rhinovirus. Children with HIV infection and severe immunocompromise may be more prone to the consequences of these infections. In addition, they may shed the offending virus longer than the HIV-uninfected individual and so should be carefully evaluated before a recommendation for attendance in group settings is made by the pediatrician.

Measles is both very contagious and may result in higher morbidity and mortality in children infected with HIV. All children with documented measles should be excluded from school or day care, and the HIV-infected contact should be referred for proper prophylaxis after either a one-time exposure or an ongoing outbreak in the community.

Varicella Zoster Virus Infections

Varicella is an extremely contagious virus, transmitted through the air, that efficiently infects susceptible contacts. Although many children now are receiving varicella zoster virus vaccine, it continues to be a problem for children with HIV and compromised immune function. These children may have more severe infection or may suffer chronic or recurrent infection.[105] Currently, only HIV-infected children with a relatively intact immune system may receive the vaccine, and its efficacy is less than in the uninfected child.

All children with acute varicella infection should be excluded from school or day care until all vesicles are crusted over. Hospitalized children with documented or suspected varicella infection should be placed into isolation immediately. Airborne and contact precautions should be instituted in addition to the standard precautions. Immunocompromised children exposed to varicella should receive varicella zoster immunoglobulin (VZIG) within 72 hours to prevent or minimize the severity of infection.[106] Those susceptible children exposed to varicella should be isolated from day 8 to day 21, if no passive immunization is given. The inoculation period should be extended to day 30 after the child receives VZIG, since it can prolong the incubation period.

Hepatitis B and C Viruses

Both hepatitis B and C are transmitted in ways similar to HIV. Children born with HIV may also be born to mothers with one or both of these viruses. All newborns should receive a complete hepatitis B vaccination series.[107] They should be serologically evaluated for immunity after vaccination is complete. Unfortunately, no vaccine is available for hepatitis C, and the risk for vertical transmission of hepatitis C is much higher if the mother is coinfected with HIV.[108] These children should be serially evaluated for infection and followed carefully if they are found to be positive. No special precautions are necessary for the day care center or school, since standard precautions should protect against transmission of hepatitis B and C.

Tuberculosis

Mycobacterium tuberculosis infection is acquired mainly by airborne transmission, and so isolation in the hospital setting is mandatory. Although pulmonary manifestations of tuberculosis are more common in adults, children should still be considered potentially contagious. Children without pulmonary manifestations are usually considered noninfectious unless the organisms could be aerosolized in another way, such as during a débridement procedure. Since the HIV-infected child may present with an atypical clinical picture and may be anergic to skin testing, the diagnosis may be delayed. Any child who is being evaluated for the possibility of tuberculosis should be placed in airborne isolation pending confirmation of the diagnosis, and precautions should be maintained until effective treatment has begun, cough has improved, and follow-up sputum smears are documented to be negative.

Outside of the hospital, children who are considered contagious should be restricted from school, day care, or other social functions until they are receiving chemotherapy, adherence to therapy is demonstrated, and the clinical symptoms have disappeared. Since children are usually infected by other close family members, all individuals in the household should be tested for tuberculosis infection or disease.

CONCLUSION

Children with HIV infection deserve the same rights to health care, privacy, and education as other children have. They can prosper from the same types of social interactions that other children are expected to enjoy. These interactions are important to the quality of life of both infected and uninfected children in the community.

Educated health care and child professionals can provide the necessary environment for all children to safely participate in community activities. It should not be expected that all HIV-infected children have been identified in the community setting, so the institution of standard precautions is of paramount importance. Although appropriate infection control precautions are universally applicable, exposure to particular pathogens may pose a special risk to HIV-infected children and must be managed in a timely fashion. For this reason, disclosure to the school or facility is encouraged; but it always remains a parental responsibility. With increasingly inclusive policies and welcoming environments, it can be expected that more parents will appropriately disclose confidential medical information to those who can use it to benefit the children in their care.

Occasionally, potentially dangerous exposures may occur in either the hospital setting or the community, and it is imperative that both health care and child care professionals understand the risks and are educated in the appropriate rapid response.

All children deserve a safe and welcoming environment, and, with the proper education and tools, both HIV-infected children and uninfected children can benefit from the educational experience provided by school and other community settings.

REFERENCES

1. AAP, Committee on Pediatric AIDS: HIV/AIDS in schools. Pediatrics 1998;101:933–935.
2. Centers for Disease Control and Prevention: Update: Universal precautions for prevention of human immunodeficiency virus, hepatitis B virus, and other bloodborne pathogens in health-care settings. MMWR 1988;37:377–382,387–388.
3. Dragic T, Litwin V, Allaway GP, et al: HIV-1 entry into CD4+ cells is mediated by the chemokine receptor CC-CKR-5. Nature 1996;381:667–673.
4. Fujikawa LS, Palestine AG, Nusenblatt RB, et al: Isolation of human T-lymphocyte virus type III from the tears of a patient with acquired immunodeficiency syndrome. Lancet 1985;2:529–530.
5. Yeung SC, Kazazi F, Randle CG, et al: Patients infected with human immunodeficiency virus type 1 have low levels of virus in saliva in the presence of periodontal disease. J Infec Dis 1993;167:803–809.
6. Ho DD, Schooley RE, Rota TR, et al: Isolation of HTLV-III from cerebrospinal fluid and neural tissues of patients with neurologic syndrome related to AIDS. N Engl J Med 1985;313:1493–1497.
7. Ho DD, Schooley RE, Rota TR, et al: HTLV-III in the semen and blood of a healthy homosexual man. Science 1984;226:451–453.
8. Thiry L, Sprecher-Goldberger S, Jonckheert T, et al: Isolation of AIDS virus from cell free breast milk of three healthy virus carriers. Lancet 1985;2:891–892.
9. Wormser GP, Bittker S, Forseter G, et al: Absence of infectious HIV type 1 in "natural" eccrine sweat. J Infect Dis 1992;165:135–138.
10. Kawashima H, Bandyopadhyay S, Rutstein R, Plotkin SA: Excretion of human immunodeficiency virus type 1 in the throat but not in urine by infected children. J Pediatric 1991;118:80–82.
11. Friedland G, Kahl P, Saltzman B, et al: Additional evidence for lack of transmission of HIV infection by close interpersonal (casual) contact. AIDS 1990;4:639–644.
12. Ho DD, Byington RE, Schooley RT, et al: Infrequency of isolation of HTLV-III virus from saliva in AIDS. N Engl J Med 1985;313:1606.
13. Stanley SK, Ostrowski MA, Justement JS, et al: Effect of immunization with a common recall antigen on viral expression in patients infected with HIV type 1. N Engl J Med 1996;334:1222–1230.
14. O'Connor TJ, Kinchington D, Kangro HO, Jeffries DJ: The activity of candidate virucidal agents, low

pH, and genital secretions against HIV-1 in vitro. Int J STD AIDS. 1995;6:267–272.
15. Willerford DM, Bwayo JJ, Hensel M, et al: HIV infection among high-risk seronegative prostitutes in Nairobi. J Infect Dis 1993;167:1414–1417.
15a. Vidmar L, Poljak M, Tomazic J, et al: Transmission of HIV-1 by human bite. Lancet 1996;347:1762.
16. Dean M, Carrington M, Winkler C, et al: Genetic restriction of HIV-1 infection and progression to AIDS by a deletion allete of the CKRS structural gene. Science 1996;273:1856–1862.
17. Menitove J (ed): Standards for Blood Banks and Transfusion Services, ed 19. Bethesda, American Association of Blood Banks, 1999.
18. Neal JJ, Fleming PL, Green TA, Ward JW: Trends in heterosexually acquired AIDS in the United States, 1988–1995. J Acquir Immune Def Syndr Hum Retrovirol 1997;14:465–474.
19. Anonymous: Needlestick transmission of HTLV-III from a patient infected in Africa. Lancet 1984;2:1376–1377.
20. DeGrurrola V, Seage GR, Mayer K, et al: Infectiousness of HIV between male homosexual partners. J Clin Epidemiol 1989;42:849–856.
21. Downs AM, de Vincenzi I: Probability of heterosexual transmission of HIV: Relationship to the number of unprotected sexual contacts. J Acquir Immune Defic Syndrome Hum Retrovirol 1996;11:388–395.
22. Mast EE, Goodman RA, Bond WW, et al: Transmission of bloodbourne pathogens during sports risk and prevention. Ann Intern Med 1995;122:283–285.
23. Peterman T, Stoneburner R, Allen JR, et al: Risk of HIV transmission from heterosexual adults with transfusion-associated infections. JAMA 1988;259:55–58.
24. Wiley J, Hershhom S, Padian NL: Heterogeneity in the probability of HIV transmission per sexual contact: The case of male to female transmission in penile-vaginal intercourse. Stat Med 1989;8:93–102.
25. Royce RA, Serata A, Cates W, Cohen M: Sexual transmission of HIV. N Engl J Med 1997;336:1072–1078.
26. Gerberding JL, Bryant-LeBlanc CE, Nelson K, et al: Risk of transmitting the human immunodeficiency virus, cytomegalovirus, and hepatitis B virus to health care workers exposed to patients with AIDS and AIDS-related conditions. J Infect Dis 1987;156:1–8.
27. Henderson DK, Fahey BJ, Willy M, et al: Risk for occupational transmission of human immunodeficiency virus type 1 (HIV-1) associated with clinical exposures. Ann Intern Med 1990;113:740–746.
28. Cardo D, Culver DH, Ciesielski CA, et al: A case-control study of HIV seroconversion in health care workers after percutaneous exposure. N Engl J Med 1997;337:1485–1490.
29. Kaplan EH, Heimer R: A model-based estimate of HIV infectivity via needle sharing. J Acquir Immune Defic Syndr 1992;5:116–118.
30. Kaplan EH: Modeling HIV infectivity: Must sex acts be counted? J Acquir Immune Defic Syndr 1990;3:55–61.
31. Abdala N, Stephens PC, Griffith BP, et al: Survival of HIV-1 in syringes. J Acquir Immune Defic Syndr Hum Retrovirol 1999;20:73–80.
32. AAP, Committee on Pediatric AIDS: Issues related to HIV transmission in schools, child care, medical settings, the home and community. Pediatrics 1999;104:318–324.
33. Kaplan JE, Oleske JM, Getchell JP, et al: Evidence against transmission of human T-lymphotrophic virus/lymphadenopathy-associated virus (HTLC-III/LAV) in families of children with the acquired immunodeficiency syndrome. Pediatr Infec Dis J 1985;4:468–471.
34. Lusher JM, Operskalski EA, Aledort LM, et al: Risk of human immunodeficiency virus type 1 infection among sexual and nonsexual household contacts of persons with congenital clotting disorders. Pediatrics 1991;88:242–249.
35. Madhok R, Gracie JA, Lowe GDO, Forbes CD: Lack of HIV transmission by casual contact. Lancet 1986;2:863.
36. Rogers MF, White CR, Sabders R, et al: Lack of transmission of immunodeficiency virus from infected children to their household contacts. Pediatrics 1990;85:210–214.
37. Centers for Disease Control and Prevention: Transmission of HIV possibly associated with exposure of mucous membrane to contaminated blood. MMWR 1997;46:620–623.
38. Centers for Disease Control and Prevention: Apparent transmission of human T-lymphotrophic virus type III/lymphadenopathy-associated virus from a child to a mother providing healthcare. MMWR 1986;35:76–79.
39. Wahn V, Kramer HH, Volt T, et al: Horizontal transmission of HIV infection between two siblings. Lancet 1986;1:694.
40. Khajoria RR: Transmission of human immunodeficiency virus through saliva after a lip bite. Case Report. Arch Intern Med 1997;157:1901.
41. Vidmar L, Poljak M, Tomazic J, et al: Transmission of HIV-1 by human bite. Lancet 1996;347:1762.
42. Baker MD, Moore SE: Human bites in children. Am J Dis Child 1987;141:1285–1290.
43. Leung AK, Robson CM: Human bites in children. Pediatr Emerg Care 1992;8:255–257.
44. Tereskerz PM, Bentley M, Jagger J: Risk of HIV-1 infection after human bites [letter to the Editor]. Lancet 1996;348:1512.
45. Tsoukas CM, Hadjis T, Shuster J, et al: Lack of transmission of HIV through human bites and scratches. J Acquir Immune Defic Syndr 1998;1:505–507.
46. Piazza M, Chirianni A, Picciotto L, et al: Passionate kissing and microlesions of the oral mucosa: Possible role in AIDS transmission. JAMA 1989;261:244–245.

47. American Academy of Pediatrics Task Force on Pediatrics AIDS: Guidelines for human immunodeficiency virus (HIV)-infected children and their foster families. Pediatrics 1992;89:681–683.
48. American Academy of Pediatrics Committee on Infectious Diseases: Health guidelines for the attendance in day-care and foster care settings of children infected with HIV. Pediatrics 1987:79:466–471.
49. American Academy of Pediatrics Task Force on Pediatric AIDS: Education of children with human immunodeficiency virus infection. Pediatrics 1991; 88:645–648.
50. Centers for Disease Control and Prevention: Update: Transmission of HIV infection during an invasive dental procedure. Florida. MMWR 1991;40:21–27, 33.
51. Robert LM, Chamberland ME, Cleveland JL, et al: Investigations of patients of health care workers infected with HIV: The Centers for Disease Control and Prevention database. Ann Intern Med 1995;122:653–657.
52. Occupational Safety and Health Administration: Hazard communication standard 1910:1200. In: Materials to Assist the Pediatric Office in Implementing the Bloodborne Pathogen, 2nd ed. Elk Grove, IL: AAP, 1994.
53. Fraser K: Someone at School has AIDS. Alexandria, VA, National Association of State Boards of Education, 1989, pp 1–35.
54. Babl F, Cooper E, Damon B, et al: HIV postexposure prophylaxis for children and adolescents. Am J Emerg Med 2000;18:1–6.
55. Centers for Disease Control and Prevention: Vigorous physical activity among high school students: United States, 1990. MMWR 1992;41:33–35.
56. Kashiwagi S, Hayashi J, Ikematsu H: An outbreak of hepatitis B in members of a high school Sumo wrestling club. JAMA 1982;248:213–214.
57. Sheridan JW: Bloodborne infection in sport. Sport Health 1992;10(suppl):1.
58. Feller AA, Flanagan TP: Point of View: HIV and competitive athletics—assessing the real risk of infection. Med Health 1996;79:362–364.
59. McGrew CA, Dick RW, Schniedwind K, et al: Survey of NCAA institutions concerning HIV/AIDS policies and universal precautions. Med Sci Sports Exerc 1993;25:917–921.
60. American Academy of Pediatrics, Committee on Sports Medicine and Fitness: Human immunodeficiency virus [acquired immunodeficiency syndrome (AIDS) virus] in the athletic setting. Pediatrics 1991;88:640–641.
61. Mast EE, Goodman RA, Bond WW, et al: Transmission of bloodbourne pathogens during sports risk and prevention. Ann Intern Med 1995;122:283–285.
62. Scott MJ, Scott MJ Jr: HIV infection associated with injections of anabolic steroids. JAMA 1989; 262:207–208.
63. Sklarek HM, Mantovani RP, Erens E, et al: AIDS in a bodybuilder using anabolic steroids. N Engl J Med 1984;311:1701.
64. Pettit L, Gee S, Beguer R: Epidemiology of sharp object injuries in a children's hospital. Pediatr Infect Dis J 1997;16:1019–1023.
65. Dominguez KL: Management of HIV-infected children in the home and institutional settings. Pediatr Clin North Am 2000;47:204–239.
66. Garner J, The Hospital Infection Control Practices Advisory Committee: Guideline for isolation precautions in hospitals. Infect Cont Hosp Epidemiol 1996;17:53–80.
67. Marcus R, Bell D, Culver D, et al: Risk of human immunodeficiency virus infection among emergency department workers. Am J Med 1993; 94:363–370.
68. Panlilio A, Welch B, Bell D, et al: Blood and amniotic fluid contact sustained by obstetric personnel during deliveries. Amer J Obstet Gynecol 1992; 167:703–708.
69. Panlilio AL, Foy DR, Edward JR, et al: Blood contacts during surgical procedures. JAMA 1991;265: 1533–1537.
70. Aoun H: When a house officer gets AIDS. Occasional Notes. N Engl J Med 1989; 321:693–696.
71. Pope M, Vetjes MG, Romani N, et al: Conjugates of dendritic cells and memory T lymphocytes from skin facilitate productive infection with HIV-1. Cell 1994;78:389–398.
72. Ruprecht RM, Bronson R: Chemoprevention of retroviral infection: Success is determined by virus inoculum and strength and cellular immunity. DNA Cell Biol 1994;13:59–66.
73. Martin LN, Murphey-Corb M, Soike KF, et al: Effects of initiation of 3-azido,3′-deoxythymidine (zidovudine) treatment at different times after injection of rhesus monkeys with simian immunodeficiency virus. J Infect Dis 1993;168:825–835.
74. Mathes LE, Polas PJ, Hayes KA, et al: Pre- and postexposure chemoprophylaxis: Evidence that 3-azido,3′-dideoxythymidine inhibits feline leukemia virus diseases by a drug-induced vaccine response. Antimicrob Agents Chemother 1992;36:2715–2721.
75. Shih C-C, Kaneshima H, Rabin L, et al: Postexposure prophylaxis with zidovudine suppresses human immunodeficiency virus type 1 infection in SCID-hu mice in a time-dependent manner. J Infect Dis 1991;163:625–627.
76. Sinet M, Desforges B, Launay O, Colin JN, Pocidalo JJ: Factors influencing zidovudine efficacy when administered at early stages of Friend virus infection in mice. Antiviral Res 1991;16:163–171.
77. Van Rompay KKA, Otsyula MG, Marthas ML, et al: Immediate zidovudine treatment protects simian immunodeficiency virus infected newborn macaques against rapid onset of AIDS. Antimicrob Agents Chemother 1995;39:125–131.

78. Hayes KA, Lafrado LJ, Erickson JG, et al: Prophylactic ZDV therapy prevents early viremia and lymphocyte decline but not primary infection in feline immunodeficiency virus-inoculated cats. J AIDS 1993;6:127–134.
79. Ruprecht RM, Chou T-C, Chipty F, et al: Interferon- and 3′-azido, 3′deoxythymidine are highly synergistic in mice and prevent viremia after acute retrovirus exposure. J AIDS 1990;3:591–600.
80. Tavares L, Roneker C, Johnston K, et al: 3′-azido-3′deoxythymidine in feline leukemia virus-infected cats: A model for therapy and prophylaxis of AIDS. Cancer Res 1987;47:3190–3194.
81. VanRompay KKA, Marthas MI, Ramos RA, et al: Simian immunodeficiency virus (SIV) infection of infant rhesus macaques as a model to test antiretroviral drug prophylaxis and therapy: Oral 3-azido-3′deoxythymidine prevents SIV infection. Antimicrob Agents Chemother 1992;36: 2381–2386.
82. McClure HM, Anderson DC, Ansari AA, et al: Nonhuman primate models for evaluation of AIDS therapy. In: AIDS: Anti HIV agents, therapies and vaccines. Ann N Y Acad Sci 1990;616:287–298.
83. Bottinger D, Johansson N-G, Samuelsson B, et al: Prevention of simian immunodeficiency virus, SIVsm, or HIV-2 infection in cynomolgus monkeys by pre- and postexposure administration of BEA-005. AIDS 1997;11:157–162.
84. Fazely F, Haseltine WA, Rodger RD, Ruprecht RM: Postexposure chemoprophylaxis with ZDV or ZDV combined with interferon-alpha: Failure after inoculating rhesus monkeys with a high dose of SIV. J AIDS 1991;4:1093–1097.
85. Connor EM, Sperling RS, Gelber R, et al: Reduction of maternal-infant transmission of human immunodeficiency virus type 1 with zidovudine treatment. N Engl J Med 1994;331:1173–1180.
86. Tsai CC, Follis KE, Sabo A, et al: Prevention of SIV infection in macaques by (R)-9-(z phosphonylmethoxypropl) adeneir. Science 1995;270: 1197–1199.
87. Bell D, Gerberding J: Human immunodeficiency virus postexposure management of healthcare workers: Report of a workshop. Am J Med 1997;102:1–3.
88. LaFon SW, Mooney BD, McMullen JP, et al: A double-blind, placebo-controlled study of the safety and efficacy of Retrovir (zidovudine, ZDV) as a chemoprophylactic agent in health care workers (HCW) exposed to HIV [Abstract 489]. In Program and Abstracts, 30th Interscience Conference on Antimicrobial Agents and Chemotherapy. Washington, DC, American Society for Microbiology, 1990, p 167.
89. Department of Health and Human Services/Henry J. Kaiser Family Foundation: Panel on clinical practices for the treatment of HIV Infection: Guidelines for the use of antiretroviral agents in HIV-infected adults and adolescents. (Available at: www.hivatis.org.) Baltimore: DHHS, 2000.
90. Coombs RW, Shapiro DE, Eastman PS, et al: Maternal viral genotypic ZDV resistance and infrequent failure of ZDV therapy to prevent perinatal transmission [Abstract 17]. In: Program and Abstracts of the Infectious Disease Society of America, 35th annual meeting. Alexandria, VA, IDSA, 1997, p 74.
91. Centers for Disease Control and Prevention: Public Health Service guidelines for management of health care worker exposure to HIV and recommendations for postexposure prophylaxis. MMWR 1998;147:1–33.
92. Forseter G, Joline C, Wormser GP: Tolerability, safety and acceptability of zidovudine prophylaxis in health care workers. Arch Intern Med 1994; 154:1745–1749.
93. Cardo DM: The most commonly asked questions about postexposure prophylaxis after occupational exposure to the HIV. Infect Dis Clin Pract 2000;9:159–163.
94. Geberding JL: Management of occupational exposures to blood-born viruses. N Engl J Med 1995;332:444–451.
95. Katz MH, Geberding JL: Postexposure treatment of people exposed to the human immunodeficiency virus through sexual contact or injection-drug use. N Engl J Med Sounding Board 1997;336:1097–1100.
96. Babl FE, Kastner B, Kharasch S, Cooper ER: The use of HIV post-exposure prophylaxis (PEP) in children and adolescents in the United States and Canada [abstract]. San Francisco, The American Pediatric Society and the Society for Pediatric Research, May, 1999.
97. Parkin JM, Murphy M, Anderson J, et al: Tolerability and side-effects of post-exposure prophylaxis for HIV infection. [research letter]. Lancet 2000;355:722–724.
98. Centers for Disease Control and Prevention: Recommendations for prevention of HIV transmission in health care settings. MMWR 1987;36 (Supp) :1–18.
99. Hospital Infection Control Practices Advisory Committee: Guidelines for isolation precautions in hospitals. J Infect Control Hosp Epidemiol 1996;17:53–80.
100. Pickering LK (ed): 2000 Red Book: Report of the Committee on Infectious Diseases, 24th ed. Elk Grove Village, IL, American Academy of Pediatrics, 2000.
101. American Academy of Pediatrics, Committee on Pediatric AIDS: Human milk, breastfeeding and transmission of HIV in the United States (RE9542) Pediatrics 1995;96:977–979.
102. Hale CM, Polder JA: The ABC's of safe and healthy child care: A handbook for child care providers.

Atlanta Department of Health and Human Services, United States Public Health Service Centers for Disease Control and Prevention Publication, 1996.

103. American Public Health Association and American Academy of Pediatrics: Caring for our children: National Health & Safety Performance Standards. Guidelines for out of home child care programs. Elk Grove, IL: AAP, 1992.

104. Chanock S, Donowitz LG, Simonds RJ: Medical issues related to provision of care for HIV-infected children in hospital, home, daycare, school and community. In Pizzo P, Wilfert K (eds): Pediatric AIDS: The Challenge of HIV Infection in Infants, Children and Adolescents. Baltimore, Williams & Wilkins, 1998, pp 645–661.

105. Shepp DH, Dandliker PS, Myers JD: Treatment of varicella-zoster virus infection in severely immunocompromised patients. N Engl J Med 1986;314:208–212.

106. Centers for Disease Control and Prevention: Prevention of varicella. Recommendations of the Advisory Committee on Immunization Practices (ACIP). MMWR 1996;45:RR-11.

107. Centers for Disease Control and Prevention: Hepatitis B virus: A comprehensive strategy for eliminating transmission in the US through universal childhood vaccination. MMWR 1991;40:1–25.

108. Thomas DL, Villano SA, Riester KA, et al: Perinatal transmission of hepatitis C virus from human immunodeficiency virus-type-1 infected mothers. J Infect Dis 1998;177:1480–1488.

HIV-Induced Central Nervous System and Developmental Abnormalities in Childhood

Pim Brouwers and Pamela Wolters

Central nervous system (CNS) disease is a significant complication of infection with HIV-1, particularly if the virus was acquired during early stages of fetal or neonatal brain development. In the majority of children, the neurologic dysfunction seems to be a direct consequence of HIV-1 infection of the CNS[1,2] that cannot be otherwise accounted for by infection of the CNS with other pathogens, neoplasm, or stroke,[3] and supporting the hypothesis that HIV is a neurotropic virus. HIV-1 is known to enter the CNS shortly after initial systemic infection[4] and has been found in the CNS of aborted fetuses of HIV-positive mothers as early as 15 weeks of gestation.[5]

The CNS abnormalities reflected in severely disabling neurologic, cognitive, and behavioral deficits have been one of the hallmark clinical presentations of pediatric AIDS. Early in the epidemic, HIV-related encephalopathy was estimated to occur in as many as 50% to 90% of children with AIDS in the United States.[6,7] More recent estimates of the prevalence of HIV-related CNS disease in children are much lower,[8-10] presumably because of earlier and more effective treatment.[11] CNS manifestations in school-aged children and adolescents in particular appear to be less frequent and less severe.

INVOLVEMENT OF THE CENTRAL NERVOUS SYSTEM

The CNS of patients with HIV-1 infection can be affected by either HIV-1 itself or, in some cases, by other infections or neoplastic disease secondary to immunodeficiency because HIV significantly reduces the host's ability to fight infection or cancer. Cerebrovascular complications also may occur, particularly in older children. Such secondary CNS complications, which may develop with coexisting HIV-1–related CNS disease but are relatively uncommon, are discussed first, and primary HIV-associated CNS complications are described second.

Central Nervous System Complications Secondary to HIV Infection

Non-HIV Central Nervous System Infections

Opportunistic infections of the CNS, whether viral, bacterial, fungal, or parasitic are infrequent in HIV-infected children as compared with adults.[12-16] Evidence of opportunistic CNS infections in cases of pediatric AIDS was only found in 10% of the cases in a multicenter autopsy series.[17] One of the reasons that opportunistic infections such as toxoplasmosis, the herpesviruses, including cytomegalovirus and herpes simplex virus,[18] and JC virus[19] are uncommon in children is that they are caused by reactivation of infections acquired earlier in life that have become latent. Accordingly, infants and children may not yet have been exposed to these organisms. In a limited number of vertically infected infants, prenatal and perinatal exposure to toxoplasmosis, cytomegalovirus, and syphilis from an infected mother may have resulted in congenital CNS infection.[20,21] However, as children with HIV-1 disease live longer, CNS opportunistic infections with these organisms may become more common, possibly as primary infections.

Central Nervous System Tumors

Primary CNS lymphoma and systemic lymphoma metastatic to the CNS are secondary complications in children with HIV-1 infection. Highly malignant CNS lymphoma was the most common cause of CNS mass lesions in an autopsy study of 31 pediatric AIDS patients,[22] although still less common than in adults with AIDS. The majority of these patients were older than 1 year of age, and they presented with mental status changes, behavioral changes, seizures, and the onset of focal neurologic signs. Neurologic deterioration is usually more rapid than in patients with HIV encephalopathy, but sometimes early signs and symptoms of CNS lymphoma can be hard to distinguish from the frequently more insidious course of HIV-1–associated encephalopathy.[23] Primary tumors commonly are multifocal and occur in deep gray structures (basal ganglia and thalamus). CT brain scans reveal isodense or hyperdense lesions that enhance after the administration of contrast material and are usually accompanied by surrounding edema. Metastatic lymphomas, however, may be located more peripherally in the CNS and may have extensive meningeal involvement. An initial partial response to cranial radiation with reduction in tumor mass has been reported, but long-term prognosis has been poor.[24]

Stroke

HIV-1 infection in children may also be complicated by cerebrovascular conditions. They can be related to HIV infection or other AIDS-associated illnesses, including cardiomyopathy. Stroke was the most common cause of focal neurologic deficits seen in an autopsy study of pediatric AIDS patients.[22] The onset of focal neurologic deficits such as hemiparesis is the most common presentation.

Strokes may be due to ischemia (secondary to thrombosis or embolism) or hemorrhage. Intracerebral hemorrhage is more common in children with immune-mediated thrombocytopenia or other bleeding disorders. Ischemic infarctions resulting in stroke have been associated with meningeal infections causing vasculitis (i.e., varicella zoster virus) and inflammation of the vessels[22,25] but have also been reported in the absence of infection and as a presenting sign.[26]

It also appears that HIV-1 may be directly implicated as a cause of cerebral arteriopathy.[27] HIV antigen has been found in endothelial cells from vessel walls of autopsied patients with strokes. There are reports of children with AIDS who have massive aneurysmal dilation of cerebral arteries such as those of the circle of Willis, sometimes with accompanying strokes.[23,28,29] An increased frequency of vascular headaches,[30] especially in adolescents with AIDS, has also been reported. Again, these observations raise the possibility that HIV-1 is associated with a vasculopathy.[31]

HIV-Related Pathology

Clinical Pathology

Children differ from adults in the pathologic spectrum of CNS HIV infection.[32] Gross examination of the CNS at autopsy of HIV-infected children often indicates low brain weight associated with acquired microcephaly.[33] Other neuropathologic abnormalities include symmetric ventricular enlargement and sulcal widening, mineralizations of the basal ganglia and frontal white matter, and myelin pallor,[6,32,34–37] particularly when the child has been encephalopathic.

Microscopically, inflammatory infiltrates composed of microglia and macrophages and multinucleated giant cells are common, especially in children with progressive encephalopathy.[32,37–39] These are found primarily in the central white matter and deep gray matter but can be detected in the neocortex. Apoptotic neurons,[40] neocortical neuronal cell loss,[41,42] or damage to dendritic processes[42] frequently are associated with these pathologic changes.

Mineralization of the walls of blood vessels in the basal ganglia and in the periventricular white matter of the frontal lobe (calcific vasculopathy) is the most common pathologic abnormality. These findings are unique to children with HIV infection and are not seen in adults.[32] Mineralizations are most frequent in small blood vessels, but they also have been noted in large arteries.[6,34,37,43,44] Basal ganglia calcifications are frequently seen together with inflammatory CNS disease.[45] White matter changes with reactive astrocytosis and myelin pallor are found in the majority of pediatric cases at autopsy and represent the second most notable abnormality.[33,34,38,46] Because myelogenesis continues through much of early childhood,[47] myelin pallor may be more difficult to appreciate in these cases.[35,37] Spinal cord involvement also is common in children with encephalopathy. Evidence of corticospinal tract degeneration was found in 75% of HIV-infected children in one study.[37] In children, the pathologic manifestations of HIV generally parallel the clinical and neuropsychological severity of the disease.[48]

Pathogenesis

The primary cause of these neurologic deficits and the underlying neuropathologic damage appears directly related to HIV-1 infection of the CNS. Using polymerase chain reaction (PCR) techniques, HIV-1 DNA has been identified in brain tissue of pediatric patients with HIV disease.[2,49] Moreover, the amount of provirus was much higher in the brain tissues of encephalopathic patients than in nonencephalopathic AIDS patients. In contrast, the levels of proviral DNA in lymph nodes and spleen were similar for both subgroups.[50] Subsequent studies have shown increased levels of HIV-1 RNA in cerebrospinal fluid (CSF) from children with abnormal CNS function compared with those with normal CNS function, whereas these subgroups did not show differences in their levels of plasma HIV-1 RNA.[1,51]

Adult studies suggest that HIV may enter the CNS shortly after systemic HIV infection.[4] The exact timing of HIV entry into the CNS in infants and children, however, is not known and may vary in subsets of patients; evidence for CNS infection of a 15-week-old fetus has been reported.[5] Most virus probably enters the CNS through HIV-infected, blood-derived macrophages.[52] The choroid plexus is a likely site of early entry.[53,54]

Productive HIV-1 infection in the brain has been identified in blood-derived macrophages, resident microglia, and multinucleated giant cells formed by the fusion of these cell types.[2,55] Limited infection of brain capillary endothelial cells[56,57] and astrocytes[58,59] also has been observed, but in vivo evidence for infection of neurons remains sparse.[55,60] Although the presence of active viral replication may be crucial for the development of HIV-associated CNS disease, the quantity of the virus per se may not be a sole determining factor for subsequent pathophysiologic changes in brain.[1]

Indirect mechanisms rather than direct killing of neurons by HIV-1 has been proposed to cause the neuropathologic condition.[38,42,61] Virus-encoded proteins such as gp-120[62,63] or viral gene products such as tat[40] and nef[64,65] as well as cytokines and other cell-derived proteins, including tumor necrosis factor-α,[66,67] metabolites of the arachidonic acid cascade,[68] nitric oxide,[69] quinolinic acid,[70] platelet-activating factor,[71] and other yet to be characterized compounds,[72] have been proposed to cause neurotoxicity and have been extensively investigated in vitro or in vivo.[73] HIV-1–infected human monocytes, however, do not seem to produce excess cytokines or neurotoxins,[74] and it has been suggested that cell-to-cell interactions between HIV-infected monocytes and other infected and noninfected cells,[68] in particular the astrocyte,[58,75] are important in the production of neurotoxins, leading to the neuropathologic condition. Current models of the development of neurologic damage in the CNS as a consequence of HIV infection have focused on the roles of excitatory amino acids as excitotoxins.[76] Deregulation of the N-methyl-D-aspartate (NMDA) receptor by excitatory amino acids as a final common pathway to abnormality has been postulated.[77] The NMDA receptor is a subtype of the glutamate receptors that mediate excitatory neurotransmission and affect synaptogenesis and synaptic plasticity in the brain. NMDA-bearing neurons are critical for long-term potentiation at the cellular level and for learning and memory at the animal and human levels.[78] NMDA deregulation, which may result from exposure to increased levels of excitotoxic factors, would lead to neural dysfunction, abnormal neural development, and neuronal death.[77] It is also possible that some virus strains may be more neurovirulent than others.[79]

When HIV enters the CNS of a fetus, infant, or child, the relation between viral invasion and persistent infection remains unclear and will undoubtedly vary with subsets of patients. The timing of HIV CNS infection during the development of the immature brain may significantly influence the neuropathogenesis and neuropathology.[80–82] The effects of latent HIV infection on the developing brain are unknown but may result in neurologic abnormalities and deficits in learning and behavior.

The importance of β-chemokines and chemokine receptors with respect to CNS manifestations has been suggested in recent studies. Chemokine receptors such as the CCR5 and the CXCR4 receptors have been found in the brain[83] and in the brains of children with AIDS.[84] Chemokines such as macrophage inflammatory protein (MIP)-1α and -1β and monocyte chemoattractant protein-1 may play a role in CNS inflammation and may influence the associated neuropathogenesis.[85] Elevated MIP-1α and MIP-1β messenger RNA expression were found in brain tissue from adult patients with AIDS dementia, compared with patients with HIV infection but without dementia.[86] Moreover, chemokine receptors have been identified as important cofactors for HIV-1 entry into target cells. The chemokine receptor (CCR5) in particular is used by macrophage tropic viruses for cell entry, and a recent study has identified that microglia, a major target for HIV infection in the CNS, expresses both CCR3 and CCR5.[87] Furthermore, these investigators found that infection of microglia by HIV-1 could be inhibited by MIP-1β, a CCR5 ligand.[87]

A second aspect of the chemokine receptors that may be important for the risk of developing HIV-associated dementia is that individuals with defective CCR5 alleles, the CCR5 Δ32 deletion, have been identified. People homozygous for this genotype seem to exhibit resistance to HIV-1 infection,[88,89] whereas infected adults and children heterozygous for this genotype may show a slower rate of progression of the disease.[90] Moreover, it has been suggested that patients with the CCR5 Δ32 heterozygous genotype may be at less risk for HIV-associated CNS manifestations.[91,91a] Thus, there may be differential genetic susceptibilities to virus infection of monocytes/macrophages and therefore of the CNS, related to chemokine receptor expression.

CLINICAL COURSE AND MANIFESTATIONS

Clinical Presentation of HIV-Related Neurobehavioral Impairments

The degree of HIV-associated CNS involvement for infants and children is variable, and the severity and prevalence of HIV-related CNS manifestations vary by the patient's stage of systemic disease, the age at which they first became symptomatic, the rate of deterioration, the severity of deficits, the number of neurobehavioral domains affected, and the patient's current age. Significantly fewer children older than 6 years of age develop CNS manifestations as compared with children under the age of 3.[8,92]

Originally, at least three profiles of neuropsychological dysfunction were recognized in infants, children, and adolescents with HIV infection[93,94]: those with encephalopathy, those with CNS compromise, and those with apparently normal functioning.

In children with HIV-related encephalopathy, most of the CNS structures and functions appear to be equally compromised, resulting in global and severe deficits in cognitive, language, motor, and social skills.[45,94] HIV-related encephalopathy can be static or progressive, and progressive encephalopathy may be further subdivided into subacute with a rapid, relentless course, or plateau with a more indolent course.[45]

The most severe form, subacute progressive encephalopathy, is almost exclusively seen in infants and young children.[6,46,95,96] These children show progressive, global deterioration, sometimes associated with the loss of previously acquired abilities and skills, resulting in a deterioration in standardized scores on formal testing.

In some children, the acquisition of new milestones has practically stopped, but previously acquired skills are not lost. In this less severe form of encephalopathy with a plateau course,[6,97–99] standardized scores on formal testing still show a significant decline.

Children with static encephalopathy continue to gain new skills and abilities, but at a slower rate than normal children. Their scores on standardized tests remain stable over time, usually somewhat below average. In some patients, static encephalopathies may stem from HIV-associated structural brain damage as a result of earlier active replication that has become quiescent and inactive.

In addition to their cognitive deficits, children with HIV-associated encephalopathy tend to have moderate to severe brain scan abnormalities (discussed later) and significant neurologic impairments such as motor abnormalities (spastic diplegia or quadriplegia and central hypotonia) and movement disorders (especially rigidity, bradykinesia, and dystonia) that affect their day-to-day functioning.[100] Abnormal eye movements, including nystagmus, impaired up-gaze, and abnormally slow saccades and pursuits, have also been reported.[12]

Other children may exhibit HIV-related CNS compromise, which is characterized by overall cognitive functioning that is typically within normal limits but with evidence of a significant decline over time in neurobehavioral functioning that remains at least in the low average range or significant impairments in selective neurodevelopmental functions.[94,101,102]

Retrospectively, patients who have shown significant improvements with antiviral therapy but who at baseline were functioning within normal limits also would be classified in this category. Children with HIV-related CNS compromise continue to have adequate functioning in school and activities of daily living. They also rarely exhibit other significant evidence of CNS disease (i.e., brain scan or neurologic abnormalities) but may have some mild to moderate brain scan abnormalities that do not seem to significantly affect their day-to-day functioning. Such mild neurologic deficits may include minor abnormalities in tone or hyperreflexia, or both, which do not affect motor function and mild cortical atrophy on imaging.

Some children exhibit apparently normal functioning in which their cognitive functioning is at least within the normal range and without evidence of significant deficits, decline in functioning or therapy-related improvements, or other neurologic abnormalities that affect functioning and can be attributed to HIV.

Finally, some children may display non–HIV-related CNS impairments. Careful review of their medical, developmental, and family history suggests that factors other than HIV disease most likely explain the majority of their neurobehavioral deficits. In utero exposure to drugs (e.g., alcohol, cocaine), prematurity, nutritional metabolic and endocrinologic abnormalities, chronic infections, psychosocial issues, and genetic factors all are confounding risk factors that could account for the deficits in functioning.[102-104] Frequently, children may have both HIV-related and non–HIV-related impairments, and determining the extent of deficits associated with the different causes is complex.

Domains of Neuropsychological Dysfunction

General Cognitive Function

Most neuropsychological and neuroimaging studies indicate that the effects of HIV disease on the CNS tend to be generalized and primarily affect brain function and structure globally.[105] Therefore, overall measures of general cognitive functioning, such as the Bayley, McCarthy, and Wechsler scales, have been found to effectively describe HIV-related CNS disease as reflected in brain imaging,[106] cerebrospinal fluid abnormalities,[70] and virologic and immunologic parameters.[1,107] General cognitive measures have also been sensitive to improvements in functioning after antiretroviral therapy.[108] As a result, the majority of research evaluating the neuropsychological functioning of infants, children, and adolescents with HIV infection has used composite measures of general cognitive function.

Studies consistently have found that infants and young children are at high risk for developing cognitive deficits associated with the effects of HIV disease. As measured by the Bayley Scales of Infant Development, infants with HIV infection exhibited impaired cognitive as well as motor development compared with uninfected infants born to HIV-positive mothers (seroreverters) or to unexposed control subjects (seronegative).[104,109-111] By 2 years of age, approximately 25% to 30% of infants with HIV infection exhibited moderate to severe cognitive deficits, as measured by standardized test scores at least two standard deviations below the mean, often with accompanying motor disabilities, while a similar percentage had mild delays.[8,104,110] A loss of previously acquired developmental skills or a significant and consistent decline in standard scores on the Mental Bayley Scales has been associated with rapid disease progression and a shorter survival time.[112]

In school-aged children and adolescents, HIV-related cognitive deficits are less prevalent and less severe than in infants and young children. In a recent multicenter clinical trial of pediatric patients naive to antiretroviral therapy, 25% of children younger than 6 years of age exhibited standard scores of less than 70 on general intelligence tests, compared with only about 9% of older, vertically infected children from 6 to 18 years of age.[8] Recent studies suggest that disease in older school-aged children and adolescents may be manifested by more subtle impairments in selective functions rather than by significant and global effects on general cognitive functioning. For example, Tardieu and colleagues[92] evaluated vertically infected school-aged children and found that they exhibited overall cognitive abilities in the average range, although some patients exhibited impairments in specific functions. In a study of children receiving neonatal blood transfusions, overall cognitive function was not significantly different between HIV-positive and HIV-negative children, but the seropositive group performed significantly worse in a few selected domains.[113] In addition, CT scan brain imaging has shown that mild cortical atrophy was more prominent anteriorly and became more global as it progressed.[80] The research findings examining specific cognitive domains in children with HIV disease are discussed in the following sections.

Language

Language is one domain that appears to be highly vulnerable to the effects of HIV disease. Children with HIV-associated encephalopathy frequently exhibit severe speech and language deficits and regression in language skills.[46,114-118] In studies administering comprehensive language tests to children with symptomatic HIV disease, expressive language was significantly more impaired than receptive language.[117,118] Although encephalopathic children had significantly greater overall language impairments compared with children without encephalopathy, the magnitude of the discrepancy between receptive and expressive language was similar for both groups. This differential deficit in expressive language may reflect a more general HIV-associated impairment of expressive behavior also found in motor skills and affect.[56] Uninfected siblings scored higher than the HIV-positive patients on both receptive and expressive language and did not show a discrepancy between these two language components.[117] In the patient group, higher overall severity ratings of CT brain scan abnormalities and poorer immune status at baseline were associated with lower receptive and expressive language scores. More specifically, a greater severity of white matter abnormalities was associated with a larger receptive-expressive discrepancy, whereas more severe cortical atrophy and basal ganglia calcifications were related to more impaired overall language function.[119] These data suggest that the observed language impairments are associated with the direct effects of HIV on the CNS rather than with the influence of environmental factors. In a longitudinal follow-up study, overall language scores declined after 24 months despite treatment with antiretroviral therapy, whereas cognitive function remained stable.[118] Coplan and associates[14] found that seven out of nine infants and young children with HIV infection exhibited significant deterioration in language without accompanying neurologic or neuroimaging abnormalities and, in some patients, prior to deterioration in global cognitive function. Several of the patients exhibiting language deterioration showed immediate improvement with initiation of antiretroviral therapy, which in some cases preceded gains in cognitive function, but incessant decline was observed in a few other patients despite treatment. These studies suggest that general cognitive tests may not be highly sensitive to changes in some selected domains or that HIV affects different domains of functioning at varying rates, indicating that specific cognitive functions such as language should be assessed longitudinally when measuring the dynamic effects of HIV on the CNS.

Attentional Deficits and Hyperactive Behaviors

Attention has many components, such as divided, focused, and sustained attention, which have been associated with different cortical and subcortical brain regions[120] and may be differentially affected in patients with pediatric HIV-related CNS disease. Attentional deficits may contribute to significant school and learning problems as well as social-emotional difficulties, so it is important to diagnose and treat them.

In children with HIV infection, behavioral ratings and assessments have indicated increased distractibility, excitability, and impulsiveness,[121–123] and an analysis of the Wechsler Intelligence Scale for Children–Revised[124] showed a relative weakness on "freedom from distractibility" factor subtests.[125] It is unclear, however, whether an increased prevalence of attentional problems and hyperactivity actually exists in these children, whether various components of attention are differentially affected, and to what degree these behavioral difficulties are directly attributable to the effects of HIV disease on the CNS.

Despite some evidence of increased prevalence of attentional problems and hyperactivity in children with HIV, most objective psychometric studies comparing children with HIV infection to those without the disease have not found significant differences between the groups.[122,126–128] For example, a comparison of HIV-positive and HIV-negative children with hemophilia revealed that deficits were found on tasks requiring sustained attention; however, these measures did not discriminate between the two groups.[128] Havens and associates (1994)[126] found high rates of disruptive behavior, including attention-deficit hyperactivity disorder, in a sample of children with HIV infection living in foster care and exposed to prenatal maternal drug use, but the rates were not significantly different from those found in control groups of seroreverters and unexposed children with comparable histories of drug exposure and foster-care placement. Similarly, hyperactive and other externalizing behaviors were found to be increased in a group of children with vertical and transfusion-acquired HIV infection as assessed by the Connors Behavior Rating Scales. A sibling comparison group, however, demonstrated a similarly elevated and, on some subscales, a higher prevalence and severity of these behaviors.[122] Thus, other causes, including those related to medical, genetic, and psychosocial variables, may contribute to these deficits.

A study comparing the performance of HIV-infected children with and without HIV-associated CNS compromise on a simple reaction time test found that the compromised patients reacted significantly more slowly and with larger variability than the noncompromised patients.[129] In a choice reaction time task, the compromised patients also had significantly longer decision times than the noncompromised patients, suggesting mental slowing that was independent from a possible motor slowing. Thus, attentional problems in children with HIV infection, particularly with sustained attention, may be evident in the later stages of the disease or in cases with clear CNS compromise.

Memory and Other Specific Cognitive Functions

Some evidence indicates that memory impairments may be a manifestation of HIV-related CNS disease in children, as reported in adults.[130,131] Deficits in visual spatial memory and immediate rote recall[99,132] as well as verbal learning and memory[133] have been documented in school-aged children with HIV infection, but such memory deficits are not consistently observed.[109,127,134] Some studies suggest that memory deficits are more frequent in children with accompanying neurologic impairment, indicative of HIV-related CNS disease.[133,135] For example, HIV-infected children with CNS compromise recalled significantly fewer words across the five learning trials and on the delayed recall of the Rey Auditory Verbal Learning Test than children without CNS compromise.[133] In addition, lower verbal learning and memory scores were associated with greater severity ratings of CT brain scan abnormalities, indicating that these deficits are related to the effects of HIV on the CNS. Other areas of cognitive functioning that may be impaired in children with HIV disease include visual scanning, cognitive flexibility,[113] and visual perception.[99,132]

Academic Achievement

Children with HIV infection may be at risk for academic difficulties associated with the effects of HIV on the CNS and frequent school absences due to acute illnesses. In studies of school-aged children with transfusion-acquired HIV infection, academic achievement scores were within the average range[113,127,134,136] but lower than expected based on intelligence test scores.[127,134,136] Similarly, in school-aged children with vertically acquired HIV infection, two thirds of the children assessed demonstrated normal school achievement as well as normal function on tests of general cognitive abilities, language, and motor functions.[92] The children with normal academic achievement had a higher percentage of CD4+ lymphocytes, indicating better immune function, than those with poorer school achievement. Thus, current studies suggest that the majority of school-aged children with HIV infection exhibit generally age-appropriate academic performance; however, they may not be learning at a level commensurate with their IQ score.

Motor Function

Impaired motor function is a frequent and often early manifestation of pediatric HIV disease. In a large multicenter clinical trial, approximately 45% of vertically infected children displayed abnormal motor function within the first year of life.[8,137] Infants and young children often exhibit impairments in both fine and gross motor development and abnormalities in muscle tone, particularly hypertonia in the upper and lower extremities or mixed tone with axial hypotonia.[98,138] Children with progressive encephalopathy exhibit the most severe motor involvement, including loss of acquired motor milestones, spastic diparesis or quadriparesis, and movement disorders such as rigidity and tremors.[46,98,139] Oral-motor functioning also may be impaired, resulting in articulation problems and feeding and swallowing difficulties.[116] In school-aged children with HIV infection, motor problems are less frequent[8,137] and less severe, although perceptual-motor skills[46,140] and higher gross motor functions of the lower extremities, such as running agility and speed,[140] may be affected.

Adaptive Functioning

In addition to evaluating neurocognitive functioning in standardized testing situations, adaptive functioning in the home environment also should be assessed to determine how the disease affects everyday behavior and quality of life. Previous research has shown a high degree of concordance between the scores on these two types of measures,[108,141] which supports the validity of using standardized testing to monitor the neurobehavioral effects of HIV disease in children.

In a study assessing adaptive behavior using a parental report measure, children with HIV-related encephalopathy exhibited greater impairments in daily functioning than children without evidence of CNS disease. After 6 months of treatment with zidovudine, children in both groups demonstrated significant improvements in the domains of communication, daily living skills, and socialization.[141] In another study, HIV-infected children with white matter abnormalities on computed tomography (CT) brain scans had significantly lower mean daily living and socialization Vineland domain scores than children without white matter abnormalities.[142] The improvement in daily functioning after antiretroviral therapy and the relation of behavioral deficits with CT brain scan abnormalities suggest that these impairments in everyday behavior are associated with the effects of HIV on the CNS.

The behavioral functioning of children with HIV disease may be influenced by the interaction of both the direct behavioral effects that are associated with the impact of HIV on the CNS and the indirect behavioral effects that refer to the psychological stresses that result from living with a life-threatening illness.[141,143] Behavioral changes should be reported to the child's health care workers so that various causes for these maladaptive behaviors can be investigated. Differentiating between direct and indirect behavioral abnormalities is often complex but is critical for selecting the appropriate medical treatments and psychosocial interventions.

Brain Imaging

Computed Tomography

Cerebral CT studies of children with HIV infection have shown remarkably consistent findings both in the earlier[44,46,95] and in the later studies.[80,144–147] Cerebral atrophy, consisting of ventricular enlargement and sulcal widening, is the most common abnormality.[80] Brain atrophy appears globally, except in the case of mild overall atrophy, when disproportionate frontal atrophy has been reported.[80] Cerebellar atrophy has also been noted in children with symptomatic HIV-1 disease, although with a lower prevalence.[80] In some infants and young children, serial head circumference measurements may show poor brain growth even when neuroimaging study findings are unremarkable.[93]

Attenuation of cerebral white matter is the second most common finding, noted in about one quarter of children with symptomatic HIV disease,[80] and the severity tends to correlate with the degree of cerebral atrophy.[6,80]

Cerebral calcifications occur less frequently and in one study were present in about one fifth of the patients.[80] Calcifications are generally symmetrical in the basal ganglia and, in more severe cases, the periventricular white matter of the frontal lobes.[6,44,46,148] When basal ganglia calcifications are a new finding, injection of contrast agents may result in enhancement of those structures.[44,46] These observations suggest that cerebral calcifications are associated with local breakdown of blood-brain barrier integrity and are consistent with the perivascular inflammation and mineralizations often seen at autopsy.[33]

Although most CT brain scan abnormalities are equally common in vertically infected and transfusion-infected children, calcifications are almost exclusively seen in vertically infected patients.[80,81] In one study,[81] CT brain scans of patients with vertically acquired disease were compared with scans of patients who acquired HIV infection through a transfusion prior to 1 year of age. Calcifications were significantly more likely in children with vertical disease than in transfused patients. Moreover, calcifications appeared at a much younger age in the vertically infected group than in the transfused group. In the group of premature infants who acquired HIV through neonatal transfusion, those who developed calcifications were born at a lower gestational age than those who did not develop calcifications.[81] The development of intracerebral calcifications may thus indicate intrauterine rather than intra- or postpartum infection and may depend in part on when the developing brain in children with HIV infection gets infected.[81]

Intracerebral calcifications tend to progress, showing increased density of existing lesions and new lesions despite treatment. Progression of calcifications occurs even when other CT brain scan abnormalities improve. These other abnormalities, such as ventricular enlargement, subarachnoid dilation, cerebellar atrophy, and white matter abnormality, tend to show comparable degrees of change.[149,150] These patterns of change in imaging variables suggest that intracerebral calcifications are relatively independent from other CNS abnormalities[80] and that, once present, they do not seem to reflect clinical disease progression in the CNS.[147]

Magnetic Resonance Imaging

Cerebral magnetic resonance imaging (MRI) studies of children with symptomatic HIV disease have been generally very similar to CT brain scan studies. In studies comparing MRI with CT, the degree of cerebral atrophy was equally identified, but CT was superior to MRI for identification of cerebral calcification.[144,145,151] MRI was better at identifying the presence of white matter abnormalities, although with the increased sensitivity of MRI, white matter abnormalities may have been detected that are of uncertain clinical significance.[142,152,153] Chamberlain[151] also found no difference in identified brain changes between CT and MRI in a longitudinal study. In symptomatic children, MRI does not appear to offer much advantage over CT with regard to the documentation of CNS involvement. MRI may be more sensitive, however, in detecting presymptomatic CNS abnormalities in mildly symptomatic and asymptomatic patients.[147,152] Quantitation of brain volumes and cerebral tissue types, such as gray and white matter, from MRI studies may help to further our understanding of structure/function relations in children with HIV infection. In a study of children with HIV-associated encephalopathy using quantitative analysis, specific patterns of brain atrophy were found[154] indicating a central atrophy primarily affecting the subcortical white matter and basal ganglia regions.

Functional Brain Imaging; Cerebral Metabolism

Proton Magnetic Resonance Spectroscopy

Magnetic resonance spectroscopy (MRS) allows for in vivo analysis of a number of metabolic components associated with the integrity of different aspects of neuronal function. Within brain regions of interest, analysis of the following metabolites is commonly conducted: (1) N-acetyl aspartate (NAA), which is inferred to be a neuron-specific molecule because it is present largely, if not entirely, within neurons, being absent in glial cultures; (2) choline-containing compounds (Cho), which are constituents of cell membranes and may be increased in demyelination; (3) creatine and phosphocreatine (Cr), which signal amplitudes and are most likely a measure of local tissue density; and (4) lactate, the presence of which may indicate active inflammation or severe tissue damage causing impaired blood perfusion and resulting ischemia.

Localized proton magnetic resonance spectra obtained from normal-appearing white matter of adults with AIDS dementia have shown a decrease in the NAA/Cr ratio, as well as an increase in relative choline concentration,[155,156] suggesting neuronal loss or dysfunction within normal-appearing cerebral white matter. In a few MRS studies of HIV-infected children, a decrease in NAA or the NAA/Cr ratio was found, particularly in children with HIV-associated CNS disease in the basal ganglia[157–159] and centrum semiovale.[160] Compared with uninfected control subjects, infected children exhibited decreases in the Cho/Cr ratio[158] and increases in the lipid signal.[160] Pavlakis and colleagues[159] investigated MRS scans before and after the initiation of antiretroviral therapy in two children with progressive encephalopathy. After treatment, the NAA/Cr ratio was improved and the lactate peak apparent at baseline disappeared. MRS clearly offers future possibilities to further document and monitor HIV-associated CNS disease and provide further insights into the neuropathogenesis of the neurobehavioral manifestations.

Positron Emission Tomography

Rottenberg and colleagues[161] were the first to describe regional abnormalities of glucose metabolism in adult patients with AIDS dementia using positron emission tomography at rest. In patients with mild dementia, increased metabolism of glucose in the basal ganglia was noted, whereas, in contrast, more severely demented patients had decreased basal ganglia metabolism, which was associated with temporal lobe hypometabolism. Temporal lobe hypometabolism appeared to be more prominent in the more severely demented patients in this study, and the degree of hypometabolism correlated with a number of neuropsychological tests of memory and attention.[161] Another study in asymptomatic HIV-positive adults showed a reduction in prefrontal glucose utilization metabolism when compared with seronegative control subjects.[162]

Unfortunately, systematic positron emission tomographic studies of children with HIV disease have not been reported. In a case study of a hemophiliac boy with symptomatic HIV infection, the positron emission tomographic scan indicated diffuse cortical hypometabolism and focal areas of markedly reduced metabolism in the right frontal and right superior temporal cortices prior to any antiretroviral treatment.[163] Following 12 weeks of zidovudine treatment, the patient's scans showed considerable improvement, with only mild abnormalities remaining in the left frontal cortex and associated improvements in neurobehavioral function.[164]

Relation of Neurobehavioral Measures to Disease Markers

Many factors (emotional, psychosocial, socioeconomic, etc) may confound the level and patterns of neurobehavioral dysfunctioning in children with HIV disease. Therefore, it is critical to validate that observed neurobehavioral abnormalities reflect the effects of HIV disease on the CNS. This can be achieved in part by showing that neurobehavioral abnormalities are related to disease markers.

In the past, the immunologic and virologic markers most widely used to define stage or progression of HIV disease have been CD4+ evaluations, as a measure of immune depletion, and serum p24 antigen levels, as a measure of viral load,[165,166] which more recently have been replaced by PCR RNA HIV-1 techniques. Early in the disease, in the asymptomatic stages, markers of immune activation such as β_2-microglobulin and neopterin have been useful.

A frequently observed relation is an increased prevalence of neurologic and neuropsychological defects in the later stages of the infection.[45,167,168] However, in infants and very young children with vertically acquired infection, neurologic abnormalities may be the first clinical signs of HIV,[10,169] and this pattern is often associated with rapidly progressive disease.

Studying the relation between CD4+ count and neurobehavioral measures is complicated in children in the first years of life because of age-related, rapid physiologic changes in absolute CD4+ count and percentage. Fortunately, formulae have been developed to correct for these changes,[170] and they were used to demonstrate that lower CD4+ values were associated with a greater degree of cognitive and language dysfunction.[107,117] In another study, changes in CD4+ values associated with the initiation of antiretroviral therapy were related to changes in neurobehavioral function.[150]

In an MRI study of 184 HIV-seropositive children with hemophilia,[152] children with more advanced disease and CD4+ cell counts less than 200 had a significantly greater prevalence of cerebral atrophy (33% prevalence) than patients who were more immune intact and had CD4+ cell counts greater than 200 (8% prevalence), even after controlling for group-related age differences. In a similar study using CT brain scans in children with symptomatic HIV disease, a significant correlation was reported between more advanced immune depletion (i.e., low CD4+ count) and a more severe degree of brain scan abnormality.[107] The associations between CT brain scan ratings and CD4+ percentage values were robust but were of similar magnitude for the different types of lesions (atrophy, calcifications, or white matter abnormalities). In a follow-up study, deterioration in cortical atrophy was associated with a decline in age-adjusted immune function (zCD4%)[150] but not with deterioration in severity of intracerebral calcifications in children starting various antiretroviral treatments.

Early studies have reported that elevations of the level of p24 antigen, a measure of viral replication, in part reflecting stage of disease, in serum and CSF are associated with the presence of encephalopathy[6,7] and a greater severity of CT brain scan abnormalities.[107]

More current methods to measure viral activity use PCR to detect and quantify HIV-1 DNA and RNA. Such studies have found that the amounts of proviral DNA in the brain tissues of encephalopathic patients are much higher than in nonencephalopathic AIDS patients, whereas levels of provirus in lymph nodes and spleen are very similar.[2,49,50] Similarly, HIV-1 RNA was more frequently detected in the CSF from children who had abnormal CNS function than in the CSF from those who did not.[1,51] Moreover, a significant correlation was found between CSF viral load determined by PCR HIV-1 RNA and degree of cortical atrophy on CT brain scan (Brouwers P, Civitello L, DeCarli C, et al: Relation between neuroimaging abnormalities and CSF viral load in children with symptomatic HIV-1 disease. Pediatrics 2000;6:390–396.).

Markers of HIV disease stage or progression, such as CD4+, p24, and RNA HIV-1 measures, have been related to neurologic functioning, as reflected by brain scan abnormalities and neurobehavioral deficits. It remains to be shown, however, that these associations reflect a causal relationship. Most likely, CD4+ measures indirectly reflect the same underlying variable, the progression and stage of HIV disease.[107] The progression of HIV-1 disease probably results in an increase in the concentration of the neuropathogenic factors responsible for HIV-associated CNS disease,[76] which were discussed earlier.

Relation of Neurobehavioral Measures to Outcome

A number of studies seem to indicate that status and changes in CNS structure and function have predictive value for further progression of HIV-1 disease. In an early longitudinal study, including CT brain scan evaluation, some children exhibited progressive cerebral atrophy, among other neurologic symptoms, and were classified with subacute progressive encephalopathy.[95] With a median duration of 19 months of follow-up, 13 of the 20 children identified as encephalopathic died, whereas none of the other patients, identified as normal or having nonprogressive encephalopathy, died.[46]

In another study, CSF quinolinic acid concentrations were related to survival in 38 children with symptomatic HIV infection. With a follow-up of 3 years, 15 of the 19 patients with the lowest CSF quinolinic acid levels at baseline were still alive, whereas only 6 of the 19 patients with the highest CSF quinolinic acid levels were still alive. Moreover, this effect of baseline CSF quinolinic acid level was independent from the immunologic status, based on CD4+ percentage, of the patient at baseline.[69]

More recent studies have shown that deterioration in neurobehavioral functioning, particularly for children younger than 30 months of age, may be highly predictive of further disease progression.[9] These changes in developmental functioning may be observed at a very global level. For example, a drop in raw score on the Bayley Scales of Infant Development between two evaluations at least 3 months apart is associated with significant disease progression and short survival.[104,112]

ASSESSMENT AND CLASSIFICATION

Periodic neurobehavioral assessments of children with HIV infection are necessary to monitor the child's functioning over time because of the high risk of developing CNS disease. These test results are also useful for identifying the child's current strengths and weaknesses and for planning rehabilitative, educational, psychological, and medical interventions in conjunction with results from other multidisciplinary team members.[102]

Methodologic Issues

Several methodologic issues need to be considered when performing multiple assessments over time in children. Children are constantly developing new skills, so interval change has to be measured against a background of normally occurring developmental growth. Socioeducational, environmental, and linguistic factors, which may affect the rate of development, also should be taken into account. The use of standardized tests with reliable norms to measure psychological functioning is therefore essential: These norms should provide reliable age norms, preferably based on small age increments, as well as reflect the socioeconomic diversity of the population through inclusion in the standardization sample.

The stability of psychological functions is another consideration, because mental development is not a continuous quantitative growth of abilities over time. For example, age-related improvements in memory may reflect both the development of different memorization strategies and an increased capacity. Although specific cognitive subfunctions may have noncontinuous and nonlinear growth, a standardized measure of overall functioning that integrates most of the neuropsychological domains tends to have such attributes. Therefore, standardized tests of overall functioning are typically chosen over narrowly defined and experimental or novel instruments to reliably document cognitive growth unless large control groups can be longitudinally evaluated at the same time.[171]

Age-scaled deviation norms are available for restricted age ranges on most of the commonly used psychometric tests for children. For example, the Bayley Scales of Infant Development[172] have an age range from 2 to 42 months. Therefore, as the child grows older, changing test instruments will be required in order to utilize age-appropriate tests and norms. Clearly, difficulties in interpreting longitudinal test results will occur if the age-appropriate test at follow-up is different from the one mandated at baseline.[173,174] The use of age-appropriate measures of overall cognitive development or general intelligence is one way to reduce interpretation problems associated with test transitions. Standard scores from such measures are relatively stable over time because of the wide range of functions assessed, and they have good validity and reliability.[175,176] When a child with stable functioning reaches the appropriate chronologic age to transfer to a test valid for an older age, then the change should be made as soon as possible. When deterioration in functioning is suspected, the test that was previously administered should be given again. For children with significant developmental delays, the transfer to a new test can be postponed if the test for the younger population assesses their delayed skills more appropriately.

Inter-test correlations and expected mean change in standard scores[177] when moving from one instrument to another are available from various studies. However, when scores lie beyond two standard deviations from the mean (e.g., for IQ scores less than 70 or greater than 130). The accuracy of such values of change are less clear.[174]

Domains of Assessment

In the assessment of children with HIV infection, the primary focus should be on which neuropsychological functions to evaluate. An optimal test battery to use for the neurodevelopmental assessment of infants, children, and adolescents with HIV disease should be designed to evaluate the wide range of abilities known to be vulnerable to the effects of HIV, including general cognitive function, language (receptive and expressive), perceptual-motor skills, attention, and memory. The second objective is to select the specific instruments with which to measure these functions that yield standard scores, account for age-related changes in development, and allow comparisons across domains of function.

The prevalence and severity of HIV-related CNS manifestations vary in infants, children, and adolescents. Moreover, pediatric HIV patients may present with varying and sometimes discordant degrees of cognitive, motor, and behavioral dysfunction, which also may have different rates of progression. Thus, the neurobehavioral domains to be assessed and the frequency of follow-up testing should be adapted for the different subgroups on the basis of these characteristics of HIV CNS disease. For example, HIV-associated CNS manifestations in school-aged children and adolescents are much less severe and may develop more slowly. Thus, assessing for more subtle changes in specific neurobehavioral functions, which develop slowly, is important.

Some of these differential subtle changes may be highlighted by comparisons among the subtest or domain scores from intelligence tests such as the component factors of the Wechsler IQ tests, including Verbal Comprehension, Perceptual Organization, Freedom from Distractibility, and Processing Speed. Differences in performance on timed and untimed subtests also may be informative. Tests that comprehensively evaluate specific abilities such as language, attention, or memory, however, also should be included in the test battery. More subtle deficits that may not be picked up by an overall general cognitive index could be identified by such tests.[118]

To evaluate the child's relevant "ecological" behaviors and quality of life in the home environment, the test battery should include measures that assess socioemotional functioning,[121] everyday adaptive behavior such as the Vineland Adaptive Behavior Scales,[178] and academic achievement such as the Wide Range Achievement Test–Revised.[179] The main functions that should be assessed in children with HIV infection and possible tests that can be used to evaluate these domains for various age groups are shown in Table 13–1.

Repeated Testing and Practice Effects

How frequently to repeat evaluations is another methodologic issue to consider. Shorter inter-test intervals will be required to assess changes in functioning when the rate of change is thought to be rapid. Longer inter-test intervals between comprehensive evaluations will be appropriate when the rate of change is thought to be slow, such as with insidious progression or preventive treatments. When inter-test intervals between comprehensive evaluations are long, interim monitoring with a smaller repeatable battery may be considered. Due to the higher risk of progressive CNS disease, younger children and infants and children with encephalopathy should be assessed more frequently than older children who display stable cognitive functioning that is at least in the average range.

Longitudinal studies require repeated testing with the possibility of practice effects when similar tests are serially administered. The child can benefit from having been in the same test situation before and thus being more familiar with the testing requirements (procedural practice effects). The child also may benefit from having seen the test materials before (material-specific practice effects). A number of factors may influence the size of practice effects. The test-retest interval is a significant determinant; the shorter the interval, the greater the practice effects. The size of the practice effect also is influenced by the child's age and rate of mental development. In younger children and infants, practice effects are limited. Practice effects will be smaller for functions on which the child experiences faster growth, because skills will be tested at the follow-up evaluation that were only emerging or not present at the previous assessment. The child's level of functioning and health status also will affect the magnitude of practice effects. Children with lower IQ scores or with medical conditions, and in particular sicker children, will have considerably smaller practice effects than healthy children with normal or superior IQ scores.[180–182] Limiting the frequency of testing is an objective to keep patients and caregivers more cooperative and motivated over time, particularly for the older children with stable cognitive function and stable disease.

Based on the previous considerations, the following general guidelines for determining repeated neurologic and neuropsychological testing for various subgroups have been suggested:[183,184] (1) infants and young children less than 2 years of age should be evaluated every 6 months because they are at high risk for developing CNS disease; (2) children from 2 to 8 years of age should be evaluated every 6 months unless they exhibit neurodevelopmental deficits, in which case they should be

Table 13-1
Neurobehavioral Functions and Associated Tests to Comprehensively Assess Infants, Children, and Adolescents with HIV Infection[†]

FUNCTION	PSYCHOMETRIC TEST	AGE RANGE*
General intelligence	Bayley Scales of Infant Development (Mental), 2nd ed. (Bayley, 1993)	1–3.5
	McCarthy Scales of Children's Abilities (McCarthy, 1972)	2.4–8.6
	Wechsler Preschool & Primary Scale of Intelligence-R (Wechsler, 1989)	3–7.3
	Wechsler Intelligence Scale for Children, 3rd ed. (Wechsler, 1991)	6–16.11
	Wechsler Adult Intelligence Scale-3rd ed. (Wechsler, 1997)	16–74
	Stanford-Binet Intelligence Scale, 4th ed. (Thorndike, et al., 1986)	2–23.11
Language	Clinical Evaluation of Language Fundamentals–3rd ed. (Semel et al., 1995)	5–16.11
	Peabody Picture Vocabulary Test-3 (Dunn & Dunn, 1997)	2.5–40
	Gardner Expressive One-Word Vocabulary Test-R (Gardner, 1990)	2–15.11
	Verbal Fluency (Spreen & Strauss, 1991)	> 25
Visuospatial	Developmental Test of Visual-Motor Integration-4R (Beery, 1997)	4–17.11
Memory and Learning	Wide Range Assessment of Memory & Learning (Sheslow, 1990)	5–17.11
	California Verbal Learning Test-Children's Version (Delis, et al., 1994)	5–16.11
	McCarthy Memory Scale (McCarthy, 1972)	2.4–8.6
	Stanford-Binet Memory Scale, 4th ed. (Thorndike, et al., 1986)	2–23
Attention	Digit Span Subtest (Wechsler et al, 1981, 1991)	≥6
	Trail Making Test (Reitan & Davison, 1974)	≥6
	Gordon Diagnostic System (Gordon, et al., 1996)	4–17
Concept formation	Ravens Progressive Matrices (Raven et al., 1984)	≥5.5
Motor function	Bayley Scales of Infant Development (Motor), 2nd ed. (Bayley, 1993)	0–3.5
	Peabody Developmental Motor Scales (Folio & Fewell, 1983)	0.5–6
	Bruininks-Oseretsky Test of Motor Proficiency (Bruininks, 1978)	>5.5
	Grooved Pegboard (Klove, 1963)	>5
Behavior	Vineland Adaptive Behavior Scales (Sparrow, et al., 1984)	0–19
	Behavior Assessment System for Children (Reynolds & Kamphaus, 1992)	2.5–19
	Conners' Rating Scales (Conners, 1989)	3–17

*Age range in years, for which the test is standardized
[†]Previously published in part in Wolters & Brouwers, 1999.

assessed every 6 months; and (3) children 8 years of age and older should be evaluated every 2 years if they exhibit stable functioning within normal limits; otherwise, annual evaluation would be recommended.

EFFECTS OF ANTIVIRAL TREATMENT ON THE CENTRAL NERVOUS SYSTEM

It has been appreciated for some time that antiretroviral therapy can improve neuropsychological dysfunction in adult and pediatric patients with HIV-1 infection.[164,185–190] In infants and children, the effect of HIV disease on neurobehavioral function has been global, and similarly the effects of treatment have typically been shown in increases in the general levels of mental abilities. It has been hypothesized that the effectiveness of various antiretroviral drugs against HIV-associated CNS disease is in part related to their ability to inhibit HIV-1 replication in relevant cells in the CNS (including macrophages and microglia).[191] Penetration of agents into the CNS is believed to be important, and a number of studies have shown that zidovudine, which penetrates relatively well, is particularly effective in the treatment of HIV-associated CNS disease.[150] Although other agents have been found to penetrate the CNS, studies documenting their effectiveness in reversing or preventing HIV-associated CNS manifestations have been limited.

The effects of zidovudine as a single drug on HIV-induced CNS disease have been studied in children[108,164] but have been most extensively documented in adults[186] with neuropsychological deficits at very high doses (1500 to 2000 mg/day), with lesser effects seen at lower doses (1000 mg/day).[188] Likewise, with didanosine, improvement in CNS symptoms has been reported in patients receiving high doses,[189,190] yet fewer data exist on its activity against HIV-associated CNS disease at lower doses. Although studies on the reversal of HIV-associated CNS disease in children have found effectiveness for zidovudine as a single agent,[108,164] studies on the prevention of such manifestations have been less clear.[137,192] Recent studies with combination therapy, although not including protease inhibitors, have shown that neurobehavioral functioning is significantly affected by the choice of antiretroviral agents, particularly for children younger than 3 years of age.[9,193]

Differential treatment effects on the CNS versus peripheral and systemic manifestations of HIV infection[194,195] highlight the fact that special attention has to be paid to the effects of antiretroviral regimens on CNS disease. Differences in pharmacokinetics and in the relevant HIV-1–infected cells to be targeted between the two compartments may require different therapies or treatment schedules. As newer HIV treatment strategies are developed, it will be particularly important to learn about their effects on the prevention or treatment of HIV-associated CNS disease.

CONCLUSION

In infants and children, neurologic complications may remain a significant cause of mortality and morbidity of HIV-1 infection.[196] The majority of these complications will be a direct consequence of HIV-1 infection of the brain, although, as these children grow older and become adolescents, the frequency of secondary complications, as seen in adults, may start to increase. Prevalence rates of HIV-associated CNS disease vary among different subgroups of HIV-infected patients, with infants and young children exhibiting more severe and more frequent CNS manifestations. Further research to define individual differences in host factors and viral factors that may identify children who are at increased risk for neurologic manifestations remains critical. Such knowledge is particularly useful because a number of studies have indicated that antiretroviral therapy may be effective in the prevention[11] and treatment of HIV-associated CNS disease.[164,186] Optimal systemic antiretroviral therapy for HIV disease, based on virologic or immunologic markers, however, may not necessarily be optimal therapy for CNS disease[194,195] because of differences in the relevant HIV-1–infected target cells[197] and differential penetration of antiviral agents into the CNS.[198]

By reducing viral replication to undetectable levels, highly active antiretroviral therapy (HAART), which uses a combination of protease and reverse transcriptase inhibitors, may significantly prolong the lives of people living with AIDS. It will be critically important to study the long-term effects of HAART on the possible development of HIV-associated CNS disease, because protease inhibitors may have only limited penetration into the CNS. Such therapies may leave the CNS relatively unprotected, particularly if no agents are included with neuroprotective action.[198] It has been suggested that increased viral replication within the CNS may play an important role in the progression to HIV encephalopathy, and the activity of the virus within the CNS may be independent of its activity in the rest of the body, at least at the later stages of the disease. These newer therapies, therefore, may not eliminate the incidence of HIV-associated CNS disease but rather delay its onset and modify its course. Adults who have been on prolonged HAART therapy and who have been without detectable serum viral load for more than 2 years still were found to have reservoirs of HIV-1.[199] It is well known that the CNS may constitute a sanctuary for disease processes, which also may be the case for HIV-1 under these conditions.

Thus, even with highly effective combination therapies, the developing brain is likely vulnerable to the effects of HIV-1, and infants and children will continue to be at risk for developing HIV-related CNS manifestations. Therefore, longitudinal neurobehavioral assessment of infants and children with HIV infection remains a significant component of the standard of care for these patients.

REFERENCES

1. Sei S, Stewart SK, Farley M, et al: Evaluation of HIV-1 RNA levels in cerebrospinal fluid and viral resistance to zidovudine in children with HIV-encephalopathy. J Infect Dis 1996;174:1200–1206.
2. Sharer LR, Saito Y, Da Cunha A, et al: In situ amplification and detection of HIV-1 DNA in fixed pediatric AIDS brain tissue. Hum Pathol 1996;27:614–617.
3. Sharer LR, Mintz M: Neuropathology of AIDS in children. In: Scaravilli F (ed). The Neuropathology of HIV Infection. Berlin, Springer-Verlag, 1993.
4. Davis L, Hjelle BL, Miller VE, et al: Early viral brain invasion in iatrogenic human immunodeficiency virus infection. Neurology 1992;42:1736–1739.
5. Lyman WD, Kress Y, Kure K, et al: Detection of HIV in fetal central nervous system tissue. AIDS 1990;4:917–920.

6. Belman AL, Diamond G, Dickson D, et al: Pediatric acquired immunodeficiency syndrome: Neurologic syndromes. Am J Dis Child 1988;142:29–35.
7. Epstein LG, Goudsmit J, Paul DS, et al: Expression of human immunodeficiency virus in cerebrospinal fluid of children with progressive encephalopathy. Ann Neurol 1987;21:397–401.
8. Englund JA, Baker CJ, Raskino C, et al: Clinical and laboratory characteristics of a large cohort of symptomatic, human immunodeficiency virus-infected infants and children. Pediatr Infect Dis J 1996;15:1025–1036.
9. McKinney RE, Johnson GM, Stanley K, et al: Randomized study of combined zidovudine-lamivudine versus didanosine monotherapy in children with symptomatic therapy-naive HIV-1 infection. The Pediatric AIDS Clinical Trials Group Protocol 300 Study Team. J Pediatr 1998;133:500–508.
10. Cooper ER, Hanson C, Diaz C, et al: Encephalopathy and progression of human immunodeficiency virus disease in a cohort of children with perinatally acquired human immunodeficiency virus infection. Women and Infants Transmission Study Group. J Pediatr 1998;132:808–812.
11. Portegies P, Enting RH, de Gans J, et al: Presentation and course of AIDS dementia complex: 10 years of follow-up in Amsterdam, The Netherlands. AIDS 1993;7:669–675.
12. Civitello LA, Brouwers P, Pizzo PA: Neurological and neuropsychological manifestations in 120 children with symptomatic human immunodeficiency virus infection [abstract]. Ann Neurol 1993;34:481.
13. Porter SB, Sande MA: Toxoplasmosis of the central nervous system in the acquired immunodeficiency syndrome. N Engl J Med 1992;327:1643–1648.
14. Krasinski K: Bacterial infections. In Pizzo PA, Wilfert CM (eds): Pediatric AIDS, 2nd ed. Baltimore, Williams & Wilkins, 1994, pp 241–253.
15. Pelton SI, Klein JO: Bacterial diseases in infants and children with infections due to human immunodeficiency virus. In Pizzo PA, Wilfert CM (eds): Pediatric AIDS: The Challenge of HIV Infection In Infants, Children, and Adolescents. Baltimore, Williams & Wilkins, 1991, pp 199–208.
16. Cohen BA, Berger JR: Neurologic opportunistic infections in AIDS. In Gendelman HE, Lipton SA, Epstein L, Swindells S (eds): The Neurology of AIDS. New York, Chapman Hall, 1998, pp 303–332.
17. Kozlowski PB, Sher JH, Dickson DW, et al: Central nervous system in pediatric HIV infection: A multicenter study. In Kozlowski PB, Snider PM, Vietze PM, Wisniewski HM: Brain in Pediatric AIDS. Basel, Karger, 1990, pp 132–146.
18. Annunziato PW, Gershon AA: Herpesvirus infections in children infected with HIV. In Pizzo PA, Wilfert CM (eds): Pediatric AIDS: The Challenge of HIV Infection in Infants, Children, and Adolescents, 3rd ed. Philadelphia, Lippincott Williams & Wilkins, 1998, pp 205–225.
19. Berger JR, Scott G, Albrecht J, et al: Progressive multifocal leukoencephalopathy in HIV-1-infected children. AIDS 1992;6:837–841.
20. Shanks GD, Redfield RR, Fischer GW: Toxoplasma encephalitis in an infant with acquired immunodeficiency syndrome. Pediatr Infect Dis J 1987;6:70–71.
21. Biggemann B, Voit T, Neuen E: Neurological manifestations in three German children with AIDS. Neuropediatrics 1987;18:99–106.
22. Dickson DW, Llena JF, Weidenheim KM: Central nervous system pathology in children with AIDS and focal neurologic signs—stroke and lymphoma. In Kozlowski P (ed): Brain Behavior and Pediatric AIDS. Basel, Karger, 1990, pp 147–157.
23. Shah SS, Zimmerman RA, Rorke LB, et al: Cerebrovascular complications of HIV in children. Am J Neuroradiol 1996;17:1913–1917.
24. Epstein LG, DiCarlo FJ Jr, Joshi VV, et al: Primary lymphoma of the central nervous system in children with acquired immunodeficiency syndrome. Pediatrics 1988;82:355–363.
25. Frank Y, Lim W, Kahn E, et al: Multiple ischemic infarcts in a child with AIDS, varicella zoster infection, and cerebral vasculitis. Pediatr Neurol 1989;5:64–67.
26. Visudtibhan A, Visudhiphan P, Chiemchanya S: Stroke and seizures as the presenting signs of pediatric HIV infection [see comments]. Pediatr Neurol 1999;20:53–56.
27. Legido A, Lischner HW, de Chadarevian JP: Stroke in pediatric HIV infection [abstract]. Pediatr Neurol 1999;21:588.
28. Park YD, Belman AL, Kim TS, et al: Stroke in pediatric acquired immunodeficiency syndrome. Ann Neurol 1990;28:303–311.
29. Husson RN, Saini R, Lewis LL, et al: Cerebral artery aneurysms in children infected with human immunodeficiency virus. J Pediatr 1992;121:927–930.
30. Civitello L: Headache in pediatric human immunodeficiency virus disease. Ann Neurol 1996;40:310.
31. Katsetos CD, Fincke JE, Legido A, et al: Angiocentric CD3(+) T-cell infiltrates in human immunodeficiency virus type 1-associated central nervous system disease in children. Clin Diagn Lab Immunol 1999;6:105–114.
32. Kure K, Llena JF, Lyman WD, et al: Human immunodeficiency virus-1 infection of the nervous system. Hum Pathol 1991;22:700–710.
33. Burns DK: The neuropathology of pediatric acquired immunodeficiency syndrome. J Child Neurol 1992;7:332–346.
34. Sharer LR, Epstein LG, Cho E, et al: Pathologic features of AIDS encephalopathy in children: Evidence for LAV/HTLV-III infection of brain. Hum Pathol 1986;17:271–284.
35. Sharer LR: Pathology of HIV-1 infection of the central nervous system: A review. J Neuropathol Exp Neurol 1992;51:3–11.

36. Michaels J, Sharer LR, Epstein LG: Human immunodeficiency virus type 1 (HIV-1) infection of the nervous system: A review. Immunodefic Rev 1988; 1:71–104.
37. Dickson DW, Belman AL, Park YD, et al: Central nervous system pathol in pediatric AIDS: An autopsy study. Acta Pathol Microbiol Immunol Scand 1989;8(suppl):40–57.
38. Budka H: Neuropathology of human immunodeficiency virus infection. Brain Pathol 1991;1:143–152.
39. Epstein LG, Sharer LR, Goudsmit J: Neurological and neuropathological features of human immunodeficiency virus infection in children. Ann Neurol 1988;23(suppl):S19–S23.
40. Gelbard HA, James HJ, Sharer LR, et al: Apoptotic neurons in brains from paediatric patients with HIV-1 encephalitis and progressive encephalopathy. Neuropathol Appl Neurobiol 1995;21:208–217.
41. Masliah E, Achim CL, Ge N, et al: Cellular neuropathology in HIV encephalitis. Res Pub Assoc Res Nerv Mental Disord 1994;72:119–131.
42. Wiley CA, Masliah E, Morey M, et al: Neocortical damage during HIV infection. Ann Neurol 1991;29:651–657.
43. Sharer LR, Cho ES, Epstein LG: Multinucleated giant cells and HTLV-III in AIDS encephalopathy. Hum Pathol 1985;16:760.
44. Belman AL, Lantos G, Horoupian D, et al: AIDS: Calcification of the basal ganglia in infants and children. Neurology 1986;36:1192–1199.
45. Brouwers P, Belman AL, Epstein L: Central nervous system involvement: Manifestations, evaluation, and pathogenesis. In Pizzo PA, Wilfert CM (eds): Pediatric AIDS: The Challenge of HIV Infection in Infants, Children, and Adolescents, 2nd ed. Baltimore, Williams & Wilkins, 1994, pp 433–455.
46. Epstein LG, Sharer LR, Oleske JM, et al: Neurologic manifestations of human immunodeficiency virus infection in children. Pediatrics 1986;78:678–687.
47. Kinney HC, Brody BA, Kloman AS, et al: Sequence of central nervous system myelination in human infancy: Patterns of myelination in autopsied infants. J Neuropathol Exp Neurol 1988;47:217–234.
48. Wiley CA, Belman AL, Dickson DW, et al: Human immunodeficiency virus within the brains of children with AIDS. Clin Neuropathol 1990;9:1–6.
49. Sei S, Kleiner DE, Kopp JB, et al: Quantitative analysis of viral burden in tissues from adults and children with symptomatic human immunodeficiency virus type 1 infection assessed by polymerase chain reaction. J Infect Dis 1994;170:325–333.
50. Sei S, Saito K, Stewart SK, et al: Increased HIV-1 DNA content and quinolinic acid concentration in brain tissues obtained from AIDS patients with HIV-encephalopathy. J Infect Dis 1995;172:638–647.
51. Pratt RD, Nichols S, McKinney N, et al: Virologic markers of human immunodeficiency virus type 1 in cerebrospinal fluid of infected children. J Infect Dis 1996;174:288–293.
52. Nottet HS, Persidsky Y, Sasseville VG, et al: Mechanisms for the transendothelial migration of HIV-1 infected monocytes into brain. J Immunol 1996;156:1284–1295.
53. Harouse JM, Wroblewska Z, Laughlin MA, et al: Human choroid plexus cells can be latently infected with human immunodeficiency virus. Ann Neurol 1989;25:406–411.
54. Falangola MF, Hanley A, Galvao-Castro B, et al: HIV infection of the choroid plexus: A possible mechanism of viral entry into the CNS. J Neuropathol Exp Neurol 1995;54:497–503.
55. Zheng J, Gendelman HE: The HIV-1 associated dementia complex: A metabolic encephalopathy fueled by viral replication in mononuclear phagocytes. Curr Opin Neurol 1997;10:319–325.
56. Moss HA, Wolters PL, Brouwers P, et al: Impairment of expressive behavior in pediatric HIV-positive patients with evidence of CNS disease. J Pediatr Psychol 1996;21:379–400.
57. Poland SD, Rice GP, Dekaban GA: HIV-1 infection of human brain-derived microvascular endothelial cells in vitro. J Acquir Immune Defic Syndrome Hum Retrovirol 1995;8:437–445.
58. Blumberg BM, Gelbard HA, Epstein LG: HIV-1 infection of the developing nervous system: Central role of astrocytes in pathogenesis. Virus Res 1994;32:253–267.
59. Tornatore C, Chandra R, Berger JR, et al: HIV-1 infection of subcortical astrocytes in the pediatric central nervous system. Neurology 1994;44:481–487.
60. Ensoli F, Wang H, Fiorelli V, et al: HIV-1 infection and the developing nervous system: Lineage-specific regulation of viral gene expression and replication in distinct neuronal precursors. J Neurovirol 1997;3:290–298.
61. Everall IP, Luthert PJ, Lantos PL: Neuronal loss in the frontal cortex in HIV infection. Lancet 1991;337:1119–1121.
62. Brenneman DE, Westbrook GL, Fitzgerald SP, et al: Neuronal cell killing by the envelope protein of HIV and its prevention by vasoactive intestinal peptide. Nature 1988;335:639–642.
63. Lipton SA, Brenneman DE, Silverstein FS, et al: Gp120 and neurotoxicity in vivo. Trends Pharmacol Sci 1995;16:122–132.
64. Blumberg BM, Epstein LG, Saito Y, et al: Human immunodeficiency virus type 1 Nef quasispecies in pathological tissue. J Virol 1992;66:5256–5264.
65. Saito Y, Sharer LR, Epstein LG, et al: Overexpression of Nef as a marker for restricted HIV-1 infection of astrocytes in postmortem pediatric central nervous tissues. Neurology 1994;44:474–481.
66. Mintz M, Rapaport R, Oleske JM, et al: Elevated serum levels of tumor necrosis factor are associated with progressive encephalopathy in children with acquired immunodeficiency syndrome. Am J Dis Child 1989;143:771–774.

67. Talley AK, Dewhurst S, Perry SW, et al: Tumor necrosis factor alpha-induced apoptosis in human neuronal cells: Protection by the antioxidant N-acetylcysteine and the genes Bcl-2 and CrmA. Mol Cell Biol 1995;15:2359–2366.
68. Gendelman HE, Lipton SA, Tardieu M, et al: The neuropathogenesis of HIV-1 infection. J Leukocyte Biol 1994;56:389–398.
69. Bukrinsky MI, Nottet HS, Schmidtmayerova H, et al: Regulation of nitric oxide synthase activity in human immunodeficiency virus type 1 (HIV-1)-infected monocytes: Implications for HIV-associated neurological disease. J Exp Med 1995;181:735–745.
70. Brouwers P, Heyes MP, Moss HA, et al: Quinolinic acid in the cerebrospinal fluid of children with symptomatic human immunodeficiency virus type 1 disease: Relationship to clinical status and therapeutic response. J Infect Dis 1993;168:1380–1386.
71. Gelbard HA, Nottet HS, Swindells S, et al: Platelet-activating factor: A candidate human immunodeficiency virus type 1-induced neurotoxin. J Virol 1994;68:4628–4635.
72. Giulian D, Vaca K, Noonan CA: Secretion of neurotoxins by mononuclear phagocytes infected with HIV-1. Science 1990;250:1593–1596.
73. Gelbard HA, Epstein LG: HIV-1 encephalopathy in children. Curr Opin Pediatr 1995;7:655–662.
74. Bernton E, Bryant H, Decoster M, et al: No direct neuronotoxicity by HIV-1 virions or culture fluids from HIV-1 infected T cells or monocytes. AIDS Res Hum Retroviruses 1992;8:495–503.
75. Tornatore C, Nath A, Amemiya K, et al: Persistent HIV-1 infection in human fetal glial cells reactivated by T-cell factor(s) or by the cytokines tumor necrosis factor alpha and interleukin 1 beta. J Virol 1991;65:6094–6100.
76. Lipton SA, Gendelman HE: Dementia associated with the acquired immunodeficiency syndrome. N Engl J Med 1995;332:934–940.
77. Lipton SA, Rosenberg PA: Excitatory amino acids as a final common pathway for neurologic disorders. N Engl J Med 1994;330:613–622.
78. Morris RGM: Selective impairment of learning and blockade of long-term potentiation by an N-methyl-D-aspartate receptor antagonist, AP5. Nature 1986;319:774–776.
79. Brengel-Pesce K, Morand P, Innocenti-Francillard P, et al: Genetic and biological analysis of variants derived from the cerebrospinal fluid of HIV type 1 subtype B- and D-infected patients with and without AIDS dementia complex. AIDS Res Hum Retrovir 1996;12:1643–1645.
80. DeCarli C, Civitello LA, Brouwers P, et al: The prevalence of computed tomographic abnormalities of the cerebrum in 100 consecutive children symptomatic with the human immune deficiency virus. Ann Neurol 1993;34:198–205.
81. Civitello L, Brouwers P, DeCarli C, et al: Calcification of the basal ganglia in children with HIV infection. Ann Neurol 1994;36:506.
82. Kerr SJ, Armati PJ, Guillemin GJ, et al: Chronic exposure of human neurons to quinolinic acid results in neuronal changes consistent with AIDS dementia complex. AIDS 1998;12:355–363.
83. Zou YR, Kottmann AH, Kuroda M, et al: Function of the chemokine receptor CXCR4 in haematopoiesis and in cerebellar development [see comments]. Nature 1998;393:595–599.
84. Vallat AV, De Girolami U, He J, et al: Localization of HIV-1 co-receptors CCR5 and CXCR4 in the brain of children with AIDS. Am J Pathol 1998;152:167–178.
85. Bell MD, Taub DD, Perry VH: Overriding the brain's intrinsic resistance to leukocyte recruitment with intraparenchymal injections of recombinant chemokines. Neuroscience 1996;74:283–292.
86. Schmidtmayerova H, Nottet HS, Nuovo G, et al: Human immunodeficiency virus type 1 infection alters chemokine beta peptide expression in human monocytes: Implications for recruitment of leukocytes into brain and lymph nodes. Proc Nat Acad Sci 1997;93:700–704.
87. He J, Chen Y, Farzan M, et al: CCR3 and CCR5 are co-receptors for HIV-1 infection of microglia. Nature 1997;385:645–649.
88. Liu R, Paxton WA, Choe S, et al: Homozygous defect in HIV-1 coreceptor accounts for resistance of some multiple-exposed individuals to HIV-1 infection. Cell 1996;86:367–377.
89. Samson M, Libert F, Doranz BJ, et al: Resistance to HIV-1 infection in Caucasian individuals bearing mutant alleles of the CCR-5 chemokine receptor gene. Nature 1996;382:722–725.
90. Buseyne F, Janvier G, Teglas JP, et al: Impact of heterozygosity for the chemokine receptor CCR5 32-Bp-deleted allele on plasma virus load and CD4 T lymphocytes in perinatally human immunodeficiency virus-infected children at 8 years of age. J Infect Dis 1998;178:1019–1023.
91. van Rij RP, Portegies P, Hallaby T, et al: Reduced prevalence of the CCR5 Delta32 heterozygous genotype in human immunodeficiency virus-infected individuals with AIDS dementia complex. J Infect Dis 1999;180:854–857.
91a. Sei S, Boler AM, Nguyen GT, et al: Protective effect of CCR5 Δ32 heterozygosity is restricted by SDF-1 genotype in children with HIV-1 infection. AIDS 2001;15:1343–1352.
92. Tardieu M, Mayaux MJ, Seibel N, et al: Cognitive assessment of school-age children infected with maternally transmitted human immunodeficiency virus type 1. J Pediatr 1995;126:375–379.
93. Belman AL: Acquired immunodeficiency syndrome and the child's central nervous system. Pediatr Clin North Am 1992;39:691–714.

94. Wolters PL, Brouwers P: Evaluation of neurodevelopmental deficits in children with HIV infection. In Gendelman HE, Lipton SA, Epstein L, Swindells S (eds): The Neurology of AIDS. New York, Chapman & Hall, 1998, pp 425–442.
95. Epstein LG, Sharer LR, Joshi VV, et al: Progressive encephalopathy in children with acquired immune deficiency syndrome. Ann Neurol 1985;17:488–496.
96. Belman AL, Ultmann MH, Horoupian D, et al: Neurological complications in infants and children with acquired immune deficiency syndrome. Ann Neurol 1985;18:560–566.
97. Belman AL: AIDS and pediatric neurology. Neurol Clin 1990;8:571–603.
98. Ultmann MH, Diamond GW, Ruff HA, et al: Developmental abnormalities in children with acquired immunodeficiency syndrome (AIDS): A follow up study. Int J Neurosci 1987;32:661–667.
99. Diamond GW, Kaufman J, Belman AL, et al: Characterization of cognitive functioning in a subgroup of children with congenital HIV infection. Arch Clin Neuropsychol 1987;2:1–16.
100. Mintz M, Tardieu M, Hoyt L, et al: Therapy improves motor function in HIV-infected children with extrapyramidal syndromes. Neurology 1996;47:1583–1585.
101. Brouwers P, Moss HA, Wolters P, et al: Developmental deficits and behavioral change in pediatric AIDS. In Grant I, Martin A (eds): Neuropsychology of HIV Infection. New York, Oxford University Press, 1994, pp 310–338.
102. Wolters PL, Brouwers P, Moss HA: HIV-1 disease in children: The effects of HIV on cognition, behavior, and learning. School Psychol Q 1995;10:305–328.
103. Bose S, Moss H, Brouwers P, et al: Psychologic adjustment of human immunodeficiency virus-infected school-age children. J Dev Behav Pediatr 1994;15:S26–S33.
104. Chase C, Vibbert M, Pelton SI, et al: Early neurodevelopmental growth in children with vertically transmitted human immunodeficiency virus infection. Arch Pediatr Adolesc Med 1995;149:850–855.
105. Brouwers P, Wolters P, Civitello L: Central nervous system manifestations and assessment. In Pizzo PA, Wilfert CM (eds): Pediatric AIDS: The Challenge of HIV Infection in Infants, Children, and Adolescents. Baltimore, Williams & Wilkins, 1998.
106. Brouwers P, DeCarli C, Civitello L, et al: Correlation between computed tomographic brain scan abnormalities and neuropsychological function in children with symptomatic human immunodeficiency virus disease. Arch Neurol 1995;52:39–44.
107. Brouwers P, Tudor-Williams G, DeCarli C, et al: Relation between stage of disease and neurobehavioral measures in children with symptomatic HIV disease. AIDS 1995;9:713–720.
108. Brouwers P, Moss H, Wolters P, et al: Effect of continuous infusion zidovudine therapy on neuropsychologic functioning in children with symptomatic human immunodeficiency virus infection. J Pediatr 1990;117:980–985.
109. Drotar D, Olness K, Wiznitzer M, et al: Neurodevelopmental outcomes of Ugandan infants with human immunodeficiency virus type 1 infection. Pediatrics 1997;100:e5.
110. Gay CL, Armstrong FD, Cohen D, et al: The effects of HIV on cognitive and motor development in children born to HIV-seropositive women with no reported drug use: Birth to 24 months. Pediatrics 1995;96:1078–1082.
111. Pollack H, Kuchuk A, Cowan L, et al: Neurodevelopment, growth, and viral load in HIV-infected infants. Brain Behav Immunity 1996;10:298–312.
112. Brouwers P, Wolters P, Moss H, et al: Encephalopathy in vertically acquired pediatric HIV disease. J Clin Exp Neuropsychol 1993;15:95.
113. Cohen SE, Mundy T, Karassik B, et al: Neuropsychological functioning in human immunodeficiency virus type 1 seropositive children infected through neonatal blood transfusion. Pediatrics 1991;88:58–68.
114. Coplan J, Contello KA, Cunningham CK, et al: Early language development in children exposed to or infected with human immunodeficiency virus. Pediatrics 1998;102:e8.
115. Condini A, Axia G, Cattelan C, et al: Development of language in 18–30-month-old HIV-1–infected but not ill children. AIDS 1991;5:735–739.
116. Pressman H: Communication disorders and dysphagia in pediatric AIDS. ASHA 1992;34:45–47.
117. Wolters P, Brouwers P, Moss H, et al: Differential receptive and expressive language functioning of children with symptomatic HIV disease and relation to CT scan brain abnormalities. Pediatrics 1995;95:112–119.
118. Wolters PL, Brouwers P, Civitello L, et al: Receptive and expressive language function of children with symptomatic HIV infection and relationship with disease parameters: A longitudinal 24-month follow-up study. AIDS 1997;11:1135–1144.
119. Wolters PL, Civitello L, Moss H, et al: Relation between specific computed tomography brain scan abnormalities and receptive and expressive language function in children with symptomatic HIV-1 infection [abstract]. J Neurovirol 1998;4:371.
120. Mirsky AF, Anthony BJ, Duncan CC, et al: Analysis of the elements of attention: A neuropsychological approach. Neuropsychol Rev 1991;2:109–145.
121. Moss HA, Brouwers P, Wolters PL, et al: The development of a Q sort behavior rating procedure for pediatric HIV patients. J Pediatr Psychol 1994;19:27–46.
122. Moss HA, Wolters PL, Brouwers P, et al: Parent report of maladaptive behaviors in children with HIV infection and their uninfected siblings. Submitted for publication, 2000.

123. Hittelman J, Willoughby A, Mendez H, et al: Neurodevelopmental outcome of perinatally-acquired HIV infection on the first 24 months of life [abstract #TUB37]. Proceedings from the VII International Conference on AIDS, Florence, Italy, 1991.
124. Wechsler D: Manual for the Wechsler Intelligence Scale for Children. New York, Psychological Corporation, 1974.
125. Brouwers P, Mohr E: A metric for the evaluation of change in clinical trials. Clin Neuropharmacol 1989;12:129–133.
126. Haven JH, Whitaker AH, Feldman JF, et al: Psychiatric morbidity in school-age children with congenital human immunodeficiency virus infection. J Dev Behav Pediatr 1994;15:S18–S25.
127. Loveland KA, Stehbens J, Contant C, et al: Hemophilia growth and development study: Baseline neurodevelopmental findings. J Pediatr Psychol 1994;19:223–239.
128. Whitt JK, Hooper SR, Tennison MB, et al: Neuropsychologic functioning of human immunodeficiency virus-infected children with hemophilia. J Pediatr 1993;122:52–59.
129. Appels M: Assessment of attentional functioning in children with HIV-1 infection. Utrecht, University of Utrecht, 1996.
130. Skoraszewski MJ, Ball JD, Mikulka P: Neuropsychological functioning of HIV-infected males. J Clin Exp Neuropsychol 1991;13:278–290.
131. Van Gorp WG, Miller EN, Satz P, et al: Neuropsychological performance in HIV-1 immunocompromised patients: A preliminary report. J Clin Exp Neuropsychol 1989;11:763–773.
132. Boivin MJ, Green SD, Davies AG, et al: A preliminary evaluation of the cognitive and motor effects of pediatric HIV infection in Zairian children. Health Psychol 1995;14:13–21.
133. Perez L, Wolters PL, Moss H, et al: Verbal learning and memory in children with HIV infection [abstract]. J Neurovirol 1998;4:362.
134. Sirois PA, Hill SD: Developmental change associated with human immunodeficiency virus infection in school-age children with hemophilia. Dev Neuropsychol 1993;9:177–197.
135. Levenson RL Jr, Mellins CA, Zawadzki R, et al: Cognitive assessment of human immunodeficiency virus-exposed children. Am J Dis Child 1992;146:1479–1483.
136. Smith ML, Minden D, Netley C, et al: Longitudinal investigation of neuropsychological functioning in children and adolescents with hemophilia and HIV infection. Dev Neuropsychol 1997;13:69–85.
137. Raskino C, Pearson D, Baker C, et al: Neurological, neurocognitive, and brain growth outcomes in HIV-infected children receiving different nucleoside antiretroviral regimens. Pediatrics 1999;104:1–10.
138. Lord D, Danoff JV, Smith MR: Motor assessment of infants with human immunodeficiency virus infection: A retrospective review of multiple cases. Pediatr Phys Ther 1995;7:9–13.
139. Belman AL: HIV-1-associated CNS disease in infants and children. In Price RW, Perry SW: HIV, AIDS and the Brain. New York, Raven Press, 1994, pp 289–310.
140. Parks RA: Occupational therapy with children who are HIV positive. In Developmental Disabilities. Rockville, MD, American Occupational Therapy Association, 1994, pp 5–6.
141. Wolters P, Brouwers P, Moss H, et al: Adaptive behavior of children with symptomatic HIV infection before and after zidovudine therapy. J Pediatr Psychol 1994;19:47–61.
142. Brouwers P, van der Vlugt H, Moss H, et al: White matter changes on CT brain scan are associated with neurobehavioral dysfunction in children with symptomatic HIV disease. Child Neuropsychology 1995;1:93–105.
143. Wiener L, Moss H, Davidson R, et al: Pediatrics: The emerging psychosocial challenges of the AIDS epidemic. Child Adolesc Soc Work J 1992;9:381–407.
144. Chamberlain MC, Nichols SL, Chase CH: Pediatric AIDS: Comparative cranial MRI and CT scans. Pediatr Neurol 1991;7:357–362.
145. Kauffman WM, Sivit CJ, Fitz CR, et al: CT and MR evaluation of intracranial involvement in pediatric HIV infection: A clinical-imaging correlation. Am J Neuroradiol 1992;13:949–957.
146. Roy S, Geoffrey G, Lapointe N, et al: Neurological findings in HIV-infected children: A review of 49 cases. Can J Neurol Sci 1992;19:453–457.
147. Brouwers P, DeCarli C, Civitello L: Brain structure and function in pediatric acquired immunodeficiency syndrome. In Lyon GR, Rumsey JM(eds): Neuroimaging: A window to the neurological foundations of learning and behavior in children. Baltimore, Paul H. Brookes Publishing, 1996, pp 183–208.
148. Price DB, Inglese CM, Jacobs J, et al: Pediatric AIDS: Neuroradiologic and neurodevelopmental findings. Pediatric Radiology 1988;18:445–448.
149. DeCarli C, Fugate L, Falloon J, et al: Brain growth and cognitive improvement in children with human immune deficiency virus-induced encephalopathy after six months of continuous infusion zidovudine therapy. J Acquir Immune Defic Syndromes 1991;4:585–592.
150. Brouwers P, DeCarli C, Tudor-Williams G, et al: Interrelations among patterns of change in neurocognitive, CT brain imaging, and CD4 measures associated with antiretroviral therapy in children with symptomatic HIV infection. Adv Neuroimmunol 1994;4:223–231.
151. Chamberlain MC: Pediatric AIDS: Longitudinal comparative MRI and CT brain imaging study. J Child Neurol 1993;8:175–181.

152. Mitchell WG, Nelson MD, Contant CF, et al: Effects of human immunodeficiency virus and immune status on magnetic resonance imaging of the brain in hemophilic subjects: Results from hemophilic growth and development study. Pediatrics 1993;91:742–746.
153. Tardieu M, Blanche W, Brunelle F: Cerebral magnetic resonance imaging studies in HIV-1 infected children born to seropositive mothers [abstract]. Paper presented at the Satellite Conference of Seventh International Conference on AIDS, Padova, Italy, 1991.
154. Scarmato V, Frank Y, Rozenstein A, et al: Central brain atrophy in childhood AIDS encephalopathy. AIDS 1996;10:1227–1231.
155. Menon DK, Ainsworth JG, Cox IJ, et al: Proton MR spectroscopy of the brain in AIDS dementia complex. J Comput Assist Tomogr 1992;16:538–542.
156. Jarvik JG, Lenkinski RE, Grossman RI, et al: Proton MR spectroscopy of HIV-infected patients: Characterization of abnormalities with imaging and clinical correlation. Radiology 1993;186:739–744.
157. Pavlakis SG, Lu D, Frank Y, et al: Magnetic resonance spectroscopy in childhood AIDS encephalopathy. Pediatr Neurol 1995;12:277–282.
158. Lu D, Pavlakis SG, Frank Y, et al: Proton MR spectroscopy of the basal ganglia in healthy children and children with AIDS. Radiology 1996;199:423–428.
159. Pavlakis SG, Lu D, Frank Y, et al: Brain lactate and N-acetylaspartate in pediatric AIDS encephalopathy. AJNR Am J Neuroradiol 1998;19:383–385.
160. Salvan AM, Lamoureux S, Michel G, et al: Localized proton magnetic resonance spectroscopy of the brain in children infected with human immunodeficiency virus with and without encephalopathy. Pediatr Res 1998;44:755–762.
161. Rottenberg DA, Moeller JR, Strother SC, et al: The metabolic pathology of the AIDS dementia complex. Ann Neurol 1987;22:700–706.
162. Pascal S, Resnick L, Barker WW, et al: Metabolic asymmetries in asymptomatic HIV-1 seropositive subjects: Relationship to disease onset and MRI findings. J Nucl Med 1991;32:1725–1729.
163. Brunetti A, Berg G, Di Chiro G, et al: Reversal of brain metabolic abnormalities following treatment of AIDS dementia complex with 3'-Azido-2',3'-Dideoxythymidine (AZT, Zidovudine): A PET-FDG study. J Nucl Med 1989;30:581–590.
164. Pizzo P, Eddy J, Falloon J, et al: Effect of continuous intravenous infusion of zidovudine (AZT) in children with symptomatic HIV infection. N Engl J Med 1988;319:889–896.
165. Butler KM, Husson RN, Lewis L, et al: CD4 status and P24 Antigenemia. Am J Dis Child 1992;146:932–936.
166. Tsoukas CM, Bernard NF: Markers predicting progression of human immunodeficiency virus-related disease. Clin Microbiol Rev 1994;7:14–28.
167. Tovo PA, de Martino M, Gabiano C, et al: Prognostic factors and survival in children with perinatal HIV-1 infection. Lancet 1992;339:1249–1253.
168. Persaud D, Chandwani S, Rigaud M, et al: Delayed recognition of human immunodeficiency virus infection in preadolescent children. Pediatrics 1992;90:688–691.
169. Scott GB, Hutto C, Makuch RW, et al: Survival in children with perinatally acquired human immunodeficiency virus type 1 infection. N Engl J Med 1989;321:1791–1796.
170. European Collaborative Study: Age-related standards for T lymphocyte subsets based on uninfected children born to human immunodeficiency virus infected women. Pediatr Infect Dis J 1992;11:1018–1026.
171. Fletcher JM, Francis DJ, Pequegnat W, et al: Neurobehavioral outcomes in diseases of childhood: Individual change models for pediatric human immunodeficiency viruses. Am Psychol 1991;46:1267–1277.
172. Bayley N: Bayley Scales of Infant Development. San Antonio, TX, Psychological Corporation, 1993.
173. Mulhern RK, Ochs J, Fairclough D: Deterioration of intellect among children surviving leukemia: IQ test changes modify estimates of treatment toxicity. J Consult Clin Psychol 1992;60:477–480.
174. Lindsey JC, O'Donnell K, Brouwers P: Methodological issues in analyzing psychological test scores in pediatric clinical trials. J Dev Behav Pediatr 2000;21:141–151.
175. Neisser U, Boodoo G, Bouchard TJ, et al: Intelligence: Knowns and unknowns. Am Psychol 1996;51:77–101.
176. Appelbaum AS, Tuma JM: Social class and test performance: Comparative validity of the Peabody with the WISC and WISC-R for two socioeconomic groups. Psychol Rep 1977;40:139–145.
177. Wechsler D: Wechsler Intelligence Scale for Children, 3rd ed. San Antonio, TX, Psychological Corporation, 1991.
178. Sparrow S, Balla D, Cicchetti D: Vineland Adaptive Behavior Scales. Circle Pines, MN, American Guidance Service, 1984.
179. Jastak S, Wilkinson G: Wide Range Achievement Test–Revised. Wilmington, DE, Jastak Associates, 1984.
180. Tuma JM, Appelbaum AS: Reliability and practice effects of WISC-R IQ estimates in a normal population. Educ Psychol Measure 1980;40:671–678.
181. Moss HA, Nannis ED, Poplack DG: The effects of prophylactic treatment of the central nervous system on the intellectual functioning of children with acute lymphocytic leukemia. Am J Med 1981;71:47–52.
182. Farwell JR, Lee YJ, Hirtz DG, et al: Phenobarbital for febrile seizures: Effects on intelligence and on seizure recurrence. N Engl J Med 1990;322:364–369.

183. Working Group on Antiretroviral Therapy and Medical Management of Infants, Children, and Adolescents With HIV Infection: Antiretroviral therapy and medical management of pediatric HIV infection. Pediatrics 1998;102:1005–1062.
184. Wolters PL, Brouwers P: Neurodevelopmental function and assessment of children with HIV-1 infection. In Zeichner S, Read J: Handbook of Pediatric HIV Care. Philadelphia, Lippincott Williams & Wilkins, 1999, pp 210–227.
185. Yarchoan R, Berg G, Brouwers P, et al: Response of human immunodeficiency virus-associated neurological disease to 3′azido-3′deoxythymidine. Lancet 1987;1:132–135.
186. Schmitt FA, Bigley JW, McKinnis R, et al: Collaboration Group: Neuropsychological outcome of zidovudine (AZT) treatment of patients with AIDS and AIDS-related complex. N Engl J Med 1988;319:1573–1578.
187. Schmitt FA, Dickson LR, Brouwers P: Neuropsychological response to antiretroviral therapy in HIV infection. In Grant I, Martin A: Neuropsychology of HIV infection: Current Research and New Directions. Oxford, Oxford University Press, 1994.
188. Sidtis JJ, Gatsonis C, Price RW, et al: Zidovudine treatment of the AIDS dementia complex: Results of a placebo-controlled trial. Ann Neurol 1993;33:343–349.
189. Yarchoan R, Pluda JM, Thomas RV, et al: Long-term toxicity/activity profile of 2′,3′-dideoxyinosine in AIDS or AIDS-related complex [see comments]. Lancet 1990;336:526–529.
190. Butler KM, Husson RN, Balis FM, et al: Dideoxyinosine in children with symptomatic human immunodeficiency virus infection. N Engl J Med 1991;324:137–144.
191. Perno CF, Yarchoan R, Cooney DA, et al: Inhibition of human immunodeficiency virus (HIV-1/HTLV-IIIBa-L) replication in fresh and cultured human peripheral blood monocytes/macrophages by azidothymidine and related 2′, 3′- dideoxynucleosides. J Exp Med 1988;168:1111–1125.
192. Brady MT, McGrath N, Brouwers P, et al: Randomized study of the tolerance and efficacy of high-versus low-dose zidovudine in human immunodeficiency virus-infected children with mild to moderate symptoms (AIDS Clinical Trials Group 128). Pediatric AIDS Clinical Trials Group. J Infect Dis 1996;173:1097–1106.
193. Englund JA, Baker CJ, Raskino C, et al: Zidovudine, didanosine, or both as the initial treatment for symptomatic HIV-infected children. N Engl J Med 1997;336:1704–1712.
194. Pizzo P, Butler K, Balis F, et al: Dideoxycytidine alone and in an alternating schedule with zidovudine in children with symptomatic human immunodeficiency virus infection. J Pediatr 1990;117:799–808.
195. Brouwers P, Henricks M, Lietzau JA, et al: Effect of combination therapy with zidovudine and didanosine on neuropsychological functioning in patients with symptomatic HIV disease: A comparison of simultaneous and alternating regimens. AIDS 1997;11:59–66.
196. Simpson DM, Berger JR: Neurologic manifestations of HIV infection. Med Clin North Am 1996;80:1363–1394.
197. Epstein LG, Gendelman HE: Human immunodeficiency virus type 1 infection of the nervous system: Pathogenetic mechanisms. Ann Neurol 1993;33:429–436.
198. Portegies P: HIV-1, the brain, and combination therapy. Lancet 1995;346:1244–1245.
199. Finzi D, Hermankova M, Pierson T, et al: Identification of a reservoir for HIV-1 in patients on highly active antiretroviral therapy. Science 1997;278:1295–1300.

14 Oral Manifestations in Pediatric HIV Infection

Catherine M. Flaitz and M. John Hicks

Oral manifestations are among the earliest and most common clinical features associated with pediatric HIV infection.[1–20] In contrast to adults, the prevalence and spectrum of oral diseases is narrower in children. In part, these differences are the result of decreased exposure at a young age to certain viruses, especially human herpesviruses and papillomaviruses, which reduces the risk for diseases such as oral hairy leukoplakia, oral warts, Kaposi's sarcoma, and lymphoma. Despite the limited range of diseases, most children will develop one or more oral manifestations of HIV infection during their disease course, similar to their adult counterparts. Furthermore, these oral diseases are prognostic markers for disease progression and immunosuppression. Because most studies have not specifically evaluated the influence of highly active antiretroviral therapy on oral disease frequency in children, it is not certain whether the significant decreases in oral lesions that are documented in adults will occur in this young age group.[5,21] Although not well recognized by most health care professionals, oral lesions account for about one quarter of hospital admissions for children with HIV infection. A summary of the most common and strongly associated oral diseases pertinent to pediatric HIV infection is outlined in Table 14–1.[1,2,6,12,17,20–29]

OROPHARYNGEAL CANDIDIASIS

The most common oral soft tissue manifestation of pediatric HIV infection is oropharyngeal candidiasis (Fig. 14–1).[1–20,28–31] Although the isolation of *Candida* species, a commensal oral cavity organism, ranges from 40% to 60% in both healthy and HIV-infected children, candidiasis is often the first clinically observable manifestation of HIV infection, with up to 72% of children developing this disease. Of significance, oropharyngeal candidiasis heralds HIV progression and immune system deterioration. In addition, concurrent oral infection is the most common clinical presentation of esophageal candidiasis, a very debilitating and symptomatic AIDS-defining condition in children.[32] Besides immunosuppression, contributing factors to mucosal superficial fungal infection include xerostomia, antibiotic and corticosteroid therapy, poor oral hygiene, and rampant dental caries.[1–20,28–31]

Until recently, the primary opportunistic fungus was considered to be *Candida albicans*, which is the most frequently cultured species in the oral cavity.[1–15,17–20] However, other pathogenic species have been identified in children, including *C. tropicalis, C. krusie, C. glabrata, C. parapsilosis, C. pseudotropicalis, C. guilliermondi,* and others.[16,28,30]

Table 14-1
Oral Manifestations Associated with Pediatric HIV Infection

Commonly associated oral lesions
  Candidiasis
    Pseudomembranous
    Erythematous
    Angular cheilitis
  Herpes simplex viral infection
  Linear gingival erythema
  Major salivary gland enlargement
  Recurrent aphthous ulcers
    Minor, major, and herpetiform

Less commonly associated oral lesions
  Bacterial infections
  Periodontal diseases
    Necrotizing ulcerative gingivitis
    Necrotizing ulcerative periodontitis
    Necrotizing stomatitis
  Viral infections (cytomegalovirus, human papillomavirus, varicella zoster virus, molluscum contagiosum)
  Xerostomia

Strongly associated oral lesions (rare in children)
  Kaposi's sarcoma
  Non-Hodgkin's lymphoma
  Oral hairy leukoplakia
  Tuberculosis-related ulcers

Oral conditions with increased severity in pediatric HIV infection
  Gingivitis and periodontitis (increased gingival and plaque indices)
  Over-retained primary teeth
  Delayed eruption of primary and permanent teeth
  Primary dentition caries

Adapted and compiled from references 2, 3, 12, 13, 19, 20, 22, 23, 24–27.

Erythematous candidiasis ranges from diffuse to patchy redness throughout the oral mucosa. At times, pinpoint to macular erythema mimics a bleeding diathesis or submucosal trauma. When the tongue is involved, there is a selective loss of filiform papillae, resulting in a red, smooth to beaded mucosal surface. A specific type of erythematous candidiasis is median rhomboid glossitis that occurs as a persistent oval patch in the midline of the dorsal tongue. Red scaling and fissuring of the lip commissures is referred to as angular cheilitis, and diffuse scaling, fissuring, and redness of the lips represents juxtavermilion candidiasis. The hyperplastic form of candidiasis is uncommon in young children, but may be observed in older children and adolescents with longstanding infection. White, rough, irregular plaques that do not rub off characterize this pattern. In contrast to pseudomembranous and erythematous forms that develop throughout the oropharyngeal region, the hyperplastic form has a predilection for the tongue and anterior buccal mucosa. Although oropharyngeal candidiasis may be asymptomatic, oral burning, taste perversion, halitosis, and dysphagia are frequent complaints. In the infant and toddler, diaper dermatitis may coexist with the oral lesions. Cutaneous involvement of the thumb or fingers may occur in children with digit-sucking habits.

Diagnosis of oropharyngeal candidiasis is usually based on clinical features and response to empirical antifungal therapy.[28] Exfoliative cytologic or biopsy examination confirms the presence of fungal organisms in the affected tissues. Definitive identification of the organism requires a culture; however, this method is not necessarily indicative of mucosal disease, because *Candida* species are common commensal organisms in the oral cavity. Fungal culture with species identification is most important when lesions are refractory to antifungal therapy. Concentration of saliva using a cytospin technique with creation of a cell block for microscopic examination allows for improved identification of yeast and hyphae, which correlates with clinically detectable oral candidiasis in HIV-infected children to a greater extent than saliva cultures alone.

Management of oropharyngeal candidiasis includes the use of topical and/or systemic antifungal agents and depends on disease severity, esophageal involvement, recurrence rate, drug compliance, the child's age, and previous history and response to antifungal therapy.[1–5,28,33–36] Nystatin, clotrimazole, ketoconazole, fluconazole,

In addition, *C. dubliniensis*, a newly emerging pathogen isolated almost exclusively in HIV-infected and oncology patients, has been found in a limited number of children.[33] Pathogenic species identification is important, especially in refractory cases, because of the differences in both susceptibility to antifungal agents and the commensal interaction with other oral microorganisms.

The clinical features of oropharyngeal candidiasis are variable, depending on the form of the disease and the affected site (see Fig. 14–1).[1–20,28–31] Pseudomembranous candidiasis or thrush presents as multifocal, creamy white papules and plaques that are nonadherent. Removal of this material often uncovers an erythematous mucosal surface.

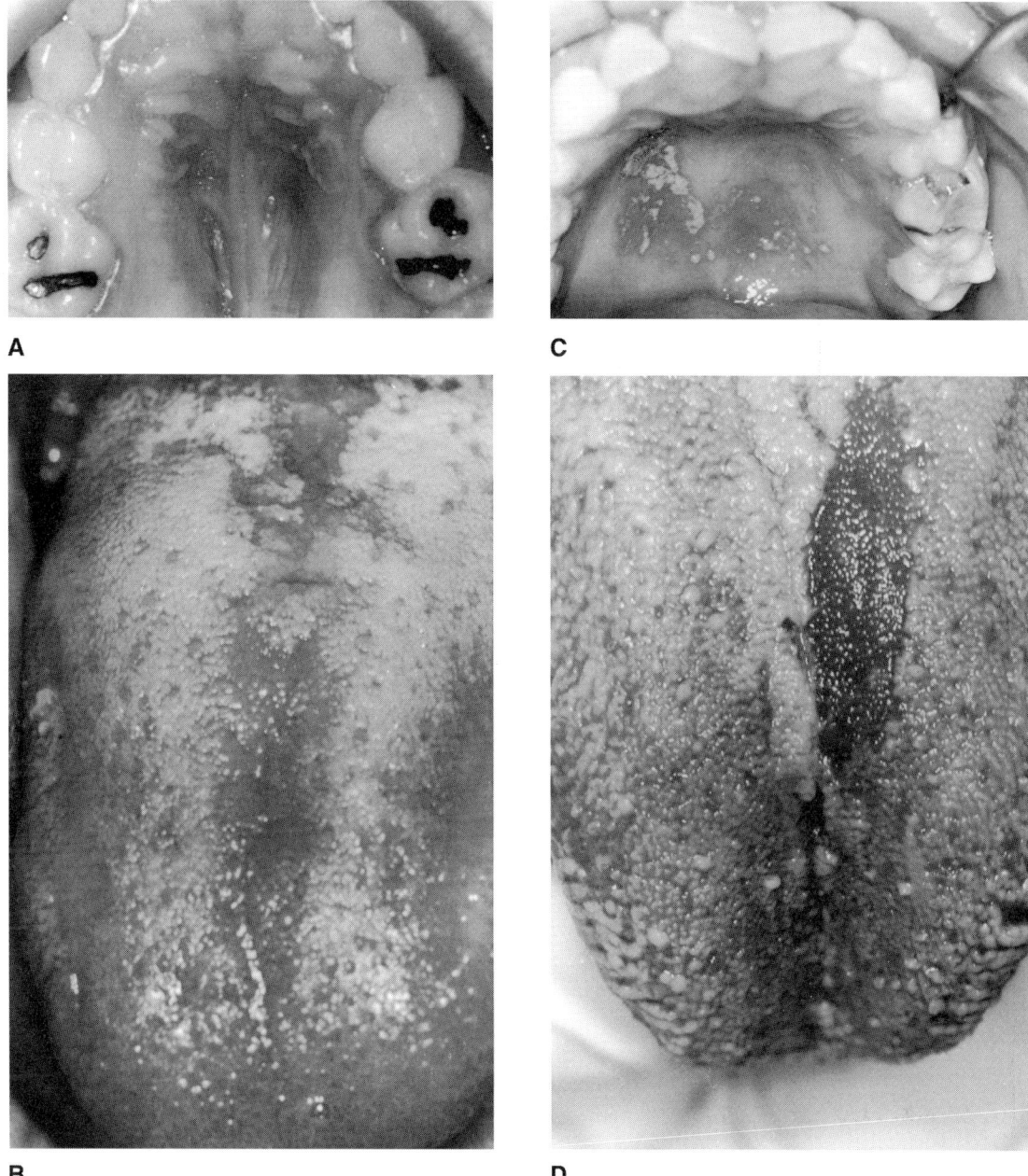

Figure 14–1. Oral candidiasis in pediatric HIV infection. Pseudomembranous candidiasis involving palate (*A*) and hypertrophic candidiasis (*B*) involving the tongue in an HIV-infected child. Erythematous candidiasis involving the palate (*C*) and median rhomboid glossitis (*D*) in another HIV-infected child.

itraconazole, and amphotericin B are examples of therapeutic agents used to manage oropharyngeal candidiasis in children.[28,34–36] When the perioral skin or lips (Fig. 14–2) are involved, topical antifungal ointments and creams are used alone or in conjunction with oropharyngeal therapy. Since angular cheilitis is coinfected frequently with *Staphylococcus aureus* (Fig. 14–2), an antibacterial ointment, such as mupirocin, may be indicated.[28,34–36] When deep fissures and cracks on the lips are observed, the combination of an antifungal and a low-potency steroid ointment may improve the healing response and decrease scarring. In general, the antifungal therapy should be continued 1 to 2 weeks after clinical resolution of the lesions. When frequent episodes are encountered,

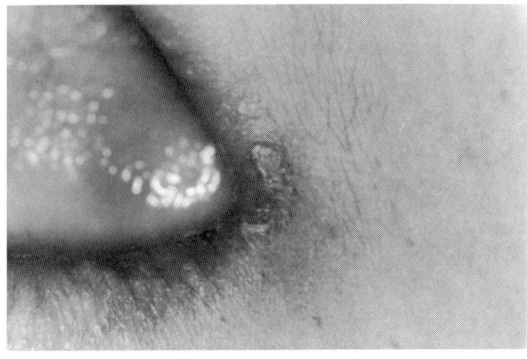 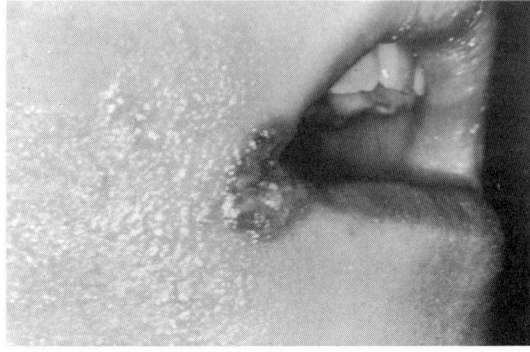

Figure 14–2. Angular cheilitis secondary to candidal infection in pediatric HIV infection (*A*) and with secondary *Staphylococcus aureus* infection (impetigo, *B*).

suppressive maintenance antifungal therapy is indicated. Candidal contamination of oral pacifiers, toothbrushes, and orthodontic appliances contributes to disease recurrence in children. Saliva transmission, especially from maternal infection, is another risk factor for recurrence in the immunocompromised child. Finally, it has been shown microscopically that deep dental caries may also act as a reservoir for *Candida* species in HIV-infected individuals.[37] Persistent or recurrent oropharyngeal candidiasis in immunocompromised patients may originate from candidal colonization of carious teeth. This emphasizes the importance of restoring carious teeth and the need for continuous caries prevention.

HERPES SIMPLEX VIRUS INFECTION

Herpes simplex virus (HSV) infection is the most common viral mucocutaneous disease affecting HIV-positive children (Fig. 14–3).[*] Similar to findings in healthy children, the majority of oral lesions are caused by HSV-1, which may produce either a primary or a recurrent infection. Herpetic lesion prevalence in pediatric HIV studies ranges from 2% to 24%, but it is likely that these figures represent an underestimation. In comparison, 33% of healthy school-aged children have had at least one episode of recurrent HSV by self-report.[38] Transmission of this disease is by saliva or direct contact with another person with a primary or recurrent HSV lesion.[*] Factors that may precipitate HSV reactivation within the trigeminal ganglion include excessive sun exposure, physical injury, febrile systemic disease, immunosuppression, emotional stress, and hormonal alterations. By definition, HIV-positive children who have two or more herpetic infection episodes within 1 year are classified as having moderately symptomatic HIV disease.[39]

Primary herpetic gingivostomatitis is a systemic viral infection with sudden onset of fever, lymphadenopathy, irritability, and malaise.[*] The classic lesions involve widespread mucosal erythema, vesicles, and painful coalescing ulcers. Although any oropharyngeal site may be affected, the gingiva and lips, including the perioral skin, are the most common sites. Excessive drooling, halitosis, and pharyngitis often accompany this oral infection. As a result of autoinoculation, ocular or digital lesions may develop, especially in children with non-nutritive sucking habits. This disease typically resolves within 14 days, but may linger for several more weeks in immunocompromised children.

Recurrent HSV infection is characterized by sudden onset of focal erythema, clustered vesicles, and coalescing ulcers that are painful (see Fig. 14–3).[†] Although a prodromal tingling and burning sensation develops prior to lesion formation, this is not a symptom that young children can identify easily. The vermilion border of the lip, perioral skin, and nasal mucosa are the most commonly involved sites. Intraorally, these lesions have a marked predilection for the gingiva and palatal mucosa. Healing is usually complete by 7 to 10 days. In some children, recurrent HSV may be responsible for the discomfort associated with tooth eruption. In

---

*See references 1–4, 7, 11, 12, 14, 16, 18, 19, 20, 29.

*See references 1–4, 7, 11, 12, 14, 16, 18, 19, 20, 29.
†See references 1–4, 7, 11, 12, 14, 26, 18, 19, 20, 29, 33, 34.

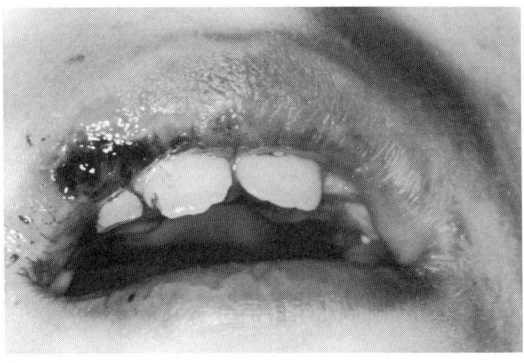 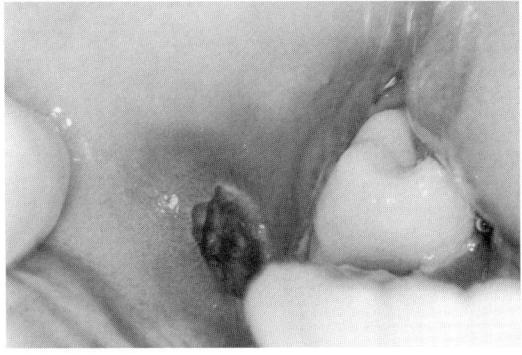

Figure 14–3. Herpes simplex ulcers of a chronic and recurrent nature in pediatric HIV infection. (*A*) Herpes simplex with crusted, hemorrhagic lesion and diffuse scarring of lip from previous herpetic lesions. (*B*) Chronic herpes simplex and cytomegaloviral ulcer with slightly scalloped but well-demarcated ulcer margins and a depressed granular base.

immunosuppressed children, the lesion pattern may be multifocal in distribution and occur on nonkeratinized mucosa. In addition, this infection may be chronic, often lasting for 4 to 6 weeks, and produce large, crateriform lesions with irregular, serpentine to scalloped margins. Coalescing vesicular to crusted lesions of the lip vermilion and perioral skin that bleed upon manipulation are characteristic when there is extraoral involvement. Although not typical for most cases of recurrent HSV, deep persistent lesions may result in significant scarring. Cytomegalovirus coinfection has been observed in these persistent oral ulcers.[40] Although not specific to HIV infection, some immunocompromised children develop an unusual disease pattern on the dorsal tongue that is referred to as geometric herpetic glossitis.[41] This painful variant appears as multiple, ulcerated fissures that radiate from the midline dorsal tongue surface. The recurrence rate is variable for herpetic lesions, but they tend to recur quite frequently in patients with severe immunosuppression.

Diagnosis of classic oral HSV infection is usually established by clinical signs and history.* Atypical lesions require additional laboratory studies, including exfoliative cytology, incisional biopsy, or tissue culture with viral isolation. Immunocytochemical and fluorescent monoclonal antibody typing can be performed on direct smears, biopsy samples, or infected cells grown in tissue culture. Superficial culture of the lesion, particularly swabbing, does not provide a definitive diagnosis, because HSV-seropositive individuals periodically shed this virus in saliva, resulting in a high false-positive rate.[40,42–44]

Although many cases of HSV are self-limiting, antiviral therapy is recommended in moderately to severely immunocompromised children and in cases in which there are frequent recurrences. Systemic acyclovir is most frequently used in children for the management of herpetic infections.[34–36,40] Lesions resistant to acyclovir have been managed effectively with foscarnet. Suppressive maintenance therapy to prevent recurrences may be indicated for some children who develop multiple episodes.

RECURRENT APHTHOUS STOMATITIS

Recurrent aphthous stomatitis (RAS) represents a recurrent, idiopathic, and noninfectious condition associated with a localized immune dysfunction (Fig. 14–4).[1–4] The prevalence of RAS in HIV-infected children ranges from 0% to 7%, similar to that in HIV-infected adults. Selected predisposing factors in children include trauma, mucosal atrophy from xerostomia and candidiasis, hematologic abnormalities, nutritional deficiencies, emotional stress, allergies, and familial predisposition. Although several microbial agents,[1–4] especially human herpesviruses,[40–44] have been implicated in the pathoetiology of these oral ulcers, a definite causal link has not been proven.

There are three clinical variations of these oral ulcers, including minor, major, and herpetiform aphthae.[1–4] These lesions present as painful ulcers of rapid onset with a marked predilection for the nonkeratinized mucosa, especially the labial and buccal mucosa, ventral tongue, and soft palate (see Fig. 14–4). More extensive cases may also involve

---

*See references 1–4, 7, 11, 12, 14, 16, 18, 19, 20, 29, 40, 41.

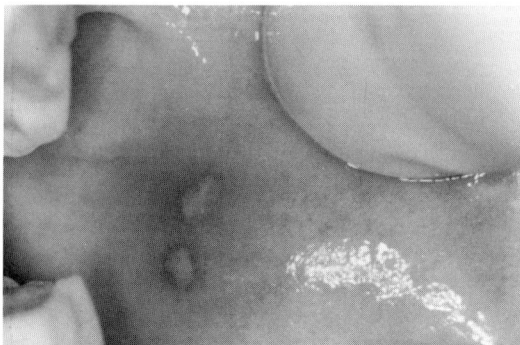

Figure 14–4. Aphthous ulcer in pediatric HIV infection involving buccal mucosa.

the pharyngeal and esophageal mucosa. In children, these painful ulcers contribute to malnutrition, dehydration, and weight loss, in addition to interfering with medication intake. Minor aphthous ulcers occur most commonly in children (see Fig. 14–4). These lesions are characterized by one to three shallow oval ulcers that are less than 5 mm in size and covered by a thin fibrinous exudate. The lesions are self-limiting and typically heal within a week without scarring. Major aphthous ulcers are often multiple, widespread, and greater than 1 cm in size. These large lesions have well-delineated to irregular borders and depressed bases and are often covered by a thick, tenacious, fibrinous exudate. Scarring is common, and healing occurs over a 2- to 6-week period in the normal host. Herpetiform aphthous ulcers are relatively uncommon in children and are characterized as numerous punctate ulcers that coalesce into larger curvilinear lesions, mimicking a viral infection. These lesions recur frequently and heal within 2 to 6 weeks. In general, RAS tends to recur more frequently in the HIV-infected child; with increased immunosuppression, major aphthous ulcers are more likely to develop.

The diagnosis of RAS is based on the site specificity of these lesions and the recurrence pattern.[1–4] Tissue cultures for viral, fungal, and mycobacterial organisms and/or incisional biopsy including the ulcer base are necessary for definitive diagnosis of persistent lesions. Cytomegaloviral infection, recrudescent herpes simplex infection, herpes zoster, histoplasmosis, mycobacterial infection, atypical bacterial infections, necrotizing periodontal disease, and non-Hodgkin's lymphoma should be included in the differential diagnosis of chronic oral ulcers. The importance of microscopic examination of lesional tissue that is refractory to empirical drug therapy cannot be overemphasized, because, with HIV infection, oral lesions may appear similar but have very disparate origins. RAS may also share similar clinical and microscopic features with drug-induced oral ulcerations. In particular, zalcitabine, abacavir, and foscarnet have been associated with oral ulcer development and resolution of ulcers after discontinuation of the medication.

Management of RAS usually involves topical corticosteroid therapy.[1–4,34–36] For severe cases, a short course of prednisone may be indicated, especially when the ulcers are multifocal and interfere with nutrition and medication intake. The addition of antifungal agents is advisable to prevent oropharyngeal candidiasis when steroids are used. Thalidomide is effective for management of RAS, especially when recurrences are frequent and severe.[44] Hematologic studies may be useful in determining whether anemia and neutropenia are contributing factors in RAS.[1–4]

OTHER ULCEROGENIC DISEASES

Cytomegalovirus may induce ulcers in those individuals with HIV, either alone or in combination with HSV.[1–4,40] This virus has a preference for endothelial cells and certain epithelial cells. The oral mucosa undergoes ulceration due to the ischemic effect associated with cytomegalovirus-infected endothelial cells and inflammatory cell recruitment to the site of infection. The number of cytomegalovirus-infected cells within the biopsy specimen may be quite few; and the ulcer may be attributed incorrectly to another infectious cause or considered nonspecific unless adequate sampling and immunocytochemistry are performed.[40] The biopsy must include the underlying lamina propria and ulcer bed for optimal cytomegalovirus detection. Recently, other herpesviruses, Epstein-Barr virus (EBV), and human herpesvirus-8, either alone or with cytomegalovirus, have been implicated in AIDS-associated oral ulcers by in situ hybridization and polymerase chain reaction.[40,45,46] Identification of a cytomegalovirus-induced oral ulcer should lead to an evaluation of the child for disseminated disease or other organ involvement, including cytomegalovirus retinitis, colitis, pneumonitis, and progressive neurologic disease.[1–4,40] Management of cytomegalovirus-induced oral ulcers typically involves the use of topical steroids, together with ganciclovir.[1–4,40,45]

Rarely, persistent oral ulcers are attributed to herpes zoster infection in children.[1,2,47] Involvement of the second and third branches of the trigeminal nerve produces oral lesions on both keratinized and nonkeratinized oral mucosa that extend to the midline. Frequently, concurrent vesicles and crusted skin lesions are found overlying the affected dental quadrant. Fever and complaints of sensitive teeth, earache, or headache are prodromal symptoms. Most cases of herpes zoster involving the trigeminal nerve heal without complications in children, except for facial skin scarring. However, there are isolated reports of osteonecrosis and spontaneous tooth loss as disease sequelae in HIV-infected adults.[47] Diagnosis is made by viral culture and direct staining of cytologic smears with fluorescent monoclonal antibodies for varicella-zoster virus. Antiviral therapy with acyclovir is recommended for herpes zoster management in immunocompromised children.[34–36]

Oral ulceration due to *Histoplasma capsulatum* is an example of a deep mycotic infection that is observed in immunocompromised individuals.[1–4] The lesion has a finely granular to beaded erythematous and ulcerated surface with irregular, firm, and rolled margins. This persistent and painful lesion may be single or multiple and is usually located on the tongue and gingival tissues. The diagnosis of histoplasmosis is made by identification of the organism in tissue sections or culture. Systemic antifungal medications are used to manage histoplasmosis, because oral lesions are a sign of disseminated disease. Blastomycosis, paracoccidioidomycosis, coccidioidomycosis, cryptococcosis, and zygomycosis are examples of other deep mycotic infections associated with chronic oral ulcers in the immunocompromised host. Owing to the high coinfection rate of HIV and tuberculosis, a mycobacterial cause for a persistent oral ulcer should be considered.[48] The diagnosis of active disease is made by identification of acid-fast bacilli in tissue sections or culture.

HOSPITALIZATION ASSOCIATED WITH ORAL LESIONS

Although oral lesions are not a common reason for hospitalization in pediatrics, 25% of HIV-infected children are admitted to hospitals because of their oral disease.[49] The most common admitting diagnosis is oral candidiasis with either candidemia or esophageal extension (57%). Major aphthae (28%) and herpes simplex virus stomatitis (15%) are the other reasons for admission. The average hospitalization attributed to oral lesions is for 3 days (range, 3–9 days). Oral lesions in HIV-infected children carry a certain degree of morbidity that is not well recognized.

HIV-ASSOCIATED PERIODONTAL DISEASE

Several periodontal conditions are associated with HIV infection and include: (1) linear gingival erythema; (2) necrotizing ulcerative gingivitis; (3) necrotizing ulcerative periodontitis; and (4) necrotizing stomatitis (Fig. 14–5).[1–6,8–20,29,43,50–54] These periodontal diseases[55–57] are not specific to HIV infection but tend to be more exaggerated in immunosuppressed individuals. In addition to these HIV-associated periodontal diseases, children are also prone to conventional gingivitis.

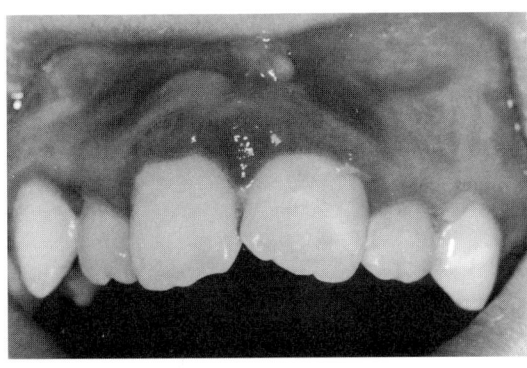
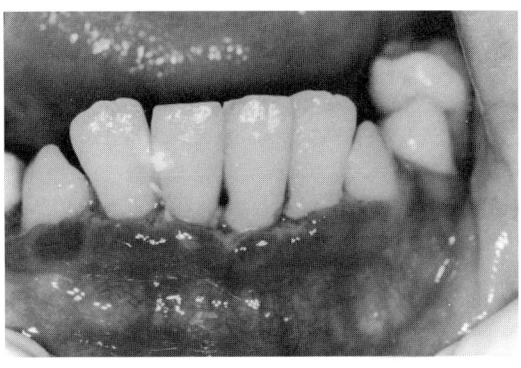

A B

Figure 14–5. Periodontal disease in pediatric HIV infection includes linear gingival erythema secondary to candidal infection (*A*) and necrotizing ulcerative periodontitis (*B*).

Linear gingival erythema (LGE) is the most common form of HIV-associated periodontal disease in HIV-infected children (see Fig. 14–5).[1–6,8–20] The prevalence of this disease varies widely in different clinical studies, ranging from 0% to 38%. Most studies that examine a young cohort of children rarely observe this disease, whereas those including adolescents from 13 to 18 years of age diagnose LGE in high numbers.[8,10] Although the microbiology of LGE has not been fully described, it is now defined as a candidal infection.[51–54] Both *C. albicans* and *C. dubliniensis* have been isolated from these lesions in both children and adults.[51] Superinfection with pathogenic bacteria due to conventional periodontitis seen in adults may explain the increased prevalence of LGE in the adolescent group.

Linear gingival erythema presents as a fiery red linear band that is 1 to 3 mm wide and involves the marginal gingiva, extending from one interdental papilla to the next (see Fig. 14–5).[1–6,8–20,51–54] Usually there is a widespread distribution, but occasionally, this entity is isolated to the gingiva adjacent to only a few teeth. Typically, this condition involves the maxillary labial gingiva in the incisor and canine regions in children. Concomitant pinpoint to diffuse erythema is observed with the adjacent attached gingiva and alveolar mucosa. The degree of erythema is disproportionally intense compared with the amount of plaque that is present on the teeth. Although bleeding with toothbrushing and spontaneous sulcular bleeding may occur with LGE, these features are uncommon. Pain is rarely noted in this atypical form of gingivitis. Critical to the diagnosis is that LGE responds minimally to plaque removal and improved oral hygiene, which distinguishes LGE from acute marginal gingivitis. Management includes appropriate antifungal treatment, because LGE represents an erythematous form of candidiasis.[51] It is important to exclude neutropenia, thrombocytopenia, and a hypersensitivity reaction, referred to as plasma cell gingivitis, in children with atypical gingivitis.

Necrotizing periodontal diseases, including necrotizing ulcerative gingivitis (NUG) and necrotizing ulcerative periodontitis (NUP), are uncommon in most HIV-infected children (see Fig. 14–5).[1–6,8–20,43,50,52–57] The prevalence of NUG is not known with certainty for children, but ranges from 0% to 11% in HIV-infected adults, while NUP has been reported in 0% to 4% of children. Although not limited to HIV disease, predisposing factors in necrotizing periodontal disease development are psychological stress, immunosuppression, malnutrition, and exposure to tobacco smoke. There is a predilection for NUG disease to occur in older adolescents and young adults in the United States and Europe when it is diagnosed in HIV-uninfected individuals. In contrast, this is a disease of the young child in developing countries, as a result of poor nutritional status, especially inadequate protein intake, and viral infection, such as measles or herpesviruses.[43] Progression of NUG to a fulminating and disfiguring disease referred to as noma or *cancrum oris* may be a lethal complication that has been described in African children. HIV-infected children from developing countries appear to be more susceptible to these necrotizing periodontal diseases.[50]

Necrotizing ulcerative gingivitis is characterized by the necrosis of one or more of the interdental papillae, pain of sudden onset, and bleeding.[1–6,8–20,52–57] Other signs and symptoms that may be present, but are not pathognomonic of NUG, include lymphadenopathy, fetid halitosis, fever, and malaise. Permanent gingival scarring with interdental papillary cratering contributes to an increased recurrence risk. Loss of gingival attachment and bone are infrequent findings but are more likely to develop with frequent recurrences of the disease. When ulceration and necrosis of the gingival tissues along with exposure and rapid destruction of alveolar bone occur, the disease is referred to as NUP (see Fig. 14–5). This more extensive disease may contribute to premature exfoliation of primary teeth and aborted development or early loss of permanent teeth. When there is extensive involvement of the alveolar bone and contiguous soft tissues, this aggressive necroulcerative lesion is referred to as necrotizing stomatitis. A declining immune system with CD4+ cell counts below 200 cells/mm^3 is associated with NUP and necrotizing stomatitis.

Microbiologic studies of NUG have demonstrated the presence of an anaerobic microflora consisting of *Treponema*, *Selenomonas*, *Prevotella intermedia*, *Fusobacterium*, and *Porphyromonas gingivalis*.[1–6,8–20,52–56] In HIV-infected individuals, *C. albicans* is commonly associated with this disease. With NUP, additional periodontopathic microorganisms are observed, similar to those in conventional periodontitis. The unique histopathologic findings of these necrotizing lesions include a thickened fibrinopurulent membrane with extensive bacterial colonization and spirochetal infiltration, overlying a lamina propria containing an acute or mixed inflammatory infiltrate with prominent hyperemia. Sequestration of variably sized alveolar bone fragments is a common finding when there is rapid bone destruction. Effacement of the underlying minor salivary glands, extensive degeneration of the striated muscle bundles, and obliterative vasculitis are additional features of necrotizing stomatitis.

Management of these necrotizing periodontal diseases requires local débridement with scaling and curettage, improved oral hygiene, and chlorhexidine gluconate oral rinse.[1–4,52–57] Short-term adjunctive use of systemic antibiotics, such as metronidazole, clindamycin, or amoxicillin with clavulanate potassium, reduces acute pain and promotes healing.[1–4] In susceptible children, an antifungal agent may be needed concurrently if systemic antibiotics are prescribed. An underlying neutropenia or coinfection with cytomegalovirus should be excluded when there is extensive tissue destruction or in cases that are refractory to treatment.

SALIVARY GLAND DYSFUNCTION

Salivary gland dysfunction in HIV-infected children presents as either xerostomia or major salivary gland enlargement (Fig. 14–6).[1–4,11–13,20,58,59] Xerostomia occurs in 15% to 35% of HIV-infected children. The cause of this condition may be HIV infection itself, therapeutic antiviral and antimicrobial drugs, prophylactic medications, antiretrovirals, γ-globulin, or lymphocytic infiltration of the major salivary glands. Reduced salivary flow results in mucosa that may become desiccated and is at higher risk for opportunistic infections, such as candidiasis, and increased caries due to lack of adequate oral clearance and inadequate remineralization of incipient caries.

Lymphocyte-mediated salivary gland disease in cases of HIV infection may be referred to as major salivary gland enlargement (parotid and/or submandibular glands, see Fig. 14–6), diffuse infiltrative lymphocytosis syndrome, or Sjögren syndrome–like disease.[1–4,11–13,20,58,59] Although the exact cause for this disease is not known, infection with EBV or HIV, or the interaction between these viruses, is suspected in the pathoetiology. Parotid gland enlargement is readily visible in 10% to 30% of children as facial masses. This oral manifestation is more common in children than in adults with

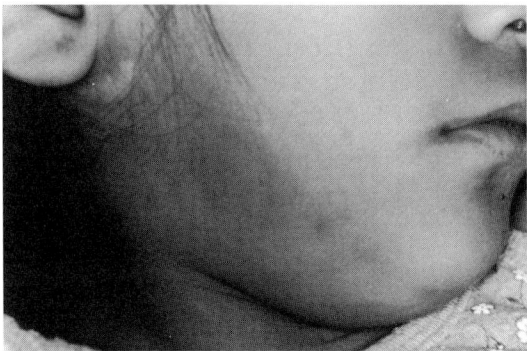

Figure 14–6. Salivary gland enlargement in pediatric HIV infection with both the submandibular and parotid glands involved.

HIV infection. However, the histopathologic appearance of lymphocyte-mediated salivary gland disease is similar in children, adolescents, and adults.[58] The swelling may be unilateral or bilateral, sometimes painful, and seen in combination with lymphoid interstitial pneumonitis and diffuse lymphadenopathy. Concurrent enlargement of the palatine tonsils may be seen, resulting in partial airway obstruction, difficulty swallowing, and sleep apnea.[58] Prior to the use of highly active antiretroviral therapy, this afebrile condition was associated with a longer median time to death than oral candidiasis (5.4 years versus 3.4 years).[59] Because mumps parotitis may also occur in HIV-infected children, this needs to be a consideration.

Diffuse infiltrative lymphocytosis syndrome of minor salivary glands can be seen in patients with HIV infection.[1–4,11–13,20,58] This disease may mimic Sjögren syndrome histologically and clinically. HIV-infected individuals do not have autoantibodies (SSA, SSB) associated with Sjögren syndrome, and the salivary glands are infiltrated by CD8+ lymphocytes rather than CD4+ lymphocytes. Diffuse infiltrative lymphocytosis syndrome is associated with an increased risk for high-grade B-cell lymphoma development. When salivary flow is reduced, the child is at risk for development of superimposed bacterial sialadenitis. In addition, superficial and deep mucoceles may develop as a result of prolonged xerostomia or blockage of the excretory ducts of the minor salivary glands.

HAIRY LEUKOPLAKIA

Hairy leukoplakia is an opportunistic infection that is caused by the Epstein-Barr virus and is a marker for increasing immunodeficiency

(Fig. 14–7).[1–4,60,61] This lesion is a common oral manifestation of HIV infection in adults, with a point prevalence of approximately 20%, whereas it is documented in only 2% of children with HIV. Although first described in conjunction with HIV infection, hairy leukoplakia has been documented in transplant recipients and in patients receiving immunosuppressive therapy. Hairy leukoplakia has a marked predilection for the lateral borders of the tongue, but is occasionally seen at other oral mucosal sites, especially the buccal mucosa. The classic clinical features are a white, thickened, corrugated patch, often with an adherent shaggy or hairy surface. Occasionally, hairy leukoplakia is more subtle and appears as an area of filmy white, thin, vertical striations or smooth-surfaced plaques. Either a bilateral or a unilateral distribution is observed that may cover a very small to extensive surface area. Although hairy leukoplakia is usually asymptomatic, tenderness, taste perversions, tongue thickening, and cosmetic embarrassment may accompany this disease. A superimposed candidal infection is associated with hairy leukoplakia in 50% of cases.

Diagnosis is based on the clinical features, in addition to the documentation of EBV infection using either tissue or cytologic samples.[1–4,60,61] The histopathologic features of hairy leukoplakia include squamous mucosa with shaggy hyperparakeratosis, acanthosis, and clusters or layers of balloon cells resembling koilocytes within the intermediate and superficial layers. There is scant to no evidence of an inflammatory cell infiltrate in the underlying connective tissue. The superficial epithelium may exhibit hyphal forms consistent with *Candida* species. EBV can be identified in the epithelial cells with immunocytochemistry and in situ hybridization. Multiple strains, recombinants, and mutant forms of EBV have been recognized in this disease, which may help to explain the increased detection of hairy leukoplakia in adults, in contrast to children, with HIV.

Although treatment is not necessary, topical podophyllin resin, antiherpetic medications, and topical retinoic acid have been used to manage symptomatic or extensive lesions.[1–4,35,36,60,61] If a candidal infection is detected, then concurrent use of antifungal therapy is recommended. Hairy leukoplakia lesions may be persistent; however, lesion regression is often noted with improvement in CD4+ counts, especially with antiretroviral therapy. Despite treatment, recurrences are common and are often associated with immune status fluctuations. Recognition of HLP is important, because it has been linked to HIV disease progression in adults. To date, neither dysplasia nor carcinoma has been associated with this tongue lesion; however, with an increased life expectancy of HIV-infected children and adults, the potential role of oncogenic EBV in oral cancer development remains unknown.

ORAL WARTS

Human papillomavirus (HPV) is responsible for a viral-induced proliferation of squamous cells that is a common cutaneous infection in healthy children and adolescents.[1–4,62] Although the prevalence of oral warts in HIV-infected children (Fig. 14–8) is not known, this disease is observed in 1% to 4% of adults with HIV. HPV-induced oral lesions associated with HIV infection include verruca vulgaris, condyloma acuminatum, focal epithelial hyperplasia, and koilocytic dysplasia. Focal epithelial hyperplasia (Heck's disease) is a benign oral cavity condition associated with HPV types 13 and 32 and is usually seen in children. These lesions appear as multiple nontender papules, plaques, and nodules with grainy, pink mucosal surfaces. The labial, buccal, and lateral tongue mucosa are most often involved, with occasional lesions on the palatal and gingival mucosa. This is the most common HPV-induced disease in HIV-infected adults, and it appears to be limited to the oral mucosa. In contrast, verruca vulgaris is typically observed with the skin, especially the hands and perioral skin. Oral mucosa involvement due to autoinoculation is uncommon and is usually limited to isolated areas of the lip vermilion, labial mucosa,

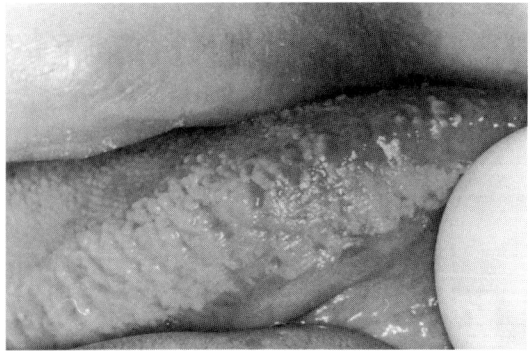

Figure 14–7. Oral hairy leukoplakia in pediatric HIV infection involving the lateral border of tongue.

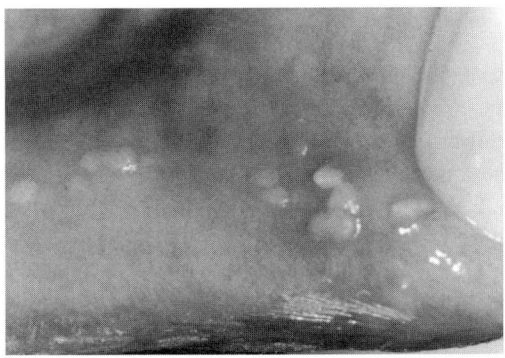

Figure 14–8. Oral wart in pediatric HIV infection involving the buccal mucosa in a child with extensive cutaneous lesions.

and anterior tongue. These lesions manifest as white, rough, conical to papillary papules or nodules. When condyloma acuminatum occurs in the oral cavity, it may develop due to sexual transmission, autoinoculation, or perinatal exposure.

Despite the high rate of cervical HPV infection in HIV-positive women, oral infection in children is rare. When they do occur intraorally, the labial mucosa, soft palate, and lingual frenum are the most frequently affected sites. The typical condyloma presents as a large, sessile, pink nodule with short, blunt surface projections. Multiple lesions may be found that tend to coalesce, forming a discrete, well-delineated enlargement. With most oral warts, conservative excision is the treatment of choice. Other methods of treatment include laser ablation, topical podophyllin resin, systemic interferon, and cimetidine. Despite aggressive therapy and the use of multiple treatment modalities, recurrences are common when oral warts are widespread. Of concern is that the long-term effect of HPV infection on the oral mucosa potentially could lead to dysplasia or malignant transformation, depending upon the HPV type (types 31, 33, and 35 represent intermediate risk; types 16 and 18 represent high risk). In HIV-infected adults, HPV-induced koilocytic dysplasia involving the oral mucosa has been described, but malignant transformation of oral warts has not been documented, in contrast to anogenital disease.

MALIGNANCY

Children with HIV infection are more susceptible to the development of certain neoplasms, and these tumors are those associated with viral transformation.[63–70] Kaposi's sarcoma occurs more frequently in HIV-infected adults, especially in men who have sex with men and in intravenous drug users. With the HIV-infected pediatric population, Kaposi's sarcoma is more common in Africa and Eastern Europe, where endemic Kaposi's sarcoma is more prevalent in the non–HIV–infected population. Human herpesvirus-8 is intimately associated with malignant transformation and is readily identified in all forms of Kaposi's sarcoma, both HIV-related and HIV-unrelated tumors. These tumors have a variable appearance, ranging from erythematous plaques to red-purple nodular lesions with surface ulcerations (Fig. 14–9). The most common oral sites are the hard and soft palates and the gingiva. Localized intraoral tumors can be managed with intralesional chemotherapy agents, such as vinblastine, with involution of the lesions and periodic maintenance therapy to avoid recurrence. Systemic chemotherapy may be necessary for more advanced disease or multiorgan involvement. Kaposi's sarcoma is associated with more advanced disease and is less common in adults since the introduction of highly active antiretroviral therapy.

Epstein-Barr virus latent infections are associated with AIDS-related lymphomas, Hodgkin's disease, Castleman's disease, multiple myeloma, and benign and malignant smooth muscle tumors in HIV infection.[63,64,66–70] This virus immortalizes B-cell lymphocytes and promotes neoplastic transformation of lymphocytes and smooth muscle cells. This allows for unopposed proliferation, with escape from cell cycle regulation. Smooth muscle tumors with episomal EBV integration are unique to pediatric HIV infection. Initial EBV infection in children occurs between the ages of 7 to 24 months. In HIV-infected children, EBV-DNA is detected in blood samples for several years at levels several hundred times greater (often >10,000 copies/0.1 mL) than those for

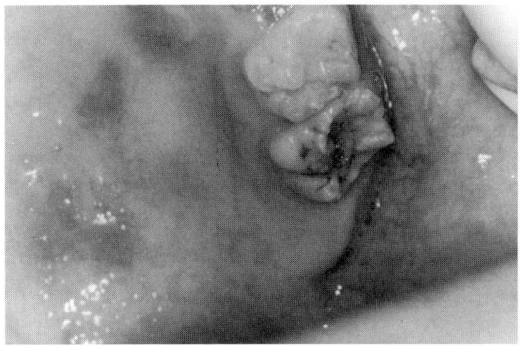

Figure 14–9. Multifocal erythematous plaques involving the hard palate characteristic for Kaposi's sarcoma in pediatric HIV infection.

EBV-infected, HIV-uninfected children. The oral cavity is a relatively common site for the development of extranodal lymphoma typically seen in people with HIV infection. Such lesions may mimic oral ulcers or manifest as nodular masses resembling Kaposi's sarcoma. Diffuse and expansile intrabony lesions may result in tooth displacement or mobility. Localized and referred pain followed by paresthesia is a common complaint when the jaws are involved.[66] Chemotherapy results in a rapid response, but maintenance therapy is necessary to avoid recurrence.

The Children's Cancer Group evaluated tumors in HIV-infected U.S. children over a 15-year period.[64,67] The distribution of tumors was 67% non-Hodgkin's lymphoma, 17% smooth muscle tumors, 8% leukemia, 5% Kaposi's sarcoma, 3% Hodgkin's lymphoma, 2% tracheal neuroendocrine carcinoma, and 2% vaginal carcinoma. Median survival is considerably reduced for patients with non-Hodgkin's lymphoma (6 months) and smooth muscle tumors (12 months). It is quite obvious that viral-associated tumors represent the vast majority of malignancies in HIV-infected children. Higher rates of cancer are anticipated in developing countries.

Currently, a small percentage (about 2%) of HIV-infected children develop cancer.[63,64,67–70] With more children living well into adolescence and early adulthood, HIV-associated malignancies will become more common in this population. It is anticipated that oral malignancies, especially lymphoma, smooth muscle tumors, leukemia, and Kaposi's sarcoma, will be more frequent in the future as the HIV-infected pediatric population grows older.

THROMBOCYTOPENIA

Bleeding diatheses secondary to thrombocytopenia is a considerable problem that has an impact on delivery of oral health care for HIV-infected children.[29,71–75] About 4% of HIV-infected children have bleeding problems associated with dental procedures; interestingly, a similar proportion of children have oral mucosa petechiae at baseline examination. During their disease course, 13% to 18% of children will have thrombocytopenia. Both antibody-mediated platelet destruction and bone marrow failure have been implicated in low platelet counts. Direct infection of megakaryocytes by HIV has also been demonstrated. More recently, it has been shown that thrombopoietin levels are markedly elevated in children with more severe thrombocytopenia. This group does not respond to steroids or immunoglobulin-mediated therapy and requires growth factors (erythropoietin, granulocyte colony-stimulating factor) to help alleviate low platelet counts. Thrombocytopenia is linked to advanced stage of disease, with as many as 52% of children with Centers for Disease Control and Prevention (CDC) C3 class disease having thrombocytopenia. It is important to determine both the quantity and the function of platelets if dental treatment is to be carried out without platelet transfusion. Oral findings associated with thrombocytopenia include spontaneous gingival bleeding (Fig. 14–10) and focal to diffuse purpura, which are most evident on the palatal and buccal mucosa. Prolonged bleeding following the exfoliation of a primary tooth or an oral surgical procedure is an indication of this problem. Hematoma formation with orofacial involvement following local anesthetic injection for dental treatment is a potentially serious sequela.

SALIVA AND HIV

Saliva is a complex fluid that lubricates and protects the oral mucosa against microbial assault and affects the development and remineralization of dental caries.[76–82] Although viral RNA, proviral DNA, and viral p24 antigens may be detected in oral fluids from most HIV-infected individuals, infectious virions are found in a small percentage (1–5%) of HIV-infected persons. This is due to the numerous protective factors in saliva, which function through several different mechanisms for the

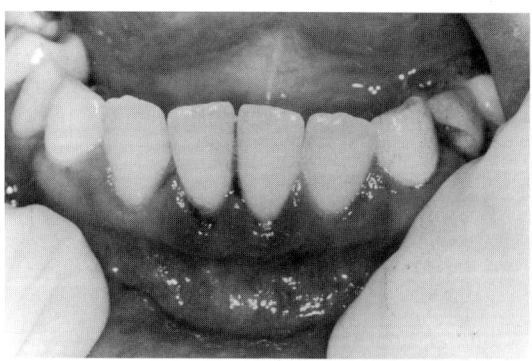

Figure 14–10. Conventional gingivitis in pediatric HIV infection with spontaneous gingival bleeding secondary to HIV-induced thrombocytopenia.

prevention of microbial disease (Table 14–2). These include immunoglobulins directed against HIV-1, high molecular weight mucins, protease inhibitors, enzymes, complement components, and other agents that inhibit viral uptake by susceptible cells. The most effective anti-HIV protein in saliva is secretory leukocyte protease inhibitor (SLPI), secreted primarily by acinar serous cells in parotid and submandibular glands. While the antiviral effect was attributed initially to SLPI's protease inhibitor function, it has been determined more recently that the major role in preventing HIV transmission is prevention of viral entry into susceptible cells. In the presence of SLPI, HIV attaches to the cell via the CD4+ receptor or other HIV receptors. However, SLPI and a 55-kD SLPI-binding protein prevent viral entry into the cell by interacting with either a chemokine coreceptor (CXCR4, CCR5) or cell surface molecules (galactosyl ceramide) associated with viral entry, viral fusion, and viral capsid uncoating.

When cells have been exposed to physiologic levels of SLPI prior to or during exposure to HIV, at least a 90% inhibition of HIV transmission occurs. SLPI is more effective at protecting cells against infection with cell-free virus than cell-associated virus. HIV-infected cells are not affected by SLPI. SLPI also inactivates the inflammatory mediators neutrophil elastase and cathepsin G. Both protease and viral entry inhibition functions remain intact, even in the acidic oral environment.

Viral production may be moderately to substantially reduced by other protease inhibitors and various proteolytic enzymes in the saliva.[76–82] Many of these inhibit viral production in cell cultures by up to 90%; however, levels greater than physiologic concentrations are generally necessary. Still, considerable inhibitory activity (about 30%) may be found with physiologic levels of protease inhibitors, such as cystatin and proteolytic enzymes. The synergistic effect of SLPI, protease inhibitors, proteolytic enzymes, and other agents probably accounts for the low level of infectious virions in saliva compared with serum and cervical and seminal fluids.

Saliva is hypotonic compared with serum and other body fluids.[82] The tonicity of saliva is one seventh that of interstitial fluids. This hypotonicity is very important in lessening the chance of oral transmission via HIV-infected mononuclear leukocytes. Saliva's tonicity induces cell lysis, and this effectively eliminates cells that could produce virions or infect other susceptible cells by cell-to-cell contact. When sterile-filtered saliva is applied to HIV-infected mononuclear leukocytes and lymphocytes for as little as 1 minute, virus production over a 24-hour period is inhibited by more than 10,000-fold, compared with two- to fivefold for salivary inhibitor proteins alone. Isotonic dilution of the saliva does adversely affect viral inhibition. With a 25% isotonic dilution, virus inhibition is

Table 14–2
Salivary Factors and Protective Mechanisms

FACTOR	MECHANISM
HIV-specific antibodies (IgA, IgG, IgM)*	Neutralize and inactivate virus
Complement (C1q)*	Bind and sequester virus
Thrombospondin†	Aggregate virus; block CD4+ binding
High molecular weight mucins*	Entrap and aggregate virus
Secretory leukocyte protease inhibitor†	Prevents virus entry; protease inhibitor
Cystatin*	Protease inhibitor
Histatin	Protease inhibitor
Statherin	Protease inhibitor
Basic proline-rich proteins	Protease inhibitor
Defensin*	Prevent virus entry
Amylase	Antimicrobial enzyme
Lactoferrin*	Binds iron
Lactoperoxidase*	Antimicrobial enzyme
Lysozyme*	Antimicrobial enzyme
Hypotonicity	Lyses cells; prevents viral replication
Salivary flow	Bathes and rinses oral cavity
Low viscosity	Promotes saliva flow

*Activity against HIV-1.
†Activity against HIV-1 at physiologic levels.
Compiled from references 76–82.

reduced to one tenth of that for undiluted saliva. No viral inhibition occurs once saliva is diluted by 75% with isotonic solutions, implying protection of infected cells from salivary lysis. The typical volume of saliva in the oral cavity is 0.75 mL, and the amount of blood necessary to partially protect infected leukocytes against salivary lysis is between 0.5 and 4.5 mL (0.25 to 2.25 mL isotonic serum). Blood volumes greater than 4.5 mL mixed with residual saliva in the oral cavity will completely inactivate the protective hypotonic effect of saliva. This is of concern for oral procedures with mild blood loss and biting episodes in an HIV-infected patient with blood shedding. In addition, HIV transmission via breastfeeding or unprotected oral sex with seminal or cervical fluid exposure is a reality due to loss of the hypotonic protective effect of saliva. In fact, 0.25 to 2.25 mL of HIV-infected breastmilk or 2.6 to 3.8 mL of HIV-infected seminal fluid inactivates the antiviral effect of saliva. With very viscous fluids such as breastmilk and seminal fluids, infected leukocytes may be protected from hypotonic saliva to a certain extent. With a salivary flow rate of 0.3 mL per minute, the hypotonicity of saliva would be affected for a minimum of 2 to 3 minutes.

A high viral load or dilution may overwhelm the protective effect of saliva.[76–82] Large amounts of blood, dilution with other body fluids such as seminal or cervical fluids during oral sex, and rinsing with isotonic solutions may affect the ability of saliva to prevent HIV transmission. This is especially important for those who practice oral sex with the false belief that HIV transmission does not occur via this route. Recent epidemiologic studies report a transmission risk of 7% with oral sex. It is also important for health care workers who may become exposed to contaminated oral fluids, especially if there is significant bleeding or dilution with isotonic solution rinsing.

Normal salivary flow and a relatively low viscosity are important factors in bathing the oral cavity with protective oral fluids and rinsing microorganisms and debris toward the gastrointestinal system.[76–82] It is well known that with HIV-infection alone, the major and minor salivary glands may be affected and result in decreased flow, leading to xerostomia and increased saliva viscosity. This produces a mucosa that is not adequately hydrated and is more susceptible to oral infections. In addition, many of the medications directed against HIV and opportunistic infections reduce salivary flow considerably.

Saliva contains a sampling of the microcosm of bacteria and fungal and viral agents within the oral cavity and provides insight into current oral infections or impending oral infections in HIV-infected persons.[30,31] The microbiologic composition of the saliva is important to determining which organisms may be associated with specific diseases that occur more commonly in patients with HIV infection. The bacterial and fungal organisms that are more common in HIV-infected patients and their relationship to oral diseases are under study. In fact, a unique organism is present in saliva in both HIV-infected and respiratory compromised children.[83] This organism is *Lautropia mirabilis*. Although no specific disease has been attributed to this organism at this time, it may serve as a marker for immunocompromise.

Perhaps more important is the ability to correlate fungal organisms by cytologic examination of saliva samples with oral candidiasis in pediatric patients.[30,31] Yeast and fungal hyphae in saliva from HIV-infected children were found in 19% of HIV-infected children and in 9% of HIV-exposed but uninfected children. In symptomatic children, salivary fungi were cytologically detected in 22% and oral candidiasis was present in 17%. With asymptomatic children, both fungi in saliva and oral candidiasis were identified in 11%. Oral candidiasis was not found in any HIV-exposed but uninfected children. With CDC immunologic categories, salivary fungi were detected in 27% of children with severe suppression, in 18% of those with moderate suppression, and in no children with no suppression. Cytologic examination of saliva provides a means to assess the presence of yeast and hyphae in the oral cavity, detect impending or existing oral candidiasis that may have been overlooked, and result in prompt antifungal therapy. Fungal cultures of saliva show similar results with both HIV-infected and HIV-exposed but uninfected children. Positive fungal cultures are found in 84% and 87% of HIV-infected and HIV-exposed but uninfected children, respectively. These results contrast dramatically with the proportion of children with clinical oral candidiasis and salivary fungi by cytologic examination in both HIV-infected and HIV-exposed uninfected children.

GINGIVAL AND PLAQUE INDICES

Gingival and periodontal disease not specifically associated with HIV infection are seen in the vast majority of HIV-infected children, and this is referred to as conventional gingivitis (see Fig. 14–10).[1–3,8–12,13,20,22,23] Of interest is the finding that CD4+ counts in HIV-infected children who have had conventional gingivitis are considerably lower (326/mm^3) than counts in HIV-infected children who have never had conventional gingivitis (727/mm^3). The prevalence of gingivitis in HIV-infected children is associated with age (6% in <1-year-olds, 55% in 1-year-olds, 85% in 2-year-olds, 87% in 3-year-olds, and 66% in 4-year-olds).

Gingival health in children is assessed by determining a gingival index at specific sites in the oral cavity.[84] A score of 0 (normal gingiva) to 3 (severe gingivitis) is assessed at each site. The total score divided by the number of sites examined yields the gingival index (GI). Few clinical investigations of gingival health using such an index have been performed with HIV-infected children.[3,12,13,19,22,23,25] In HIV-infected children with a mean age of 6.3 years, only 32% were found to have normal gingiva (GI = 0). Approximately one half of the HIV-infected children had mild gingival inflammation (GI = 0.1 to 1.0), while one fifth had moderate gingival inflammation (GI = 1.1 to 2.0) and the remaining 2% had severe gingival inflammation (GI = 2.1 to 3.0). Increasing gingival indices were associated with more extensive primary and permanent dentition caries. With oral candidiasis and oral ulcers, the mean GI was increased by 2.3-fold and 4.5-fold, respectively.

Dental plaque is a critical component in caries development and is associated with gingival inflammation (Fig. 14–11).[84] The association between plaque accumulation and oral candidiasis in HIV-infected children is well recognized.[3,12,13,19,22,23,25] In 2- and 3-year-olds with HIV infection, plaque is present in 91% of children with oral candidiasis. Plaque accumulation is assessed using a plaque index (PI). Assigning a score of 0 to 3 (none to severe plaque deposit) at selected tooth sites and then dividing the total score by the number of sites determines this index. PIs have not been analyzed to a significant degree in HIV-infected children. In a 48-month longitudinal study, the mean PI for HIV-infected children was fourfold greater than that for HIV-exposed, uninfected children. With HIV-infected children, approximately one half had mild plaque accumulations (PI = 0.1 to 1.0), one quarter had moderate plaque accumulations (PI = >1.0 to 2.0), 5% had severe plaque accumulations (PI = 2.1 to 3.0), and 20% had no plaque detected (PI = 0). There was a trend toward increased PIs for HIV-infected children with lower CD4+ percentages (<15%, 15% to 24%), moderate to severe immunosuppression, and moderate to severe symptoms. When oral candidiasis or oral ulcers were present, the mean PI was increased by 1.5-fold.

OVER-RETAINED PRIMARY TEETH AND DELAYED ERUPTION OF PRIMARY AND PERMANENT TEETH

In HIV-infected children, there is a tendency for the primary teeth to be retained past the expected exfoliation time (Fig. 14–12).[1,3,12,20,29] Over-retention of primary teeth in one study population occurred in 25% of children regardless of gender. At the same time, permanent tooth eruption was delayed in slightly more than 40% of HIV-infected children. Lower CD4+ counts are

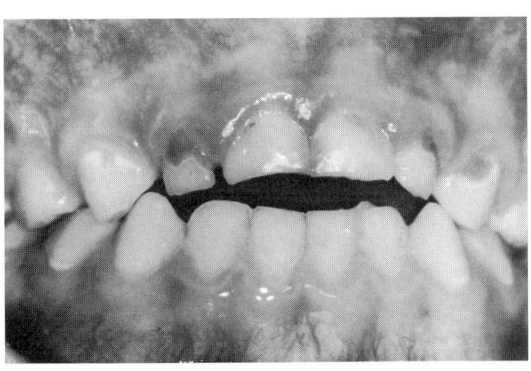
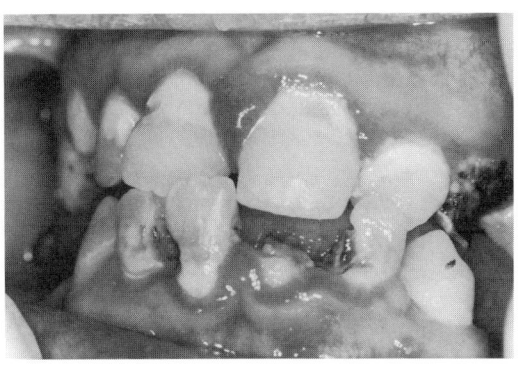

A   B

Figure 14–11. Extensive dental caries in the primary (A) and permanent (B) dentitions and marked dental plaque accumulation in pediatric HIV infection.

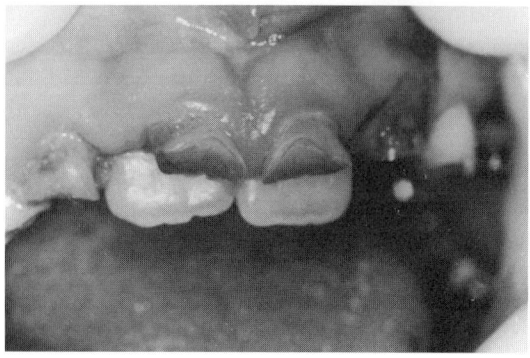

Figure 14–12. Over-retention of primary maxillary central incisors with delayed palatal eruption of permanent maxillary central incisors in pediatric HIV infection.

linked to delayed dental development. At 3 years of age, two fewer primary teeth have erupted in HIV-infected children with mean CD4+ counts of less than 200/mm^3 compared with those HIV-infected children with mean CD4+ counts of 800/mm^3 or more. This phenomenon may be associated with failure to thrive, delayed growth, and endocrine dysfunction that are known to occur in HIV-infected children. The consequences of this on the primary dentition would be an extended period of exposure to caries development. While in the permanent dentition, delayed eruption may result in a longer preeruption maturation period and a decreased exposure time for caries development compared with the general pediatric population. This would initially reflect a lower caries experience in the permanent dentition than age-matched HIV-negative children.

DENTAL CARIES

Although soft tissue lesions have been the primary focus of many dental studies, caries is a more prevalent disease in the HIV-infected population (see Fig. 14–11).[6–9,11,12,13,15,20,24–27,29] Caries in the primary and permanent dentitions affects at least 70% of HIV-infected children in the United States (Table 14–3). Because of the young age of most HIV-infected children, the primary dentition has been studied more thoroughly. With the primary dentition in the general pediatric population, there are four distinct caries patterns: (1) anterior caries involving smooth surfaces, (2) posterior caries, (3) pit and fissure caries, and (4) caries-free. With the HIV-infected group, the anterior caries pattern is over-represented compared with HIV-negative children (see Fig. 14–11). This pattern of caries is also known as early childhood caries and has carried the name nursing bottle or baby bottle tooth decay. In the HIV population, this caries pattern may result from poor oral hygiene practices, inappropriate use of a nursing bottle containing high-sucrose liquids at bedtime, or ad lib medications containing high sucrose content, xerostomia induced by HIV infection or medications, the need for high caloric and carbohydrate/sucrose diets, and saliva alterations in viscosity, cytokines, protease inhibitors, and immunoglobulins. Early childhood caries affects almost one third of HIV-infected children compared with less than 5% of the general pediatric population. In addition, rampant or extensive caries involving at least 10 primary tooth surfaces may be seen in almost one half of HIV-infected young children.

Primary dentition caries in HIV-infected children from developed countries is substantially higher than that for the general pediatric population (see Table 14–3).[3,6–9,11,12,13,15,20,24–27,29] In the United States, 2- to 9-year-old HIV-infected children have a greater than twofold increase in the number of tooth surfaces and teeth involved by caries compared with the same age group of uninfected children.[85] The proportion of caries-free children in the 5- to 9-year-old age group is reduced by 40% in those with HIV infection in the United States. In the United Kingdom, the primary dentition is affected to an even greater extent in HIV-infected children than in the United States.

Caries in the mixed primary and permanent dentitions show similar trends for children with HIV infection (see Table 14–3).[12,24–27,29] When HIV-infected children are compared with their HIV-negative siblings, caries in the primary dentition are increased by greater than twofold, whereas caries in the permanent dentition are similar between these groups. The number of caries-free HIV-infected children is 40% less when compared with their HIV-negative siblings. For those children older than 6 years of age, HIV infection is associated with a threefold increase in primary dentition caries and similar permanent dentition caries prevalence. Remarkably, only 7% of HIV-infected children older than 6 years of age were caries-free, whereas one third of their HIV-negative siblings older than 6 years of age were caries-free.

Because of the young age of the perinatally HIV-infected children, relatively few children with permanent dentitions have been available for

Table 14–3
Dental Caries Experience in Pediatric HIV Infection

STUDY GROUP	TEETH AFFECTED, N		CARIES-FREE, %
Primary Dentition Caries			
Baylor College of Medicine HIV-Infected Children	dfs	dft	
2 to 9 year olds	7.0	3.7	57
<2 year-olds	0.9	na	87
2 to 4 year-olds	2.7	3.0	65
5 to 9 year-olds	14.4	4.5	32
United States NHANES III National Survey (general pediatric population)			
2 to 9 year olds	3.1	1.4	62
2 to 4 year-olds	1.2	0.6	83
5 to 9 year-olds	4.1	1.9	50
United Kingdom HIV-Infected Children	dmfs	dmft	
≤ 6 year-olds	10.2	4.0	31
6 to 11 year-olds	17.9	4.9	31
New Jersey HIV-Infected Children			
2 to 5 year-olds	8.2	na	na
6 to 11 year-olds	13.9	na	na
New Jersey HIV-Negative Household Peers			
2 to 5 year-olds	3.5	na	na
6 to 11 year-olds	5.0	na	na
Mixed Primary and Permanent Dentition Caries			
New Jersey HIV-Infected Children‡	deft	DMFT	
All children	3.8	1.0	34
3 to 6 year-olds	3.2	0	46
>6 year-olds	5.7	1.3	7
New Jersey HIV-Negative Siblings‡			
All Children	1.5	1.0	56
3 to 6 year-olds	2.0	1.0	58
>6 year-olds	1.7	1.6	33
United Kingdom HIV-Infected Children		dmft/DMFT	
> 5 year-olds		1.8	na
5 year-olds		4.2	na
6 to 7 year-olds		6.9	na
8 to 11 year-olds		4.6	na
All children		4.4	37
Permanent Dentition Caries			
Baylor College of Medicine HIV-Infected Children	DMFS	DMFT	
5 to 11 year-olds	1.5	0.8	72
United States NHANES III National Survey (general pediatric population)			
5 to 11 year-olds	0.9	0.6	74
United Kingdom HIV-Infected Children			
6 to 11 year-olds	1.5	0.9	31

dfs, decayed, filled primary tooth surfaces; dft, decayed, filled primary teeth; deft, decayed, extracted, filled primary teeth; dmfs, decayed, missing, filled primary tooth surfaces; dmft, decayed, missing, filled primary teeth; DMFS, decayed, missing, filled permanent tooth surfaces; DMFT, decayed, missing, filled permanent teeth; na, not available/done.
Compiled from references 13, 24–27, 85.

epidemiologic study.[12,24–27,29] Most clinical studies have shown a similar caries experience in the permanent dentition between HIV-infected and the general pediatric populations (see Table 14–3). In a limited U.S. population of 5- to 11-year-old HIV-infected children, caries in the permanent dentition was increased from 0.6 decayed, missing, filled permanent tooth surfaces (DMFS; see Table 14–3) to 0.9 DMFS in HIV-infected children; however, caries-free status in the permanent dentition was similar.[24] It is well known that in HIV-infected children there is delayed eruption of the permanent teeth and over-retention of the primary teeth. This would lead to an artifactually low caries rate initially in the HIV-infected population compared with HIV-negative children. It is anticipated that as the teeth erupt on a slower time course, the HIV population would eventually experience caries at a higher rate than the uninfected population, similar to that noted for the primary dentition in HIV infection (see Fig. 14–11). This may be especially true considering that salivary gland dysfunction, either due to HIV infection or due to continuing xerostomia-inducing medications, would be even greater than in younger HIV-infected children.

Caries in HIV-infected children from developing countries may be even more devastating. A recent clinical study of dental caries in Romanian children (mean age, 8.8 years) demonstrated the association of caries development and HIV infection.[29] In these HIV-infected children, primary dentition caries was increased by 25% over 8-year-old Romanian school children. In the permanent dentition, caries was increased by 3.5-fold. In addition, the number of caries-free HIV-infected children was 43% lower compared with 8-year-old Romanian school children.[86] This dramatic increase in caries in both the primary and permanent dentition of Romanian HIV-infected children occurred in the absence of treatment with antiretroviral agents and other prophylactic medications.

Immunosuppression is associated with increased caries prevalence in the primary dentitions of children with HIV infection.[24] At the end of a 2-year period, the number of carious surfaces had increased by twofold and by 5.5-fold in the CDC moderate and severe immunologic categories, respectively, compared with the CDC no-immunosuppression category. Caries-free children in the CDC moderate and severe immunosuppressed categories were decreased by 14% and 22%, respectively, when compared with the CDC no-immunosuppression category. When CD4+ percentage groups were compared, similar caries increases were seen in HIV-infected children with low CD4+ percentages. Carious surfaces in the primary dentition were increased by 2.5-fold and 3.1-fold in the 15% to 24% CD4+ and less than 15% CD4+ groups, respectively, compared with the greater than 25% CD4+ group.

ORAL HEALTH

HIV-infected children have considerable oral disease, including soft tissue lesions, salivary gland dysfunction, and dental caries. Severe caries, such as those seen in children with HIV infection, affects the quality of life and overall well-being dramatically.[87] Toothaches, oral intake limitations, hampered growth, and sleep disturbances due to pain are very common complaints in the general pediatric population with marked caries. Appropriate dental care alleviates these complaints in more than 85% of affected children. Because of growth retardation, failure to thrive, increased nutritional demands, immunocompromise, salivary dysfunction, and high sucrose-containing medications, maintenance of optimal oral health is especially important for HIV-infected children. Although access to dental care has improved, renewed emphasis on oral health importance needs to be relayed to care providers. Less than 30% of children who have been referred for dental care complete the prescribed dental treatment.[88] Scheduled regular dental examinations and treatment will prevent certain oral diseases and allow for interventional therapy for soft tissue lesions, salivary gland dysfunction, and dental caries, which will have an impact on the overall health and well-being of the HIV-infected child. Integration of dental health professionals knowledgeable in HIV-associated oral conditions and in preventive and therapeutic oral health practices is crucial to the medical management of pediatric HIV infection.

REFERENCES

1. Ramos-Gomez FJ: Oral aspects of HIV infection in children. Oral Diseases 1999;3:S31–S35.
2. Ramoz-Gomez FJ, Flaitz C, Catapano P, et al: Classification, diagnostic criteria, and treatment recommendations for orofacial manifestations in HIV-

infected pediatric patients. J Clin Pediatr Dent 1999;23:85–96.
3. Ramos-Gomez FJ, Petru A, Hilton JF, et al: Oral manifestations and dental status in paediatric HIV infection. Int J Paediatr Dent 2000;10:3–11.
4. Ramos-Gomez FJ, Hilton JF, Canchola AJ, et al: Risk factors for HIV-related orofacial soft-tissue manifestations in children. Pediatr Dent 1996;18:121–126.
5. Flanagan MA, Barasch A, Koenigsberg SR, et al: Prevalence of oral soft tissue lesions in HIV-infected minority children treated with highly active antiretroviral therapies. Pediatr Dent 2000;22:287–291.
6. Flaitz C, Hicks J, Cron S, et al: Oral lesions in pediatric HIV infection: A longitudinal study [IADR Abstracts]. J Dent Res 2000;79:152.
7. Kline MW: Oral manifestations of pediatric human immunodeficiency virus infection: A review of the literature. Pediatr 1996;97:380–388.
8. Howell RB, Jandinski JJ, Palumbo P, et al: Oral soft tissue manifestations and CD4 lymphocyte counts in HIV-infected children. Pediatr Dent 1996; 18:117–120.
9. Del Toro A, Berkowitz R, Meyerowitz C, Frenkel LM: Oral findings in asymptomatic (P-1) and symptomatic (P-2) HIV-infected children. Pediatr Dent 1996;18:114–116.
10. Barasch A, Safford MM, Catalanotto FA, et al: Oral soft tissue manifestations in HIV-positive vs. HIV-negative children from an inner city population: A two-year observational study. Pediatr Dent 2000; 22:215–220.
11. Chigurupati R, Raghavan SS, Studen-Pavlovich DA: Pediatric HIV infection and its oral manifestations: A review. Pediatr Dent 1996;18:106–113.
12. Atkinson JC: Oral cavity and associated structures. In Moran C, Mullick FG (eds): Systemic Pathology of HIV Infection and AIDS in Children. Washington DC. AFIP/AMR Press, 1997, pp 55–71.
13. Gelbier M, Lucas VS, Zervou NE, et al: A preliminary investigation of dental disease in children with HIV infection. Int J Paediatr Dent 2000;10:13–18.
14. Ferguson FF, Berentsen B, Nachman S: Experiences of a pediatric dental program for HIV-positive children: Oral manifestations and dental diseases observed in 58 children. In Greenspan JS, Greenspan D (eds): Oral Manifestations of HIV Infection. Chicago, Quintessence Publishing, 1995, pp 240–246.
15. Kozinetz CA, Carter AB, Simon C, et al: Oral manifestations of pediatric vertical human immunodeficiency virus infection. AIDS Patient Care STDs 2000;14:89–94.
16. Moniaci D, Cavallari M, Greco D, et al: Oral lesions in children born to HIV-1 positive women. J Oral Pathol Med 1993;22:8–11.
17. EC Clearinghouse on Oral Problems Related to HIV Infection and WHO Collaborating Centre on Oral Manifestations of the Immunodeficiency Virus: Classification and diagnostic criteria for oral lesions in HIV infection. J Oral Pathol Med 1993; 22:289–291.
18. Nicolatou O, Theodoridou M, Mostrou G, et al: Oral lesions in children with perinatally acquired human immunodeficiency virus infection. J Oral Pathol Med 1999;28:49–53.
19. Fonesca R, Cardoso AS, Pomarico I: Frequency of oral manifestations in children infected with human immunodeficiency virus. Quintessence Int 2000; 31:419–422.
20. Valdez IH, Pizzo PA, Atkinson JC: Oral health of pediatric AIDS patients: A hospital-based study. ASDC J Dent Child 1994;61;114–118.
21. Patton LL: Sensitivity, specificity and positive predictive value of oral opportunistic infections in adults with HIV/AIDS as markers of immune suppression and viral burden. Oral Surg Oral Med Oral Pathol Oral Radiol Endod 2000;90:182–188.
22. Flaitz C, Carter B, Hicks J, et al: Gingival health in pediatric HIV infection: A longitudinal study. Pediatr Dent 2000;22:240.
23. Vierla AR, Ribeiro de Souza IP, Modesto A, et al: Gingival status of HIV+ children and the correlation with caries incidence and immunologic profile. Pediatr Dent 1998;20:169–172.
24. Hicks MJ, Flaitz CM, Carter AB, et al: Dental caries in pediatric human immunodeficiency virus infection: A longitudinal study. Pediatr Dent 2000; 22:359–364.
25. Elderidge K, Gallagher JE: Dental caries prevalence and dental health behaviour in HIV infected children. Int J Paediatr Dent 2000;10:19–26.
26. Howell RB, Jandinski J, Palumbo P, et al: Dental caries in HIV-infected children. Pediatr Dent 1992;14:370–371.
27. Tofsky N, Nelson EM, Lopez RN, et al: Dental caries in HIV-infected children versus household peers: Two-year findings. Pediatr Dent 2000;22:207–214.
28. Flaitz CM, Hicks MJ: Oral candidiasis in children with immune suppression: Clinical appearances and therapeutic considerations. ASDC J Dent Child 1999;85:161–166.
29. Flaitz CM, Wullbrandt B, Sexton J, et al: Prevalence of orodental findings in HIV-infected Romanian children. Pediatr Dent 2000;23:44–50.
30. Flaitz CM, Hicks MJ, Carter AB, et al: Saliva technique for cytologic, microbiologic and viral evaluation in pediatric HIV infection. ASDC J Dent Child 1998;65:318–324.
31. Hicks MJ, Carter AB, Rossmann SN, et al: Detection of fungal organisms in saliva from HIV-infected children: A preliminary cytologic analysis. Pediatr Dent 1998;20:162–168.
32. Chiou CC, Groll AH, Gonzalez CE, et al: Esophageal candidiasis in pediatric acquired immunodeficiency

33. Brown DM, Jabra-Rizk MA, Falker WA, et al: Identification of *Candida dubliniensis* in a study of HIV-seropositive pediatric dental patients. Pediatr Dent 2000;22:234–238.
34. Flaitz CM, Baker KA: Treatment approaches to common symptomatic oral lesions in children. Dent Clin North Am 2000;44:671–696.
35. Nielsen K: Pediatric HIV infection. HIV Clinical Management, volume 12. Available at www.medscape.com/medscapeHIV/clinicalMgmt. December 24, 1999 (accessed September 24, 2000).
36. Abrams EJ: Opportunistic infections and other clinical manifestations of HIV disease in children. Pediatr Clin North Am 2000;47:79–108.
37. Jacob LS, Flaitz CM, Nichols CM, Hicks MJ: Role of dentinal carious lesions in the pathogenesis of oral candidiasis in HIV infection. J Am Dent Assoc 1998;129:187–194.
38. Kleinman DV, Swango P, Pindborg JJ: Epidemiology of oral mucosal lesions in United States schoolchildren: 1986–87. Community Dent Oral Epidemiol 1994;22:243–253.
39. Caldwell MB, Oxtoby MJ, Simonds RJ, et al: 1994 Revised classification system for human immunodeficiency virus infection in children less than 13 years of age. MMWR 1994;43:1–10.
40. Flaitz CM, Nichols CM, Hicks MJ: Herpesviridae-associated persistent mucocutaneous ulcers in acquired immunodeficiency syndrome: A clinicopathologic study. Oral Surg Oral Med Oral Pathol Oral Radiol Endod 1996;81:433–441.
41. Cohen PR, Kazi S, Grossman ME: Herpetic geometric glossitis: A distinctive pattern of lingual herpes simplex virus infection. Southern Med J 1995;88:1231–1235.
42. Knaup B, Schunemann S, Wolff MH: Subclinical reactivation of herpes simplex virus type 1 in the oral cavity. Oral Microbiol Immunol 2000;15:281–283.
43. Contreras A, Falker WA, Enwonwu CE, et al: Human herpesviridae in acute necrotizing ulcerative gingivitis in children in Nigeria. Oral Microbiol Immunol 1997;12:259–265.
44. Calabrese L, Fleischer AB Jr: Thalidomide: Current and potential clinical applications. Am J Med 2000;108:487–495.
45. Syrjanen S, Leimola-Virtanen R, Schmidt-Westhausen A, Reichart PA: Oral ulcers in AIDS patients frequently associated with cytomegalovirus (CMV) and Epstein-Barr virus (EBV) infections. J Oral Pathol Med 1999;28:204–209.
46. Flaitz CM, Jin Y-T, Hicks MJ, et al: Kaposi's sarcoma-associated herpesvirus-like DNA sequences (KSHV/HHV-8) in oral AIDS-Kaposi's sarcoma: A PCR and clinicopathologic study. Oral Surg Oral Med Oral Pathol Oral Radiol Endod 1997;83:259–264.
47. Chindia ML: HIV-associated fulminating herpes zoster infection with alveolar necrosis and tooth exfoliation: A case report. Dental Update 1997;24:126–128.
48. Chan SP, Birnbaum J, Rao M, Steiner P: Clinical manifestation and outcome of tuberculosis in children with acquired immunodeficiency syndrome. Pediatr Infect Dis J 1996;15:443–447.
49. Hauk M, Berkowitz RJ, Moss M, et al: Hospitalization associated with oral lesions in perinatally HIV-infected children. Pediatr Dent 1997;19:484–485.
50. Souby R, Taelman H, Banyangiliki V, et al: Necrotizing periodontal disease in HIV-1 infected patients: A 4-year study in Kigali, Rawanda. In Greenspan JS, Greenspan D (eds): Oral manifestations of HIV infection: Proceedings of the Second international workshop on the oral manifestations of HIV infection. Carol Stream, IL, Quintessence, 1995, pp 60–67.
51. Velegraki A, Nicolatou O, Theodoridou A, et al: Paediatric AIDS-related linear gingival erythema: A form of erythematous candidiasis? J Oral Pathol Med 1999;28:178–182.
52. Robinson PG: Treatment of HIV-associated periodontal disease. Oral Dis 1997;3:S238–240.
53. Holmstrom P, Westergaard J: HIV infection and periodontal disease. Periodontol 2000 1998;18:37–46.
54. Lamster IB, Grbic JT, Mitchell-Lewis DA, et al: New concepts regarding the pathogenesis of periodontal disease in HIV infection. Ann Periodont 1998;3:62–75.
55. Armitage GC: Development of a classification system for periodontal diseases and conditions. Ann Periodontol 1999;4:1–6.
56. Novak MJ: Necrotizing ulcerative periodontitis. Ann Periodontol 1999;4:74–77.
57. Rowland RW: Necrotizing ulcerative gingivitis. Ann Periodontol 1999;4:65–73.
58. Chetty R, Vaithilingum M, Thejpal R: Epstein-Barr virus status and the histopathological changes of parotid gland lymphoid infiltrates in HIV-positive children. Pathology 1999;31:413–417.
59. Katz MH, Mastucci MT, Leggott PJ, et al: Prognostic significance of oral lesions in children with perinatally acquired immunodeficiency virus infection. Am J Dis Child 1993;147:45–48.
60. Triantos D, Porter SR, Scully C, Teo CG: Oral hairy leukoplakia: Clinicopathologic features, pathogenesis, diagnosis, and clinical significance. Clinical Infect Dis 1997;25:1392–1396.
61. Greenspan JS, Greenspan D, Palefsky JM: Oral hairy leukoplakia after a decade. Epstein-Barr Virus Report 1995;2:123–128.
62. Flaitz CM, Felefli S: Human papillomavirus and oral disease. In Sterling JC, Tyring SK (eds): Human Papillomavirus: Clinical and Scientific Advances. London, Arnold Publishers, 2000.

63. Meuller BU: Cancers in children infected with human immunodeficiency virus. Oncologist 1999;4:309–317.
64. Granovsky MO, Mueller BU, Nicholson HS, et al: Cancer in human immunodeficiency virus-infected children: A case series from the Children's Cancer Group and the National Cancer Institute. J Clin Oncol 1998;16:1729–1735.
65. Berkowitz R, Frenkel LM: Cancer in the HIV-infected child. Pediatr Dent 1996;18:127–128.
66. Willard CC, Foss RD, Hobbs TJ, Auclair PL: Primary anaplastic large cell (Ki-1 positive) lymphoma of the mandible as the initial manifestation of acquired immunodeficiency syndrome in a pediatric patient. Oral Surg Oral Med Oral Pathol Oral Radiol Endod 1995;80:67–70.
67. Abuzaitoun OR, Hanson IC: Organ-specific manifestations of HIV disease in children. Pediatr Clin North Am 2000;47:109–125.
68. Parmley RT: Evolution of AIDS and AIDS-related malignancies in pediatric pateints in the United States. J Nihon Univ Sch Dent 1997;39:8–11
69. McClain KL, Leach CT, Jensen HV, et al: Association of Epstein-Barr virus leiomyosarcomas in children with AIDS. N Engl J Med 1995;332:12–18.
70. McClain KL, Joshi VJ, Murphy SB: Cancers in children with HIV infection. Hematol Oncol Clin North Am 1996;10:1189–1201.
71. Aquino MZ, Sato KH, Kamikawa J, et al: Thrombocytopenia in HIV-infected children [abstract Mo.B.1293]. Int Conf AIDS 1996;11:105.
72. Piancastelli J, Puga A, Gutierrez L, et al: Thrombocytopenia in HIV-infected children: A retrospective review. Conf Retroviruses Opportunistic Inf 1996;3:150.
73. Costa R, Serban M, Isac A, et al: Thrombocytopenia in paediatric HIV infection [abstract 32160]. Int Conf AIDS 1998;12:552.
74. Young G, Loechelt B, Rakusan TA, et al: Thrombopoietin levels in HIV-associated thrombocytopenia in children. J Pediatr 1998;133:765–769.
75. Rigaud M, Leibobitz E, Quee CS, et al: Thrombocytopenia in children infected with human immunodeficiency virus: Long-term follow-up and therapeutic considerations. J AIDS 1992;5:450–455.
76. Shugars DC, Alexander AL, Fu K, Freel SA: Endogenous salivary inhibitors of human immunodeficiency virus. Arch Oral Biol 1999;44:445–463.
77. Shugars DC, Slade GD, Patton LL, Fiscus SA: Oral and systemic factors associated with increased levels of human immunodeficiency virus type 1 RNA in saliva. Oral Surg Oral Med Oral Pathol Oral Radiol Endod 2000;89:432–440.
78. Shugars DC: Endogenous mucosal antiviral factors of the oral cavity. J Infect Dis 1999;179:S431–435.
79. Shugars DC, Wahl SM: The role of the oral environment in HIV-1 transmission. J Am Dent Assoc 1998;129:851–858.
80. Skott P, Lucht E, Julander I, et al: Salivary sIgA response in HIV-1 infection. J AIDS 1999;21:73–80.
81. Shugars DC, Sauls SL, Weinberg JB: Secretory leukocyte protease inhibitor blocks infectivity of primary monocytes and mononuclear cells with both monocytotrophic and lympocytotrophic strains of human immunodeficiency virus type 1. Oral Dis 1997;3:S70–72.
82. Baron S, Poast J, Cloyd MW: Why is HIV rarely transmitted by oral secretions? Saliva can disrupt orally shed, infected leukocytes. Arch Intern Med 1999;159:303–310.
83. Rossmann SN, Wilson RH, Hicks J, et al: Isolation of *Lautropia mirabilis* from oral cavities of human immunodeficiency virus-infected children. J Clin Microbiol 1998;36:1756–1760.
84. Alaluusua S, Malmivirta R: Early plaque accumulation: A sign for caries risk in young children. Community Dent Oral Epidemiol 1994;22:273–276.
85. Kaste LM, Selwitz RH, Oldakowski RJ, et al: Coronal caries in the primary and permanent dentition of children and adolescents 1–17 years of age: United States, 1988–1991. J Dent Res 1996;76(Spec Iss):631–641.
86. Petersen PE, Danila I, Dalean A, et al: Oral health status among schoolchildren in Romania, 1992. Community Dent Oral Epidemiol 1994;22:90–93.
87. Low W, Tan S, Schwartz S: The effect of severe caries on the quality of life in young children. Pediatr Dent 1999;21:325–326.
88. Broder HL, Russell SL, Varagiannis E, Reisine ST: Oral health perceptions and adherence with dental treatment referrals among caregivers of children with HIV. AIDS Educ Prev 1999;11:541–551.

15

Cutaneous Manifestations in Pediatric HIV Infection

Timothy Dilon Daniel and Moise L. Levy

As the HIV/AIDS pandemic continues, increasing numbers of the world's pediatric population are becoming infected with the virus. According to the World Health Organization, in 1999 the number of children younger than 15 years of age who were infected with HIV throughout the world was 1.3 million.[1] In the United States, there were 12,969 children and adolescents younger than 19 years of age living with HIV as of December 2000.[2] Between the years 1982 to 1995, 6984 cases of pediatric AIDS were reported.[3] Thus, there has been a doubling of the incidence of HIV within the last 3 years. Most of the pediatric population is infected via vertical transmission from the mother.[3] The increasing incidence of HIV infection worldwide, coupled with the use of highly active antiretroviral therapy in developed countries, has resulted in an estimated more than 1.2 million children younger than 15 years currently living with HIV/AIDS.[1]

Several studies have shown that the prevalence of cutaneous disorders in adult HIV-positive patients is more than 85%.[4–6] A recent study revealed a similar prevalence of cutaneous disorders in children with HIV/AIDS. In particular, the prevalence of cutaneous disorders in HIV-infected children was 89%.[7] Infectious origins account for 75% of these cutaneous disorders, and inflammatory origins account for most of the remainder. With the advent of antiviral combination therapy regimens for HIV, cutaneous lesions once resistant to treatment are now being controlled.[8,9] Thus, the prevalence of skin lesions in HIV patients may decrease in future studies.[10]

The cutaneous lesions of HIV/AIDS patients are typically severe exacerbations or manifestations of chronic typical skin disorders that would otherwise be benign or regress spontaneously in the immunocompetent population.[6,7,11–17] As discussed in earlier chapters, HIV destroys the CD4+ lymphocytes, resulting in a deficit in the immune system. Moreover, recent evidence shows that the subsets of T helper cells Th1 and Th2 can more adequately explain the pathogenesis of most inflammatory cutaneous diseases. In advanced stages of HIV infection, in which the viral load is high and the CD4+ count is low, Th2 cells are the predominant helper cells. It is during this period that an atypical cutaneous manifestation occurs.[11] The severity and frequency of occurrence of the cutaneous lesions correlate with the CD4+ cell count.[12,18] These skin lesions are generally more difficult to treat.

It is important for caretakers to be familiar with cutaneous manifestations in HIV/AIDS pediatric patients, since these represent the first sign of HIV infection. Moreover, early identification of these lesions may lead to early treatment of HIV infection and prevent the sequelae of opportunistic diseases.

This chapter discusses the cutaneous complications associated with HIV/AIDS in the pediatric population but does not address oral diseases. The different dermatologic problems are classified into broad categories of infectious, inflammatory, neoplastic, vascular, iatrogenic/hypersensitivity, and nutritional deficiency. Although the categories may overlap, such classifications are used to help focus the discussion. Within each category, the lesions will be explored based on their type, incidence or prevalence, pathogenesis or etiology, diagnosis, and treatment.

INFECTIOUS

Viral

Herpes Simplex Virus

In one study of 85 HIV-infected pediatric patients, herpes simplex virus was the most common viral infection. The prevalence was more than 21%, and most patients had frequent or chronic herpes simplex virus infection.[7] Although most of the lesions in HIV pediatric patients tend to be located in the oral cavity as herpetic gingivostomatitis, they can occur on any skin surface.[14] Perioral, malar, nasal and finger tips, and perianal skin are other common sites.[19] Recurrences are most common on the vermilion border of the lip.[20] These lesions tend to occur as groups of vesicles on an erythematous base and are more severe than in immunocompetent patients. They are typically painful and may progress to pustules, erosions, and ulcers or become encrusted (Figs. 15–1 and 15–2).[21] Histologically, they manifest as intraepidermal acantholytic vesicles, multinucleated giant keratinocytes with intranuclear inclusions.

Diagnosis is made clinically and confirmed by Tzanck smear, viral culture, or antigen detection. A thymidine kinase inhibitor such as acyclovir, famciclovir, or valacyclovir is the recommended first-line therapy. For acyclovir-resistant herpes simplex virus, continuous infusion of acyclovir or intravenous foscarnet is recommended.[11,21] Cool compresses or sitz baths, topical anesthetics such as 2% to 5% lidocaine gel or ointment, and pramoxine ointment or gel can be helpful local treatment. In cases in which ulcers may become infected, topical or systemic antibiotics may be added.[11]

Varicella Zoster Virus

The manifestations of varicella zoster virus in pediatric HIV patients can include primary varicella, severe herpes zoster, and chronic varicella. Varicella zoster virus infection can also cause disseminated disease in pediatric AIDS patients.[19] Primary varicella can occur with or without complications of pneumonia, hepatitis, pancreatitis, or central nervous system involvement.[13,21] In one prospective study of 11 HIV-infected pediatric patients with hemophilia, all patients developed herpes zoster over a 5-year period.[22]

Primary varicella is characterized initially as papules, which progress to vesicles on an erythematous base, giving the appearance of "dew drops on a rose petal" (Fig. 15–3). These vesicles may rapidly become pustules, then rupture and form crust or ulcers. Papules, vesicles, pustules, and crust can also occur concomitantly. The lesions of zoster have a very similar appearance to those of primary varicella, but they tend to occur along one, two, or more contiguous dermatomes (Fig. 15–4). Bullae, nodules, and hyperkeratotic plaques can also be found in patients with chronic zoster.[13,23]

The histology, diagnosis, and treatment of varicella zoster virus lesions are similar to what has been described previously for herpes simplex.

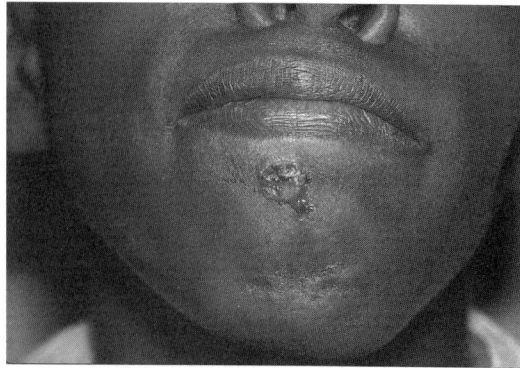

Figure 15–1. A vesicle on the chin of a patient with herpes simplex virus.

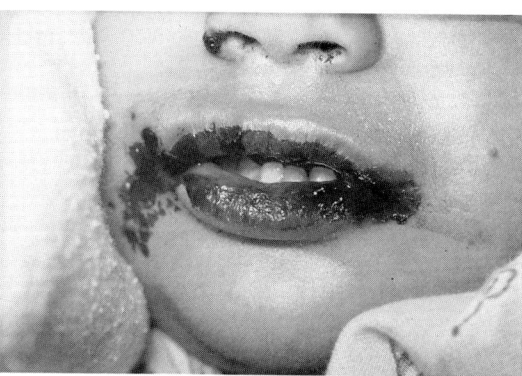

Figure 15–2. Crusting and hemorrhage on the lips and face of a young girl with herpes simplex virus type 1 infection.

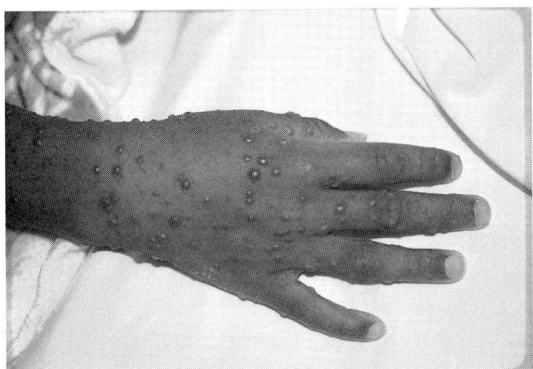

Figure 15–3. Multiple tense vesicles on the hand of a patient infected with varicella.

Molluscum Contagiosum

In one study, 14% of the pediatric patients with HIV infection developed skin lesions of molluscum contagiosum.[7] The DNA pox virus that causes molluscum contagiosum is the largest virus known to affect humans. There are three theories explaining the virulent activity of the virus that causes molluscum contagiosum.[11] The first theory states that the viral genes cause the production of defective MHC-1 surface proteins, which compete with the assembly of normal MHC-1 molecules from the host genes. The lymphocytes are therefore forced to spare the virus-infected cells. The second theory suggests that the virus secretes proteins that compete with the host chemokines and thus inhibit the inflammatory response around the infection site. The third theory states that the virus produces proteins that protect the infected cells from degradative substances secreted by the cell, such as peroxide.

The lesions of molluscum contagiosum are characterized by dome-shaped translucent papules (1–2 mm), nodules (5–10 mm), and tumors (>1 cm) (Fig. 15–5). The papules often contain a central umbilication. Most of the lesions are found on the face, trunk, and extremities, and there can be more than 100 lesions per patient.[20] Microscopic examination of smears of the contents of the papules typically reveals intracytoplasm. They appear as single, ovoid, eosinophilic structures.

Although the diagnosis is typically clinical, in some instances, biopsy or cytologic examination is done to rule out other similar-appearing lesions, such as cutaneous cryptococcosis or pneumocystosis, and to confirm the diagnosis.[11,21] Cryotherapy or cantharidin are useful first lines of therapy. The lesions are frozen with liquid nitrogen every 1 to 2 weeks. Cantharidin is applied every 3 to 4 weeks. Electrodesiccation or laser surgery is used in cases refractory to cryotherapy.[11] Curettage, topical tretinoin, topical 5-fluorouracil, topical podophyllin, and trichloroacetic acid (25% to 50%) peels, imiquimod, and cidofovir have also been recommended as effective therapy.[21,24,25] Even with these therapies, molluscum infections in HIV patients tend to progress and persist for months to years or recur, causing significant cosmetic problems, especially on the face. However, the use of highly active antiretroviral therapy often causes regression of the lesions as the CD4+ count increases.[26]

Human Papillomavirus

Human papillomavirus (HPV) infection has been shown to occur in about 8% to 10% of pediatric HIV patients. A variety of HPV types show different clinical manifestations. The cutaneous nongenital types, flat warts (verrucae plana), and common warts (verrucae vulgaris) covering most

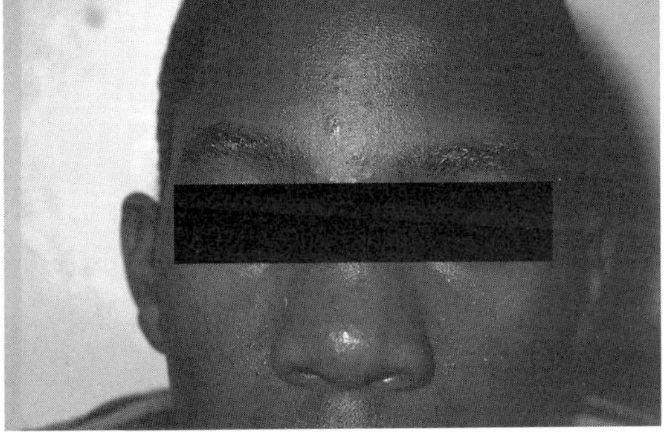

Figure 15–4. Linear vesiculation and crusting typical of herpes zoster.

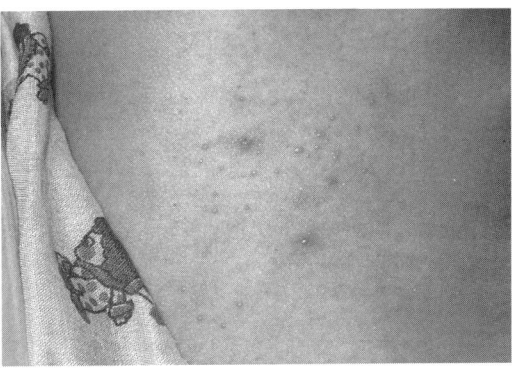

Figure 15–5. Dome-shaped papules typical of molluscum contagiosum.

of the face and body have been observed.[27] The flat warts are associated with HPV 1, 2, 3, and 4. Verruca vulgaris is associated with HPV 3, 5, 8, and 10.[11] The mucosal type, condylomata acuminata, has been observed frequently in HIV-infected children and tends to occur in the anogenital region.[19,28] These are associated with HPV 6, 16, 18, 31, and 33. There is a higher incidence of epithelial lesions with these strains, and they are potential malignant precursors.[11]

Flat warts are characterized by sharply defined round, oval, or polygonal flat papules (1 to 5 mm) of skin color or light brown. They are most prevalent on the face and upper trunk (Fig. 15–6). Common warts are typically firm papules (1–10 mm) of skin color with a hyperkeratotic and clefted surface. These are seen more frequently in the periungual regions, although any skin surface can be involved.[11] The lesions of condyloma acuminata are characterized by soft, fleshy, sessile papules with a smooth or rough surface. They can range in size from minute papules to cauliflower-like masses of skin color. They tend to involve the mucosal surfaces of the external genitalia and perianal and oral sites. Histologically, these lesions manifest koilocytosis, hyperkeratosis, and acanthosis. Atypical keratinocytes may also be seen in evolving carcinoma in situ.

Diagnosis of HPV infections is usually clinical. Biopsies are used to rule out malignancies associated with such infections. The HPV type can be determined by DNA in situ hybridization, polymerase chain reaction, or immunoperoxidase stain for HPV antigens. These lesions are treated with cryotherapy using liquid nitrogen, topical agents such as trichloroacetic or salicylic acid, podophyllin, podophyllotoxin, imiquimod, or ablative surgery.[29] Topical or intralesional cidofovir may also be useful.[30,31]

Cytomegalovirus

Although the cytomegalovirus can be isolated from almost 60% of pediatric AIDS patients, cutaneous manifestations of cytomegalovirus infection in pediatric AIDS patients are rare.[3,7] During a 5-year study of 85 HIV pediatric patients, only 2% developed cutaneous lesions as a result of cytomegalovirus infection. Disseminated cytomegalovirus infection commonly manifests as disorders of the internal organs resulting in pneumonia, encephalitis, hepatitis, gastritis, colitis, or chorioretinititis.[3] Cutaneous lesions from cytomegalovirus infections in pediatric AIDS patients are characterized by ulcers, pustules, vesicles, and verrucous and palpable purpuric papules. The legs, arms, and perineum are the common sites of predilection.[7,13]

The diagnosis of cytomegalovirus disease is made by isolation of the virus via culture or detection of viral antigens.[3] Biopsy can aid in such diagnosis and will show infection of fibroblasts and endothelial cells in the dermis, with intracytoplasmic and intranuclear inclusions. The overlying epidermis may become ulcerated.[11] Intravenous ganciclovir and foscarnet are used either alone or in combination for antiviral treatment of cytomegalovirus.[11,21]

Epstein-Barr Virus

The typical cutaneous manifestation of Epstein-Barr virus infection in HIV patients is oral hairy leukoplakia (Fig. 15–7).[11,21] Although common in adults, the disease is rare in HIV-positive children.[7] Oral hairy leukoplakia is discussed in Chapter 14.

Bacterial

Severe and recurrent bacterial infection is common in pediatric AIDS patients.[3,32] The defect in humoral immunity occurs early in the course of HIV infection and precedes defects in cell-mediated immunity. The reason that this sequence of defects occurs primarily in children and the mechanism by which it occurs are unknown.[14,19,32] Being unable to elicit effective antibody response,

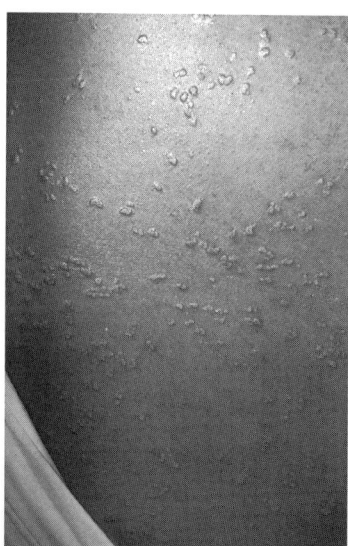

Figure 15–6. Multiple flat-topped, skin-colored papules with slightly verrucous surfaces.

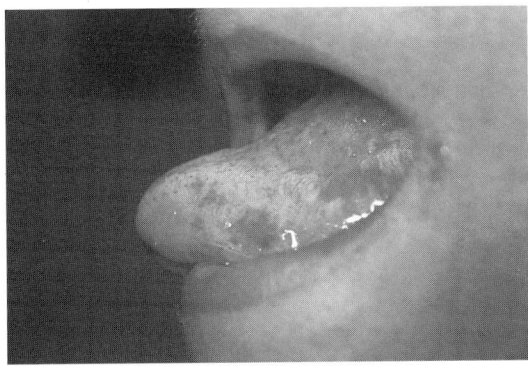

Figure 15–7. Lacey white plaques on the lateral surface of the tongue typical of hairy leukoplakia.

pediatric AIDS patients are very susceptible to recurrent bacterial infections, which are usually severe or atypical.[14,19] Bacterial sepsis with resulting dermatologic manifestations, including purpura and petechiae, has been seen in HIV-infected children.[14] The most frequently isolated organisms from the blood of patients with bacteremia are *Streptococcus pneumoniae*, *Haemophilus influenzae* type b, and *Salmonella*.[19,30] Patients with staphylococcal infections present most often with skin manifestations.

Staphylococcus aureus

Staphylococcal skin infections in pediatric HIV-positive children are the most common bacterial dermatologic infection.[14,19] Although staphylococcal infections also occur in immunocompetent children, recurrence and dissemination are more common in pediatric HIV patients.[3,11] The nares are most often the initial site of colonization.[11] These skin infections usually manifest superficially as impetigo or folliculitis or more deeply as cellulitis, abscess, or ecthyma.[11,14,19,21,32]

Lymphangitis may also be seen. Staphylococcal impetigo is seen as either localized or widespread erythematous crusted papules. Alternatively, an erythematous painful macule that can develop a vesicle or bulla and rupture is seen.[11] Staphylococcal folliculitis is characterized by widespread acneiform papules and pustules. They can be pruritic and therefore associated with excoriation.[11] *Staphylococcus aureus* cellulitis is characterized as a warm, erythematous, edematous, shiny plaque or patch with well defined borders.

Clusters of gram-positive bacteria can be seen histologically in lesions caused by staphylococcal infection. A histologic specimen from impetigo typically reveals subcorneal vesicles, acantholytic cells, spongiosis, and a dermal perivascular infiltrate of lymphocytes and neutrophils.[11,33] The histology of folliculitis shows suppuration in the dermis, especially around or within the hair follicles.[11] Abscesses are seen to involve the hair follicles extending to the deep dermis and subcutis.[33]

Localized superficial staphylococcal infections can be treated with mupirocin or other suitable topical antibiotics. Penicillinase-resistant penicillins, first-generation cephalosporins, clindamycin, or ciprofloxacin may be indicated with more extensive involvement. With recurrent disease, rifampin, mupirocin, or both can be added to the nares.[11,21] For severe infections, an initial course of intravenous antibiotics followed by oral antibiotics may be required.[21] Incision and drainage may also be indicated for some infections.[21] Monthly prophylaxis with intravenous immunoglobulin has been recommended for HIV pediatric patients with recurrent bacterial infections.[3,19]

Mycobacteria

Mycobacterial infections have been reported in both adult and pediatric AIDS patients. These infections are due to *Mycobacterium tuberculosis* as well as the atypical or environmental mycobacteria.[34–36] The morphology of such lesions is varied and can include crusted nodules, inflammatory papules or nodules, plaques, follicular papules, and ulcerations (Figs. 15–8 and 15–9). Such lesions, if unresponsive to empiric therapies, require skin biopsy for culture and histopathologic examination. Histologic examination of biopsy specimens may show hyperkeratosis, acanthosis, and papillomatosis with granulomatous inflammation. In immunocompromised patients, granulomatous inflammation is seen less than in hosts with normal immunity. Abscesses may be seen often in immunocompromised patients, with suppurative granulomas being most common, according to one review.[13,37]

Pseudomonas aeruginosa

Cutaneous infections with *Pseudomonas aeruginosa* have also been seen in pediatric HIV patients.[20,32] These skin lesions can be seen with or without septicemia and are most common in HIV patients with neutropenia.[21] Folliculitis, otitis externa, and ecthyma gangrenosum are the typical manifestations of pseudomonas infection of the skin.[14,20] Sites of inoculation can be any break in the mucocutaneous barriers, including intravenous or central venous lines.[33] Similar to lesions caused

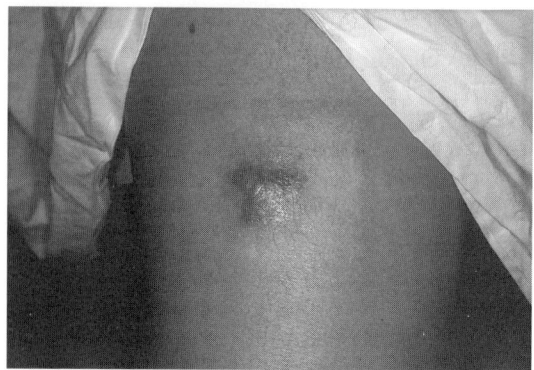

Figure 15–8. A fluctuant nodule on the thigh of a patient from which *Mycobacterium chelonei* was grown.

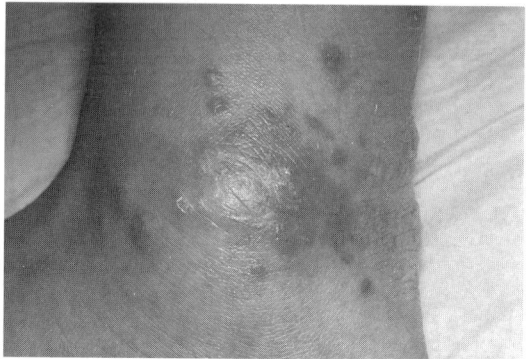

Figure 15–9. Inflammatory papules and a plaque on the ankle of a child with culture proven *Mycobacterium marianum* infection.

by *Staphylococcus aureus*, firm erythematous papules and nodules with localized necrosis or ulcers with adherent necrotic central crust may be seen.[11,14] They can be single or multiple on any part of the body but are most common in intertriginous areas.[33] Histologically, a vasculitis without thrombosis is seen with deficient neutrophils at the infection site.[33]

Pseudomonas skin infections can be suspected clinically and confirmed by culture of exudate or biopsy of a lesion.[11, 33] Oral antibiotics such as ciprofloxacin can be used to treat folliculitis resulting from pseudomonas infections. Deep-seated infections require appropriate intravenous antibiotic coverage. For some lesions, surgical excision may be necessary.[21]

Bacillary Angiomatosis

Although the papulonodular vasculitic lesions resulting from *Bartonella henselae* infections have been observed in HIV- infected adults, no case has yet been reported in pediatric HIV-positive patients.[3] One case was reported in an immunocompromised pediatric patient on chemotherapy. These lesions, associated with cat scratches or bites, can be anticipated in pediatric HIV patients.[3,13]

Fungal

Candidiasis

Candida albicans infection is the most common mucocutaneous fungal infection seen in pediatric HIV patients.[7,19] In particular, 56% of the 85 children studied over 5 years in one study developed a mucocutaneous candidal infection.[7] Another study of 36 pediatric AIDS and AIDS-related complex patients revealed that 75% of those children suffered from persistent mucocutaneous candidiasis.[38] Persistent oral candidiasis that occurs without prior antibiotic use is used as an AIDS-defining illness in pediatric patients.[39] In children with HIV, more than 93% will develop oral candidiasis at some time in their illness.[7] The frequent occurrence of candidal infections in HIV patients is related to diminished lymphocyte numbers. Additionally, candidal spores propagate in the environment.[7] Oral candidal infections are discussed more fully in Chapter 14. Cutaneous candidal infections in HIV pediatric patients tend to involve the intertriginous areas, including the neck folds, diaper area, and axillae.[13,14] The intertriginous lesions are characterized initially as papules and pustules on an erythematous base. Eventually, the pustules may erode, resulting in central confluent erosions on erythematous patches with marginal scaling and "satellite" pustules at the periphery.[33] Paronychial and nail involvement resulting from candidiasis also occurs.[13] These lesions usually present as painful swelling with erythema, especially over the proximal or lateral nail folds. White purulent exudate, discoloration of nail, and onychodystrophic nail can also occur.[33]

Diagnosis is made by clinical features and confirmation with microscopy or culture. Microscopically, a positive potassium hydroxide (KOH) scraping should reveal pseudohyphae and yeast forms. Mild superficial cutaneous, genital, and nail infections of candida in HIV pediatric patients can be treated with topical antifungals, such as the azoles.[21,42] Topical corticosteroids can be added for a short period to reduce the inflammatory component.[42] For recalcitrant widespread or severe superficial candidal infection, an oral regimen such as fluconazole or itraconazole is recommended.[42]

Dermatophytes

Tinea and widespread onychomycosis have been observed in HIV-infected children.[7,16] In the study by El Hachem and associates[7] with 85 HIV-infected children, 6% developed tinea infections and 5% developed onychomycosis infections over a 5-year period. Compared with HIV-negative patients, the incidence or prevalence of tinea infections in HIV-positive patients is about the same. However, the severity, recurrence, and refractory nature to treatment are greater in HIV-positive patients.[21,40] Tinea infections occur over the usual cutaneous sites.[7,16,21] The incidence of onychomycosis is higher in HIV-positive patients compared with the general population.[21] Onychomycosis, in contrast to candidal infections, typically involves only the nail and does not tend to cause paronychia.[40] Trichophyton rubrum is the most common dermatophyte isolated from this site of infection.[14,16,40] These dermatophytes synthesize keratinases, which digest keratinocytes and allow the fungi to exist in the keratin. Nails infected with fungi tend to become opaque and thickened and may split or crumble.[40] The characteristic skin lesion is an erythematous plaque with scale, central clearing, and a raised periphery, often consisting of tiny vesicles.[33,40] If the lesion involves hair-bearing areas, it may appear as a chronic plaque-like form of folliculitis (Fig. 15–10).[40] Sometimes, the lesions of the toewebs and soles of the feet and, less frequently, the palms of the hands can manifest as chronic maceration, scaling, blistering, and thickening of the skin.[33,40]

Dermatophytosis is diagnosed by clinical findings and confirmed by observing hyphae on microscopic examination of a KOH scraping or by isolating the dermatophyte from a culture of the lesion. For mild cases of tinea corporis, tinea cruris, tinea faciei, tinea manuum, tinea pedis, and superficial white or mild distal subungual onychomycosis, topical antifungals such as the imidazoles or allylamines are recommended.[21,41,43] If the lesions are severe or recalcitrant to topical agents, or for treating hyperkeratotic areas of the palms and soles proximal or onychomycosis, systemic therapy with an oral agent is recommended. Griseofulvin, itraconazole, or terbinafine are recommended oral antifungals.[41,44]

Histoplasmosis

Histoplasmosis is caused by the fungus *Histoplasma capsulatum*. Primary cutaneous inoculation is rare.[45] Disseminated histoplasmosis with cutaneous involvement in adult patients as young as 21 years old has been reported.[46] The prevalence of mucocutaneous lesions in adult HIV patients with disseminated histoplasmosis is between 11% and 20%, as compared with 6% in immunocompetent patients with disseminated histoplasmosis.[46,47] Since disseminated histoplasmosis has been reported in pediatric HIV patients, cutaneous manifestations can be expected.[47] The lesions are protean, with erythematous papules and nodules, macules, and patches being most common.[11,46] Plaques, pustules, fistulae, folliculitis, and herpes-like lesions have been seen, but less frequently.[11,46,47] The sites of predilection include the face, arms, trunk, and legs.[11,46] Biopsy of the lesion reveals oval *H. capsulatum* organisms in the dermis. Diffuse dermal infiltrates of histiocytes, neutrophils, and leukocytoclasis are also seen.[11]

Since the lesions are protean, a biopsy of representative lesions using periodic acid-Schiff or methenamine stains can help establish the diagnosis. Cultures of representative lesions confirm the diagnosis.[40,46] Acute cases can be treated with amphotericin or itraconazole and chronic cases with itraconazole or fluconazole.[21]

Cryptococcosis

Cryptococcosis is caused by the ubiquitous encapsulated fungus, *Cryptococcus neoformans*. Cryptococcal infection in HIV pediatric patients is rare, with a prevalence of about 1.4% as compared with 6% to 10% in adults.[48] Extrapulmonary cryptococcal infections occur in about 6% of HIV adult patients and 1% of pediatric patients.[49] Cutaneous lesions occur in 10% to 15% of patients with cryptococcosis.[50] Cutaneous cryptococcal infection

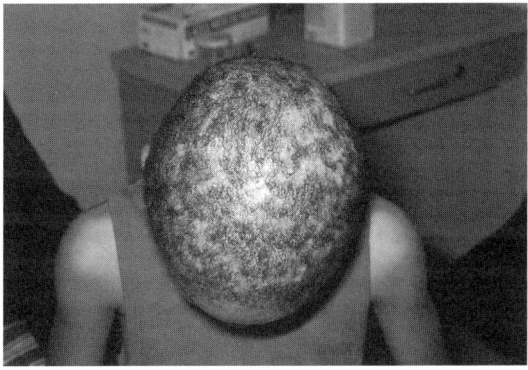

Figure 15–10. Diffuse scale and alopecia on a patient with tinea capitis.

mimicking molluscum contagiosum infection in an HIV-positive pediatric patient has been reported.[50] These lesions tend to be polymorphous, appearing as erythematous papules, nodules, pustules, granulomas, ulcers, cellulitis, or abscesses of the skin and thus are difficult to diagnose clinically.[10,21,48–50] A pale appearance of the dermis due to the presence of numerous cryptococci and minimal inflammatory reaction is the typical histologic appearance.[21,50]

The diagnosis of cutaneous cryptococcosis is suggested by microscopic examination of material scraped from a lesion, applied to a slide, and stained with KOH, periodic acid-Schiff, or methenamine silver stain to visualize the budding cryptococci. Appropriate fungal culture of biopsy specimens or swabs from ulcers or pustules can confirm the diagnosis. Patients without symptoms and limited disease can be treated with fluconazole or itraconazole. More severe disease can be treated initially with amphotericin with or without flucytosine and followed by fluconazole or itraconazole as maintenance therapy.

Aspergillosis

Although several cases of primary and invasive cutaneous aspergillus have been reported in HIV-infected pediatric patients, the prevalence in a 7-year study of 473 HIV-positive children was less than 0.5%.[51,52] Primary cutaneous aspergillosis is rare but must be considered in the differential diagnosis of skin lesions occurring beneath adhesive tapes or at catheter sites. Early diagnosis can prevent dissemination of the infection, which can result in death.[51,53] The most common organisms cultured are *Aspergillus fumigatus* and *Aspergillus glaucus*. Invasive aspergillosis is difficult to diagnose, and cutaneous involvement may aid in early diagnosis and treatment.[52] Cutaneous aspergillosis can present as solitary or multiple papules, plaques, tender nodules, and post-traumatic non-healing ulcers (Fig. 15–11).[51–53]

Diagnosis of cutaneous aspergillosis is made by examination of biopsy specimens stained with methenamine silver or periodic acid-Schiff to detect hyphal elements.[51–53] KOH examination of fresh smears may reveal the typically broad hyphae. A culture of the tissue can confirm the presence of *Aspergillus*. Surgical débridement or resection along with antifungal chemotherapy such as amphotericin or itraconazole is recommended for lesions of primary cutaneous aspergillus.[51–54] Amphotericin B is recommended for the invasive infections.[52]

Parasitic Disorders

Scabies

Sarcoptes scabiei infestation is a very common childhood disease. When occurring in HIV-positive children, it can be more severe and atypical forms are observed.[7,16] Scabies was seen to occur in 5% of 85 HIV-positive children who were followed over 5 years.[7] In addition to papules and vesicles seen in typical cases (Fig. 15–12), crusted or Norwegian scabies also manifest with fissuring and hyperkeratosis. Although these severely pruritic lesions are most prominent on the extensor surfaces of extremities, palms, soles, buttocks, and scalp, they can involve entire surface of the skin.[7,10,16] The histologic appearance is of a superficial and mid-to-deep perivascular and interstitial infiltrate of lymphocytes with numerous eosinophils. When crusting is prominent, the epidermis is hyperplastic and numerous sarcoptic mites can be seen in the cornified layer.

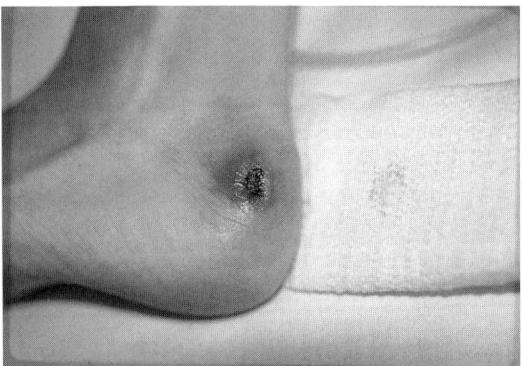

Figure 15–11. An ulcerated nodule with a dark eschar from which aspergillosis was diagnosed.

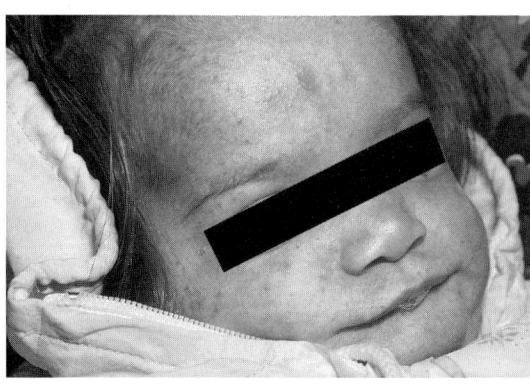

Figure 15–12. Multiple pinpoint scaling and erythematous papules on a young child with scabies.

The diagnosis of scabies is made by microscopic examination of the scrapings from active lesions, which should reveal mites and ova. Scrapings can be treated with KOH or mineral oil prior to examination. Lindane lotion or 5% permethrin cream applied to the total body surface (including under the nails) for 8 to 12 hours is the recommended first-line treatment. It is generally recommended to repeat the application in 1 week. Occasionally, multiple treatments are required, especially when there are recurrences. Oral ivermectin has been shown to be an effective treatment. Clothing and linen must be laundered and other household contacts treated. Antipruritic agents and topical steroids to diminish the inflammation are usually given as adjunctive therapy.[10,11]

Acanthamoeba

A few cases of *Acanthamoeba* infection with cutaneous involvement have been reported in pediatric HIV patients.[55,56] The infection is more common in adult HIV patients. Cutaneous *Acanthamoeba* infection is characterized initially by tender erythematous subcutaneous nodules, which can drain purulent material and after enlargement may develop into a nonhealing ulcer (Fig. 15–13).[21,55,56] The infection can disseminate to involve the central nervous system, sinuses, bone, and other organs.[21,56] The histologic examination can reveal a granulomatous reaction with areas of acute inflammation and necrosis in the deep dermis of the skin. Amoebic trophozoites and cysts resembling histiocytes may also be seen.[21,55,56] In addition to histopathology, culturing the organism from affected tissue can aid in the diagnosis. The diagnosis can be further confirmed by indirect immunofluorescence.[55,56]

There is no universal treatment for *Acanthamoeba* infection. Multiple-drug therapy that includes intravenous pentamidine, oral sulfadiazine, fluconazole, and flucytosine is recommended.[21,55]

Demodicidosis

The term demodicidosis or demodicosis is used to describe the papulopustular lesions caused by infestation of the *Demodex* mites. The species *Demodex folliculorum* and *Demodex brevis* are obligate parasites of the human pilosebaceous unit.[57] Demodicosis is rare in children, but a few cases in HIV-pediatric patients have been reported.[57–59] Cases in children with lymphocytic leukemia have also been reported.[60] The lesions may be more frequent in HIV-positive children than in immunocompetent children. Erythematous papules, pustules, and patches with pityriasis-like scales can be seen (Fig. 15–14).[57–59] They are found predominantly on the face, especially the nasolabial folds and cheeks. The histopathologic appearance consists of perifollicular granulomatous infiltrate and epithelioid tubercles encased by lymphocytes and plasma cells. Some demodectic mites can be seen in the follicular infundibuli.[57–59]

Because these lesions are clinically similar to a perioral dermatitis or rosacea, the diagnosis of demodicidosis must be confirmed by the presence of numerous *Demodex* mites in skin scrapings or histologic examination of a skin biopsy sample (Fig. 15–15).[57–59] Topical metronidazole and oral erythromycin have been shown to be effective treatments.[57–59] In one report, a 1% lindane lotion was also an effective therapy.[61] Ivermectin may also be used.

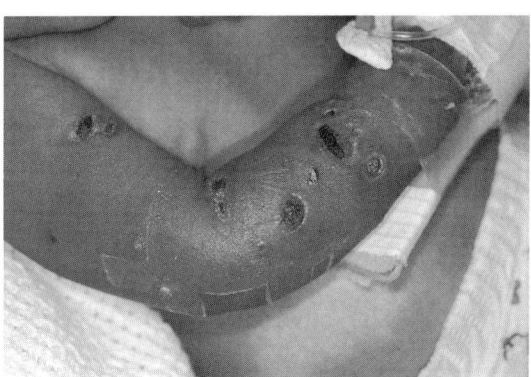

Figure 15–13. Ulcerated and crusted nodules representing infection with *Acanthamoeba*.

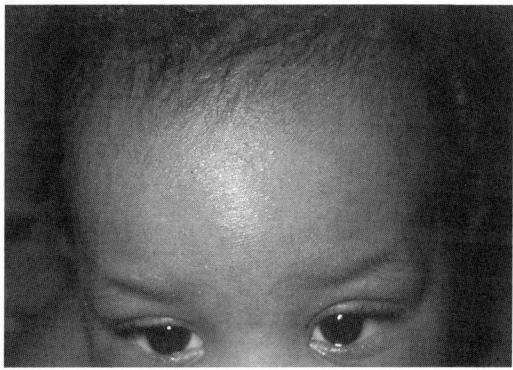

Figure 15–14. Multiple follicular papules on a child with demodicidosis.

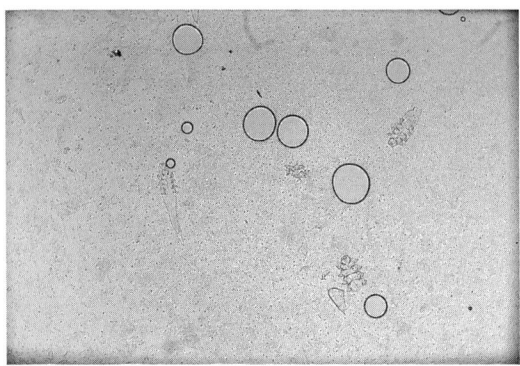

Figure 15–15. A microscopic examination showing multiple *Demodex* mites.

INFLAMMATORY DISEASES

Seborrheic Dermatitis

In adult HIV patients, seborrheic dermatitis is the most common dermatologic problem observed, with an estimated prevalence of 46% to 83% as compared to 1% to 3% in the general population.[62–65] Although a generalized cutaneous eruption with features of seborrheic dermatitis is said to be common in pediatric HIV patients,[14,20] in one study of pediatric HIV patients, the incidence of seborrheic dermatitis was only 6%.[7] Although there is no proven cause of seborrheic dermatitis, the severity of the rash correlates with the progression of the HIV disease and Th1/Th2 ratio.[14,64,65] Diffuse or confluent pink to red recalcitrant scaly plaques with slight induration involving the face and scalp are some of the characteristics of seborrheic dermatitis.[10,20] A generalized erythroderma or scaly erythematous patches involving the trunk, scalp, and extremities have also been seen. The rash can also manifest as erosive intertrigo, especially in the postauricular and nasolabial folds and perineum.[20] Histologically, psoriasiform hyperplasia of the epidermis with mounds of neutrophil-containing parakeratosis around the ostia of the infundibulum of the hair follicles is seen. Deeper lymphocytic inflammation of the sebaceous gland and scattered necrotic keratinocytes are also observed.[10,64,65]

Diagnosis is usually made by clinical findings. The lesions are treated with topical corticosteroids and, at times, antifungal creams.[10,21] Therapies including topical sulfur, phenol, and saline solution (for scalp use), and shampoos containing, tar, salicylic acid, sulfur, selenium sulfide, and zinc pyrithione are also recommended treatment. Patient education is necessary to inform them about the chronicity of the skin disease.[21]

Eosinophilic Folliculitis

A pediatric case of HIV-associated eosinophilic folliculitis was recently reported.[66] This eosinophilic folliculitis is different from infantile eosinophilic pustular folliculitis (infantile Ofuji disease) in immunocompetent patients or HIV-associated infectious folliculitis.[66–68] The prevalence of eosinophilic folliculitis is not known.[21] Nevertheless, this pruritic chronic sterile skin eruption tends to occur in HIV patients with CD4+ counts less than 200 cells/mm^3 and is therefore a good marker of advanced immunodeficiency.[10,21,66] The pathogenesis is not fully known. However, it is speculated that normally innocuous follicular antigens such as *Pityrosporum* yeast, *Demodex* mites, corynebacteria, and staphylococci may become antigenic in a Th2-dominant milieu and secondarily cause HIV eosinophilic folliculitis.[10]

The typical clinical features of HIV eosinophilic folliculitis include pruritic folliculocentric urticarial papules on the face, neck, upper trunk, and proximal extremities. The papules measure between 3 and 5 mm in diameter and can coalesce to plaques. Excoriation and crusting are often seen.[10,66] Numerous collections of eosinophils in the infundibular area of hair follicles and of the isthmus characterize the histology. In addition, perifollicular infiltrates of lymphocytes, eosinophils, mast cells, and, sometimes, neutrophils are seen. Epidermal hyperplasia, hypergranulosis, and hyperkeratosis as evidence of lichen simplex chronicus secondary to pruritus are usually seen.

The clinical findings, eosinophilia elevated serum IgE levels, and skin biopsy are important criteria for diagnosing eosinophilic folliculitis. To exclude other causes of folliculitis such as infectious diseases, examination for mites, Gram stain, bacterial and fungal culture, Tzanck smear, viral culture, and KOH examination of pustule content may be performed. Several different modes of therapy have been tried, with limited success.[10,21,66] Topical therapies, including antibiotics, corticosteroids, and permethrin, have been used. Phototherapy with ultraviolet B (UVB) radiation and psoralen plus ultraviolet A (PUVA) have also been used, primarily in adults. Systemic antihistamines, corticosteroids, itraconazole, isotretinoin, dapsone, and metronidazole have all been advocated to treat HIV eosinophilic folliculitis.[10,21,66]

Patient education is highly recommended, since the disease is incurable but treatable. Additionally, symptoms and number of lesions may wax and wane.[21]

Atopic Dermatitis

In two separate studies, atopic dermatitis in HIV pediatric patients has been reported to occur with frequencies of 25% and 50%.[7,69] In the study showing a 25% incidence of atopic dermatitis, this incidence was noted to be similar to that seen in healthy children.[7] There is contradictory information regarding the IgE levels in HIV children with atopic dermatitis. In one study, the IgE level was high in 50% of atopic HIV children, and another study found no difference in IgE levels compared with a control group not infected with HIV.[7,70] Allergic rhinitis, asthma, and hyperlinear palms are associated with atopic dermatitis.[10,70] In newly diagnosed HIV pediatric patients, atopic dermatitis tends to present shortly after seroconversion in patients without prior atopic symptoms or as a recurrence of previously quiescent atopic disease.[71,72] The typical lesions consist of erythematous patches and plaques with associated scaling, crusting, and, in some cases, lichen simplex chronicus. Pruritus is common. Severe recurrent forms with erythroderma occasionally occur. The histologic appearances reveal superficial perivascular infiltrate of lymphocytes and eosinophils with epidermal hyperplasia and foci of spongiosis.

Severe pruritus and a history of atopy aid in making the diagnosis, which can be confirmed by a biopsy. The treatment for atopic dermatitis in HIV patients includes avoidance of irritants and application of emollients and topical corticosteroid preparations.[10] Recombinant interferon-γ was used to treat HIV-related atopic dermatitis in one study of six adult patients, and a good response was observed.[72] The application of newer topical immunomodulators is yet to be examined in these patients.

Psoriasis

No increased incidence of psoriasis is seen in HIV patients. However, the manifestations of psoriasis in HIV patients tend to be more severe and recalcitrant as compared with immunocompetent patients.[10,16,21] Even though the incidence of psoriasis in childhood is believed to be generally underestimated, several cases of psoriasis have been reported in HIV pediatric patients.[7,16,73] Both plaque and guttate psoriasis are observed in pediatric HIV patients.[7,16] Psoriasis in HIV pediatric patients may manifest as erythematous hyperkeratotic plaques, with thick silvery scales or guttate papules and plaques located preferentially on the extensor surfaces, trunk, face, and scalp (Fig. 15–16).[10,16,21,73] Onycholysis, pitting, and subungual hyperkeratosis may also be seen.[10,21] Pruritus is common. The histologic features seen in HIV-associated psoriasis are similar to those seen in psoriasis of non-HIV patients. Diffuse parakeratosis containing neutrophils, acanthosis with elongation of rete ridges, and thinning of the suprapapillary plate and dilated tortuous blood vessels have been observed.[10,73] Spongioform pustules in the epidermis are seen in patients with pustular psoriasis.[10]

The diagnosis is made by the clinical picture and confirmed by a biopsy, with findings as described earlier.[10,73] Topical therapy for psoriasis includes emollients, keratolytics, corticosteroids, tar, anthralin, vitamin D_3 derivatives, and 5-fluorouracil. Corticosteroids, 5-fluorouracil, and cyclosporine can also be injected intralesionally. Although phototherapy and photochemotherapy have been shown to be effective in treating psoriasis, there are interesting concerns about the use of light treatment in HIV patients and its immunosuppressive effects.[20,71] Systemic treatment such as with antifungals, antibiotics, retinoids, vitamin D_3 analogues, methotrexate, hydroxyurea, and cyclosporine have shown effectiveness in treating psoriasis. Combinations of these therapies have been used and have been shown to be effective.[21,74] Cryosurgery, laser surgery, and superficial shaving of lesions have also been used with some measure of success.[73] Patient

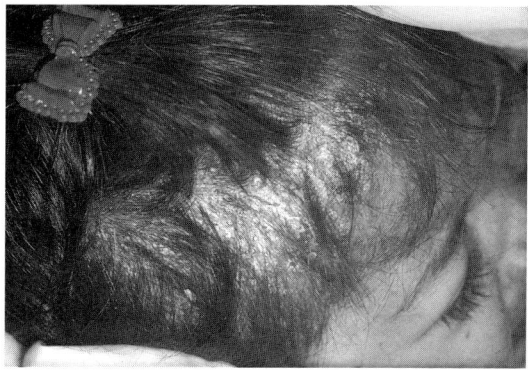

Figure 15–16. Adherent white crust with erythema on the scalp of a young girl with psoriasis.

education about the chronicity and precipitating factors of psoriasis is necessary.

Granuloma Annulare

Although granuloma annulare (GA) has been reported in HIV patients as young as 20 years old, a thorough Medline search failed to locate any report of GA in pediatric HIV patients.[75–78] Most adult HIV patients with GA have generalized GA and less localized lesions.[75] Multiple discrete flesh-colored or erythematous dermal papules, annular dermal plaques, and nodules are the most common features seen.[75–77] Histologic examination of GA generally shows normal epidermis with a focal area of fibrinoid necrosis in the dermis. This focus of necrobiosis is surrounded by macrophages and lymphocytes in an interstitial, palisading, or mixed pattern.[75–76] Although the origin of GA is unknown, precipitating factors that include UV light, insect bites, trauma, and neoplasm have been proposed.

The diagnosis of GA is made by clinical findings and confirmed by a biopsy of one of the lesions. In some HIV patients with GA, spontaneous resolution of the lesions has been observed.[76,77] Intralesional triamcinolone, topical corticosteroids under occlusion, dapsone, niacinamide, chloroambucil, and PUVA phototherapy have been used to treat GA lesions with some measure of success.[76]

Vitiligo and Alopecia Areata

Both vitiligo and alopecia areata (AA) have been reported in pediatric HIV patients.[7,79,80] The extremities, face, scalp, chest, and neck are the most common sites of predilection for the vitiligo. The alopecia can occur anywhere on the scalp or at other hair-bearing sites.[7] Although the mechanism for these autoimmune skin diseases in pediatric HIV patients is unknown, some theories have been proposed.[79,80] One theory is that HIV induces nonspecific polyclonal B cell activation with resulting autoantibody production. Another theory involves the activation of cells or production of cytokines by HIV-infected cells, which results in the formation of cellular cytotoxic agents against melanocytes. Direct infection with consequential destruction of the melanocytes by HIV has also been proposed.[80]

The diagnoses of these disorders are made by clinical appearance. In some cases, typical histopathologic features of AA can be seen by scalp biopsy. The treatments, though not uniformly successful, usually consist of topical corticosteroids, intralesional corticosteroids (for AA), topical irritants (tars, anthralin), dinitrochlorobenzene, squaric acid dibutyl ester, diphenylcyclopropenone (for AA), and others.

Hyperpigmentation and Eruptive Dysplastic Nevi

In a study of 145 HIV patients observed over a period of 1 year, 104 of the patients were found to have a mucocutaneous disorder, half (54) of whom, had hyperpigmentation. Hyperpigmentation was the most common skin manifestation in this study.[81] The increased pigmentation was diffuse, although it was especially seen in sun-exposed areas, such as the face and limbs. Eruptive dysplastic nevi, that is, an increase in the formation of multiple new histologically atypical nevi over a short time period, has been reported in pediatric HIV patients.[82] These nevi are typically oval or rounded in shape, with sizes varying from 3 mm to 7 cm and with colors varying from light brown to black. They are most commonly located on the trunk, neck, and upper extremities. Poorly circumscribed nests of melanocytes with few atypical cells, bridging of rete ridges, mild papillary fibroplasia, and a lymphocytic infiltrate of the dermis are some of the histologic features seen in these nevi.[82]

The diagnosis of these lesions is made by clinical examination in addition to the findings seen upon biopsy. Severely atypical lesions should be completely excised, and such patients should be followed closely for the increased risk of development of melanoma.

NEOPLASTIC

Kaposi Sarcoma

Kaposi sarcoma (KS) is a malignant vascular neoplasm believed to be caused by the human herpesvirus type 8, also called KS-associated herpesvirus. Hormonal and genetic factors may also be involved in the pathogenesis.[10] The incidence of KS in both adult and pediatric patients has increased concomitantly with the advent of HIV.[83] KS is the most common malignancy in adult HIV patients but is very infrequent in pediatric

HIV patients.[84] In a retrospective study looking at KS in pediatric patients in Zambia during a 13-year period from Jan 1980 through Dec 1992, there were 85 cases of KS in children younger than 14 years. Eighty percent of those patients were HIV positive. Moreover, the lymphadenopathic form accounted for 79% and the mucocutaneous form for 11% of all the cases of pediatric KS seen.[83] An increase in the incidence of the mucocutaneous form has been noted to coincide with the onset of the HIV epidemic.[83] There have been several other reported cases of cutaneous KS in pediatric HIV patients; however, the incidence of cutaneous KS in pediatric patients overall is considered low or rare.[85–88]

The clinical features of cutaneous KS consist of pink, red, brown, purple, or black macules, patches, nodules, or plaques.[10,21,83–87] The type of lesions seen depends on the stage of KS. At the early stage, faint pink macules and patches with symmetrical or asymmetrical borders are seen, which can progress at a later stage to darker lesions with scales and then to raised plaques, papules, or nodules.[11,21,89] These lesions tend to occur at sites of trauma and may be localized or generalized or may form a zosteriform pattern. The legs, feet, trunk, nose, scalp, and hard palate are common sites of predilection.[10,21] Individual lesions, groups of lesions, or coalesced groups of lesions varying from a few millimeters to 10 cm in diameter can be seen.[10,20,81,89] Pruritus or pain may be associated with these lesions.[10]

Findings on biopsy specimens depend on the stage of the lesions. Early patch lesions show thin-walled vascular spaces of irregular outline with proliferation of spindle-shaped endothelial cells surrounding the blood vessels. Extravasation of erythrocytes and hemosiderin are present in the tissue.[10,86] The plaque stage shows more diffuse interstitial proliferation of irregular slit-like spaces with extravasated erythrocytes, plasma cells, and hemosiderin deposits. Eosinophilic hyaline globules may also be seen.[10,89] In the nodular stage, spindle cells in sheets and fascicles with atypical cytologic features and mitoses are seen. Slit-like vascular spaces with extravasated erythrocytes may be observed.[10,31] The diagnosis of KS is based on typical clinical findings with the histopathologic features.[10,83–87]

Local therapies have been shown to be effective in treating isolated or sporadic lesions.[10,21] Cryotherapy with liquid nitrogen treatment every 2 to 4 weeks is usually the first option of local treatment. Intralesional vinblastine within 2- to 4-week intervals or vinblastine via iontophoresis has been shown to be effective against small lesions. Radiation therapy or surgical procedures such as excision, CO_2 laser, and pulsed-dye laser have also been shown to be effective in some cases. Systemic therapy has been used for aggressive or symptomatic disease.[10,21] In particular, biologic response modifiers such as interferon-α, interleukin-2, and intravenous immunoglobulin have been used. Chemotherapeutic agents used either alone or in combinations have demonstrated efficacy in the treatment of KS.[10,21] These agents include the vinca alkaloids, including vinblastine and vincristine, the anthracyclines such as liposomal doxorubicin and daunorubicin, the podophyllotoxins such as etoposide and teniposide, and antibiotics such as bleomycin.

Lymphoma

Although most cases of lymphomas in HIV pediatric patients tend to involve visceral sites, lymphomas involving the skin in these patients have also been reported.[19,84,89] Such lesions may represent secondary metastases and not primary sites.[19,88] The exact incidence of cutaneous involvement of lymphomas is not known. Lesions of non-Hodgkin and Hodgkin lymphoma are typically pink to purple papules or nodules.[10] Cutaneous T cell lymphomas in these patients manifest as widespread plaques that may progress to erythroderma. These lesions can be found on the head, neck, trunk, or extremities.[10,21]

Histologically, cutaneous lymphomas demonstrate a diffuse infiltrate of atypical monomorphic lymphoid cells predominantly within the dermis and subcutaneous fat.[10] Lesions due to Hodgkin disease show an inflammatory infiltrate, with atypical cells having a Reed-Sternberg appearance. Psoriasiform hyperplasia of the epidermis with a band-like infiltrate of atypical lymphocytes is the histologic feature of T cell lymphoma.[10]

Correlation of the clinical appearance of skin lesions and histologic features is the typical mode of diagnosis. Flow cytometry and DNA probes are employed to further characterize and subtype the neoplasm.[10] Chemotherapy has been used to treat these neoplasms, but their effectiveness must be weighed against their ability to further suppress the immune system of these already immunocompromised patients.[10,21] Chemotherapeutic agents that have been used include methotrexate, prednisone, bleomycin, adriamycin, cyclophosphamide, and vincristine.[10,88]

VASCULAR

Leukocytoclastic Vasculitis

There are several reports of cutaneous leukocytoclastic vasculitis in pediatric HIV patients.[7,20,91] This skin disorder manifests as pruritic erythematous papules located primarily on the lower extremities. They may also be found on the trunk and neck. Moreover, papules are purpuric and palpable and some may have necrotic centers.[20,90] In addition, diffuse infiltrates of neutrophils and occasional eosinophils and lymphocytes are seen in the underlying dermis. Leukocytoclasia, hemorrhage, and focal vessel wall fibrinoid necrosis are also seen histologically.[90] Elevated immunoglobulins such as IgE may be seen in the serum.[90]

The diagnosis of this type of vasculitis can often be made by clinical findings and confirmed with a skin biopsy. The pruritus associated with this disorder can be controlled with systemic antihistamine and topical steroids.[90] Generally, no specific treatment for the skin lesions has been recommended, since the vasculitis usually resolves spontaneously.

Thrombocytopenic Purpura

In one study of 140 children with symptomatic HIV infection, 19 of those children (13%) had thrombocytopenia.[91] There are other case reports of pediatric HIV patients with thrombocytopenia, which included both idiopathic thrombocytopenia purpura and thrombotic thrombocytopenia purpura.[92,93] The patients usually present with ecchymoses and petechia, often due to minor trauma. Other common presenting complaints include bleeding episodes such as gastrointestinal hemorrhage and epistaxis, fever, and mental status changes.[91,92] Decreased platelet count, increased platelet antibodies, schistocytes, target cell, and fragmented red blood cells are seen by analysis of blood.[92]

The diagnosis of thrombocytopenic purpura is made by clinical suspicion and platelet count. Depending on the type of thrombocytopenia, whether idiopathic thrombocytopenia purpura or thrombotic thrombocytopenia purpura, plasmapheresis, intravenous immunoglobulin, steroids, and vincristine may be helpful in managing the acute episode.[91,92]

IATROGENIC/HYPERSENSITIVITY SYNDROME

Drug Reaction

There is a high incidence of adverse cutaneous drug reactions in HIV patients that is greater than in the normal population.[93–97] In some studies, the incidence of cutaneous drug reactions in HIV patients ranges between 50% and 69%.[93,95] The higher incidence in HIV patients than in the normal population can be partially attributed to the more frequent use of multiple drug regimens for prolonged periods in HIV patients. Within pediatric HIV patients, there are several case reports of adverse cutaneous drug reactions.[19,20,85,97–99] Two studies report incidences of 12% and 16% of HIV-positive children who developed adverse drug reactions.[7,20] Trimethoprim-sulfamethoxazole is the most frequent cause of adverse reaction in HIV pediatric patients.[3,95] The cutaneous eruptions occur 5 to 10 days after the initiation of trimethoprim-sulfamethoxazole therapy.[20,98] A diffuse maculopapular, blanchable, erythematous, pruritic rash involving the trunk and extremities is the most common cutaneous manifestation.[19,20,85,97–99] However, erythema multiforme, Stevens-Johnson syndrome, and toxic epidermal necrolysis have also been observed.[3,19,85,99] Histologically, a superficial perivascular inflammatory infiltrate of lymphocytes with scattered eosinophils is observed.[10] In addition, the dermoepidermal junction may show vacuolar alteration and individual necrotic keratinocytes.[10]

Adverse drug reactions are diagnosed by the patient's history along with clinical findings and a biopsy. Discontinuing the use of the offending drug, if known, and replacing it with an alternate medication is essential to the management of severe drug reactions. Mild maculopapular eruptions without mucous membrane involvement or cutaneous necrosis do not require such. Desensitization to antibiotics such as trimethoprim-sulfamethoxazole has been shown to be successful in some cases of urticaria.[10]

Photosensitivity Eruptions

An adult patient with chronic photosensitivity to both UVA and UVB and resulting erythema, scale, and edema of his scalp, neck, face, and dorsal surface of his hands and forearms after sun exposure has been reported.[100] The patient's serum and urine porphyrins, antinuclear antibodies, anti-Ro, anti-La, anti-Sm, anti-RNP antibodies, and Venereal Disease Research Laboratory (VDRL) findings were all negative. No pediatric case of this disorder associated with HIV has been reported.

Porphyria Cutanea Tarda

More than 70 cases of porphyria cutanea tarda (PCT) associated with HIV have been reported.[100–103] In addition to HIV, toxic hepatic factors such as hepatitis C, alcoholism, and hepatotoxic drug use appear to trigger PCT in HIV patients by compromising an already abnormal porphyrin biosynthetic pathway in the liver.[101,102] Patients with overt PCT develop vesicles, bullae, ulcers, and skin fragility on areas exposed to the sun.[101,102] Diagnosis of PCT is made by clinical features and elevated urinary and fecal porphyrins.[98,99] Fluorescence of urine under Wood's light can also be seen. Avoiding sunlight, alcohol, and estrogen can help decrease the skin lesions of PCT. Therapeutic phlebotomy or chloroquine when phlebotomy is contraindicated has been successfully used to cause clinical and biochemical remission.[33,101]

NUTRITIONAL DEFICIENCIES

Pellagra, Scurvy, and Acrodermatitis Enteropathica

It is not uncommon for children with HIV/AIDS, especially those in developing countries, to suffer nutritional deficiencies.[104] The cause of the nutritional deficit may result from decreased oral intake and malabsorption that tends to occur with HIV infection.[15,20] These nutritional deficiencies can have many cutaneous manifestations. Flaky, erythematous-fissured skin sites and alopecia as evidence of kwashiorkor in pediatric HIV patients have been reported.[16] Hyperpigmented, verrucous lesions were seen on the legs of an HIV-positive child that were shown by skin biopsy to be consistent with pellagra, zinc deficiency, or acrodermatitis enteropathica.[104] Another child was diagnosed with scurvy after presenting with a petechial eruption of the lower legs and bleeding of the gums. Tong and associates[105] reported a child with an orofacial lesion and other cutaneous features consistent with acrodermatitis enteropathica whose eruptions responded to treatment with zinc supplements (Fig. 15–17).

The diagnoses of these cutaneous eruptions due to nutritional deficiencies are made by clinical findings and quantitative serum evaluation of the nutrient. Treatment requires replacement of the deficient nutrients orally or parenterally.[16,105]

CONCLUSION

HIV infection allows for florid and atypical manifestation of many common cutaneous diseases. Some of these skin diseases, such as histoplasmosis and Kaposi sarcoma, are not commonly seen in immunocompetent patients. Because the skin can serve as a window to systemic diseases, early diagnosis of skin disorders may allow quick recognition of diseases such as HIV infection and other disseminated infections associated with HIV. As highly active antiretroviral therapy continues to improve HIV patients' immune status and decrease their viral load, fewer and less extreme dermatologic manifestations may result.

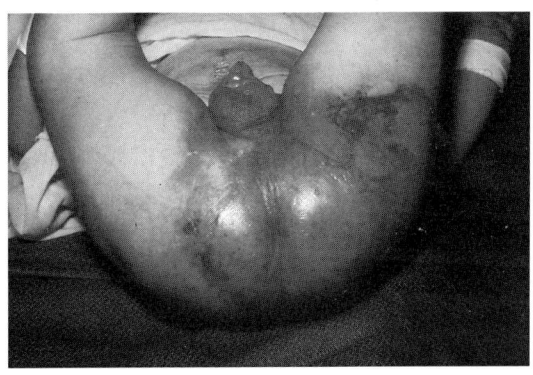

Figure 15–17. An erosive inflammatory perianal dermatitis in a patient with zinc deficiency.

REFERENCES

1. Joint United Nations Programme on HIV/AIDS (UNAIDS). Report on the global HIV/AIDS epidemic. June 2000.
2. Center for Disease Control and Prevention. HIV/AIDS Surveillance Report, Vol 12, December 2000.
3. Domachowske J: Pediatric human immunodeficiency virus infection. Clin Microbiol Rev 1996; 9(4): 448–68.
4. Uthayakumar S, Nandwani R, Drinkwater T: The prevalence of skin disease in HIV infection and its relationship to the degree of immunosuppression. Br. J. Dermatol 1997; 137: 595–98.
5. Coldiron BM, Bergstresser PR: Prevalence and clinical spectrum of skin disease in patients infected with human immunodeficiency virus. Arch Dermatol 1989; 125: 357–361.
6. Samet JH, Skelton HG, Yeager J et al: Dermatologic manifestations in HIV- infected patients: A primary care perspective. Mayo Clin Proc 1999; 74: 658–660.
7. El Hachem M, Bernardi S, Giuseppe P, et al: Mucocutaneous manifestations in children with HIV infection and AIDS. Pediatr Dermatol 1998; 15(6): 429–434.
8. Conant MA: HIV related skin diseases clear with combination therapy. West J Med 1998; 169(4): 225–26.
9. Evans TY, Tyring SK: Advances in antiviral therapy in dermatology. Dermatol Clin 1998; 16(2): 409–419.
10. Aftergut K, Cockerell CJ: Update on the cutaneous manifestations of HIV infection. Clinical and Pathologic Features. Dermatol Clin 1999; 17: 445–471.
11. Porras B, Costner M, Friedman-Kien AE, et al: Update on cutaneous manifestation of HIV infection. Med Clin North Am 1998; 82(5): 1033–1080.
12. Smith KJ, Skelton HG, Yeager J, et al: Cutaneous findings in HIV-1-positive patients: A 42-month prospective study. J Am Acad Dermatol 1994; 31(5): 746–54.
13. Prose NS: Cutaneous manifestations of pediatric HIV infection. Pediatr Dermatol 1992; 9(4): 326–28.
14. Zuckerman G, Metron M, Bernstein LJ, et al: Neurological disorders and dermatologic manifestations in HIV- infected children. Pediatr Emerg Care 1991; 7(2): 99–105.
15. Nance KV, Smith ML, Joshi VV: Cutaneous manifestations of acquired immunodeficiency syndrome in children. Int J Dermatol 1991; 30(8): 531–39.
16. Prose NS: Mucocutaneous disease in pediatric human immunodefiency virus infection. Pediatr Clin North Am 1991; 38(4): 977–90.
17. Torre D, Zeroli C, Fiori GP, et al: Dermatologic manifestations of AIDS in children. Pediatrician 1991; 18(3): 195–203.
18. Munoz-Perez MA, Rodriquez-Pichardo A, Camacho F, et al: Dermatological findings correlated with CD4 lymphocyte counts in a prospective 3 year study of 1161 patients with human immunodeficiency virus disease predominantly acquired through intravenous drug abuse. Br J Dermatol 1998; 139(1): 33–9.
19. Straka BF, Whitaker DL, Morrison SH, et al: Cutaneous manifestations of the acquired immunodeficiency syndrome in children. J Am Acad Dermatol 1988; 18: 1089–1102.
20. Prose NS, Mendez H, Menikoff H, et al: Pediatric human immunodeficiency virus infection and its cutaneous manifestations. Pediatr Dermatol 1987; 4(2): 67–74.
21. Rico MJ, Myers SA, Sanchez MR: Guidelines of care for dermatologic conditions in patients infected with HIV. Guidelines/Outcomes Committee. American Academy of Dermatology. J Am Acad Dermatol 1997; 37(3 Pt 1): 450–72.
22. Verroust F, Lemay D, Laurian Y: High frequency of herpes zoster in young hemophiliacs [letter]. N Engl J Med 1987; 316: 166–7.
23. Grossman M: Chronic hyperkeratotic herpes zoster and human immunodeficiency virus infection. J Am Acad Dermatol 1993; 28: 306–308.
24. Calista D, Boschini A, Landi G: Resolution of disseminated molluscum contagiosum with highly active anti-retroviral therapy (HAART) in patients with AIDS. Eur J Dermatol 1999; 9(3): 211–3.
25. Skinner Jr RB, Ray S, Talanin NY: Treatment of molluscum contagiousum with topical 5% imiquimod cream. Pediatr Dermatol 2000; 17(5):420.
26. Toro JR, Wood LV, Patel NK, et al: Topical cidofovir: A novel treatment for recalcitrant molluscum contagiosum in children infected with human immunodeficiency virus 1. Arch Dermatol 2000; 136(8):983–5.
27. Prose NS, vonKnebel Doeberitz C, Miller S, et al: Wide spread flat warts associated with human papilloma virus type 5: A cutaneous manifestation of human immunodeficiency virus infection. J Am Acad Dermatol 1990; 23: 978–81.
28. Forman A, Prendiville J: Association of human immunodeficiency virus seropositivity and extensive perineal condylomata acuminata in a child. Arch Dermatol 1988; 124: 1010–1011.
29. Drake LA, Dinehart SM, Farmar ER, et al: Guidelines of care for warts: Human papilloma virus. J AM Acad Dermatol 1995; 32: 98–103.
30. Baker GE, Tyring SK: Therapeutic approaches to papillomavirus infection. Dermatol Clin 1997;15: 331–40.
31. Hengge JR, Tietze G: Successful treatment of recalcitrant condyloma with topical cidofovir. Sex Transm Infect 2000;76:143.
32. Berstein LJ, Krieger BZ, Novick B, et al: Bacterial infection in the aquired immunodeficiency syndrome of children. Pediatr Infect Dis 1985; 4: 472–5.

33. Fitzpatrick TB, Johnson RA, Wolf K, et al: Color atlas and synopsis of clinical dermatology: Common and serious diseases, 3rd Edition, McGraw Hill Co, 1997.
34. Friedli A, Krischer J, Hirschel B, et al: An annular plaque due to myocobacterium haemophilum infection in a patient with AIDS. J Am Acad Dermatol 2000; 43:913–915.
35. Cureo N, Pagerols X, Gomez L, et al: Mycobacterium Kansasii infection limited to the skin in a patient with AIDS. Br J Dermatol 1996;135:324–6.
36. Antinori S, Galimberti L, Tadini et al: Tuberculosis cutis miliaris disseminata due to multidrug visit and Mycobacterium tuberculosis in AIDS patients. Eur J Microbiol Infections Dis 1995;14:911–14.
37. Bartralot R, Pujol RM, Garcia-Patos V, et al: Cutaneous infections due to nontuberculous mycobacteria; histopathological review of 28 cases. Comparative study between lesions observed in immunosuppressed patients and normal hosts. J Cutan Pathol 2000;27:124–9.
38. Shannon KM; Ammann AJ: Acquired immune deficiency syndrome in childhood. J Pediatr 1985: 106:332–42.
39. Berkowitz CD: AIDS and parasitic infections, including pneumocystis carinii and cryptosporidium. Pediatr Clin North Am 1985;32:933–52
40. Drake LA, Dinehart SM, Farmer ER, et al: Guidelines of care for superficial mycotic infections of the skin: Mucocutaneous candidiasis. J Am Acad Dermatol 1996; 34(1):110–115.
41. Odom RB, Berger TG: The cutaneous manifestations of AIDS. Current Concepts—UpJohn 1990;1–33.
42. Drake LA, Dinehart SM, Farmer ER, et al: Guidelines of care for superficial mycotic infections of the skin: Tinea corporis, tinea cruris, tinea faciei, tinea mannum and tinea pedis. J Am Acad Dermatol 1996; 34(2):282–286.
43. Drake LA, Dinehart SM, Farmer ER, et al: Guidelines of care for superficial mycotic infections of the skin: Onychomycosis. J Am Acad Dermatol 1996; 34(1):116–121.
44. Drake LA, Dinehart SM, Farmer ER, et al: Guidelines of care for superficial mycotic infections of the skin: Tinea capitis and tinea barbae. J Am Acad Dermatol 1996; 34(2):290–294.
45. Knobler RM: Human immunodeficiency virus infection. Dermatol Clin 1989; 7:369.
46. Cohen PR, Grossman ME, Silvers DN: Disseminated histoplasmosis and human immunodeficiency virus infection. Int J Dermatol 1991; 30: 614–622.
47. The Latin American AIDS Pathology Study Group. Opportunistic infections in pediatric HIV infection: A study of 74 autopsy cases in Latin America. Pediatric Pathol Lab Med 1997; 17(4): 569–576.
48. Abadi J, Nachman S, Kressel AB, et al: Cryptococcosis in children with AIDS. Clin Infect Dis 1999; 28(2): 309–313.
49. Leggiadro RJ, Kline MW, Hughes WT: Extrapulmonary cryptococcosis in children with acquired immunodeficiency syndrome. Pediatr Infect Dis J 1991; 10: 658–662.
50. Jimenez-Acosta F, Casado M, Borbujo J, et al: Cutaneous cryptococcosis mimicking molluscum contagiosum in a hemophiliac with AIDS. 1987; 12: 446–450.
51. Walsh TJ: Editorial Response: Primary cutaneous aspergillosis—an emerging infection among immunocompromised patients. Clin Infect Dis 1998; 27: 453–457.
52. Shetty D, Giri N, Gonzalez CE, et al: Invasive aspergillosis in human immunodeficiency virus-infected children. Pediatr Infect Dis J, 1997; 16: 216–221.
53. Arikan S, Uzun O, Cetinkaya Y, et al: Primary cutaneous aspergillosis in human immunodeficiency virus-infected patients: Two cases and review. Clin Infect Dis 1998; 27: 641–643.
54. van Burik JH, Colven R, Spach DH: Itraconazole therapy for primary cutaneous aspergillosis in patients with AIDS. Clin Infect Dis 1998; 27: 643–644.
55. Selby DM, Chandra RS, Rakusan TA, et al: Amebic osteomyelitis in a child with acquired immunodeficiency syndrome: A Case Report. Pediatr Pathol Lab Med 1998; 18(1): 89–95.
56. Friedland LR, Raphael SA, Deutsch ES: Disseminated acanthamoeba infection in a child with symptomatic human immunodeficiency virus infection 1992; 11: 404–407.
57. Patrizi A, Neri I, Chieregato C: Demodicidosis in immunocompetent young children: Report of Eight Cases. Dermatology 1997; 195: 239–242.
58. Sanchez-Viera M, Hernanz JM, Sampelayo, T: Granulomatous rosacea in a child infected with the human immunodeficiency virus. J Am Acad Dermatol 1992; 27: 1010–1011.
59. Bario J, Lecona M, Hernanz JM: Rosacea-like Demodicosis in an HIV-positive child. Dermatology 1996; 192: 143–145.
60. Ivy SP, Mackall CL, Gore L, et al: Demodicidosis in childhood acute lymphoblastic leukemia; an opportunistic infection occurring with immunosuppression. J Pediatr 1995;127(5):751–4.
61. Ashack RJ, Frost ML, Norins AL: Papular pruritic eruption of demodex folliculitis in patients with acquired immunodeficiency syndrome. J Am Acad Dermatol 1989;21:3067.
62. Eisenstat B, Wormser GP: Seborrheic dermatitis and butterfly rash in AIDS (letter). N Eng J Med. 1984; 311: 358–364.
63. Mathes BM, Douglass MC: Seborrheic dermatitis in patients with acquired immunodeficiency syndrome. J Am Acad Dermatol. 1985; 13: 947–951.

64. Kaplan MH, Sadick N, McNutt SN, et al: Dermatologic findings and manifestations of acquired immunodefiency syndrome (AIDS). J Am Acad Dermatol 1987; 16(3): 485–509.
65. Monika Froschl HG, Land ML: Seborrheic dermatitis and atopic eczema in human immunodeficiency virus infection. Semin Dermatol 1990; 9(30): 230–232.
66. Pratistadevi KR, Nilesh M, Ncoza CD: et al: HIV-associated eosinophilic folliculitis in an infant. Am J Dermatopathol 1999; 21(3):241–246.
67. Fearfield LA, Rowe A, Francis N, et al: Itchy folliculitis and human immunodeficiency virus infection: clinicopathological and immunological features, pathogenesis and treatment. Br J Dermatol 1999; 141(1): 3–11.
68. Buezo GF, Fraga J, Abajo P: HIV-associated eosinophilic folliculitis and follicular mucinosis. Dermatology 1998; 197(2): 178–180.
69. Fisher B, Warner L: Cutaneous manifestations of the acquired immunodeficiency syndrome. Int J Dermatol 1987; 26: 615–630.
70. Ellaurie M, Rubinstein A, Rosentreich DL: IgE levels in pediatric HIV-1 infection. Ann Allergy Asthma Immunol 1995; 75(4): 332–336.
71. Ball L, Harper J: Atopic eczema in HIV-seropositive haemophiliacs. Lancet 1987; 2: 627–628.
72. Parkin JM, Eales LJ, Galazka AR, et al: Atopic manifestations in the acquired immune deficiency syndrome: response to recombinant interferon gamma. Br Med J 1987; 294: 1185–1186.
73. McAleer P, Chu P, White SM, et al: Psoriasis associated with human immunodeficiency virus in an infant. Pediatr Dermatol 1999; 16(2): 144–145.
74. Drake LA, Ceilley RI, Cornelison RL, et al: Guidelines of care for psoriasis. J Am Acad Dermatol 1993; 28: 632–637.
75. Toro JR, Chu P, Yen TS, et al: Granuloma annulare and human immunodeficiency virus infection. Arch Dermatol 1999; 135: 1341–1346.
76. Calista D, Landi G: Disseminated granuloma annulare in acquired immunodeficiency syndrome: Case Report and Review of the Literature. Cutis 1995; 55: 158–160.
77. Ghadially R, Sibbald RG, Walter JB et al: Granuloma annulare in patients with human immunodeficiency virus infections. J Am Acad Dermatol 1989; 20: 232–235.
78. Cohen PR: Granuloma annulare: A mucocutaneous condition in human immunodeficiency virus-infected patients. Arch Dermatol 1999; 135: 1404–1407.
79. Duvic M, Rapini R, Hoots WK, et al: Human immunodeficiency virus-associated vitiligo: expression of autoimmunity with immunodeficiency. J Am Acad Dermatol 1987; 17(4): 656–662.
80. Cho M, Cohen PR, Duvic M: Vitiligo and alopecia areata in patients with human immunodeficiency virus infection. South Med J 1995; 88(4): 489–491.
81. Jing W, Ismail R: Mucocutaneous manifestations of HIV infection: a retrospective analysis of 145 cases in a Chinese population in Malaysia. Int J Dermatol 1999; 38: 457–463.
82. Duvic M, Rapini RP, Levy ML, et al: Eruptive dysplastic nevi associated with human immunodeficiency virus infection. Arch Dermatol 1989; 125: 397–401.
83. Athale UH, Patil PS, Chintu C, et al: Influence of HIV epidemic on the incidence of Kaposi's sarcoma in Zambian children. J Acquir Immune Defic Syndr Hum Retrovirol 1995; 8(1): 96–100.
84. McClain KL, Joshi VV, Murphy SB: Cancers in children with HIV infection. Hematol Oncol Clin North Am 1996; 10(5): 1189–1201.
85. Gutierrez-Ortega P, Hierro-Orozco S, Sanchez-Cisneros R: Kaposi's sarcoma in a 6-day-old infant with human immunodeficiency virus. Arch Dermatol 1989; 125: 432–433.
86. Prose NS: HIV infection in children. J Am Acad Dermatol 1990; 22(6): 1223–1231.
87. Orlow SJ, Cooper D, Petrea S: AIDS-associated Kaposi's sarcoma in Romanian children. J Am Acad Dermatol 1993; 28(3): 449–453 .
88. Nadal D, Caduff R, Frey E, et al: Non-hodgkin's lymphoma in four children infected with the human immunodeficiency virus. Cancer 1994; 73(1): 224–230.
89. Connor E, Boccon-Gibod L, Joshi V, et al: Cutaneous acquired immunodeficiency syndrome-associated Kaposi's sarcoma in pediatric patients. Arch Dermatol 1990; 126: 791–793.
90. Chren MM, Silverman RA, Sorensen RU, et al: Leukocytoclastic vasculitis in a patient with human immunodeficiency virus. J Am Acad Dermatol 1989; 21: 1161–1164.
91. Ellaurie M, Burns ER, Berstein LJ, et al: Thrombocytopenia and human immunodeficiency virus in children. Pediatrics 1988; 82(6): 905–908.
92. Prasad VK, Kim IK, Farrington K, et al: TTP following ITP in an HIV-positive boy. J Pediatr Hematol Oncol 1996; 18(4): 384–386.
93. Dover JS, Johnson RA: Cutaneous manifestations of human immunodeficiency virus infection. Arch Dermatol 1991; 127: 1383–1391, 1549–1558.
94. Bigby M, Jick S, Jick H, et al: Drug-induced cutaneous reactions: a report from the Boston Colaborative Drug Surveillance Program on 15,438 consecutive inpatients, 1975 to 1982. JAMA 1986; 256: 3358–3363.
95. Coopman SA, Johnson RA, Platt R, et al: Cutaneous disease and drug reactions in HIV infection. N Eng J Med 1993; 328(23): 1670–1674.
96. Bayard PJ, Berger TG, Jacobson MA: Drug hypersensitivity reactions and human immunodeficiency disease. J Acquired Immune Defic Syndr 1992; 5: 1237–1257.
97. De Raeve L, Song M, Van Maldergem L: Adverse cutaneous drug reactions in AIDS. B J Dermatol 1988; 119: 521–523.

98. Chanock SJ, Luginbuhl LM, McIntosh K, et al: Life-threatening reaction to trimethoprim/sulfamethoxazole in pediatric human immunodeficiency virus infection. Pediatrics 1994; 93(3): 519–521.
99. Hira SK, Wadhawan D, Kamanga J, et al: Cutaneous manifestations of human immunodeficiency virus in Lusaka, Zambia. J Am Acad Dermatol 1988; 19(3): 451–457.
100. Toback AC, Longley J, Cardullo AC, et al: Severe chronic photosensitivity in association with acquired immunodeficiency syndrome. J Am Acad Dermatol 1986; 15(5): 1056–1057.
101. Mansourati FF, Stone VE, Mayer KH: Porphyria cutanea tarda and HIV/AIDS: a review of pathogenesis, clinical manifestations and management. Int J STD AIDS 1999; 10(1): 51–56.
102. Hogan D, Card RT, Ghadially R, et al: Human immunodeficiency virus infection and porphyria cutanea tarda. J Am Acad Dermatol 1989; 20(1): 17–20.
103. Lobato MN, Berger TG: Porphyria cutanea tarda associated with the acquired immunodeficiency syndrome. Arch Dermatol 1988; 124: 1009–1010.
104. Penneys NS, Hicks B: Unusual cutaneous lesions associated with acquired immunodeficiency syndrome. J Am Acad Dermatol 1985; 13: 845–852.
105. Tong TK, Andrew LR, Abey A: Childhood acquired immune deficiency syndrome manifesting as acrodermatitis enteropathica. J Pediatr 1986; 108: 426–428.

16

Gastrointestinal Illness and Wasting in Pediatric Patients with HIV Infection

Colleen M. Hadigan and Harland S. Winter

GASTROINTESTINAL COMPLICATIONS OF HIV INFECTION AND TREATMENT

HIV-infected children frequently develop gastrointestinal disorders, both as a consequence of HIV infection and immunodeficiency and as a complication of HIV treatment. Chronic or recurrent diseases result in undernutrition, from either malabsorption or insufficient caloric intake. Recognition of gastrointestinal disorders among HIV-infected children is critical to providing appropriate treatment and to minimizing the negative impact on growth and development so often associated with these illnesses. Furthermore, malnutrition contributes to impaired immune function and, in the setting of HIV infection, may have a profound impact on disease progression,[1] morbidity, and mortality.

Anorexia

There are many potential causes of depressed appetite and food refusal among HIV-infected children. The mouth is the point of introduction of food and often can be the source of difficulty. Discomfort associated with chewing may decrease oral intake and may be the presenting symptom of an oral infection such as thrush or stomatitis in a young child. Previous studies have demonstrated oral candidal infections in up to 72% of HIV-infected children;[2] the prevalence has been estimated at 11% to 20% among asymptomatic children.[3] Similarly, herpes simplex virus (HSV), linear gingival erythema, and recurrent aphthous ulcers are common oral lesions associated with pediatric HIV infection. Medications, such as didanosine and zalcitabine, also are associated with aphthous ulcers. Other causes of anorexia, such as Kaposi sarcoma, non-Hodgkin lymphoma, oral hairy leukoplakia, and tuberculosis, are rarely seen in pediatric patients.

The development of orofacial manifestations of HIV infection may be an early sign of disease progression in children. Careful inspection of the mouth will identify oral lesions that may substantially interfere with adequate caloric intake. Therefore, patients need to receive routine dental examinations. Identification of oral lesions and their management are summarized in Table 16–1. Prompt eradication of infection and control of pain will minimize the negative impact of oral lesions on caloric intake.

Increased disease activity and elevation of circulating cytokines such as tumor necrosis factor may also diminish appetite.[4] The use of appetite stimulants such as megestrol acetate has been studied in the adult HIV-infected population with AIDS wasting and increases both weight and caloric intake. In a retrospective review of 19 children with HIV and growth failure, Clarick and associates[5] found that megestrol acetate treatment resulted in weight gain but not in linear growth. Because one potential side effect of megestrol acetate is the development of diabetes mellitus, the use of megestrol acetate should be avoided in

Table 16-1
Oral Lesions Associated with HIV-2 Infection

ORAL LESION	EVALUATION	MANAGEMENT

Candidiasis
  Pseudomembranous
  Erythematous
  Angular cheilitis
	Candida spp. detected in culture or cytology smear	Nystatin, clotrimazole, fluconazole, ketoconazole

Herpes simplex virus	Presumptive diagnosis or HSV DNA hybridization	Usually self-limited Acyclovir
Recurrent aphthous ulcer	Ulcers w/ pseudomembrane and erythematous halo response to steroid therapy	Topical steroid therapy Flucinonide
Linear gingival erythema	Fiery red linear band of the gingiva, possibly *Candida*	Oral hygiene, plaque removal

children with fat redistribution, insulin resistance, hyperlipidemia, or lipodystrophy.

Dysphagia and Odynophagia

Difficulty swallowing (dysphagia) and pain with swallowing (odynophagia) can result in marked decrease or complete cessation of food intake among HIV-infected children. These symptoms are likely to be associated with infection or inflammation of the esophagus. Ulceration of the esophagus may be due to acid reflux, but among symptomatic children with AIDS, infectious causes such as *Candida* species, cytomegalovirus, and HSV should also be considered. In 1996, the Centers for Disease Control and Prevention (CDC) reported candidiasis of the esophagus as an AIDS-indicator condition in 13% (87/678) of US infants and children younger than 13 years of age with AIDS.[6] Prior to more effective antiretroviral therapies, Miller and colleagues[7] demonstrated that 70% of symptomatic children with HIV infection had abnormal histologic findings following an upper gastrointestinal endoscopy and biopsy. Antiretroviral medications such as zidovudine and zalcitabine have been associated with pill-induced esophagitis and should also be considered as a possible cause of pain or difficulty with swallowing. Current recommendations for adults with HIV infection who have thrush and symptoms of esophagitis are to provide empiric therapy for candidal esophagitis. One study demonstrated that therapy with fluconazole was safe and effective and resulted in a 75% response in symptoms. If no response is noted within 3 to 5 days, then endoscopy is recommended for further evaluation.[8] Although a barium swallow may be useful in the assessment of candidal esophagitis and esophageal ulcers in adults, this technique is considerably less sensitive in children and therefore may fail to detect clinically significant ulceration and esophageal disease.

Upper gastrointestinal endoscopic examination of the esophagus with biopsy is recommended for the diagnostic evaluation of HIV-infected children who have persistent symptoms of dysphagia or odynophagia. The presence of multiple adherent white-yellow plaques, which may be confluent and involve the entire length of the esophagus, helps identify esophageal candidiasis; however, diagnosis of *Candida* infection requires identification of yeast forms on endoscopic mucosal biopsy or brushing. The presence of *Candida* does not exclude the possibility of additional esophageal infection, and as many as 25% of HIV-infected adults with esophageal candidiasis are coinfected.[8] Cytomegalovirus esophagitis may appear as one or more discrete ulcers with well defined margins. Cytomegalovirus may be identified by characteristic intranuclear inclusions on mucosal biopsies and further confirmed by immunohistochemical staining for, or culture of, cytomegalovirus on mucosal biopsies. The endoscopic appearance of HSV esophagitis is variable and includes diffuse, erosive esophagitis characterized by multiple small superficial ulcerations or numerous small vesicles. Biopsy, cytology, and culture, as well as immunohistochemical staining, will confirm HSV infection.

In most patients, candidal esophagitis can be treated readily with oral fluconazole (3–6 mg/kg once daily, maximum 200 mg), but for patients with severe disease or those who have failed oral therapy, intravenous amphotericin B may be necessary.[9] Infections and ulceration caused by cytomegalovirus and HSV should be treated with antiviral therapy (ganciclovir, acyclovir, and foscarnet). Selection of antiviral agent or agents, dose, and duration should be determined by the severity of immunodeficiency and the extent of viral infection (e.g., concurrent identification of cytomegalovirus retinitis or infection of the cerebrospinal fluid).

Abdominal Pain

Children with HIV infection who present with complaints of abdominal pain may be experiencing pain resulting from infections or side effects of medication specific to HIV. Nevertheless, the differential diagnosis should include potentially serious causes of abdominal pain in otherwise healthy children. For example, abdominal pain in the setting of vomiting or decreased bowel sounds on physical examination should alert the physician to possible bowel obstruction or appendicitis. Radiographic and surgical evaluation and treatment should be considered when appropriate.

In addition to the many causes of abdominal pain in young children not infected with HIV, pancreatitis may be a serious cause for abdominal pain among children with HIV infection. The development of pancreatitis has been associated with increased mortality in children within months following diagnosis.[10] Cytomegalovirus and, less commonly, cryptosporidium may infect the epithelium of the biliary tract, causing inflammation that may eventually lead to obstruction of the pancreatic duct. Antiretroviral medications, particularly didanosine, have been recognized as contributing to the development of pancreatitis among HIV-infected children, but this is relatively uncommon. The use of other medications for the prevention and treatment of opportunistic infections, such as pentamidine and isoniazid, are more frequently associated with an increased risk of pancreatitis. The diagnosis of pancreatitis among symptomatic patients with HIV infection may be difficult. Salivary amylase elevations are not uncommon among HIV-infected individuals, and the measurement of total serum amylase has been shown to be a poor indicator of clinical pancreatitis in this population.[11,12] Therefore, if pancreatitis is suspected, serum amylase should be fractionated to detect elevation of pancreatic amylase or serum lipase should be determined. If the patient is currently being treated with a medication known to cause pancreatitis, discontinuation should be considered. All forms of enteral nutrition can exacerbate pancreatitis and prolong recovery time, and therefore prompt initiation of parenteral nutritional support is important to avoid significant malnutrition as a complication of the disease. Treatment of pancreatitis, even in cases in which a viral infection is believed to be the cause, is primarily supportive.

Abdominal pain is a commonly reported side effect of many of the medications used to treat children with HIV infection and its complications (Table 16–2). When a patient presents with complaints of abdominal pain, the recent medication history should be reviewed to help identify a possible

Table 16–2
Gastrointestinal Toxicity of Medications Commonly Used in the Treatment of HIV-Infected Children

Abdominal Pain
Didanosine (ddI)
Lamivudine (3TC)
Indinavir
Ritonavir
Saquinavir
Azithromycin
Clarithromycin
Fluconazole
Diarrhea
Didanosine (ddI)
Lamivudine (3TC)
Nelfinavir
Saquinavir
Acyclovir
Foscarnet
Atovaquone
Azithromycin
Clarithromycin
Fluconazole
Itraconazole
Nausea
Didanosine (ddI)
Lamivudine (3TC)
Indinavir
Ritonavir
Saquinavir
Acyclovir
Foscarnet
Atovaquone
Azithromycin
Clarithromycin
Cotrimazole
Fluconazole
Itraconazole
Ketoconazole

Major toxicities indicated among the most frequent for antiretroviral, antiviral, and treatment and prevention of opportunistic infections.[9]

causal agent, and medications should be adjusted whenever possible to minimize these side effects. As with oral and esophageal pain, untreated chronic abdominal pain may result in significantly diminished caloric intake and eventual malnutrition among children with HIV infection.

Diarrhea

Diarrhea is a common clinical manifestation of HIV infection and a frequently reported side effect of a number of the medications used to treat children with HIV infection (see Table 16–2). Historically, the incidence of diarrhea has been a clinical marker of a declining immune system and of viral load progression. The differential diagnosis of diarrhea in the HIV-infected child includes common enteric pathogens, opportunistic infections such as *Mycobacterium avium-intracellulare* and cytomegalovirus, *Clostridium difficile* colitis associated with antibiotic use, and conditions of malabsorption such as lactose intolerance and pancreatic insufficiency. In addition, common causes of diarrhea among otherwise healthy children, such as milk or soy protein intolerance, postinfectious enteritis, and inflammatory bowel disease, must also be considered when the clinician evaluates an HIV-infected child with chronic diarrhea.

Enteric pathogens should be suspected initially in the child who presents with acute diarrhea. Stool samples should be obtained to test for the presence of *Salmonella, Shigella, Yersinia, Campylobacter, Giardia lamblia, C. difficile,* and *Escherichia coli*. Infection by *M. avium-intracellulare* and *Cryptosporidium* may be difficult to diagnose, as the organisms may not be identifiable in the stool during the early stage of infection. In addition, mucosal biopsy may be necessary to determine the presence of viral pathogens such as HSV and cytomegalovirus. Therefore, while stool culture is the first-line diagnostic approach for identification of the enteric pathogens, colonoscopic evaluation and biopsy may be indicated to assist in the diagnosis and management of the patient with HIV infection and diarrhea. Treatment of enteric pathogens should be guided by the identification of the specific pathogen.

In the child with chronic diarrhea and no identifiable enteric pathogen, malabsorption and drug toxicity should be considered. The presence of reducing substance or fecal fat in a stool sample is suggestive of carbohydrate and fat malabsorption, respectively. Lactose intolerance can be confirmed by noninvasive lactose hydrogen breath testing. As many as 40% of HIV-infected children without an identified enteric pathogen demonstrated lactose malabsorption[13] and, in one series, lactose malabsorption was associated with weight loss.[14] The relationship among symptoms of diarrhea, nutritional status, and lactose malabsorption is not always causal, and therefore the potential impact of diet restriction on overall caloric intake must be weighed carefully when one contemplates a lactose-free diet. The identification of fat malabsorption should be followed by a careful assessment of pancreatic function and evaluation for previously unrecognized pancreatitis. Because restriction of fat may have serious nutritional consequences, benefits from a low-fat diet should be documented.

Nausea and Vomiting

Nausea and vomiting frequently accompany conditions associated with abdominal pain previously covered in this chapter (e.g., pancreatitis) and are frequently reported side effects of medications used in children with HIV infection (see Table 16–2). Not only is persistent nausea a strong appetite suppressant, but vomiting can also result in significant caloric loss as well as diminished food intake. Because nausea and vomiting can seriously affect the nutritional status of children with HIV infection, recognition and treatment of all the causes of nausea and vomiting are important to maintaining the child's health.

Infectious gastritis may cause nausea and vomiting in children with HIV infection. Gastric inflammation and mucosal injury may result from infection with *Helicobacter pylori, Cryptosporidium,* and *Candida*. In particular, chronic use of acid suppression therapy may be permissive to *Candida* and increase the risk of candidal gastritis. Cytomegalovirus and HSV have also been identified as pathogens causing gastritis in HIV-infected patients. Upper gastrointestinal endoscopy and biopsy may be useful in establishing the diagnosis and discriminating among infectious causes.

Gastrointestinal Bleeding

Gastrointestinal bleeding is not a common complication of HIV infection in children, but when present may be attributable to HIV-related conditions. Opportunistic infections such as cytomegalovirus may lead to ulceration of the upper gastrointestinal tract, which can manifest with clinically significant bleeding, hematemesis, and melena. Furthermore, patients who present with a gastrointestinal bleed should be evaluated for possible coagulopathy, which among severely malnourished children can result from vitamin K deficiency. Tumors of the gastrointestinal tract are rare in the pediatric population, including Kaposi sarcoma, the most common HIV-associated tumor of the gastrointestinal tract. Leiomyoma and leiomyosarcoma have been reported in HIV-infected children in association with Epstein-Barr virus infection.[9] If they occur, these tumors may also result in gastrointestinal blood loss. Patients who present with hematemesis of unclear origin should be evaluated by a gastroenterologist, and upper endoscopy should be considered.

Gastrointestinal bleeding from the distal small intestine and colon may present as bloody diarrhea or bright red blood per rectum and may result from colonic infection. *Salmonella* and *Shigella*, common pathogens causing bacterial colitis in HIV-infected patients, typically manifest with bloody diarrhea. Cytomegalovirus may cause mucosal inflammation and vasculitis resulting in bloody stool without diarrhea. *C. difficile* colitis may also manifest with bloody diarrhea and should be included in the differential diagnosis of the chronically hospitalized child or in the setting of recent antibiotic therapy. Stool specimens should be obtained and cultured for bacterial pathogens (*Salmonella*, *Shigella*, *Yersinia*, and *Campylobacter*), ova, and parasites and sent for detection of *C. difficile* toxin. If these studies are unrevealing and symptoms persist, colonoscopy should be performed to further evaluate the source of bleeding. Biopsies of the mucosa help identify cytomegalovirus by observing characteristic intranuclear inclusions or by mucosal immunohistochemical staining.

Hepatitis and Jaundice

Children with HIV infection frequently have elevations in serum aminotransferase levels. HIV infection itself is known to cause hepatomegaly and elevated aminotransferase levels. The differential diagnosis includes other infectious causes (hepatitis B, hepatitis C, *M. avium-intracellulare* infection, Epstein-Barr virus, cytomegalovirus) and drug toxicity (rifabutin, isoniazid, fluconazole, itraconazole, ketoconazole, rifampin, Bactrim, lamivudine, stavudine, zalcitabine, nevirapine, and ritonavir). Hepatitis B does not usually cause hepatocellular injury in the HIV-infected child. Recent investigation of vertical transmission of HIV and hepatitis C has demonstrated that the rate of infection of hepatitis C is significantly higher in children with HIV coinfection compared with babies who are exposed to hepatitis C alone. The rate of hepatitis C cotransmission varies depending on the study, but the range is 22.5% to 40% in HIV-coinfected infants versus 3.2% to 7.5% in non–HIV-infected infants.[15–17] Therefore, infants born to HIV- and hepatitis C–coinfected mothers are at considerable risk of acquiring hepatitis C.

Chronic, progressive liver disease is uncommon among HIV-infected children, but if transaminase elevation persists for several months, percutaneous liver biopsy may help determine the cause of the elevation and assess the extent of hepatocellular damage. While hepatotoxicity may necessitate discontinuation of an antiretroviral agent, potential hepatotoxic medications such as fluconazole, frequently used to treat HIV-infected children, may also contribute to liver injury.

The child with HIV infection and jaundice should be evaluated for obstruction of the common bile duct or cholestatic hepatitis. Common bile duct obstruction can be caused by gallstones or may result from fibrosis, inflammation, or injury of the biliary tract. Ultrasonography of the liver, gallbladder, and biliary tree should be performed in the evaluation of jaundice. *Cryptosporidium* can infect the bile duct and lead to inflammation of the bile duct epithelium and acalculous cholecystitis. Symptoms of acute cholecystitis include fever, right upper quadrant abdominal pain, and tenderness. Cytomegalovirus infection can cause similar symptoms and therefore should be considered in the differential diagnosis of jaundice, fever, and right upper quadrant abdominal pain.

NUTRITION

In the past decade, the advent of combination antiretroviral therapy has revolutionized the management of HIV-infected children in the United States. As a result of immune reconstitution and the decreased incidence of opportunistic infections, children with perinatally acquired HIV infection are now living longer. Despite significant reductions in maternal-infant transmission in the United States in the past decade, there has been a significant increase in the number of children living with HIV infection. Advances in antiretroviral therapy, however, have not uniformly resulted in improvement in nutrition and growth in HIV-infected children. In the United States in 1998, the HIV wasting syndrome rose from the fifth to the second most common AIDS-defining illness in children.[18] The evaluation and management of growth and nutrition in the child infected with HIV remains one of the most difficult challenges for physicians and health care providers in the years ahead.

The association between growth failure and morbidity and mortality in HIV disease among infants and children is well established, especially in developing countries, and continues to be an area of active investigation. In the Women and Infants Transmission Study (WITS), HIV-infected and uninfected children born to HIV-positive women had serial anthropometric measurements; HIV-infected children weighed less (−0.71 kg) and were shorter (−2.25 cm) at 18 months of age than uninfected children.[19] In addition, data from the Mothers and Infants Cohort Study demonstrated that the severity of disease is associated with the degree of growth failure and stunting and that growth failure typically precedes progression of HIV disease.[20] In this study, a prospective cohort of 161 unexposed infants was compared with 148 exposed, uninfected infants and 49 HIV-infected infants. Among the HIV-infected infants, children in the lowest quartile for weight growth velocity were more likely to have HIV disease progression compared to those in the highest weight growth velocity quartile. In addition, the HIV-infected children with early, severe disease had the lowest body mass index and rapidly diverged from the other groups, beginning at 3 months of age. These studies demonstrate that growth disturbance is often evident early in HIV-infected children and may be the first clinical sign of disease progression.

Despite advances in antiretroviral therapy, the association between growth failure and HIV disease has persisted. Carey and colleagues[21] examined weight and height growth velocity among 1338 HIV-infected children between the ages of 3 months and 18 years and found that growth velocity was an independent predictor of mortality even after adjusting for antiretroviral therapy, CD4+ T-cell count, and age. Viral load and energy intake are inversely related, and the rate of growth and energy intake are directly related to HIV replication. This suggests that in children with HIV-associated growth failure, caloric intake may be insufficient to maintain normal growth.[22] Therefore, careful assessment of growth parameters and nutritional monitoring remain an essential aspect in caring for the health of an HIV-infected child.

Assessment of Growth and Nutrition

Infant Growth and Nutrition

The most easily acquired and perhaps most important information used to assess the growth and nutritional status of an infant is serial measurement of weight, height, and head circumference. Slow weight gain and accrual of height may be the earliest indication of malnutrition in a young infant with HIV infection and should be evaluated during routine pediatric visits. Growth velocity is greatest in the first 3 months of life and declines over the subsequent 18 months. Evidence of delayed growth in height or weight signals the need for careful evaluation and close follow-up.

Assessment of caloric intake is an integral part of the evaluation of growth and nutrition in a child. Although the accuracy of dietary recall and dietary records may be limited, trained dietary staff can estimate caloric intake and determine whether daily energy and protein requirements are being met. Table 16–3 outlines the Recommended Dietary Allowances (RDAs) of protein and energy during the first 18 months of life.[23] When interviewing a parent or guardian to estimate caloric intake, it is important to include not only a comprehensive review of the quantities and types of foods consumed but also the details of formula and food preparation, nonformula beverage consumption, and snacks. Also, symptoms of poor appetite, nausea, vomiting, and diarrhea should be reviewed. Nausea and vomiting are common side effects of many of the antiretroviral medications and may contribute significantly to malnutrition and poor growth in the HIV-infected child owing to decreased caloric intake as well as calories lost from vomiting.

Table 16–3
Recommended Daily Allowances of Calories and Protein Intake for Children According to Age[23]

AGE, y	KILOCALORIES/kg		PROTEIN, g/kg	
0–0.5	108		2.2	
0.5–1	98		1.6	
1–3	102		1.2	
4–6	90		1.1	
7–10	70		1.0	
	Males	Females	Males	Females
11–14	55	47	1.0	1.0
15–18	45	40	0.9	0.8

The child's home environment is a critical factor in determining the availability of adequate and appropriate nutrition. Parental HIV infection and AIDS, including malnutrition, can have a devastating impact on the financial and physical capability of a family to acquire and deliver appropriate nutrition to an infant. Seemingly simple tasks such as food shopping and food choices may be difficult for many families. When such obstacles are identified, home nursing and social services are needed to provide additional support to the child and family.

Childhood and Adolescence: Growth Evaluation

Although growth is most rapid in the first 2 years of life, concern for growth and nutrition does not end for the HIV-infected child in infancy. Growth failure and delayed puberty are serious complications of HIV infection in children and adolescents.[24–26] Gertner and coworkers,[26] in a prospective study of HIV-infected boys (ages 10–12 years) with hemophilia, found statistically significant decreases in height among HIV-infected (n = 188) versus non–HIV-infected (n = 120) boys. These boys also had a delayed rate of change in Tanner stage after the age of 13 years compared to non-HIV-infected control subjects. These data highlight the continued importance of careful monitoring of weight and height development as well as nutrition throughout childhood and adolescence for children with HIV infection.

Serial measurements of height and weight are essential for tracking growth in school-aged children. These measurements can be used to calculate height and weight growth velocity as well as body mass index (weight in kg/height in m^2) and provide a reasonable assessment of growth and nutritional status (Table 16–4). In children with decreased height velocity, determination of bone age is important. Among HIV-infected boys in the hemophilia study with decreased height velocity, delayed bone age accounted for 35% of the variation observed in height.[26] During routine health care visits, appropriate Tanner staging should be documented to follow pubertal development. If decreased growth or delayed puberty is identified, a thorough dietary history of caloric and nutrient intake should be obtained.

Assessment of body composition also may provide evidence for growth or developmental delay. While simple anthropometric measurements are readily available tools for the evaluation of lean body mass, more sensitive and reproducible methods to determine body composition, fat free mass (FFM), and body fat distribution are being adapted for use in HIV-infected children. When normative data are available, techniques such as bioelectrical impedance analysis, dual energy x-ray absorptiometry, cross-sectional computed tomography, and magnetic resonance imaging can be used to characterize body composition and to identify specific abnormalities associated with HIV-related growth failure and AIDS wasting in the pediatric population. Arpadi and colleagues[25] reported body composition alterations among HIV-infected prepubertal children with growth failure. Both boys and girls (ages 4–11 years) with a 12-month height velocity at the fifth percentile or less for age had normal fat stores but diminished FFM. Surprisingly, boys with HIV infection and normal growth parameters also had decreased FFM. This preferential decrease in FFM is not only consistent with observations in adults with AIDS-related weight loss and wasting[27] but also supports previous reports of decreased muscle mass among children with perinatally acquired HIV infection.[24] Treatment with nutritional support alone does not appear to restore lean body mass and correct the alteration in body composition.[28]

HIV Wasting

As previously stated, severe wasting is a common AIDS-defining illness and was reported as an AIDS-indicator condition in 17% of children with AIDS in 1996. Wasting is defined by the CDC as (1) weight loss of 10% or more of pre-illness body weight; (2) downward crossing of at least two percentile lines on the weight-for-age chart (e.g., going from the 50th to the 25th and then to the 5th percentile) in a child 1 year of age or older; or (3) weight-for-height less than the 5th percentile on two consecutive measurements at least 30 days apart.[29]

Table 16–4
Age of Peak Height and Weight Growth Velocity

	AGE OF PEAK HEIGHT VELOCITY	AGE OF PEAK WEIGHT VELOCITY
Females	12.5 ± 1.5	12.4 ± 1.4
Males	13.8 ± 1.1	13.9 ± 0.5

Values established for adolescents in the US (years ± standard deviation).[26]

There is no single mechanism responsible for AIDS wasting. Many HIV-related conditions, such as esophageal infection, recurrent fevers, and medication-induced nausea and vomiting, are associated with diminished energy intake. Especially in Africa and Asia, the impaired health of the child's primary provider may be a barrier to adequate food intake. There are limited data in HIV-infected children to link AIDS wasting to diminished caloric intake. In two studies in which caloric intake was measured in HIV-infected children, most children received calories and nutrients at or above the RDA, and there was no direct correlation between energy intake and nutritional status.[30,31] However, in these studies, patients were assessed early in the course of infection[28] and symptomatic patients were below the RDA for energy intake.[31]

More recently, dietary intake in children with HIV infection and impaired growth was determined by 24-hour recall and direct observation. There was no difference in energy intake between HIV-infected patients with normal growth and those with impaired growth.[32] However, in a subset of children who met criteria for AIDS wasting, significantly less energy was consumed as compared with patients with other patterns of impaired growth. Long-term decreased energy intake, as well as diminished intake during periods of acute illness, are likely contributing factors to AIDS wasting in children.

Increased energy expenditure has also been proposed in the pathogenesis of AIDS wasting. The majority of data to support increased energy expenditure among patients with HIV infection has come from studies in adults. More recently, sophisticated measurements of total energy expenditure among HIV-infected adults and children have been performed using doubly labeled water.[32,33] These studies have failed to demonstrate a "hypermetabolic" state among patients with HIV infection and impaired growth or wasting.

Intestinal dysfunction and nutrient malabsorption are other important contributors to wasting and malnutrition among HIV-infected children. Infectious enteritis, malnutrition, and potentially direct effects of HIV virus may cause injury to the intestinal epithelium, resulting in impaired nutrient absorption. This intestinal epithelial injury, regardless of its origin, is manifested as steatorrhea, carbohydrate and iron malabsorption, and increased intestinal permeability.[12,33,34] Estimates of the prevalence of intestinal dysfunction were as high as 60% to 80% in the era of HIV management prior to the development of highly active antiretroviral therapy,[34] and malabsorption must be considered in the evaluation of all children with HIV infection and wasting.

Lipodystrophy

A lipodystrophy syndrome, characterized by fat redistribution, dyslipidemia, and insulin resistance, has been increasingly recognized among adults with HIV infection receiving combination antiretroviral therapy. Patients who are affected by this syndrome may develop marked accumulation of abdominal and dorsocervical fat, substantial loss of peripheral subcutaneous fat, or a combination of both regional fat accumulation and atrophy. These physical characteristics are associated with metabolic disturbances, including hyperinsulinemia, hypertriglyceridemia, low high-density lipoprotein cholesterol, and increased incidence of diabetes and impaired glucose tolerance.[35]

Although the exact mechanism responsible for these findings is not known, both protease inhibitors and nucleoside reverse transcriptase inhibitors have been shown to potentially contribute to the development of certain components of this syndrome.[36,37] Lipodystrophy is an area of active investigation with a focus on the underlying causal mechanisms, the potential long-term morbidity and mortality of the associated metabolic abnormalities and increased risk of cardiovascular disease, and potential approaches to the treatment of lipodystrophy.

Less is known about lipodystrophy in children with HIV infection who are on combination antiretroviral therapy. Arpadi and colleagues[38] performed a 5-year longitudinal study of 28 prepubertal children with HIV infection who were receiving antiretroviral therapy. They found that 29% of children demonstrated changes in regional fat distribution consistent with lipodystrophy (i.e., increased truncal fat and lipoatrophy of the arms or legs as assessed by repeated dual energy x-ray absorptiometry). These changes, as well as increases in triglyceride levels, were associated with exposure to protease inhibitors. These preliminary findings suggest that lipodystrophy and the metabolic complications documented in adults may also be common among children. Long-term use of combination antiretroviral therapy and the development of lipodystrophy among children may confer serious complications such as increased risk of diabetes, central obesity, and cardiovascular disease. Additional research and clinical investigation are needed to fully establish the incidence and prevalence of lipodystrophy among the pediatric HIV population and to determine the potential mediating effects of growth and puberty on its development.

Vitamin and Mineral Deficiencies

Vitamin and mineral deficiencies and their contribution to the progression of HIV/AIDS have been the topic of intense investigation, particularly in developing nations. The nutritional assessment of an HIV-infected child should include evaluation for possible vitamin and mineral deficiencies. For example, general malnutrition, malabsorption, and excess losses may combine to create a condition of chronic iron deficiency anemia, which, if corrected, may have a dramatic impact on improving the child's health.

Vitamin A deficiency has received a significant amount of attention because of its role in HIV transmission and disease progression. Worldwide, vitamin A deficiency affects 50 million children under the age of 5 years, and 350,000 children develop blindness each year from vitamin A deficiency. Vitamin A deficiency among pregnant HIV-infected women has been associated with increased vertical transmission.[39,40] However, vitamin A deficiency is relatively rare in the United States and, in this population, may play no significant role in transmission. Vitamin A deficiency is also associated with impaired immune function, including diminished antibody production and impaired secretory epithelial function in the gut and respiratory tract. By this mechanism, vitamin A deficiency may contribute to disease progression and mortality among HIV-infected patients. In a trial of vitamin A supplementation conducted in Tanzania, HIV-infected children experienced a 63% reduction in all causes of mortality with vitamin A supplementation compared with placebo.[41] Although this is compelling evidence in support of vitamin A supplementation, vitamin A deficiency is relatively uncommon among HIV-infected children in North America, and vitamin A concentrations appear not to be related to mortality in this population.[42]

Deficiencies of other micronutrients have been assessed as potential contributors to HIV disease progression, morbidity, and mortality. While some studies have failed to identify significant deficiencies or associations between deficiencies and severity of disease,[42,43] others have demonstrated such links. For example, selenium deficiency has been associated with increased risk of mortality,[44] and HIV-infected children with vitamin B_{12} and zinc deficiencies have lower CD4+ counts.[45] There is currently no consensus about the use of routine vitamin and mineral supplementation in HIV-infected children to exceed the RDA; however, all HIV-infected children, particularly those children presenting with impaired growth or malnutrition, should be observed for clinical signs and symptoms of vitamin and mineral deficiencies. When the use of a multivitamin or mineral supplement is being considered, supplementation doses should be reviewed with a registered dietician or physician familiar with age-appropriate RDA guidelines.

Strategies for Nutritional Management

Gastrostomy Tube

In almost all circumstances, it is preferable that children receive the recommended amount of energy and nutrients through the consumption of a well-balanced diet. However, there are numerous reasons why this is often difficult or impossible to achieve in an HIV-infected child. For example, opportunistic infections of the mouth and esophagus, nausea and vomiting associated with antiretroviral medications, and anorexia may all interfere with a child's ability to eat and drink what is necessary for optimal growth and general health.

The use of short-term nasogastric tube feeding and the placement of a gastrostomy tube may help overcome these challenges in feeding HIV-infected children.[24,46] Miller and colleagues[46] demonstrated that the use of gastrostomy tube feeding resulted in increased weight and increased weight-for-height Z-scores in a cohort of 23 children with HIV infection. Although this study did not demonstrate significant improvement in linear growth, other important benefits in health care, such as decreased rates of hospitalization and reduced mortality rates among children who gained weight with gastrostomy tube feeding, were noted. Gastrostomy tube placement should be considered when oral dietary supplementation has failed and a child is below 80% of standard weight or weight-for-height. A period of nasogastric tube feedings may be beneficial to demonstrate that direct gastric feeding will be tolerated and successful prior to gastrostomy tube placement. Gastrostomy tubes and buttons may be placed safely endoscopically or by using radiographic techniques. Insertion should not be performed in a neutropenic child.

More recently, gastrostomy tubes have been successfully employed for administration of antiretroviral medication in children.[47] Placed either for combined use in nutritional supplementation and medication delivery, or solely to improve adherence to medication regimens, Shingadia and colleagues[47] show that gastrostomy tubes may markedly decrease the time to administer medications and improve adherence in young children. Gastrostomy tube placement was well tolerated. In this series of 17 children, only one child developed a mild stomal cellulitis that resolved with antibiotic therapy. The additional benefit of improved medication delivery and compliance may make gastrostomy tube placement more readily acceptable to the patient and family when it is being considered for nutritional purposes.

Parenteral Nutrition

Total parenteral nutrition (TPN) is available as an alternative strategy for nutritional support but is reserved for those children who demonstrate persistent malnutrition despite aggressive attempts to maximize oral and enteral nutrition. Candidates for TPN include patients with chronic pancreatitis, nausea and vomiting not controlled by antiemetic therapy, severe chronic malabsorption, and biliary tract disease or gastrointestinal obstruction. TPN requires placement of a central venous catheter, and the inherent risks of catheter placement and subsequent infection must be considered prior to initiation. Few data are available on the specific use of TPN and its associated risks in HIV-infected children. In adults with HIV infection, TPN therapy has been shown to promote weight gain by increasing both fat and, in some patients, lean body mass.[48,49] In one series on the use of TPN in adults with AIDS, the risk of catheter-related sepsis was 0.12 per 100 days of treatment, which is similar to the rates observed in patients receiving TPN for malignancy.[50] However, if TPN is initiated in a patient with HIV infection, meticulous monitoring of the TPN and the catheter site by a health professional is necessary to minimize the risk of infection while providing optimal nutrition. In addition, planning the reintroduction of enteral feedings as soon as possible once TPN has been initiated will minimize the patient's time on TPN. When medically acceptable, even small amounts of oral feeding during TPN may provide significant psychosocial benefits to the patient.

Nutritional support of the HIV-infected child should begin at birth and continue throughout the life of the child. Effective nutrition should consider the needs of not only the child but also the family. On a global scale, the responsibility for insuring that families have access to food falls on governmental and nongovernmental agencies that must continue to advocate access for all to balanced nutrition.

ACKNOWLEDGMENT

This work was supported in part by NIH grants K23-DK02844 and T32-DK07703.

REFERENCES

1. Bogden J, Kemp F, Han S, et al: Status of selected nutrients and progression of human immunodeficiency virus type 1 infection. Am J Clin Nutr 2000;72:809–815.
2. Ramos-Gomez FJ, Flaitz C, Catapano P, et al: The Collaborative Workgroup on Oral Manifestations of Pediatric HIV Infection, Oral AIDS Center, University of California, San Francisco: Classification, diagnostic criteria and treatment recommendations for orofacial manifestations in HIV-infected pediatric patients. J Clin Pediatr Dent 1999;23:85–95.
3. Ferguson F, Berensten B, Nachman S: Experiences of pediatric dental program for HIV positive children. In Greenspan JS, Greenspan D (eds): Oral Manifestations of HIV Infection. Proceedings of the Second International Workshop on the Oral Manifestations of HIV Infection, January 31–February 3, 1993, San Francisco, CA. Chicago, Quintessence Publishing, 1993, pp 240–246.
4. Miller TL: Nutritional aspects of pediatric HIV infection. In Walker WA, Watkins JB (eds): Nutrition Pediatrics: Basic Science and Clinical Applications, 2nd ed. Hamilton, Ontario, BC Decker, 1997, pp 534–550.
5. Clarick RH, Hanekom WA, Yogev R, Chadwick EG: Megestrol acetate treatment of growth failure in children infected with human immunodeficiency virus. Pediatrics 1997;99:354–357.
6. Centers for Disease Control and Prevention: HIV/AIDS Surveillance Report. MMWR 1996;8:1–39.
7. Miller TL, Martin SR, Cooper ER, et al: Gastrointestinal inflammation and carbohydrate intolerance in HIV infected children. Pediatr Res 1990;27:650.
8. Wilcox CM: Current concepts of gastrointestinal disease associated with HIV infection. Clin Persp Gastroenterol 2000;3:9–17.
9. National Pediatric and Family HIV Resource Center, Working Group on Antiretroviral Therapy and Medical Management of Infants, Children, and Adolescents with HIV Infection: Antiretroviral therapy and medical management of pediatric HIV infection. Pediatrics 1998;102:1005–1063.

10. Miller TL, Winter HS, Luginbuhl LM, et al: Pancreatitis in pediatric human immunodeficiency virus infection. J Pediatrics 1992;120:223–227.
11. Konecny P: Hyperamylasemia in asymptomatic HIV patients. Ann Clin Biochem 1997;43:259–262.
12. Hancock MR, Smith NA, Hawkins DA, et al: Biochemical assessment of pancreatic disease in human immunodeficiency virus infected men. J Clin Pathol 1997;50:674–676.
13. Miller TL, Orav EJ, Martin SR, et al: Malnutrition and carbohydrate malabsorption in children with vertically transmitted human immunodeficiency virus infection. Gastroenterology 1991;100:1296–1302.
14. Yolken RH, Hart W, Oung I, et al: Gastrointestinal dysfunction and disaccharide intolerance in children infected with human immunodeficiency virus. J Pediatrics 1991;118:359–363.
15. Mazza C, Ravaggi A, Rodella A, et al, for the Study Group of Vertical Transmission: Prospective study of mother to infant transmission of hepatitis C virus (HCV) infection. J Med Virol 1998;54:12–19.
16. Papevangelou V, Pollack H, Rochford G, et al: Increased transmission of vertical hepatitis C virus (HCV) infection to human immunodeficiency virus (HIV)-infected infants of HIV- and HCV-coinfected women. J Infect Dis 1998;178:104–152.
17. Zanetti AR, Tanzi E, Romano L, et al: A prospective study on mother-to-infant transmission of hepatitis C virus. Intervirology 1998;41:208–212.
18. Lindegren ML, Steinberg S, Byers RH: Epidemiology of HIV/AIDS in children. Pediatr Clin N Am 2000;47:1–20.
19. Moye J, Rich KC, Kalish LA, et al, for the Women and Infants Transmission Study Group: Natural history of somatic growth in infants born to women infected by human immunodeficiency virus. J Pediatr 1992;128:58–69.
20. Muenz LR, Landesman S, Moye J, et al: Weight and weight change in HIV-1-infected infants: A prospective study in the first two years of life. The Mothers and Infants Cohort Study. Paper presented at the NICHD/PACTG Workshop on Growth, Nutrition, and Metabolic Complications in HIV infected children, Washington, DC, May 2000.
21. Carey VJ, Yong FH, Fenkel LM, McKinney RE: Pediatric AIDS prognosis using somatic growth velocity. AIDS 1998;12:1361–1369.
22. Arpadi S, Cuff P, Kotler D, et al: Growth velocity, fat-free mass and energy intake are inversely related to viral load in HIV-infected children. J Nutr 2000;130:2498–2502.
23. National Research Council: Recommended Daily Allowances, 10th ed. Washington, DC, National Academy Press, 1989.
24. Miller T, Evans S, Orav EJ, et al: Growth and body composition in children with human immunodeficiency virus-1 infection. Am J Clin Nutr 1993;57:588–592.
25. Arpadi SM, Horlick MNB, Wang J, et al: Body composition in prepubertal children with human immunodeficiency virus type 1 infection. Arch Pediatr Adolesc Med 1998;142:688–693.
26. Gertner JM, Kaufman FR, Danfield SM, et al: Delayed somatic growth and pubertal development in human immunodeficiency virus-related hemophiliac boys: Hemophilia growth and development study. J Pediatr 1994;124:497–502.
27. Kotler DP, Wang J, Pierson RN: Body composition in patients with acquired immunodeficiency syndrome. Am J Clin Nutr 1985;42:1155–1165.
28. Hendersen RA, Saavedra JM, Perman JA, et al: Effect of enteral tube feeding on growth of children with symptomatic human immunodeficiency virus infection. J Pediatr Gastroenterol Nutr 1994;18:429–434.
29. Grunfeld C, Feingold KR: Metabolic disturbances and wasting in the acquired immunodeficiency syndrome. N Engl J Med 1992;327:329–337.
30. Miller TL, Evans S, Morris V, et al: Prospective study of the alterations in growth and nutritional requirements in HIV infected children. Gastroenterology 1991;100:A538.
31. Zuin G, Comi D, Fontana M, et al: Energy and nutrient intakes in HIV-infected children. Pediatr AIDS HIV Infect Fetus Adolesc 1994;5:159–161.
32. Johann-Liang R, O'Neill L, Cervia J, et al: Energy balance, viral burden, insulin-like growth factor-1, interleukin-6 and growth impairment in children with human immunodeficiency virus. AIDS 2000;14:683–690.
33. Guarino A, Albano F, Tarallo L, et al: Intestinal malabsorption in HIV-infected children: Relationship with diarrhea, failure to thrive, enteric microorganisms and immune impairment. AIDS 1993;7:1435–1440.
34. Castaldo A, Tarallo L, Palomba E, et al: Iron deficiency and intestinal malabsorption in HIV disease. J Pediatr Gastroenterol Nutr 1996;22:359–363.
35. Hadigan C, Meigs JB, Corcoran C, et al: Characterization of metabolic abnormalities and cardiovascular disease risk factors in HIV-infected men and women with the lipodystrophy syndrome. Clin Inf Dis 2001;32:130–139.
36. Walli RK, Herfort O, Michl GM, et al: Treatment with protease inhibitors associated with peripheral insulin resistance and impaired oral glucose tolerance in HIV-1 infected patients. AIDS 1998;12:F167–F173.
37. Carr A, Miller J, Law M, Cooper D: A syndrome of lipoatrophy, lactic acidaemia and liver dysfunction associated with HIV nucleoside analogue therapy: Contribution to protease inhibitor-related lipodystrophy syndrome. AIDS 2000;14:F25–F32.
38. Arpadi SM, Cuff PA, Horlick MB, et al: Changes in regional body fat and serum triglycerides and cholesterol in HIV-infected children. Antiretroviral Therapy 2000;5(suppl):14.

39. Semba RD, Miotti PG, Chiphangwi JD, et al: Maternal vitamin A deficiency and mother-to-child transmission of HIV-1. Lancet 1994;343:1593–1597.
40. Greenberg BL, Semba RD, Vink PE, et al: Vitamin A deficiency and maternal-infant transmission of HIV in two metropolitan areas in the United States. AIDS 1997;11:325–332.
41. Fawzi WW, Mbise RL, Hertmark E, et al: A randomized trial of vitamin A supplements in relation to mortality among human immunodeficiency virus-infected and uninfected children in Tanzania. Pediatr Infect Dis J 1999;18:127–133.
42. Read JS, Bethel J, Harris DR, et al: Serum vitamin A concentrations in a North American cohort of human immunodeficiency virus type-1-infected children. National Institute of Child Health and Human Development Intravenous Immunoglobulin Clinical Trial Study Group. Pediatr Infect Dis J 1999;18:134–142.
43. Henderson RA, Talusan K, Hutton N, et al: Serum and plasma markers of nutritional status in children infected with the human immunodeficiency virus. J Am Dietetic Assoc 1997;97:1377–1381.
44. Campa A, Shor-Posner G, Indacochea F, et al: Mortality risk in selenium-deficient HIV-positive children. J Acquir Immune Defic Syndr Hum Retrovirol 1999;20:508–513.
45. Baum MK, Shor-Posner G, Lu Y, et al: Micronutrients and HIV-1 disease progression. AIDS 1995;9:1051–1056.
46. Miller T, Awnetwant EL, Evans S, et al: Gastrostomy tube supplementation for HIV-infected children. Pediatrics 1995;96:696–702.
47. Shingadia D, Viani RM, Yogev R, et al: Gastrostomy tube insertion for improvement of adherence to highly active antiretroviral therapy in pediatric patients with human immunodeficiency virus. Pediatrics 2000;105:e80.
48. Kotler DP, Tierney AR, Culpepper-Morgan JA, et al: Effect of home total parenteral nutrition on body composition patients with acquired immunodeficiency syndrome. J Parent Ent Nutr 1990;14:454–458.
49. Ireton-Jones CS, Stiller DL: Evaluation of outcomes for patients with AIDS receiving home total parenteral nutrition. Nutrition 1998;14:731–735.
50. Singer P, Rothkopf MM, Kvetan V, et al: Risks and benefits of home parenteral nutrition in the acquired immunodeficiency syndrome. J Parent Ent Nutr 1991;15:75–79.

17

Abnormal Cardiovascular Function in HIV-Infected Infants and Children

Marcie J. Keesler, Stacy D. Fisher, and Steven E. Lipshultz

HIV-associated illnesses were responsible for the deaths of approximately 510,000 children worldwide in 1998.[1] Before the era of highly active antiretroviral therapy, approximately 50% of children living with HIV infection survived until the age of 9 years.[2] As the number of children living longer with HIV infection increases, a significant number will experience related cardiovascular complications. HIV-infected children with increased longevity are more likely to succumb to cardiac complications or a wasting syndrome.[3] Tables 17–1 and 17–2 summarize retrospective and cross-sectional studies of cardiovascular abnormalities in pediatric HIV infection, showing the prevalence and extent of associated disease.

A majority of children infected with HIV were exposed by vertical transmission of the virus in the perinatal period. Transmission of HIV from mother to child has been estimated at 15% to 35% in children born to mothers who are HIV infected.[4] Transmission rates can be reduced below 8% with the use of antiretroviral therapy in the second and third trimesters of pregnancy in infected women.[4] Cardiac complications associated with HIV infection range from subclinical electrocardiographic changes to cardiomyopathy and sudden death. In children without treatment, approximately 10% to 25% will have a course that is characterized by encephalopathy, pneumonia, and death.[5] In a recent study of 68 HIV-infected children (48 with vertical transmission, 20 infected by transfusion of blood products), 28% experienced serious cardiac events after AIDS diagnosis. During follow-up, 43 of the 68 children died and 35% of those who died had known cardiac dysfunction.[6]

Predictors of cardiac complications associated with HIV infection in children include encephalopathy, wasting, decreased CD4+ count, and prior history of a serious cardiac event. Predictors of overall mortality include encephalopathy, wasting, and a low age-adjusted CD4+ count.[6] Figure 17–1 illustrates the estimated length of time to a serious cardiac event from the time of AIDS diagnosis in an HIV-infected child.

RAPID PROGRESSORS AND NON-RAPID PROGRESSORS

Children up to 2 years of age who are infected with HIV can be classified as either rapid progressors or non-rapid progressors based on their symptoms and immunologic status. Those children who are classified as rapid progressors have an AIDS-defining condition other than lymphoid interstitial pneumonia/pulmonary lymphoid hyperplasia or severe immunosuppression in the first year of life.[7]

Rapid disease progression has been associated with a higher mortality rate. Changes in cardiac and pulmonary function in rapid progressors include increased respiratory rate, increased heart rate, and decreased fractional shortening on serial echocardiographic measurements.[8] Figure 17–2 illustrates the cumulative mortality among 93 HIV-1–infected

Table 17-1
Retrospective Studies of Cardiovascular Abnormalities in Pediatric Patients with HIV Infection

STUDY	PATIENTS, n	PATIENT CHARACTERISTICS	TESTING MODALITY	MAJOR FINDINGS
Domanski et al[80]	137	All ages and risk factors 1 mo–5 years	ECHO	Cardiomyopathy, 14% (19/137) 6% average decrease in fractional shortening
Al-Attar et al[6]	68	All ages and risk factors All with AIDS Reviewed since AIDS diagnosis	Survival study	Serious cardiac event, (CHF, tamponade, CVA, arrest) 28% (19/68) 35% (15/43) of deaths in setting significant of cardiac disease (encephalopathy, male sex, wasting predictive of cardiac death)
Grenier et al[42]	95	4 mo–12 years 15 HIV+; 80 HIV+ with symptoms Reviewed for average of 10 mo	ECHO	Echocardiographic abnormalities, 25% (24/95) Increased left ventricular contractility, 75% (18/24) Cardiomyopathy, 87.5% (21/24) 92% of deaths had abnormal heart Cardiac cause for 25% (3/12) of deaths
Tripp et al[81]	129	All ages	ECHO	Cardiomyopathy, 9% (11/129) Pericardial effusion, 2% (2/129)
Luginbuhl et al[38]	81	Mean age, 4.1 years Mean follow-up, 1.8 years 8 HIV+; 73 HIV+ with symptoms	ECHO	Chronic CHF, 10% (8/81) Transient CHF, 10% (8/81) Cardiopulmonary arrest, 9% (7/81) 33% (10/30) of deaths with cardiac dysfunction
Mast et al[82]	45	0–8 years All with autopsy or Echocardiogram	ECHO/chest radiograph 21 autopsied	Pericardial effusion, 58% (26/45) Tamponade, 8% (2/26) Normal chest radiograph, 50% (13/26) Ventricular dilation or hypertrophy, 43% (9/21)

CHF, congestive heart failure; CVA, cerebrovascular accident; ECHO, echocardiography.

Table 17-2
Cross-Sectional Studies of Cardiovascular Involvement in Pediatric Patients with HIV Infection

STUDY	PATIENTS, n	PATIENT CHARACTERISTICS	TESTING MODALITY	MAJOR FINDINGS
Nogueira et al[83]	32	Children infected with HIV ages 3 mo–13 years 90% perinatal transmission 69% with symptoms	ECHO/electro-cardiography	Total abnormalities, 47% (15/32); 73% (11/15) cases pulmonary hypertension 27% (4/15) cases LV dysfunction
Kavanaugh-McHugh et al[16]	61	HIV-infected children	ECHO	Total abnormalities, 70% (43/61) LV dilation, 30% (18/61) LV dysfunction, 18% (11/61) RV dilation, 18% (11/61) Pericardial effusion, 51% (31/61)
Kavanaugh-McHugh et al[43]	88	Echocardiogram on enrollment and at 6-mo intervals	ECHO	Ventricular dilation, 34% (30/88) Pericardial effusion, 16% (14/88) Decreased ventricular function, 20% (18/88) Atrial dilation, 11% (10/88)
Issenberg et al[44]	22	6 mo–6 years 12 AIDS, 10 ARC	ECHO	LV dilation/dysfunction, 45% (10/22) RV dilation, 9% (2/22) Pericardial effusion, 18% (4/22)
Sherron et al[45]	23	4–48 mo All with ARC or AIDS	ECHO	LV dysfunction, 74% (17/23) Decreased fractional shortening, 65% (15/23) Pericardial effusion, 18% (4/22) Pulmonary artery hypertension, 17% (4/23)
Lindvig et al[84]	24	All with AIDS	ECHO	Total abnormalities, 54% (13/24) RV diameter, >26 mm, 37.5% (9/24) Dilated left atrium or left ventricle, 12.5% (2/24) Pericardial effusion, 21% (5/24)

ARC, AIDS-related condition; ECHO, echocardiography, LV, left ventricular; RV right ventricular.

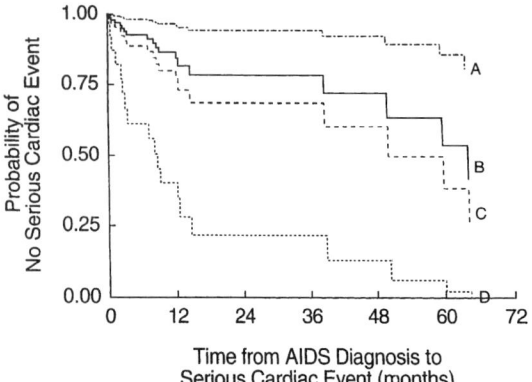

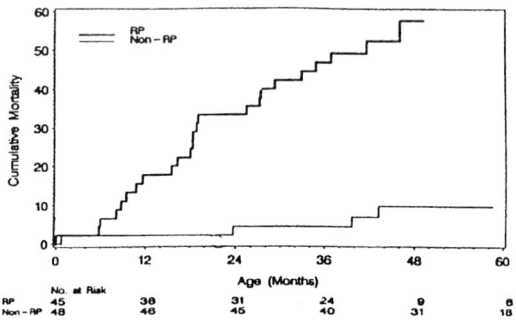

Figure 17–1. Time to occurrence of a serious cardiac event (transient and chronic congestive heart failure, hypotension, severe dysrhythmia, cardiac tamponade, cerebrovascular accident associated with hemodynamic instability, and cardiac arrest) in AIDS patients in 1992. The curve A represents AIDS patients with no wasting and no prior cardiac events. The curve marked B represents AIDS patient with no wasting but with a history of prior cardiac events. The curve marked C represents AIDS patients with wasting and no prior cardiac events. The curve marked D represents AIDS patients with wasting and a history of prior cardiac events. (From Al-Attar I, Orav EJ, Exil V, et al: Predictors of cardiac morbidity and related mortality in children with the acquired immune deficiency syndrome. Pediatr Res 1995;37:169A).

Figure 17–2. Cumulative mortality by age among 93 HIV-1–infected children (45 rapid progressors and 48 non-rapid progressors). (From Shearer WT, Lipshultz SE, Easley KA, et al: Alterations in cardiac and pulmonary function in pediatric rapid human immunodeficiency virus type 1 disease progressors. Pediatrics 2000;1:1–8.)

children (45 rapid progressors and 48 non-rapid progressors). The 5-year cumulative mortality rate for rapid progressors is significantly higher as the child ages. Rapid progressors were also found to have higher HIV-1 RNA burden and lower CD8+ (cytotoxic) T cell counts than non-rapid progressors. Subclinical cardiac and pulmonary functional abnormalities are present in rapid progressors and contribute to reported poor outcomes.[8] Clinical considerations and intervention for rapid progressors are different than for non-rapid progressors because of increased rates of early morbidity and mortality.

FETAL AND CONGENITAL CARDIOVASCULAR EFFECTS OF HIV INFECTION

In the United States, approximately 7000 children are born to HIV-infected women annually, and vertical transmission is responsible for up to 95% of cases of infection in children younger than 4 years of age.[9] The environment in the presence of maternal HIV infection may affect the fetal cardiovascular system, whether or not the newborn is infected with HIV. The multicenter Pediatric Pulmonary and Cardiac Complications of HIV Infection (P^2C^2 HIV) study performed echocardiography on 174 fetuses of HIV-infected mothers and found significant differences in cardiovascular structure and function from fetuses of non–HIV-infected women.[10] These differences were found irrespective of the presence or absence of HIV infection in the newborn. The fetuses of HIV-infected mothers had increased right and left ventricular wall thickness and reduced left ventricular dimensions compared with normal control fetuses. Twenty-two of the fetuses who were later confirmed to be HIV-infected were compared with 123 fetuses of HIV-infected mothers who were ultimately HIV negative, and left ventricular diastolic dimension was found to be significantly increased in the HIV-infected children.

Congenital cardiovascular malformations were found in 5 of 175 children with perinatally acquired HIV infection.[11] Abnormalities included an atrial septal defect, tetralogy of Fallot, tricuspid atresia, a ventricular septal defect, and a ventricular septal defect associated with pulmonic stenosis. The P^2C^2 HIV study reported a high prevalence (12.3%) of congenital cardiovascular malformations in children born to mothers who are HIV-infected.[12] Rates were 5 to 10 times higher than reported in population-based epidemiologic studies but not higher than in normal populations similarly screened.[12]

Maternal factors, including intravenous drug use, confound evaluation of HIV influence on cardiac development. Fetal development in a mother infected with HIV often involves other hostile environmental factors, such as smoking and low socioeconomic status, nutritional deficits, coinfections, and illicit and prescribed drug use, which affect heart development and function regardless of the HIV status of the child.

ABNORMAL CARDIAC GROWTH

Left ventricular hypertrophy is commonly found in children infected with HIV. Ventricular dilation evokes compensatory hypertrophy over time, resulting in a significant increase in left ventricular mass. The mean cardiac weight in HIV-infected children has been reported to be 184% higher than in uninfected children.[13] In children infected with HIV, the magnitude of left ventricular hypertrophy is inadequate to reduce peak systolic wall stress to normal. Increased wall stress results in increasing ventricular dilation and eventual decreased left ventricular function.[14]

LEFT VENTRICULAR DYSFUNCTION

Left Ventricular Systolic Dysfunction

Left ventricular dysfunction is common among HIV-infected children and is emerging as a prominent manifestation of HIV infection.[15] Table 17–3 summarizes prospective studies of cardiovascular involvement related to left ventricular dysfunction. Left ventricular abnormalities of structure and function in HIV-infected children are more likely to persist and to be symptomatic than right ventricular abnormalities or pericardial effusions.[16] Results from the P^2C^2 HIV study of 130 vertically infected children revealed that 25% had a fractional shortening more than two standard deviations below normal. Forty-two percent of these patients had depressed contractility and reduced left ventricular performance.[17] Left ventricular fractional shortening is a significant independent predictor of overall mortality, even after adjustment for age, height, CD4+ count, and progressive neurologic disease.[17] Reduced left ventricular fractional shortening and increased wall thickness were also found to be predictive of an increased rate of mortality independent of CD4+ count and encephalopathy in a study of 193 HIV-infected children.[18] Figure 17–3 illustrates cumulative survival rates of HIV-infected children with reduced fractional shortening or altered left ventricular mass or end-diastolic dimension.

The prevalence of decreased left ventricular function (fractional shortening ≤25%) was 5.7%, with a 2-year cumulative incidence of 15.3% among 205 vertically infected children.[19] The 2-year cumulative incidence of decreased left ventricular fractional shortening was 10.7% in the HIV-infected

Table 17–3
Prospective Studies of Cardiovascular Involvement in Pediatric Patients with HIV Infection

STUDY	PATIENTS, n	PATIENT CHARACTERISTICS	FOLLOW-UP	MAJOR FINDINGS
Lipshultz[18]	193	Vertical transmission Mean age, 2.1 years	5 years	Depressed LVFS ($P \leq .001$) and increased wall thickness ($P \leq .004$) predictors in increased mortality
Starc et al[19]	205	Vertical transmission Enrolled at median age 22 months	2 years	Prevalence of decreased LV function 5.7%; 2 years cumulative incidence, 15.3%
Lipshultz[15]	196	Vertical transmission Median age, 2.1 years	2 years	Depressed LVFS correlated with immunodysfunction at baseline but not longitudinally
Haddad Herdy et al[85]	25	Children with AIDS Ages 3 mo–11 years		Dilated CM in 32% (8/25) (6 asymptomatic); 20% (5/25) with pericardial effusion
Starc et al[47]	86 HIV+ 419 HIV– born to + mothers	Vertical transmission Followed since birth	1.1 years (mean)	LVFS < 19% = 1.7% (9/505) LVFS < 25% = 8.6% (42/505) LVEDD (Z-score > 1.5) = 5.8% Cardiomegaly (by radiography) = 13.7%
Lipshultz et al[66]	34	Vertical transmission	4.1 mo (mean)	LVFS initially depressed and remained so

Continued

Table 17-3
Prospective Studies of Cardiovascular Involvement in Pediatric Patients with HIV Infection
Continued

STUDY	PATIENTS, n	PATIENT CHARACTERISTICS	FOLLOW-UP	MAJOR FINDINGS
Lipshultz[17]	130	Followed since birth Vertical transmission	4.1 mo (mean)	LV contractility depressed LVEDD increased (P<.003) Initially depressed contractility 42% (55/130) Initially increased LV afterload 20% (26/130) Initially decreased fractional shortening 25% (32/130) Follow-up: progressive deterioration of LV performance with reduced contractility and increased afterload ($P < .02$)
Ruga et al[86]	41	Vertical transmission 1 mo–8 years	14.1 mo	Dilated cardiomyopathy 10% (4/41) LV hypertrophy by ECG 29% (12/41) Decreased LVFS 5% (2/41)
Dollfus et al[87]	31	3 mo–10 years All HIV+ with symptoms All on zidovudine	3–23 mo	Dilated cardiomyopathy 32% (10/31) Severe heart failure 6% (2/31)
DeSimone et al[88]	20	Vertical transmission Followed since birth	3.7 years	LV dilatation 10% (2/20) Gallop rhythm 5% (1/20)
Lipshultz et al[13]	31	3 mo–22.5 years 11 HIV+; 20 HIV+ with symptoms	Variable	New/progressive changes in 84% (16/19) patients followed with ECG LV/RV hypertrophy = 48% (15/31) Decreased contractility = 26% (8/31) Increased contractility = 32% (10/31) Pericardial effusion = 26% (8/31)

CM, cardiomyopathy; ECG, electrocardiogram; LV, left ventricular; LVEDD, left ventricular end-diastolic dimension; LVFS, left ventricular fractional shortening; RV, right ventricular.

children, compared with 3.1% in the HIV-uninfected children.[19] Approximately 10% of HIV-infected children had congestive heart failure or were treated with cardiac drugs over a 2-year period.[19] Figure 17-4 shows the cumulative incidence of an initial episode of decreased left ventricular fractional shortening in HIV-infected and noninfected children. Depressed left ventricular function correlated with a low CD4+ count at baseline but not longitudinally, suggesting that the CD4+ cell count may not be a useful surrogate marker of HIV-associated left ventricular dysfunction.[15]

Malnutrition and wasting are associated with an increased rate of cardiovascular mortality in HIV-infected children.[6] An inverse relationship between heart rate and nutritional status in HIV-infected children suggests an increased basal metabolic rate in which malnutrition, altered cardiac muscle mass, and left ventricular dysfunction are interdependent.[20]

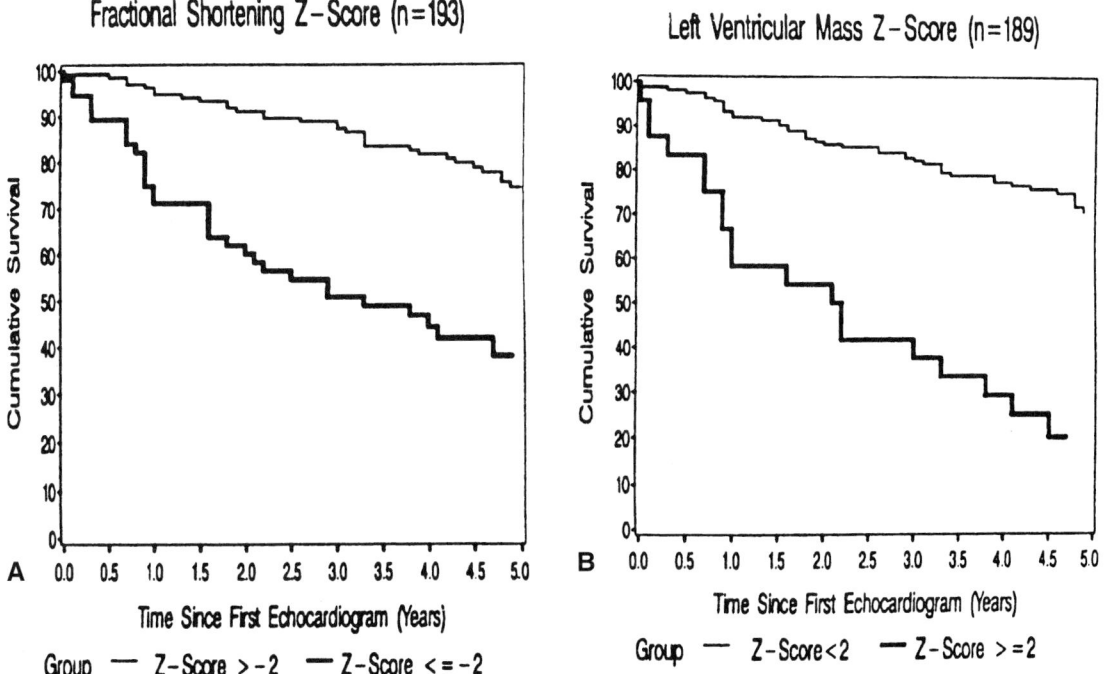
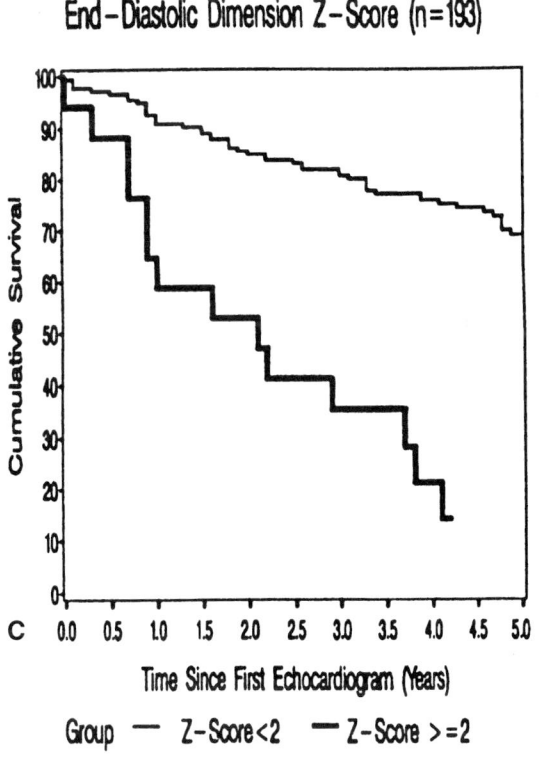

Figure 17–3. Kaplan-Meier cumulative survival for 193 HIV-infected children according to baseline clinical characteristics and baseline echocardiographic measurements. A, Fractional shortening; B, left ventricular mass; C, end-diastolic dimension. (From Lipshultz SE, Easley KA, Orav EJ, et al: Cardiac dysfunction and mortality. The prospective P^2C^2 HIV multicenter study. Circulation 2000;102:1542–1548.)

Left Ventricular Diastolic Dysfunction

Unpublished data from the P²C² HIV study compared echocardiographic parameters of children infected with HIV with those of a control population, children not infected with HIV. Children with HIV had Doppler flow patterns consistent with impaired relaxation. These differences persisted from the perinatal period through 10 years of follow-up. Left ventricular diastolic dysfunction indicated a significant risk for congestive heart failure and death in children infected with HIV and may explain symptoms of congestive heart failure in children with normal left ventricular systolic function.

MYOCARDITIS

Myocarditis is a common cause of left ventricular systolic dysfunction. Dilated cardiomyopathy may be related to a direct action of HIV on the myocardial tissue or to an autoimmune process induced by HIV alone or in conjunction with coinfecting viruses.[21] Histologic examination of postmortem myocyte biopsy samples revealed myocarditis in 11 of 32 HIV-infected children and borderline myocarditis in another 13 children, whereas control samples had no evidence of inflammation.[22] Adenovirus and cytomegalovirus were the most common viruses found by polymerase chain reaction, and an association was suggested between the presence of viral nucleic acids in the myocardium and the development of myocarditis, dilated cardiomyopathy, or congestive heart failure in HIV-infected children.[22] *Toxoplasma gondii*, coxsackievirus group B, Epstein-Barr virus, cytomegalovirus, adenovirus, and HIV nucleic acids within myocytes have been found in myocardial biopsy specimens.[23]

Right ventricular biopsy performed on 76 adult patients within 1 month of the diagnosis of cardiomyopathy revealed evidence of myocarditis in 63, HIV nucleic acid sequences in cardiac myocytes in 58, and active myocarditis in 36. In the 36 patients with active myocarditis, 9 had coexisting viral infections (coxsackievirus group B [$n = 6$], cytomegalovirus [$n = 2$], or Epstein-Barr virus [$n = 1$]).[21]

HIV-related cardiomyopathy often cannot be associated with any specific opportunistic infection. Approximately 40% of patients have not experienced an opportunistic infection before the onset of cardiac symptoms.[24] Infections present are not necessarily related to cardiomyopathy. HIV-infected children had a cumulative Epstein-Barr virus infection rate similar to that of HIV-uninfected children.[25] Alternatively, cytomegalovirus infection was similar in HIV-infected and uninfected infants. At 6 months of age, HIV-infected children had higher rates of cytomegalovirus infection, and rates continued to increase and diverge from those in uninfected children through 4 years of age.[26] Those children who acquired cytomegalovirus infection within 18 months of life had a significantly higher rate of cardiomyopathy than those with HIV without cytomegalovirus infection.

Autopsy and biopsy results have revealed only scant and patchy inflammatory cell infiltrates in the myocardium.[27] HIV virions appear to infect myocardiocytes in patchy distributions. The infected cells, however, are not surrounded by an inflammatory response, and no clear association has been made between the infection and functional disability.

Myocardial biopsy may be clinically helpful, as lymphocytic infiltrates suggesting myocarditis or treatable opportunistic infections would permit aggressive therapy of an underlying pathogen or consideration of intravenous immunoglobulin therapy.

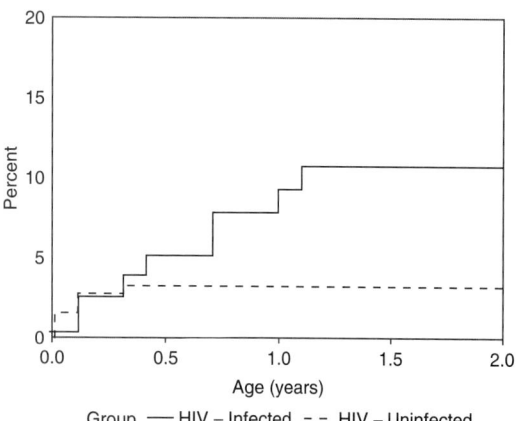

Figure 17–4. Kaplan-Meier cumulative incidence of an initial episode of decreased left ventricular fractional shortening (≤25%) in HIV-infected and noninfected children over the first 2 years of life ($P = .01$; log-rank test). (From Starc TJ, Lipshultz SE, Kaplan S, et al: Cardiac complications in children with human immunodeficiency virus infection. Pediatrics 1999;104:e14).

HIV-ASSOCIATED VASCULAR DISEASE

Vasculitis has been described in up to 23% of 148 HIV-infected individuals by muscle, peripheral nerve, or skin biopsy.[28] Clear evidence of increased vascular disease in children with HIV is available. Suspicious clinical signs include fever of unknown origin, unexplained multisystem disease, unexplained arthritis or myositis, glomerulonephritis, peripheral neuropathy (especially mononeuritis multiplex) or unexplained gastrointestinal, cardiac, or central nervous system ischemia.

The most common reported types of vasculitis in HIV-infected patients include degenerative lesions such as arteriopathy, inflammatory lesions, and atherosclerotic lesions. The most devastating effects of HIV-associated vascular disease occur due to involvement of the coronary or cerebral vessels. Inflammatory arterial lesions have been described on pathologic examination of brains of children with encephalopathy.[29] Fibrocalcific lesions in the intima and media resulting in luminal narrowing of small and medium arterioles have been described in the heart and other organs in HIV-infected children.[29]

Aneurysmal coronary dilation has been described in at least three HIV-infected children and has been associated with myocardial infarction.[30,31] Cerebral aneurysms have been associated with stroke and have been reported in seven HIV-infected children.[31] These reported aneurysms have not been associated with infectious causes. Aneurysms in the abdominal aorta, aortic arch, and other arteries are well described and often linked with infectious agents such as *Mycobacterium tuberculosis*, *Staphylococcus*, and *Salmonella*.

Systemic necrotizing vasculitis, hypersensitivity vasculitis, Henoch-Schönlein purpura, lymphomatoid granulomatosis, and primary central nervous system angiitis are the most commonly reported inflammatory lesions diagnosed in HIV-infected patients. Often a specific type of vasculitis cannot be diagnosed. Antibiotic and antiretroviral agents, including penicillin, trimethoprim-sulfamethoxazole, and amoxicillin, are the most commonly implicated agents in cases of vasculitis, especially drug hypersensitivity vasculitis, among AIDS patients. Other drugs commonly implicated include griseofulvin and amitriptyline.

Accelerated atherosclerosis and premature cerebrovascular disease have been described in autopsy studies of patients without traditional coronary atherosclerotic risk factors.[32] Both protease inhibitor therapy and chronic inflammatory states have also been associated with these findings.

Mild and nonprogressive aortic root dilation was seen by echocardiographic evaluation in children 2 to 9 years of age with vertically transmitted HIV infection (unpublished data from the P²C² HIV study). Long-term follow-up of aortic root size on sequential echocardiograms will be important as life expectancy increases in patients with chronic HIV infection. If further dilation of the root occurs on sequential examinations, transesophageal echocardiography or computer tomography should be performed to evaluate the ascending aorta and aortic arch.

The pathogenesis of HIV-associated vascular disease is unclear, and theories include a role of HIV itself, drug reactions, and other infectious causes. HIV antigen deposited in the vessel wall in a case of leukocytoclastic vasculitis suggests the direct role of HIV in the pathogenesis of the vasculitis.[33]

Aggressive treatment approaches involve immunosuppressive therapy, a search for related infectious causes, and antimicrobial prophylaxis.

AUTONOMIC DYSFUNCTION

Syncope and presyncope, inappropriate hypotensive or hypertensive responses, diminished sweating, diarrhea, and bladder dysfunction are clinical signs of autonomic dysfunction in HIV-infected individuals. Formal testing has shown that heart rate variability, Valsalva ratio, cold pressor testing, and hemodynamic responses to isometric exercise, tilt table testing, and standing showed that autonomic dysfunction occurred in patients with AIDS-related complex and was pronounced in patients with AIDS. Patients with HIV-associated encephalopathy or neuropathy had the most pronounced abnormalities.[34]

Hemodynamic abnormalities, dysrhythmias, unexplained arrest, and sudden death are common in observed children with HIV, especially when acute deterioration, intervention, or encephalopathy is present.[30,35,36] An interesting observation is that enhancement of the autonomic nervous system in some patients is the key abnormality on formal testing where an exaggerated response may be detrimental.[34]

The cause of autonomic dysfunction in patients with HIV infection is largely unexplained. Inflammatory changes in cardiac conduction tissue and peripheral nerves have been described in deceased HIV-infected children with autonomic dysfunction.[13,37] Because encephalopathy has been associated with cardiac disease and death in children, a related mechanism of central nervous system and nervous tissue destruction (vasculitis or immune mediated) is hypothesized.[38–40]

DYSRHYTHMIAS AND ELECTROCARDIOGRAPHIC ABNORMALITIES

Electrocardiographic abnormalities are diverse and highly prevalent among HIV-infected children. Frequently observed abnormalities are tachycardia described in 49% to 70% and ventricular hypertrophy in 20% to 30% of HIV-infected children.[13,39,41–43] Tables 17–4 and 17–5 list cross-sectional and longitudinal studies using electrocardiography or Holter monitoring to evaluate pediatric AIDS patients. Key abnormalities are listed. Rhythm disturbances include marked sinus arrhythmia, atrial ectopy, and ventricular arrhythmias.[38,41,43] However, studies described have not been able to control for the prenatal environment and factors such as cocaine exposure, which have been shown to affect the electrocardiogram. These studies do represent a population of children with HIV who would routinely be encountered.

PERICARDIAL DISEASE

Pericardial disease should be suspected in patients with clinical signs of dyspnea out of proportion to pulmonary disease or when cardiomegaly is present on chest radiograph.

A prevalence rate of 16% to 26%[13,43–46] and a 1-year cumulative incidence rate of 0.6%[47] for pericardial effusion in HIV-infected children have been documented.[48] The discrepancy in prevalence and incidence rates likely reflects different stages of HIV infection in patients studied. Pericardial effusions are less frequent in children than in adults and tend to be small and asymptomatic. Cases of pericardial tamponade or effusions related to sudden death have been reported in children.

In a longitudinal study, pericardial effusion occurred in 51% of HIV-infected children but was transient on serial echocardiography in more than half.[16] Effusions are often associated with systemic disease or other cardiac abnormalities, such as

Table 17–4
Cross-Sectional Studies of Electrocardiographic Abnormalities in Pediatric Patients with HIV Infection

STUDY	PATIENTS, n	PATIENT CHARACTERISTICS	MAJOR FINDINGS
Kavanaugh-McHugh et al[43]	88	Children with symptomatic HIV infection	Electrocardiographic abnormalities, 51% Ventricular hypertrophy, 17% ST/T changes, 33% Conduction abnormalities, 48% Atrial enlargement, 5% Rhythm disturbances, 24%
Lipshultz et al[13]	30	3 mo–22.5 years 11 HIV+; 20 HIV+ with symptoms	Sinus tachycardia, 77% (23/30) Left ventricular hypertrophy, 37% (11/30) Right ventricular hypertrophy, 13% (4/30) ST/T changes, 50% (15/30) Atrial ectopy, 40% (12/30) Ventricular ectopy, 30% (9/30) Normal, 7% (2/30)
Issenberg et al[44]	22	6 mo–6 years	Electrocardiographic abnormalities, 55% (12/22) Ventricular hypertrophy, 36% (8/22) Right bundle branch block, 5% (1/22)

Table 17-5
Longitudinal Studies of Electrocardiographic Abnormalities in Pediatric Patients with HIV Infection

STUDY	PATIENTS, n	PATIENT CHARACTERISTICS	FOLLOW-UP	MAJOR FINDINGS
Saidi et al[65]	205; 463	HIV-1–infected older than 28 days; HIV-1–uninfected enrolled during pregnancy or during the first 28 days	5 years	Incidence of second-degree atrioventricular block, supraventricular or ventricular tachycardia, 13% (27/205)
Grenier et al[42]	95	4 mo–12 years	10 mo (mean) Range 1–24 mo (retrospective)	30% (24/80) with AIDS had ECG changes; Ventricular hypertrophy, 21% (20/95); Right bundle branch block: atrial flutter, prolonged QTc, frequent VPBs, 1% (1/95); Nonspecific ST/T changes, 6% (6/95)
Luginbuhl et al[38]	81	Mean age at entry, 1.5 years; 8 HIV+; 38 ARC; 35 AIDS	2.1 years (mean) (retrospective)	Tachycardia, 64% (52/81); Bradycardia, 11% (9/81); Atrial ectopy, 25% (20/81); Premature junctional beats, 4% (3/81); VPBs, 15% (12/81); Marked sinus arrhythmia, 17% (14/81); Ventricular tachycardia, 2% (2/81); Ventricular fibrillation, 1% (1/81)
Tripp et al[81]	129	All ages		Myocardial dysfunction, or ECG changes 14% (18/129); 19% (17/90) surviving to 3 years
DeSimone et al[88]	20	All vertically infected	3.7 years (mean) (prospective)	ST/T changes, 20% (4/20)
Lipshultz et al[35]	105	All with AIDS		Tachycardia, 47% (49/105); Bradycardia, 7% (7/105); Marked sinus arrhythmia, 15% (16/105), including 30% of patients with unexpected arrest; High-grade ventricular ectopy, 5% (5/105), including 30% of patients with unexpected arrest
Kavanaugh-McHugh et al[43]	88	All symptomatic with HIV	Prospective	Rhythm disturbances, 24% (21/88); Conduction abnormalities, 48% (42/88); Ventricular hypertrophy, 17% (15/88); ST/T changes, 33% (29/88); Atrial enlargement, 5% (4/88)

ECG, electrocardiographic; VPBs, ventricular premature beats.

malignancy. Infection is a common cause of effusion, and the infectious agents reported in children include *Staphylococcus aureus, Mycobacterium avium-intracellulare, Staphylococcus epidermidis, Pseudomonas aeruginosa, Enterococcus,* and cytomegalovirus. *Mycobacterium tuberculosis* as a cause of pericardial effusion has been widely described in adults but has not yet been reported in children with HIV infection.

Pericardial effusion does occur more frequently late in HIV disease and may be part of a generalized serous effusive process involving pleural and peritoneal surfaces as well. Enhanced cytokine production in the later stages of HIV disease may be causative. Other causes include uremia from HIV-associated nephropathy or drug-induced nephrotoxicity.

Pericardiocentesis had a diagnostic yield of 36% and often supplied unexpected diagnostic information with therapeutic implications.[49] If pericardiocentesis is performed for diagnostic or therapeutic purposes, aspirate should be sent for bacterial, fungal, protozoal, and viral culture examination and for cytology.

In adults, fibrinous pericarditis is also well described. Pericardial disease in adults is clearly associated with an increased mortality rate, even when effusion is transient.[50,51] Similar evaluation of children with pericardial disease has not been performed.

CARDIOVASCULAR TUMORS

Malignancy, particularly B cell lymphoma, is common in late-stage HIV disease. Cardiac malignancy is generally metastatic in origin. Primary cardiac malignancy is rare and is generally due to lymphoma. Cardiac lymphoma is highly symptomatic and rapidly progressive; patients present with dyspnea, right-sided heart failure, myocardial infarction, tachyarrhythmias, conduction abnormalities, or superior vena cava syndrome.[52] Systemic multiagent chemotherapy with or without concomitant radiation or surgery has been beneficial in some patients, but overall the prognosis is grave.

Kaposi sarcoma involving the heart was described with a 1% incidence in a series of 565 autopsies of patients with AIDS.[53] Kaposi sarcoma is associated with human herpesvirus type 8 and chiefly affects adult male homosexual individuals infected with HIV. The tumor is an endothelial cell neoplasm with a predilection in the heart for subpericardial fat around the epicardial coronary arteries. More recent studies show no invasion of the epicardial coronary arteries, possibly due to effects of antiretroviral or chemotherapeutic therapies. Kaposi sarcoma affecting the heart is generally asymptomatic and an incidental finding at autopsy.

Leiomyosarcoma, associated with Epstein-Barr virus, is a rare, malignant tumor of smooth muscle origin with an increased incidence in HIV-infected children. Leiomyosarcomas often involve the arterial wall and are chiefly noncardiac.[54,55] An intracardiac mass in late-stage HIV disease is associated with a uniformly poor prognosis.

PULMONARY HYPERTENSION

Pulmonary hypertension in patients with HIV disease has been described as both a primary and a secondary process. More commonly, pulmonary hypertension results from recurrent bronchopulmonary infections, obliterative vascular disease of the lung from intravenous drug use, left ventricular dysfunction, or thromboembolic disease. Pulmonary hypertension found on screening echocardiographic examination or right heart catheterization should prompt further investigation for treatable pulmonary infection.

Primary pulmonary hypertension has been described in a disproportionate number of HIV-infected adults and children, primarily in case reports. In one prospective study of HIV-infected individuals with pulmonary symptoms, 6 of 70 (8%) were diagnosed with primary pulmonary hypertension.[56] Primary pulmonary hypertension occurs in about 0.5% of hospitalized adults with AIDS.[57] Autopsy and biopsy specimens suggest injury due to mediator release elsewhere in the body rather than direct HIV endothelial infection in lung arterioles.[58,59]

HIV-infected patients with pulmonary hypertension presented earlier and with less functional disability than non–HIV-infected patients with pulmonary hypertension in one study.[60] Prognosis and response to therapy were similar to prognosis and response in non–HIV-infected patients with pulmonary hypertension. Ten of the 20 HIV-infected patients died within 1 year after the diagnosis of pulmonary hypertension. Of the 10 who died, 8 had no illness related to HIV infection, and CD4+ count was unrelated to survival.

Therapy includes anticoagulation, if appropriate in consideration of comorbidities, and vasodilator agents as tolerated. Vasodilator agents, including prostacyclin, should be started under close monitoring using a Swan-Ganz catheter to guide titration of therapy.

Diagnosis, Monitoring, and Therapy of Cardiovascular Complications in HIV-Infected Children

Cardiac disease in HIV-infected children is often asymptomatic or masked by systemic illness in which the signs and symptoms are attributed to another cause.[13,61,62] A thorough cardiovascular history and physical examination should be conducted in all HIV-infected patients to differentiate symptomatic from asymptomatic patients. Worrisome symptoms in pediatric patients include syncope, chest pain, changes in feeding patterns, diaphoresis with activity or feeding, growth failure, respiratory difficulties, evidence of poor perfusion, peripheral edema, diastolic filling sounds or an S3 gallop on examination, and hepatomegaly.[48]

Laboratory, echocardiographic, and electrocardiographic assessments are often useful in further defining and evaluating patients for cardiovascular disease. Laboratory evaluation may include assessment of selenium and carnitine levels in a search for reversible causes of left ventricular dysfunction. Serum markers of cardiac muscle damage are relatively limited, whereas troponin assays are more sensitive and specific for myocardial injury than creatine phosphokinase muscle-brain isoenzyme in infants and children. Markers are useful in the setting of left ventricular dysfunction.

Echocardiography provides a quantitative assessment of cardiac structure and function and provides specific information for clinical care. Assessment of left ventricular dimensions and fractional shortening and parameters of diastolic function and for structural abnormalities, vegetations, thrombi, intracardiac masses, pericardial thickening or effusion, and coronary dilation or aneurysms is noninvasively performed with echocardiography. Echocardiography is more sensitive and specific for detecting cardiac disease in HIV-infected children than either chest radiograph or electrocardiography.[63]

Electrocardiography may reveal abnormalities of heart rhythm or conduction, chamber enlargement, ischemia, or nonspecific ST and T-wave changes. A prospective study of HIV-infected individuals with normal echocardiograms and abnormal electrocardiograms showed that 14% developed new echocardiographic abnormalities in a 22-month follow-up period, suggesting earlier manifestations of cardiovascular disease by electrocardiograms.[64] Holter monitoring and cardiac event recorders are useful in the evaluation of cardiac symptoms or abnormalities on electrocardiograms or echocardiograph. Identified arrhythmias tend to be benign in HIV-infected children; therefore, routine Holter monitoring is not indicated.[65]

Asymptomatic patients should undergo echocardiography as a baseline, then yearly, and electrocardiography every 2 years.[48] Patients with serious noncardiac illness should undergo echocardiography and electrocardiography as a baseline, then echocardiography every 8 months, and electrocardiography every year.[48] Patients with cardiac symptoms should have a formal cardiac assessment, including baseline echocardiography, electrocardiography, and Holter monitoring, and should begin directed therapy.[48]

Pericardiocentesis may be beneficial for both diagnostic and therapeutic purposes in patients with pericardial effusion. Patients with pericardial effusion and clinical signs of tamponade such as elevated jugular venous pressure, dyspnea, hypotension, tachycardia, and pulsus paradoxus or echocardiographic signs of tamponade such as valvular inflow respiratory variation by continuous wave Doppler, septal bounce, right ventricular diastolic collapse, and a large effusion should undergo pericardiocentesis for both diagnostic and therapeutic purposes.

Patients with evidence of pericardial effusion without tamponade physiology should be evaluated for treatable opportunistic infections and for evidence of malignancy. Highly active antiretroviral therapy should be considered if not already instituted. Repeat echocardiography is recommended after 1 month unless clinical symptoms of tamponade develop in the interim.

Endomyocardial biopsy may be clinically helpful in the evaluation of left ventricular dysfunction, as it may reveal lymphocytic infiltrates suggesting myocarditis or treatable opportunistic infections (by special stains). Diagnosis permits aggressive therapy of a specific underlying pathogen.

In patients with left ventricular dysfunction, serum troponin assays may be helpful and elevations should stimulate consideration of cardiac catheterization or endomyocardial biopsy or both. Myocarditis proven by biopsy should prompt consideration of therapy with intravenous immunoglobulin. Cytomegalovirus inclusions on the biopsy specimen warrant antiviral therapy, and abnormal mitochondria may encourage consideration of a "drug holiday" from zidovudine or other potentially cardiotoxic agents. Repeat ultrasonographic examination after 2 weeks of therapy should be performed to allow a more aggressive approach if left ventricular dysfunction persists or worsens, and to encourage continued therapy if improvement has occurred.[48]

Monthly immunoglobulin infusions in HIV-infected pediatric patients have been associated with minimized left ventricular dysfunction, an increase in left ventricular wall thickness, and a reduction in peak left ventricular wall stress on echocardiogram, suggesting that both impaired myocardial growth and left ventricular dysfunction may be immunologically mediated.[66] The apparent efficacy of immunoglobulin therapy may be the result of immunoglobulins removing cardiac autoantibodies or dampening the secretion or effects of cytokines and cellular growth factors. Immunomodulatory therapy may be helpful in special circumstances or in children with declining left ventricular function.

Patients should be evaluated for nutritional status. If deficiencies are found, they should receive supplements. Supplementation with selenium, carnitine, multivitamins, or all three may be helpful, especially in anorexic patients or in those with wasting or diarrhea syndromes. Other therapy of left ventricular systolic dysfunction is symptomatic and includes diuretics, digoxin, and angiotensin-converting enzyme inhibitors as tolerated. Angiotensin-converting enzyme inhibitors may be difficult for HIV-infected patients to tolerate because of low systemic vascular resistance, and mortality benefits are not clear.

Complications of Therapy for HIV

The increased use of potent antiretroviral medications and the concept of highly active antiretroviral therapy, which generally combines three or more agents and usually includes a protease inhibitor, has clearly increased the quality of life and life span of HIV-infected patients.[67-70] Protease inhibitors, particularly when used with combination therapy or highly active antiretroviral therapy, are associated with lipodystrophy, fat wasting and redistribution, and metabolic abnormalities. Protease inhibitors have been associated with hyperlipidemia, body fat redistribution, insulin resistance, and the development of increased atherosclerotic risk profiles.[71-73] HIV-infected patients treated with protease inhibitors have reported substantial decreases in total body fat with peripheral lipodystrophy (fat wasting of the face, limbs, and buttocks) and relative conservation or enhancement of central adiposity (truncal obesity, breast enlargement, and "buffalo hump") in comparison with patients who have not received protease inhibitors.[73] Lipid alterations associated with protease inhibitors include higher triglyceride, total cholesterol, insulin, lipoprotein(a), and C-peptide levels and lower high-density lipoprotein levels (all promoting an atherogenic profile).[71-73] Insulin requirements in insulin-dependent diabetic patients notably increase 70% on average with the addition of a protease inhibitor.

Lipid abnormalities were found to be protease inhibitor specific in patients on protease inhibitors compared with their own baseline (pretreatment) nonfasting serum values.[72] Protease inhibitor therapy increased lipoprotein(a) by 48% in patients with pretreatment elevated values (>20 mg/dL). In some cases, switching protease inhibitors may reverse both elevations in triglyceride levels and abnormal fat deposition.

Zidovudine has been implicated in skeletal muscle myopathies.[74,75] In culture, zidovudine causes a dose-dependent destruction of human myotubules.[75] Carnitine deficiency resulting from impaired oxidative metabolism due to mitochondrial dysfunction has also been described by biochemical analysis of muscle biopsy specimens from affected patients.[76]

Cardiac muscle myopathies have been suggested due to mitochondrial abnormalities in cardiac muscle cultured cells treated with zidovudine in vitro.[77] This has not been evident in clinical data. A recent study of a group of children born to HIV-infected mothers found no association between zidovudine exposure in the perinatal period and the presence of left ventricular structural and functional abnormalities through 14 months of age.[78] Rare patients with left ventricular dysfunction, however, have improved with cessation of zidovudine therapy.

Intravenous pentamidine is used for therapy of *Pneumocystis carinii* pneumonia in patients intolerant of trimethoprim-sulfamethoxazole. Cases of torsades de pointes and refractory ventricular tachycardia have been associated with this therapy.[4,48,79] Management recommendations for the use of intravenous pentamidine are outlined in Figure 17–5.

Multiple medication reactions and interactions have occurred during the treatment of HIV infection. Medication reactions are a significant cause of cardiac emergencies in HIV-infected patients. Several cardiovascular effects of drugs used in the therapy of HIV-infected patients include orthostatic hypotension, ventricular tachycardia, or torsades de pointes with erythromycin; orthostatic hypotension or anaphylaxis with trimethoprim-sulfamethoxazole; hypertension or arrhythmia with amphotericin B; reversible cardiac failure with foscarnet; ventricular tachycardia and hypotension with ganciclovir; arrhythmia, cardiomyopathy, or myocardial infarction with vincristine; orthostatic hypotension with interferon-α; hypotension, arrhythmia, or sudden death with interleukin-2; and cardiomyopathy with systemic corticosteroids. Interactions with digoxin and warfarin are common, and individual drug effects should be evaluated before institution or addition of any new therapy.

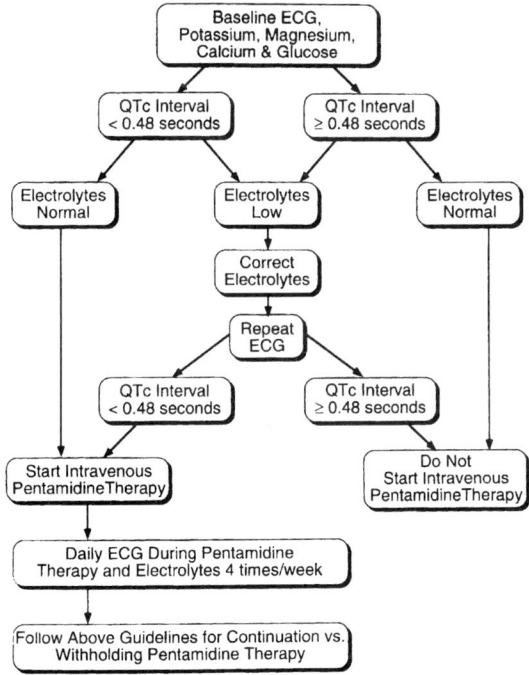

Figure 17–5. Recommendations for HIV-infected patients starting intravenous pentamidine treatment. (From Moorthy LN, Lipshultz SE: Cardiovascular monitoring of HIV-infected patients. In Lipshultz SE (ed): Cardiology in AIDS. New York, Chapman & Hall, 1998, p 345. Data based on Eisenhauer MD, Eliasson AH, Taylor AJ, et al: Incidence of cardiac arrhythmias during intravenous pentamidine therapy in HIV-infected patients. Chest 1994;105:389–395.)

CONCLUSION

As HIV-infected patients survive longer, related cardiovascular manifestations are emerging as a major source of morbidity and mortality. Complications related to the infection itself, the comorbid infections, and current therapies all have an impact on the cardiovascular system. Predictors of cardiovascular morbidity and mortality are discussed in Table 17–6, including low CD4+ T lymphocyte count, encephalopathy, and wasting, which are all markers of late-stage HIV infection. Monitoring and early therapy of cardiovascular risk factors and symptoms related to HIV infection will help to increase longevity and improve quality of life.

REFERENCES

1. Centers for Disease Control and Prevention: Basic Statistics-International Projections Statistics. [Web Page] 1998; http://www.cdc.gov/nchstp/hiv_aids/statsinternat.html.
2. Tovo PA, De Martino M, Gabiano C, et al: Prognostic factors and survival in children with perinatal HIV-1 infection. The Italian Registry for HIV Infections in Children. Lancet 1992;339:1249–1253.
3. Langston C, Cooper E, Goldfarb J, et al: Human immunodeficiency virus–related mortality in infants and children. Data from the Pediatric Pulmonary and Cardiovascular Complications of Vertically Transmitted HIV (P^2C^2) study. Pediatrics 2001; 107:328–338.
4. Connor EM, Sperling RS, Gelber R, et al: Reduction of maternal infant transmission of human immunodeficiency virus type 1 with zidovudine treatment. N Engl J Med 1994; 331:1173–1180.
5. Wilfert CM, Wilson C, Luzuriaga K, Epstein L: Pathogenesis of pediatric human immunodeficiency virus type 1 infection. J Infect Dis 1994; 170:286–292.
6. Al-Attar I, Orav J, Exil V, et al: Predictors of cardiac morbidity and related mortality in children with acquired immune deficiency syndrome [abstract]. Pediatr Res 1995; 37:169A.
7. Kline MW, Paul ME, Bohannon B, et al: Characteristics of children surviving five years of age or older with vertically acquired human immune deficiency infection. Pediatr AIDS HIV Infect 1995; 6:350–353.
8. Shearer WT, Lipshultz SE, Easley KA, et al: Alterations in cardiac and pulmonary function in pediatric rapid human immunodeficiency virus type 1 disease progressors. Pediatrics 2000; 105:1–8.
9. Mofenson L: Epidemiology and determinants of vertical HIV transmission. Semin Pediatr Infect Dis 1994; 5:252–265.

10. Hornberger LK, Lipshultz SE, Easley KA, et al: Cardiac structure and function in fetuses of human immunodeficiency virus [abstract]. J Am Coll Cardiol 1995; 25:30A.
11. Vogel RL, Alboliras ET, McSherry GD, et al: Congenital heart defects in children of human immunodeficiency virus positive mothers [abstract]. Circulation 1988; 78: II17.
12. Lai WW, Lipshultz SE, Easley KA, et al: Prevalence of congenital cardiovascular malformations in children of human immunodeficiency virus infected women. J Am Coll Cardiol 1998; 32:1749–1755.
13. Lipshultz SE, Chanock S, Sander SP, et al: Cardiovascular manifestations of human immunodeficiency virus infection in infants and children. Am J Cardiol 1989; 63:1489–1497.
14. Lipshultz SE, Colan SD, Grenier MA: Left ventricular dysfunction in HIV-infected infants and children. In Lipshultz S (ed): Cardiology in AIDS, 1st ed. New York, Chapman and Hall, 1998, pp 141–152.
15. Lipshultz SE, Easley KA, Orav J, et al: Left ventricular structure and function in children infected with human immunodeficiency virus: The prospective P^2C^2 HIV multicenter study. Circulation 1998; 97:1246–1256.
16. Kavanaugh-McHugh A, Hutton N, Holt E, et al: Echocardiographic abnormalities in pediatric HIV infection: Prevalence and serial changes [abstract]. Pediatr Res 1992; 31:166A.
17. Lipshultz SE: Pediatric Pulmonary and Cardiovascular Complications of Vertically Transmitted HIV Infection study group. Progressive cardiac dysfunction in HIV-infected children [abstract]. Proc Int Conf AIDS 1993; 9:48.
18. Lipshultz SE, Easley KA, Orav EJ, et al: Cardiac dysfunction and mortality in HIV-infected children. The prospective P^2C^2 HIV multicenter study. Circulation 2000, 102:1542–1548.
19. Starc T, Lipshultz SE, Kaplan S: Cardiac complications in children with human immunodeficiency virus infection. Pediatrics 1999; 104:1–9.
20. Hoffman MA, Lipshultz SE, Miller TL: Malnutrition and cardiac abnormalities in the HIV-infected patient. In Miller TL (ed): Nutritional Aspects of HIV Infection. New York, Oxford University Press, 1999, pp 137–139.
21. Barbaro G, DiLorenzo G, Grisorio B, Barbarini G: Incidence of dilated cardiomyopathy and detection of HIV in myocardial cells of HIV-positive patients. Gruppo Italiano per lo Studio Cardiologico dei Pazienti Affetti da AIDS. N Engl J Med 1998; 339:1093–1099.
22. Bowles NE, Kearney DL, Ni J, et al: The detection of viral genomes by polymerase chain reaction in the myocardium of pediatric patients with advanced HIV disease. J Am Coll Cardiol 1999; 34:857–865.
23. Acierno LJ: Cardiac complications in acquired immunodeficiency syndrome (AIDS): A review. J Am Coll Cardiol 1989; 13:1144–1154.
24. Herskowitz A, Willoughby SB, Vlahov D, et al: Dilated heart muscle disease associated with HIV infection. Eur Heart J 1995; 16:50–55.
25. Jenson H, McIntosh K, Pitt J, et al: Natural history of primary Epstein-Barr virus infection in children of mothers infected with human immunodeficiency virus type 1. J Infect Dis 1999; 179:1395–1404.
26. Kovacs A, Schluchter M, Easley K, et al: Cytomegalovirus infection and HIV-1 disease progression in infants born to HIV-1-infected women. N Engl J Med 1999; 341:77–84.
27. Herskowitz A: Cardiomyopathy and other symptomatic heart diseases associated with HIV infection. Curr Opin Cardiol 1996; 11:325–331.
28. Gherardi RK, Amiel H, Martin-Mondiere C: The spectrum of vasculitis in human immunodeficiency virus-infected patients: A clinicopathologic evaluation. Arthritis Rheum 1993; 36:1164–1174.
29. Joshi VV, Pawel B, Conner E, et al: Arteriopathy in children with acquired immune deficiency syndrome. Pediatr Pathol 1987; 7:261–275.
30. Bharati S, Lev M: Pathology of the heart in AIDS. Prog Cardiol 1989; 2:261–272.
31. Starc TJ, Joshi VV: Vascular disease in HIV infection. In Lipshultz S (ed): Cardiology in AIDS, 1st ed. New York, Chapman and Hall, 1998, pp 209–222.
32. Paton P, Tabib A, Lorie R, et al: Coronary artery lesions and human immunodeficiency virus infection. Res Virol 1993; 144:225–231.
33. Potashner W, Patterson B, Karasik A, et al: Leukocytoclastic vasculitis with HIV infection [letter]. J Rheumatol 1990; 17:1104–1107.
34. Freeman R, Roberts MS, Friedman LS, Broadbridge C: Autonomic function and human immunodeficiency virus infection. Neurology 1990; 40:575–580.
35. Lipshultz SE, Luginbuhl LM, Saul JP, et al: Dysrhythmias, unexpected arrest and sudden death in pediatric HIV infection [abstract]. Circulation 1991; 84:II-660.
36. Lipshultz SE, Luginbuhl LM, McIntosh K, Orav EJ: Cardiac morbidity and mortality in children with symptomatic HIV infection [abstract]. Circulation 1992; 86:I-362.
37. Bharati S, Lev M: Conduction system in children with acquired immunodeficiency syndrome. Chest 1989; 96:406–413.
38. Luginbuhl LM, Orav EJ, McIntosh K, Lipshultz SE: Cardiac morbidity and related mortality in children with HIV infection. J Am Med Assoc 1993; 269: 2869–2875.
39. Lobato MN, Caldwell B, Ng P, Oxtoby MJ: Encephalopathy in children with perinatally

acquired human immunodeficiency virus infection. J Pediatr 1995; 126:710–715.
40. Villa A, Cruccu V, Foresti V, et al: HIV-related functional involvement of autonomic nervous system. Acta Neurol 1990; 12:14–18.
41. Lipshultz SE, Orav EJ, Sanders SP, et al: Cardiac structure and function in children with human immunodeficiency virus infection treated with zidovudine. N Engl J Med 1992; 327:1260–1265.
42. Grenier MA, Karr SS, Rakusan TA, Martin GR: Cardiac disease in children with HIV: Relationship of cardiac disease to HIV symptomatology. Pediatr AIDS HIV Infect Fetus Adolesc 1994; 5:174–178.
43. Kavanaugh-McHugh AL, Ruff AJ, Rowe SA, et al: Cardiac abnormalities in a multicenter interventional study of children with symptomatic HIV infection. Pediatr Res 1991; 29:176A.
44. Issenberg HJ, Charytan M, Rubinstein A: Cardiac involvement in children with acquired immune deficiency [abstract]. Am Heart J 1985; 110:710.
45. Sherron P, Pickoff AS, Ferrer PL, et al: Echocardiographic evaluation of myocardial function in pediatric AIDS patients [abstract]. Am Heart J 1985; 110:710.
46. Mast HL, Haller JO, Schiller MS, Anderson VM: Pericardial effusion and its relationship to cardiac disease in children with acquired immunodeficiency syndrome. Pediatr Radiol 1992; 22:548–551.
47. Starc TJ, Lipshultz SE, Easley K, et al: Cardiac complications in HIV infected children: The NHLBI P^2C^2 study [abstract]. Pediatr Res 1995; 37:189.
48. Moorthy LN, Lipshultz SE: Cardiovascular monitoring of HIV infected patients. In Lipshultz S (ed): Cardiology in AIDS. New York, Chapman & Hall, 1998, pp 345–384.
49. Hsia J, Ross AM: Pericardial effusion and pericardiocentesis in human immunodeficiency virus infection. Am J Cardiol 1994; 74:94–96.
50. Blanchard DG, Hagenhoff C, Chow LC, et al: Reversibility of cardiac abnormalities in human immunodeficiency virus (HIV)-infected individuals: A serial echocardiographic study. J Am Coll Cardiol 1991; 17:1270–1276.
51. Heidenreich P, Eisenberg M, Kee L, et al: Pericardial effusion in AIDS. Circulation 1995; 92:3229–3234.
52. Jenson HB, Pollock BH: Cardiac cancers in HIV-infected patients. In Lipshultz S (ed): Cardiology in AIDS. New York, Chapman & Hall, 1998, pp 255–263.
53. Klatt EC, Nichols L, Noguchi TT: Evolving trends revealed by autopsies of patients with the acquired immunodeficiency syndrome: 565 autopsies in adults with the acquired immune deficiency syndrome, Los Angeles, Calif, 1982–1993. Arch Pathol Lab Med 1994; 118:884–890.
54. Chadwick EG, Connor EJ, Hanson IC, et al: Tumors of smooth muscle origin in HIV-infected children. J Am Med Assoc 1990; 263:3182–3184.

55. McClain KL, Leach CT, Jenson HB, et al: Association of Epstein-Barr virus with leiomyosarcomas in children with AIDS. N Engl J Med 1995; 332:12–18.
56. Speich R, Jenni R, Opravil M, Pfab M, Russi EW: Primary pulmonary hypertension in HIV infection. Chest 1991; 100:1268–1271.
57. Himelman RB, Dohrmann M, Goodman P, et al: Severe pulmonary hypertension and cor pulmonale in the acquired immunodeficiency syndrome. Am J Cardiol 1989; 64:1396–1399.
58. Mette SA, Palevsky HI, Pietra GG, et al: Primary pulmonary hypertension in association with human immunodeficiency virus infection. A possible viral etiology for some forms of hypertensive pulmonary arteriopathy. Am Rev Respir Dis 1992; 145:1196–1200.
59. Coplan NL, Shimony RY, Ioachim HL, et al: Primary pulmonary hypertension associated with human immunodeficiency viral infection. Am J Med 1990; 89:96–99.
60. Petitpretz P, Brenot F, Azarian R, et al: Pulmonary hypertension in patients with human immunodeficiency virus infection: Comparison with primary pulmonary hypertension. Circulation 1994; 89:2722–2727.
61. Herskowitz A, Baughman KL: Effect of HIV infection on the heart. Heart Dis 1994; 24:495–504.
62. Himelman RB, Chung WS, Chernoff DN, et al: Cardiac manifestations of human immunodeficiency virus infection: A two dimensional echocardiographic study. Am Coll Cardiol 1989; 13:1030–1036.
63. Lipshultz SE: Cardiovascular manifestations of pediatric HIV infection. In Pizzo PA, Wilfert CM (eds): Pediatric AIDS: The Challenge of HIV Infection in Infants, Children, and Adolescents, 2nd ed. Baltimore, Williams & Wilkins, 1994, pp 483–511.
64. Hsia J: Cardiovascular consequences of AIDS. In Lipshultz SE (ed): Cardiology and Coexisting Disease. New York, Churchill Livingstone, 1994, pp 349–370.
65. Saidi AS, Moodie DS, Lipshultz SE, et al: Electrocardiography and 24-hour electrocardiographic ambulatory recording (Holter monitor) studies in children infected with human immunodeficiency virus type 1. Pediatr Cardiol 2000; 21:189–196.
66. Lipshultz SE, Orav EJ, Sanders SP, Colan SD: Immunoglobulins and left ventricular structure and function in pediatric HIV infection. Circulation 1995; 92:2220–2225.
67. Mocroft A, Vella S, Benfield TL, et al: Changing patterns of mortality across Europe in patients infected with HIV-1. EuroSIDA Study Group. Lancet 1998; 352:1725–1730.
68. Palella FJ, Delaney KM, Moorman AC, et al: Declining morbidity and mortality among patients with advanced human immunodeficiency virus

infection. HIV Outpatient Study Investigators. N Engl J Med 1998; 338:853–860.
69. Vittinghoff E, Scheer S, O'Malley P, et al: Combination antiretroviral therapy and recent declines in AIDS incidence and mortality. J Infect Dis 1999; 179:717–720.
70. Detels R, Munoz A, McFarlane G, et al: Effectiveness of potent antiretroviral therapy on time to AIDS and death in men with known HIV infection duration. Multicenter AIDS Cohort Study Investigators. J Am Med Assoc 1998; 280:1497–1503.
71. SoRelle R: Vascular and lipid syndromes in selected HIV-infected patients. Circulation 1998; 98: 829–830.
72. Periard D, Telenti A, Sudre P, et al: Atherogenic dyslipidemia in HIV-infected individuals treated with protease inhibitors. The Swiss Cohort Study. Circulation 1999; 100:700–705.
73. Carr A, Samaras K, Burton S, et al: A syndrome of peripheral lipodystrophy, hyperlipidaemia and insulin resistance in patients receiving HIV protease inhibitors. AIDS 1998; 12:51–58.
74. Cupler EJ, Danon MC, Jay C, et al: Early features of zidovudine-associated myopathy: Histopathological findings and clinical correlations. Acta Neuropathol 1995; 90:1–6.
75. Lamperth L, Dalakas MC, Dagani F, et al: Abnormal skeletal and cardiac muscle mitochondria induced by zidovudine (AZT) in human muscle in vitro and in an animal model. Lab Invest 1991; 65:742–751.
76. Wharton JM, Demopoulos PA, Goldschlager N: Torsades de pointes during administration of pentamidine isothionate. Am J Med 1987; 83:571–576.
77. Lewis W, Grupp IL, Grupp G, et al: Cardiac dysfunction occurs in the HIV-1 transgenic mouse treated with zidovudine. Lab Invest 2000; 80:187–197.
78. Lipshultz SE, Easley KA, Orav EJ, et al: Absence of cardiac toxicity of zidovudine in infants. N Engl J Med 2000; 343:759–805.
79. Eisenhauer MD, Eliasson AH, Taylor AJ, et al: Incidence of cardiac arrhythmias during intravenous pentamidine therapy in HIV-infected patients. Chest 1994; 105:389–395.
80. Domanski MJ, Sloas MM, Follmann DA, et al: Effect of zidovudine and didanosine treatment on heart function in children infected with human immunodeficiency virus. J Pediatr 1995; 127:137–146.
81. Tripp ME, McKinney RE, Katz SL: Cardiac complications of human immunodeficiency virus (HIV) infection in children (abstract). Pediatr Res 1993; 33:185A.
82. Mast HL, Haller JO, Schiller MS, Anderson VM: Pericardial effusion and its relationship to cardiac disease in children with acquired immunodeficiency syndrome. Pediatr Radiol 1992; 22:548–551.
83. Nogueira G, Macedo AJ, Paixao A, et al: Cardiovascular morbidity in children with human immunodeficiency virus infection. Acta Medica Portuguesa 1998; 11:1051–1057.
84. Lindvig K, Nielsen TL, Videboek R, Pedersen C: Echocardiographic screening in 24 consecutive AIDS patients. Dan Med Bull 1990; 37:449–451.
85. Haddad Herdy GV, Leite MM, Lopes VG, et al: Cardiac changes in children with AIDS. Arq Bras Cardiol 1997; 68:273–277.
86. Ruga E, Cozzani S, Secchieri S, et al: Cardiac abnormalities and HIV infection: Follow-up of forty-one pediatric patients (abstract). Int Conf AIDS 1993; 9:463.
87. Dollfus C, Bancillon A, Tillous-Borde I, Lasfargues G: Cardiac abnormalities and immunologic status in children with HIV infection treated with zidovudine (abstract). Int Conf AIDS 1993; 9:463.
88. De Simone L, Galli L, Manetti A, et al: Long-term cardiac follow-up in children with perinatal HIV-1 infection (abstract). Int Conf AIDS 1992; 8:B205.

Depression of Blood Cells in HIV-Infected Children and Adolescents

Patrick S. Sullivan, Donna T. Beck, Michael Rosenberg, and Joanna Dobroszycki

All three major blood cell lineages are depressed in persons with HIV infection and progressive HIV disease, leading to anemia, thrombocytopenia, and leukopenia. These conditions occur commonly in HIV-infected children and adults and are associated with poor clinical outcomes: anemia is associated with more rapid progression to AIDS[1]; and anemia,[2–5] thrombocytopenia,[2,6] and leukopenia[7] in HIV-infected persons have been shown to be associated with decreased survival. Thus, understanding the mechanisms of suppression of blood cells by HIV and clinical approaches to the management of these hematologic manifestations is important.

Several general principles are common to the suppression of all three cell lines (Fig. 18–1). First, the occurrence and severity of anemia, thrombocytopenia, and leukopenia are related to the stage of HIV disease, and therapy that decreases viral replication may result in significant improvement in hematologic indices. Second, deficiencies of red blood cells, platelets, and white blood cells have many possible causes, and in many patients deficiencies are the consequence of multiple mechanisms. Third, it is important to systematically identify treatable, underlying causes of deficiencies in blood cell populations and to treat identifiable reversible causes before considering growth factor therapy.

Relatively few studies focus on suppression of blood cell production by HIV in children; however, some data are available from published results of clinical trials. There is a larger body of literature addressing suppression of blood cell production in adults, and in many cases the results of these studies can be reasonably assumed to be pertinent to children.

GENERAL MECHANISMS OF SUPPRESSION OF BLOOD CELL PRODUCTION

A variety of in vitro and in vivo data document that the production of blood cells is vulnerable to suppression at the level of the bone marrow in persons with HIV infection. The role of direct infection of hematopoietic progenitor cells in HIV-related myelosuppression is controversial; however, several lines of evidence suggest that decreased numbers of hematopoietic precursor cells and inhibition of precursor cells may play roles in the pathogenesis of HIV-related anemia, neutropenia, and thrombocytopenia.[8] In general, suppression may occur as a consequence of direct infection of hematopoietic precursor cells[9,10] or of bone marrow stromal and endothelial cells,[11–13] or because of the inhibitory effects of cytokines produced during HIV infection and replication.[14,15] Additionally, suppression of blood cell production may occur because of replacement of bone marrow by malignant cells (myelophthisis), by infection of the marrow with other pathogens, or by administration of myelosuppressive drugs.

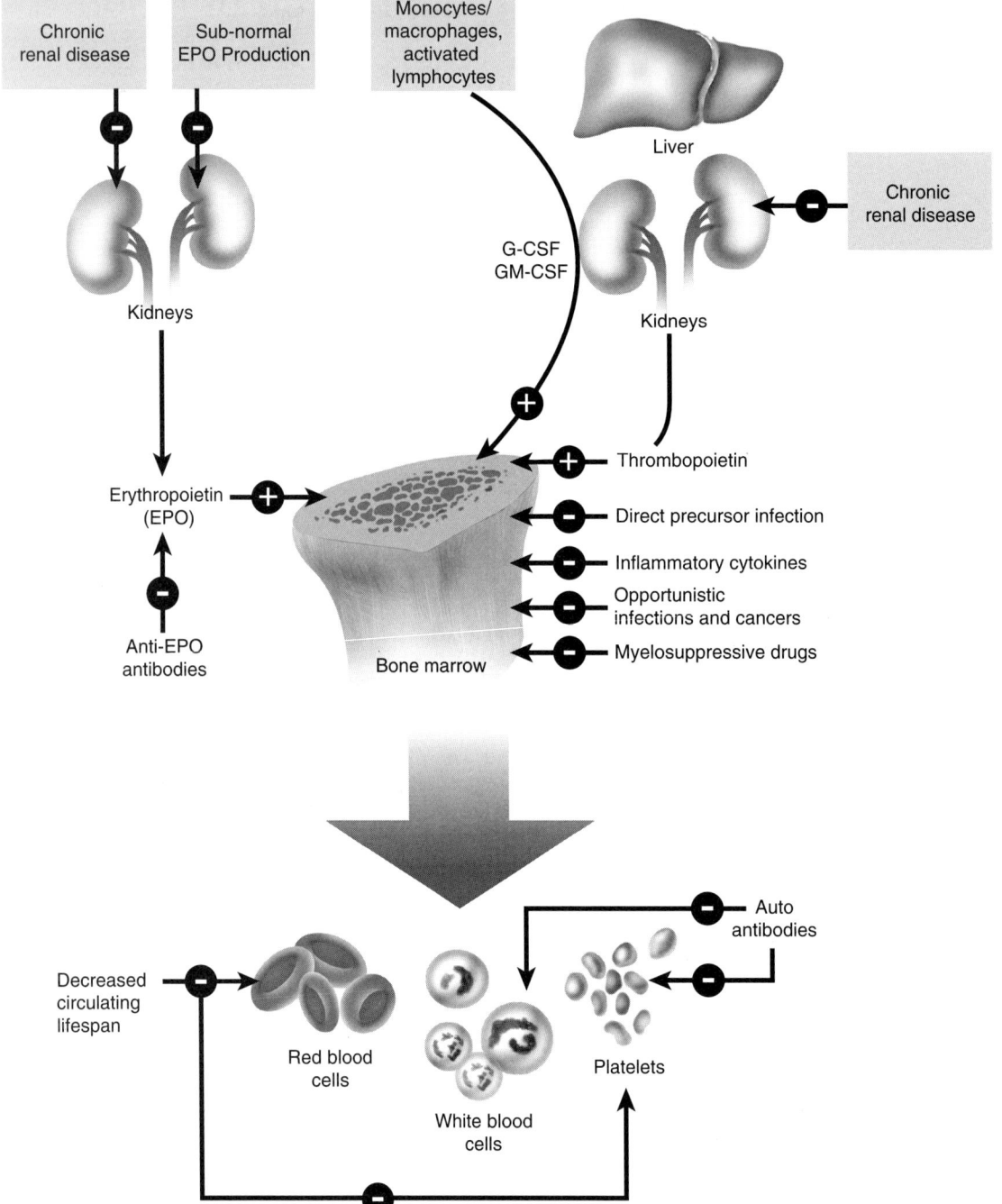

Figure 18–1. Factors positively (+) and negatively (−) affecting blood cell production in children and adolescents with HIV infection.

Direct Infection of Hematopoietic Precursor Cells

HIV has been identified in the bone marrow in megakaryocytes[16–19] and pluripotent CD34+ hematopoietic precursor cells.[9,10] Receptor molecules associated with HIV binding and internalization, including CD4,[9,10,20,21] CXCR-4, and CCR-5,[22,23] have also been identified in progenitor cells, including erythrocytic precursor cells.[21] However, the role of internalized HIV in precursor cells is not clear,[24,25] and studies comparing the isolation of HIV from progenitors in anemic versus nonanemic or thrombocytopenic versus nonthrombocytopenic HIV-infected persons have not been reported.

Cytokine-Mediated Suppression of Hematopoiesis

HIV infection and progressive HIV disease result in the excessive production of inflammatory cytokines, some of which are myelosuppressive.[26] Elevated serum concentrations of tumor necrosis factor-α, interferon-1α,[27,28] and interferon-γ;[29] neopterin;[29] and human transforming growth factor-β[30] have been reported in HIV-infected persons, especially those with advanced HIV disease. Tumor necrosis factor-α and transforming growth factor-β inhibit colony formation of hematopoietic precursor cells in vitro;[15] transforming growth factor-β inhibits CD34+ precursor cells.[14] Neopterin and interferon-γ have been associated with low hemoglobin concentration among persons with HIV infection.[29]

Invasive Bone Marrow Disease

The bone marrow may be affected by many generalized invasive disease processes. Some cancers, including lymphomas, may physically displace bone marrow. Some opportunistic pathogens, including *Mycobacterium avium-intracellulare* complex and *Histoplasma capsulatum*,[31–33] may also infect bone marrow, resulting in myelosuppression. Parvovirus B19 infection has also been associated with marrow infection, pure red blood cell aplasia, and pancytopenia.[34–39]

Prescription of Myelosuppressive Drugs

Many drugs used to treat HIV infection or to prevent opportunistic illnesses are associated with myelosuppression. Notably, ganciclovir[40] and foscarnet[41] can cause generalized bone marrow suppression. Trimethoprim-sulfamethoxazole has been reported to cause acute marrow toxicity, although the incidence of trimethoprim-sulfamethoxazole–associated hematopoietic effects is probably low.[42] Furthermore, drugs may affect specific cell lineages; zidovudine has been known since early clinical trials to suppress red blood cell production in children and adults.[43,44]

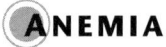

ANEMIA

Occurrence

Anemia is the most common hematologic manifestation of HIV infection, with the exception of CD4+ lymphocytopenia.[45] Studies in children entering clinical trials indicate a cross-sectional prevalence of 23% to 48%,[46,47] and the cumulative prevalence among HIV-infected 12-month-old infants is 37%.[2] Studies in adults have demonstrated that the occurrence of anemia is significantly correlated with stage of HIV disease: in one large observational study,[4] the prevalence of anemia was 28% to 31% among persons with HIV infection and no AIDS diagnosis, 51% to 52% among persons with AIDS diagnosed only by CD4+ T-lymphocyte count less than 200 cells/μL or CD4+ T-lymphocyte percentage less than 14%, and 77% to 87% among persons with AIDS diagnosed by clinical criteria. In another report, the prevalence of anemia in a cohort of 6725 patients with a median CD4+ T-lymphocyte count of 201 cells/mm³ was 59%.[5] Studies of incidence indicate that the strongest predictors of anemia among HIV-infected adults and adolescents are clinical AIDS diagnosis and CD4+ T-lymphocyte count less than 200 cells/mm.[3,4] The incidence of anemia among adults is higher among women and African Americans.[4]

Significance

Few survival studies for HIV-infected children with anemia are available. In one small study, the hazard of death associated with anemia was 2.2 to 3.1 among HIV-infected children younger than 12 months of age.[2] In another, a hematocrit less than 25% was associated with poor clinical outcome.[48] Further studies are needed to evaluate the impact of anemia on survival among children.

More data are published on survival for HIV-infected anemic adults, with results from three large observational studies demonstrating that anemia is associated with shorter survival.[49] In carefully controlled analyses, anemia emerged as a significant predictor of survival, even when controlling for other important prognostic factors. The hazard of death was 1.4 to 3.8 times greater for HIV-infected persons who developed anemia in two cohorts:[3,4] in another analysis, the hazard of death associated with a 1 g/dL decrease in hemoglobin (1.57) was comparable to the risk of a doubling of HIV RNA concentration, or a 50% decrease in CD4+ T-lymphocyte count.[5] Even if anemia is a marker for severe HIV disease, the fact that it has prognostic value in addition to CD4+ T-lymphocyte count and HIV RNA level suggests that it could be a marker for some aspect of disease progression not measured by CD4+ T-lymphocyte count and viral load. Although the results of these observational studies do not prove that anemia is causally related to decreased survival, the consistency among the studies suggests that the relationship is important.

Etiology

There are numerous potential causes of anemia (Table 18–1), and multiple mechanisms of anemia may be important for an individual patient. A thorough laboratory evaluation is important to evaluate whether the anemia is regenerative, whether iron deficiency[50] or vitamin B12 deficiency[51] is present, whether macrocytosis is present, and whether endogenous erythropoietin concentrations are appropriate for the degree of anemia.[52,53] This laboratory evaluation will help the clinician address treatable causes of anemia and evaluate the likelihood of success of erythropoietin therapy.

Zidovudine administration consistently results in decreased hemoglobin concentrations in a significant proportion of HIV-infected patients.[43,44,46,54,55] Among children, up to 67% of patients administered intravenous zidovudine develop anemia,[46] and this effect is dose dependent. Zidovudine-induced anemia is usually associated with macrocytosis,[55] and anemia may be a dose-limiting toxicity for some patients.[56]

Evaluation of anemia should also include consideration of opportunistic illnesses, including disseminated *M. avium-intracellulare* complex and histoplasmosis,[31–33] other bone marrow infections such as Parvovirus B19,[34–38] and myelophthisic disease associated with lymphoma. Bone marrow aspiration and biopsy are important for the diagnostic evaluation of anemia for which no other cause is identified or when multiple cell lineages are affected.[57,58] In addition, the blood smears of HIV-infected children arriving from countries with endemic malaria should be examined for the presence of malaria parasites. Owing to widespread chloroquine resistance, treatment of falciparum malaria should include agents active against these resistant strains, such as quinine and clindamycin.

Nutritional deficiencies may also be important causes of anemia in children. Compared with adults, iron deficiency plays a more important role in anemia pathogenesis for children; in one study of 71 HIV-infected children, 48% had abnormally low basal serum iron concentrations.[50] The high prevalence of iron deficiency may be related to diet or to intestinal malabsorption secondary to gastrointestinal infections or HIV-mediated enteropathy.[50] Children with iron deficiency commonly have microcytic, hypochromic anemia[59]; serum iron, ferritin, transferrin saturation, and marrow iron stores may be low. Ingestion of potentially toxic concentrations of environmental lead among HIV-infected infants and toddlers living in older dwellings containing lead-based paint may also contribute to anemia, both by competing with iron for gastrointestinal uptake and by inhibiting crucial enzymes involved in erythropoiesis. Vitamin B_{12} deficiency in children is associated with megaloblastic anemia and hypersegmented neutrophils,[51,60] whereas in HIV-infected adults, vitamin B_{12} deficiency may result in hyposegmentation of neutrophils.[61]

Increased destruction of red blood cells may be the result of immune-mediated hemolysis. Autoimmune hemolytic anemia may be drug-induced or occur secondary to another infection. Although a high proportion of HIV-infected persons have red blood cell–associated antibodies,[62–65] overt hemolysis is rare,[66] and the presence of cold agglutinins[67] or a

Table 18–1
Causes of Anemia in Children with HIV Infection

Causes of decreased production:
- Cytokine-mediated suppression secondary to TNF, IL-1, TGF-β release, IFN-γ, and neopterin.
- Secondary to bone marrow infection with Parvovirus B19, Mycobacterium avium-intracellulare, fungal infection
- Secondary to direct infection/effects of HIV on marrow progenitor cells
- Iatrogenic (toxicity related to zidovudine, ganciclovir, trimethoprim-sulfamethoxazole, others)
- Myelophthisis (especially associated with lymphoma)
- Maturational problems associated with nutritional deficiencies (folate, B12, iron deficiency)
- Anemia of chronic (HIV) disease

Causes of increased destruction:
- Autoimmune hemolytic anemia
- Acute hemolysis associated with G6-PD deficiency
- Hemolytic uremic syndrome
- Disseminated intravascular coagulation
- Hemoglobinopathy (sickle cell anemia, others)

Causes of increased loss of erythrocytes:
- Bleeding associated with thrombocytopenia
- Gastrointestinal bleeding secondary to GI disease

positive direct antiglobulin test[68] is not usually associated with anemia. However, circulating erythrocyte lifespan may be shortened in persons with HIV infection.[69] Occasional cases of classic autoimmune hemolytic anemia and hemolytic uremic syndrome have been described.[70–72]

One readily preventable cause of hemolysis is drug-induced hemolysis associated with glucose-6-phosphate dehydrogenase deficiency; this metabolic abnormality is more prevalent among African American children and those of Mediterranean descent.[73] For children with glucose-6-phosphate dehydrogenase deficiency, hemolysis may be induced by administration of trimethoprim-sulfamethoxazole,[74] dapsone,[75] or other medications that place oxidative stress on the erythrocyte. Screening children for glucose-6-phosphate dehydrogenase deficiency before prescription of these drugs allows prevention of drug-induced hemolysis. Additionally, infections such as salmonellosis may induce hemolysis in the setting of glucose-6-phosphate dehydrogenase deficiency.[76]

Increased loss of red blood cells may occur secondary to thrombocytopenia or to hemorrhagic colitis associated with cytomegalovirus infection.[77] Occult blood loss into the intestinal lumen should be considered for patients with regenerative anemia.

Anemia may be related to defects in erythropoietin production, half-life, or action. Endogenous erythropoietin concentrations in persons with HIV infection may be lower than expected for the degree of anemia.[52] Autoantibodies to erythropoietin may also decrease the effects of endogenous or exogenous erythropoietin.[78]

The anemia of HIV disease (anemia of chronic disease) is multifactorial and is a manifestation of the cytokine effects, decreased erythrocyte production, and shortened erythrocyte lifespan discussed herein. In the absence of other specific causes, the anemia of chronic disease is the most common clinical cause of anemia in children with HIV infection.

Therapy and Prophylaxis

Underlying nutritional deficiencies and infectious diseases should be identified, treated, and prevented when possible. For example, in a group of 401 adults, prescription of prophylaxis for *M. avium* complex led to decreases in the number of *M. avium* infections and in transfusion requirements.[79] For patients with suspected zidovudine-induced anemia, the clinician may want to consider reducing the zidovudine dose, as zidovudine-associated anemia is dose-dependent,[80] or switching to an alternate antiretroviral regimen with less bone marrow toxicity. In our experience, aggressive treatment of underlying HIV infection with highly active antiretroviral therapy alone is often effective in reversing anemia (M. Rosenberg and J. Dobroszycki, personal observation).

Treatments of symptomatic anemia may include blood transfusion or erythropoietin therapy. Empiric blood transfusions are generally avoided[81] but are appropriate in the setting of severe acute blood loss or hemodynamic instability. Several studies indicate that blood transfusion may be associated with shorter survival among HIV-infected anemic patients.[3,82] Following transfusion, immune activation may result in transient increases in plasma viral load,[83] decreased natural killer cell activity,[84] and decreased lymphocyte response in mixed culture.[85] Although causality is not clear and the need for blood transfusion may be a marker for severe disease, prior receipt of transfusions has been associated with increased incidence of cytomegalovirus disease, bacterial infections, and HIV wasting syndrome.[86] The clinician must weigh the short-term benefits of blood transfusion with the potential long-term detrimental effects of this treatment.

Erythropoietin therapy may be more appropriate for the treatment of chronic or less severe acute anemia.[87] It is indicated for treatment of zidovudine-induced anemia,[88] but patients with anemia of HIV disease may also respond to erythropoietin therapy.[89] Studies from adults indicate that those anemic patients with endogenous erythropoietin concentration of less than 500 mU are more likely to respond to erythropoietin therapy,[90] although clinical response to erythropoietin may occur in patients with high endogenous serum erythropoietin concentrations.[91] A starting dose of 50 U/kg three times per week is recommended,[88] although higher doses may be required in some children.[92] Iron supplementation should be prescribed concurrently because increasing red blood cell production may quickly exhaust iron stores.[93] For some children, even high concentrations of erythropoietin do not stimulate red blood cell production, perhaps because of the presence of antierythropoietin autoantibodies.[78]

THROMBOCYTOPENIA

Occurrence

Thrombocytopenia has long been recognized in association with HIV infection and was defined as a category B clinical condition in the HIV surveillance case definition of 1993.[94] Among children, thrombocytopenia (defined by a platelet count of less than 50,000/mm³) was reported in 8% of 388 children with hemophilia and HIV infection,[95] and 8 of 43 children (19%) in a clinical trial of dideoxyinosine monotherapy.[47] Thrombocytopenia may occur as the sole presenting initial manifestation of HIV infection in children.[96,97]

The cumulative incidence of thrombocytopenia in a group of 75 HIV-infected infants was 19% by 1 year.[2] In the Centers for Disease Control and Prevention (CDC)–sponsored Pediatric Spectrum of HIV Disease study, a clinical cohort study, the 1-year incidence of thrombocytopenia through 1994 was 2.1%, with higher incidence among children with AIDS. In this cohort, incident thrombocytopenia was associated with AIDS, CD4+ class 2 or class 3, splenomegaly, and concurrent anemia (CDC, 1995).

Platelet count has been inversely correlated with viral load in adults.[98,99] Among adults and adolescents, thrombocytopenia has been reported to occur in 9% to 37% of HIV-infected persons (prevalence)[100–103] and has been reported to occur more commonly among persons with more advanced stage of HIV disease,[6,100] among white men,[6,100] among older persons,[6,100] and among injecting drug users.[6,103] In a large observational cohort study,[6] the 1-year incidence of thrombocytopenia among adults was 4.9% and was correlated with stage of HIV disease: the incidence was 1.7% among persons with HIV infection but not AIDS, 3.1% among persons with AIDS defined only by immunologic criteria, and 8.7% among persons with at least one AIDS-defining opportunistic illness.

Significance

Although the degree of thrombocytopenia may be variable in HIV-infected thrombocytopenic persons and clinically evident bleeding usually occurs only when platelet counts drop below 20,000/mm³, several lines of evidence suggest that HIV-related thrombocytopenia is important clinically. In three adult cohorts, 28% to 81% of persons with HIV-related thrombocytopenia had clinical signs of bleeding.[100,101,104] Thrombocytopenia has been associated with increased risk of death among HIV-infected children with hemophilia[95] and HIV-infected children younger than 12 months of age.[2] In a large cohort of adults,[6] 5.4% of persons with an antemortem diagnosis of thrombocytopenia had thrombocytopenia or a bleeding manifestation listed as a contributing cause of death. In the same cohort, thrombocytopenia was associated with a 70% increase in the risk of death in a survival analysis.[6]

Etiology

A list of causes of thrombocytopenia in children with HIV infection is presented in Table 18–2. HIV-related thrombocytopenia in children shares many features with classic immune-mediated thrombocytopenia. The mean circulating platelet half-life in patients with HIV-related thrombocytopenia is lower than in patients without HIV infection or HIV-infected persons with no thrombocytopenia[105,106]; for example, in one study, the circulating platelet half-life was 87 hours in HIV-infected thrombocytopenic patients and 232 hours in control subjects. Sporadic cases of thrombotic thrombocytopenic purpura also occur.[107,108]

A large proportion of children with HIV infection may have elevated platelet-associated immunoglobulins.[59,109] The mechanism of immune destruction of platelets is likely related to antigenic mimicry of platelet antigens by HIV, with the resulting production of antibodies with antiplatelet binding capacity. Specifically, cross-reactivity has been demonstrated between the glycoprotein 120 of HIV and the glycoprotein IIIa of platelets.[110–112] Antibody-coated

Table 18–2
Causes of Thrombocytopenia in Children with HIV Infection

Causes of decreased platelet production
- Cytokine-mediated myelosuppression secondary to TNF, IL-1, and TGF-β release
- Secondary to bone marrow infection with Parvovirus B19 (usually pancytopenia) or other viral infections
- Secondary to direct infection/effects of HIV on megakaryocytes
- Iatrogenic (toxicity related to zidovudine, ganciclovir, trimethoprim-sulfamethoxazole, others)
- Myelophthisis (especially associated with lymphoma)

Causes of shortened platelet circulating half-life
- HIV-related thrombocytopenia (similar to autoimmune thrombocytopenic purpura)
- Disseminated intravascular coagulation
- Thrombotic thrombocytopenic purpura/hemolytic uremic syndrome

platelets are subject to premature removal from circulation by the reticuloendothelial system; the major site of platelet sequestration is usually the spleen.[113] As in classic immune-mediated thrombocytopenia, bone marrow aspirates from patients with HIV-related thrombocytopenia usually reveal evidence of appropriately increased megakaryocyte populations.[114]

Decreased thrombopoietin production does not appear to be a major causative factor in HIV-related thrombocytopenia.[115] Both HIV-infected thrombocytopenic and nonthrombocytopenic patients have serum thrombopoietin concentrations greater than concentrations in HIV-uninfected persons.[116] The elevation of serum thrombopoietin concentration appears to parallel progression of HIV disease.[117] For patients with active liver disease, serum thrombopoietin concentrations may be inappropriately low for the degree of thrombocytopenia.[98]

Direct infection of megakaryocytes with HIV has been demonstrated by *in situ* hybridization,[16,17,118] and the expression of CD4+ receptors by megakaryocytes[119,120] suggests that specific HIV-receptor interactions may mediate the internalization of HIV by megakaryocytes. Megakaryocytes from the marrow of HIV-infected persons also may exhibit structural abnormalities such as denuded megakaryocyte nuclei.[121] Although the significance of direct infection of megakaryocytes by HIV is still unclear, direct suppression of platelet production by this mechanism remains a theoretical cause of thrombocytopenia.[122]

Treatment

Because other infections or cancer can serve as an underlying cause of thrombocytopenia, a thorough evaluation to identify underlying infections and malignancies should be conducted and any identified infection treated. In general, optimizing the antiretroviral treatment regimen may be important to reducing virus load (and therefore antigenic stimulus) for HIV-related thrombocytopenia.[98,123–125] In recent years, we have identified at least six perinatally infected children with chronic HIV-related thrombocytopenia that resolved upon initiation of highly active antiretroviral therapy (M. Rosenberg and J. Dobroszycki, personal observation).

Patients with very low platelet counts or clinically evident bleeding may require other interventions to replace lost platelets or to decrease the rate of platelet destruction. Available interventions include platelet transfusion (reserved for patients with life-threatening bleeding or those undergoing surgery), administration of immunosuppressive doses of corticosteroids,[126–128] splenectomy,[113,129] splenic irradiation,[128] administration of intravenous immunoglobulins,[128,130,131] and administration of anti–red blood cell Rh factor D antibody preparations.[132] In general, these interventions result in improvement in thrombocytopenia in 17% to 58% of patients,[127,128] but in many cases the elevations in platelet counts are not sustained over time.

Administration of corticosteroids seems counterintuitive in patients with significant immunosuppression related to HIV disease, but a study of six children administered short-course prednisone found that there were no detrimental effects attributable to corticosteroid administration.[133] Splenectomy of adults with HIV-related thrombocytopenia and hypersplenism has produced favorable response rates, without an increased incidence of infections during follow-up[113,129]; splenectomy may also have other benefits for HIV-infected patients, such as decreased splenic sequestration of CD4+ T lymphocytes.[134] Splenic irradiation may result in transient increases in platelet count, but long-term results of this therapy have been consistently disappointing.[135–140]

Thrombopoietin has recently been cloned and sequenced and may eventually be available for clinical use in the treatment of patients with thrombocytopenia.[141] It is not clear whether recombinant human thrombopoietin will have a role in the management of HIV-associated thrombocytopenia in children; however, evidence from thrombocytopenic chimpanzees infected with HIV suggests that thrombopoietin therapy to correct platelet counts in thrombocytopenic HIV-infected patients may eventually be possible.[142]

LEUKOPENIA/NEUTROPENIA

Occurrence

The prevalence of leukopenia has been documented in HIV-infected children entering clinical trials; 26% to 38% of study participants had total white blood cell counts of less than 3000 cells/mm³.[46,47] Among adults with HIV infection, 57% to 76% may be leukopenic.[45] In a large clinical cohort,[7] the 1-year incidence of leukopenia (defined as total white blood cell count <2500/mL) among HIV-infected adults was 14%, with a higher incidence among persons with CD4+ T-lymphocyte counts less than 200 cells/mm³ and persons with clinical AIDS. In regression modeling for adults, the factors most strongly associated with leukopenia were low CD4+ T-lymphocyte count, diagnosis of at least one AIDS-defining opportunistic illness, female sex, and prescription of zalcitabine and trimethoprim-sulfamethoxazole.[7]

Leukopenia may be due to lymphocytopenia, neutropenia, or both. Progressive CD4+ lymphocytopenia is the hallmark of HIV infection, and lymphocytopenia is more common among persons with at least one AIDS-defining opportunistic illness diagnosis than among persons without clinical AIDS. Reference ranges for absolute lymphocyte counts and CD4+ T-lymphocyte counts are higher for children than for adults.[143,144]

Significance

Profound neutropenia (absolute neutrophil count <500 cells/mm³) has been associated with increased incidence of bacterial infections,[145] bacterial septicemia[146,147] and an increased risk of infection of implantable ports.[148] Leukopenia,[7] but not neutropenia,[149] has been demonstrated to be an independent predictor of survival by regression analysis, whereas CD4+ lymphocytopenia is clearly associated with increased risk of death.[150] HIV infection may also result in neutrophil dysfunction, including deficiencies in chemotaxis,[151] phagocytosis,[152,153] bacterial killing,[154] and oxidative burst capacity.[155]

Etiologies

Causes of leukopenia include many of the mechanisms of decreased hematopoiesis discussed elsewhere in this chapter (Table 18–3). Of specific importance is the myelosuppressive effect of zidovudine administration. In children, up to 43% of children administered zidovudine may develop neutropenia, and suppression of white blood cell production may be a dose-limiting effect of this drug.[56] Marrow toxicity from other drugs, such as ganciclovir,[40] may also be important iatrogenic causes of decreased white blood cell production.

Antineutrophil antibodies may be observed with low frequency in patients with HIV infection,[156–158] and the prevalence of such antibodies is higher among patients with more advanced stages of HIV disease. However, it is not clear that autoimmune neutropenia is always associated with the presence of antineutrophil antibodies in children.[159]

Table 18–3
Causes of Leukopenia in Children with HIV Infection

Causes of decreased white blood cell production
- Cytokine-mediated myelosuppression secondary to TNF, IL-1, and TGF-β release
- Secondary to bone marrow infection with Parvovirus B19 (usually pancytopenia)
- Secondary to direct infection/effects of HIV on hematopoietic precursor cells
- Other viral infections (e.g., cytomegalovirus)
- Iatrogenic (toxicity related to zidovudine, ganciclovir, trimethoprim-sulfamethoxazole, others)
- Myelophthisis (especially associated with lymphoma)

Causes of decreased white blood cell circulating half-life
- Autoimmune leukopenia
- Disseminated intravascular coagulation

Treatment

In general, optimization of antiretroviral therapy may result in correction of leukopenia without any other intervention. As with other cytopenias, careful evaluation for underlying infectious diseases or cancers that might affect the bone marrow is important, and underlying disease processes should be treated. For patients with profound neutropenia, careful monitoring of body temperature and clinical status are important so that, if fever or other manifestations of infection occur, antibiotic therapy may be instituted promptly.

The use of white blood cell–specific growth factors to promote myelopoiesis has been somewhat controversial. It is well established that the use of granulocyte-macrophage colony stimulating factor (GM-CSF) is effective in reversing severe neutropenia in children[160] and adults.[161–163] The use of GM-CSF has been somewhat limited in the past because of concerns that activation of immune cells could result in increased HIV replication.[164–166] However, data from in vitro and in vivo settings suggest that the use of GM-CSF is not associated with increased HIV RNA level.[167–169] GM-CSF may also have desirable effects in HIV-infected persons beyond stimulation of increased white blood cell numbers. For example, GM-CSF may increase the antiretroviral efficacy of zidovudine and stavudine.[165,170,171] GM-CSF may also be associated with increased numbers of CD34+ precursors in bone marrow[172] and with improved function of monocytes, macrophages, and neutrophils.[173–178]

Granulocyte-colony stimulating factor (G-CSF) has also been shown to improve white blood cell counts in pediatric patients with zidovudine-related neutropenia, allowing these patients to continue to take therapeutic doses of zidovudine.[160] A starting dose of 5 µg/kg/day is recommended,[179] although doses ranging from 1 to 20 µg/kg/day have been used. In adults, administration of G-CSF, but not GM-CSF, has been associated with improved survival among neutropenic HIV-infected persons.[163] Chronic G-CSF therapy appears to be safe and well tolerated, as only one case of disseminated intravascular coagulation has been described in association with its use.[180] G-CSF is used extensively in our pediatric HIV outpatient clinic for the management of drug, infection, and HIV-related neutropenia (M. Rosenberg and J. Dobroszycki, personal communication). The dose required to maintain normal white blood cell counts is variable and must be individualized for each patient.

CONCLUSIONS

Deficiencies in red blood cells, platelets, and white blood cells are common problems for children with HIV infection. Many cases are caused by the direct and indirect effects of HIV infection itself, and other cases are attributable to concurrent infections, side effects of pharmacologic therapy, or immunologic mechanisms. The approach to diagnosis and therapy should be (1) to identify and treat underlying causes; (2) to optimize antiretroviral therapy; and (3) if no improvement results, to consider the use of growth factor therapy or secondary interventions such as intravenous immunoglobulin.

The epidemiology of hematologic manifestations of HIV infection in children is incompletely described, and further attention should be given to studies or analyses of existing data to document the impact of these problems on children with HIV infection. Until such data are available, reasonable extrapolations from studies of adults with HIV infection provide some insight into the problem of depression of blood cells in HIV-infected children.

REFERENCES

1. Morfeldt-Manson L, Bottiger B, Nilsson B, von Stedingk LV: Clinical signs and laboratory markers in predicting progression to AIDS in HIV-1 infected patients. Scand J Infect Dis 1991;23:443–449.
2. Forsyth BW, Andiman WA, O'Connor T: Development of a prognosis-based clinical staging system for infants infected with human immunodeficiency virus. J Pediatr 1996;129:648–655.
3. Moore RD, Keruly JC, Chaisson RE: Anemia and survival in HIV infection. J Acquir Immune Defic Syndr Hum Retrovirol 1998;19:29–33.
4. Sullivan PS, Hanson DL, Chu SY, et al: Epidemiology of anemia in human immunodeficiency virus (HIV)-infected persons: Results from the multistate adult and adolescent spectrum of HIV disease surveillance project. Blood 1998;91:301–308.
5. Mocroft A, Kirk O, Barton SE, et al: Anaemia is an independent predictive marker for clinical prognosis in HIV-infected patients from across Europe. EuroSIDA study group. AIDS 1999;13:943–950.
6. Sullivan PS, Hanson DL, Chu SY, et al: Surveillance for thrombocytopenia in persons infected with HIV: Results from the multistate Adult and Adolescent Spectrum of Disease Project. J Acquir Immune Defic Syndr Hum Retrovirol 1997;14:374–379.
7. Sullivan PS, Chu SY, Jones JL, et al: Epidemiology of hematologic manifestations of HIV infection [Abstract 2222]. Blood 1995;86:559A.
8. Stella CC, Ganser A, Hoelzer D: Defective in vitro growth of the hemopoietic progenitor cells in the acquired immunodeficiency syndrome. J Clin Invest 1987;80:286–293.
9. Carr JM, Ramshaw HS, Li P, Burrell CJ: CD34+ cells and their derivatives contain mRNA for CD4 and human immunodeficiency virus (HIV) co-receptors and are susceptible to infection with M- and T-tropic HIV. J Gen Virol 1998;79:71–75.
10. Zauli G, Furlini G, Vitale M, et al: A subset of human CD34+ hematopoietic progenitors express low levels of CD4, the high-affinity receptor for human immunodeficiency virus-type 1. Blood 1994;84:1896–1905.
11. Bahner I, Kearns K, Coutinho S, et al: Infection of human marrow stroma by human immunodeficiency virus-1 (HIV-1) is both required and sufficient for HIV-1-induced hematopoietic suppression in vitro: Demonstration by gene modification of primary human stroma. Blood 1997;90:1787–1798.
12. Schwartz GN, Kessler SW, Rothwell SW, et al: Inhibitory effects of HIV-1-infected stromal cell layers on the production of myeloid progenitor cells in human long-term bone marrow cultures. Exp Hematol 1994;22:1288–1296.
13. Moses AV, Williams S, Heneveld ML, et al: Human immunodeficiency virus infection of bone marrow endothelium reduces induction of stromal hematopoietic growth factors. Blood 1996;87:919–925.
14. Zauli G, Vitale M, Gibellini D, Capitani S: Inhibition of purified CD34+ hematopoietic progenitor cells by human immunodeficiency virus 1 or gp120 mediated by endogenous transforming growth factor beta 1. J Exp Med 1996;183:99–108.

15. Geissler RG, Ottmann OG, Eder M, et al: Effect of recombinant human transforming growth factor beta and tumor necrosis factor alpha on bone marrow progenitor cells of HIV-infected persons. Ann Hematol 1991;62:151–155.
16. Zucker-Franklin D, Cao YZ: Megakaryocytes of human immunodeficiency virus-infected individuals express viral RNA. Proc Natl Acad Sci U S A 1989;86:5595–5599.
17. Louache F, Bettaieb A, Henri A, et al: Infection of megakaryocytes by human immunodeficiency virus in seropositive patients with immune thrombocytopenic purpura. Blood 1991;78:1697–1705.
18. Voulgaropoulou F, Pontow SE, Ratner L: Productive infection of CD34+ cell-derived megakaryocytes by X4 and R5 HIV-1 isolates. Virology 2000;269:78–85.
19. Sakaguchi M, Sato T, Groopman JE: Human immunodeficiency virus infection of megakaryocytic cells. Blood 1991;77:481–485.
20. Louache F, Debili N, Marandin A, et al: Expression of CD4 by human hematopoietic progenitors. Blood 1994;84:3344–3355.
21. Cleveland RP, Liu YC: CD4 expression by erythroid precursor cells in human bone marrow. Blood 1996;87:2275–2282.
22. Deichmann M, Kronenwett R, Haas R: Expression of the human immunodeficiency virus type-1 coreceptors CXCR-4 (fusin, LESTR) and CKR-5 in CD34+ hematopoietic progenitor cells. Blood 1997;89:3522–3528.
23. Kowalska MA, Ratajczak J, Hoxie J, et al: Megakaryocyte precursors, megakaryocytes and platelets express the HIV co-receptor CXCR4 on their surface: Determination of response to stromal-derived factor-1 by megakaryocytes and platelets. Br J Haematol 1999;104:220–229.
24. Koka PS, Jamieson BD, Brooks DG, Zack JA: Human immunodeficiency virus type 1-induced hematopoietic inhibition is independent of productive infection of progenitor cells in vivo. J Virol 1999;73:9089–9097.
25. Zauli G, Capitani S: HIV-1-related mechanisms of suppression of CD34+ hematopoietic progenitors. Pathobiology 1996;64:53–58.
26. Means RT Jr: Cytokines and anaemia in human immunodeficiency virus infection. Cytokines Cell Mol Ther 1997;3:179–186.
27. Maury CP, Lahdevirta J: Correlation of serum cytokine levels with haematological abnormalities in human immunodeficiency virus infection. J Intern Med 1990;227:253–257.
28. Moldawer LL, Marano MA, Wei H, et al: Cachectin/tumor necrosis factor-alpha alters red blood cell kinetics and induces anemia in vivo. FASEB J 1989;3:1637–1643.
29. Fuchs D, Zangerle R, Denz H, Wachter H: Inhibitory cytokines in patients with anemia of chronic disorders. Ann N Y Acad Sci 1994;718:344–346.
30. Allen JB, Wong HL, Guyre PM, et al: Association of circulating receptor Fc gamma RIII-positive monocytes in AIDS patients with elevated levels of transforming growth factor-beta. J Clin Invest 1991;87:1773–1779.
31. Horsburgh CR Jr: *Mycobacterium avium* complex infection in the acquired immunodeficiency syndrome. N Engl J Med 1991;324:1332–1338.
32. Ellaurie M, Rubinstein A: Elevated tumor necrosis factor-alpha in association with severe anemia in human immunodeficiency virus infection and *Mycobacterium avium intracellulare* infection. Pediatr Hematol Oncol 1995;12:221–230.
33. Kurtin PJ, McKinsey DS, Gupta MR, Driks M: Histoplasmosis in patients with acquired immunodeficiency syndrome: Hematologic and bone marrow manifestations. Am J Clin Pathol 1990;93:367–372.
34. Nigro G, Gattinara GC, Mattia S, et al: Parvovirus-B19-related pancytopenia in children with HIV infection. Lancet 1992;340:115.
35. Koch WC, Massey G, Russell CE, Adler SP: Manifestations and treatment of human Parvovirus B19 infection in immunocompromised patients. J Pediatr 1990;116:355–359.
36. Griffin TC, Squires JE, Timmons CF, Buchanan GR: Chronic human parvovirus B19-induced erythroid hypoplasia as the initial manifestation of human immunodeficiency virus infection. J Pediatr 1991;118:899–901.
37. Frickhofen N, Abkowitz JL, Safford M, et al: Persistent B19 parvovirus infection in patients infected with human immunodeficiency virus type 1 (HIV-1): A treatable cause of anemia in AIDS. Ann Intern Med 1990;113:926–933.
38. Abkowitz JL, Brown KE, Wood RW, et al: Clinical relevance of parvovirus B19 as a cause of anemia in patients with human immunodeficiency virus infection. J Infect Dis 1997;176:269–273.
39. Naides SJ, Howard EJ, Swack NS, et al: Parvovirus B19 infection in human immunodeficiency virus type 1-infected persons failing or intolerant to zidovudine therapy. J Infect Dis 1993;168:101–105.
40. Faulds D, Heel RC: Ganciclovir: A review of its antiviral activity, pharmacokinetic properties and therapeutic efficacy in cytomegalovirus infections. Drugs 1990;39:597–638.
41. Chrisp P, Clissold SP: Foscarnet: A review of its antiviral activity, pharmacokinetic properties and therapeutic use in immunocompromised patients with cytomegalovirus retinitis. Drugs 1991;41:104–129.
42. Keisu M, Wiholm BE, Palmblad J: Trimethoprim-sulphamethoxazole-associated blood dyscrasias. Ten years' experience of the Swedish spontaneous reporting system. J Intern Med 1990;228:353–360.
43. Englund JA, Baker CJ, Raskino C, et al: Zidovudine, didanosine, or both as the initial treatment for symptomatic HIV-infected children. AIDS Clinical Trials Group (ACTG) Study 152 Team. N Engl J Med 1997;336:1704–1712.

44. Richman DD, Fischl MA, Grieco MH, et al: The toxicity of azidothymidine (AZT) in the treatment of patients with AIDS and AIDS-related complex. A double-blind, placebo-controlled trial. N Engl J Med 1987;317:192–197.
45. Perkocha LA, Rodgers GM: Hematologic aspects of human immunodeficiency virus infection: Laboratory and clinical considerations. Am J Hematol 1988;29:94–105.
46. Pizzo PA, Eddy J, Falloon J, et al: Effect of continuous intravenous infusion of zidovudine (AZT) in children with symptomatic HIV infection. N Engl J Med 1988;319:889–896.
47. Butler KM, Husson RN, Balis FM, et al: Dideoxyinosine in children with symptomatic human immunodeficiency virus infection. N Engl J Med 1991;324:137–144.
48. Ellaurie M, Burns ER, Rubinstein A: Hematologic manifestations in pediatric HIV infection: Severe anemia as a prognostic factor. Am J Pediatr Hematol Oncol 1990;12:449–453.
49. Moore RD: Human immunodeficiency virus infection, anemia, and survival. Clin Infect Dis 1999;29:44–49.
50. Castaldo A, Tarallo L, Palomba E, et al: Iron deficiency and intestinal malabsorption in HIV disease. J Pediatr Gastroenterol Nutr 1996;22:359–363.
51. Remacha AF, Riera A, Cadafalch J, Gimferrer E: Vitamin B-12 abnormalities in HIV-infected patients. Eur J Haematol 1991;47:60–64.
52. Spivak JL, Barnes DC, Fuchs E, Quinn TC: Serum immunoreactive erythropoietin in HIV-infected patients. JAMA 1989;261:3104–3107.
53. Camacho J, Poveda F, Zamorano AF, et al: Serum erythropoietin levels in anaemic patients with advanced human immunodeficiency virus infection. Br J Haematol 1992;82:608–614.
54. McKinney RE Jr, Maha MA, Connor EM, et al: A multicenter trial of oral zidovudine in children with advanced human immunodeficiency virus disease. The Protocol 043 Study Group. N Engl J Med 1991;324:1018–1025.
55. Fischl MA, Richman DD, Hansen N, et al: The safety and efficacy of zidovudine (AZT) in the treatment of subjects with mildly symptomatic human immunodeficiency virus type 1 (HIV) infection. A double-blind, placebo-controlled trial: The AIDS Clinical Trials Group. Ann Intern Med 1990;112:727–737.
56. Blanche S, Duliege AM, Navarette MS, et al: Low-dose zidovudine in children with a human immunodeficiency virus type 1 infection acquired in the perinatal period. Pediatrics 1991;88:364–370.
57. Northfelt DW, Mayer A, Kaplan LD, et al: The usefulness of diagnostic bone marrow examination in patients with human immunodeficiency virus (HIV) infection. J Acquir Immune Defic Syndr 1991;4:659–666.
58. Costello C, Rule S, Shanson D, Mir N: Bone-marrow diagnosis of opportunistic infections in HIV disease. AIDS 1992;6:1559–1560.
59. Sandhaus LM, Scudder R: Hematologic and bone marrow abnormalities in pediatric patients with human immunodeficiency virus (HIV) infection. Pediatr Pathol 1989;9:277–288.
60. Remacha AF, Cadafalch J: Cobalamin deficiency in patients infected with the human immunodeficiency virus. Semin Hematol 1999;36:75–87.
61. Burkes RL, Cohen H, Krailo M, et al: Low serum cobalamin levels occur frequently in the acquired immune deficiency syndrome and related disorders. Eur J Haematol 1987;38:141–147.
62. McGinniss MH, Macher AM, Rook AH, Alter HJ: Red cell autoantibodies in patients with acquired immune deficiency syndrome. Transfusion 1986;26:405–409.
63. Toy PT, Reid ME, Burns M: Positive direct antiglobulin test associated with hyperglobulinemia in acquired immunodeficiency syndrome (AIDS). Am J Hematol 1985;19:145–150.
64. Bordin JO, Kerbauy J, Souza-Pinto JC, et al: Quantitation of red cell-bound IgG by an enzyme-linked antiglobulin test in human immunodeficiency virus-infected persons. Transfusion 1992;32:426–429.
65. Bolton-Maggs PH, Rogan PD, Duguid JK, et al: Cold agglutinins in haemophiliac boys infected with HIV. Arch Dis Child 1991;66:732–733.
66. De Angelis V, Biasinutto C, Pradella P, Errante D: Mixed-type auto-immune haemolytic anaemia in a patient with HIV infection. Vox Sang 1995;68:191–194.
67. Ciaffoni S, Luzzati R, Roata C, et al: Presence and significance of cold agglutinins in patients with HIV infection. Haematologica 1992;77:233–236.
68. De Angelis V, Biasinutto C, Pradella P, et al: Clinical significance of positive direct antiglobulin test in patients with HIV infection. Infection 1994;22: 92–95.
69. Hollinger FB, Mouneimne Y, Lahart C, et al: Life span of circulating membrane CD4 inserted into the plasma membranes of autologous red blood cells of HIV-infected subjects. J Acquir Immune Defic Syndr Hum Retrovirol 1995;9:126–132.
70. Telen MJ, Roberts KB, Bartlett JA: HIV-associated autoimmune hemolytic anemia: Report of a case and review of the literature. J Acquir Immune Defic Syndr Hum Retroviral 1990;3:933–937.
71. Rapoport AP, Rowe JM, McMican A: Life-threatening autoimmune hemolytic anemia in a patient with the acquired immune deficiency syndrome. Transfusion 1988;28:190–191.
72. Esforzado N, Poch E, Almirall J, et al: Hemolytic uremic syndrome associated with HIV infection. AIDS 1991;5:1041–1042.
73. Petrakis NL, Wiesenfeld SL, Sams BJ, et al: Prevalence of sickle-cell trait and glucose-6-phosphate dehydrogenase deficiency. N Engl J Med 1970;282:767–770.
74. Allen SD Jr, Wilkerson JL: The importance of glucose-6-phosphate dehydrogenase screening in a urologic practice. J Urol 1972;107:304–305.

75. Todd P, Samaratunga IR, Pembroke A: Screening for glucose-6-phosphate dehydrogenase deficiency prior to dapsone therapy. Clin Exp Dermatol 1994;19:217–218.
76. Constantopoulos A, Economopoulos P, Kandylas J: Fulminant diarrhoea and acute haemolysis due to G.-6-P.D. deficiency in salmonellosis. Lancet 1973;1:1522.
77. Grant HW: Patterns of presentation of human immunodeficiency virus type 1-infected children to the paediatric surgeon. J Pediatr Surg 1999;34:251–254.
78. Sipsas NV, Kokori SI, Ioannidis JP, et al: Circulating autoantibodies to erythropoietin are associated with human immunodeficiency virus type 1-related anemia. J Infect Dis 1999;180:2044–2047.
79. Kravcik S, Toye BW, Fyke K, et al: Impact of *Mycobacterium avium* complex prophylaxis on the incidence of mycobacterial infections and transfusion-requiring anemia in an HIV-positive population. J Acquir Immune Defic Syndr Hum Retrovirol 1996;13:27–32.
80. Fischl MA, Parker CB, Pettinelli C, et al: A randomized controlled trial of a reduced daily dose of zidovudine in patients with the acquired immunodeficiency syndrome. The AIDS Clinical Trials Group. N Engl J Med 1990;323:1009–1014.
81. American College of Physicians: Practice strategies for elective red blood cell transfusion. Ann Intern Med 1992;116:403–406.
82. Vamvakas E, Kaplan HS: Early transfusion and length of survival in acquired immune deficiency syndrome: Experience with a population receiving medical care at a public hospital. Transfusion 1993;33:111–118.
83. Mudido PM, Georges D, Dorazio D, et al: Human immunodeficiency virus type 1 activation after blood transfusion. Transfusion 1996;36:860–865.
84. Kaplan J, Sarnaik S, Gitlin J, Lusher J: Diminished helper/suppressor lymphocyte ratios and natural killer activity in recipients of repeated blood transfusions. Blood 1984;64:308–310.
85. Blumberg N, Triulzi DJ, Heal JM: Transfusion-induced immunomodulation and its clinical consequences. Transfus Med Rev 1990;4:24–35.
86. Sloand E, Kumar P, Klein HG, et al: Transfusion of blood components to persons infected with human immunodeficiency virus type 1: Relationship to opportunistic infection. Transfusion 1994;34:48–53.
87. Henry DH, Beall GN, Benson CA, et al: Recombinant human erythropoietin in the treatment of anemia associated with human immunodeficiency virus (HIV) infection and zidovudine therapy. Overview of four clinical trials. Ann Intern Med 1992;117:739–748.
88. Prescribing information for Epogen epoietin alfa for injection. In Medical Economics editors: Physicians' Desk Reference. Montvale, NJ, Medical Economics Company, 1998.
89. Henry DH, Jemsek JG, Levin AS, et al: Recombinant human erythropoietin and the treatment of anemia in patients with AIDS or advanced ARC not receiving ZDV. J Acquir Immune Defic Syndr 1992;5:847–848.
90. Fischl M, Galpin JE, Levine JD, et al: Recombinant human erythropoietin for patients with AIDS treated with zidovudine. N Engl J Med 1990;322:1488–1493.
91. DaCosta NA, Hultin MB: Effective therapy of human immunodeficiency virus-associated anemia with recombinant human erythropoietin despite high endogenous erythropoietin. Am J Hematol 1991;36:71–72.
92. Mueller BU, Jacobsen F, Jarosinski P, et al: Erythropoietin for zidovudine-associated anemia in children with HIV infection. Pediatric AIDS HIV Infect 1994;5:169–173.
93. Hotta T, Ogawa H, Saito A, Ito A: Iron balance following recombinant human erythropoietin therapy for anemia associated with chronic renal failure. Int J Hematol 1991;54:195–200.
94. Centers for Disease Control and Prevention: 1993 Revised classification system for HIV infection and expanded surveillance case definition for AIDS among adolescents and adults. MMWR Morb Mortal Wkly Rep 1992;41:1–19.
95. Ehmann WC, Rabkin CS, Eyster ME, Goedert JJ: Thrombocytopenia in HIV-infected and uninfected hemophiliacs. Multicenter Hemophilia Cohort study. Am J Hematol 1997;54:296–300.
96. Labrune P, Blanche S, Catherine N, et al: Human immunodeficiency virus-associated thrombocytopenia in infants. Acta Paediatr Scand 1989;78:811–814.
97. Saulsbury FT, Boyle RJ, Wykoff RF, Howard TH: Thrombocytopenia as the presenting manifestation of human T-lymphotropic virus type III infection in infants. J Pediatr 1986;109:30–34.
98. Ciernik IF, Cone RW, Fehr J, Weber R: Impaired liver function and retroviral activity are risk factors contributing to HIV-associated thrombocytopenia. Swiss HIV Cohort Study. AIDS 1999;13:1913–1920.
99. Levy S, Geny A, Partisani M, et al: Correlation between platelet number and viral load in HIV-1 infection. AIDS 1997;11:1399–1400.
100. Sloand EM, Klein HG, Banks SM, et al: Epidemiology of thrombocytopenia in HIV infection. Eur J Haematol 1992;48:168–172.
101. Finazzi G, Mannucci PM, Lazzarin A, et al: Low incidence of bleeding from HIV-related thrombocytopenia in drug addicts and hemophiliacs: Implications for therapeutic strategies. Eur J Haematol 1990;45:82–85.
102. Landonio G, Cirasino L, Prete A, et al: Thrombocytopenia (TP) in HIV infection. Eur J Haematol 1993;50:239–240.
103. Mientjes GH, van Ameijden EJ, Mulder JW, et al: Prevalence of thrombocytopenia in HIV-infected

and non-HIV infected drug users and homosexual men. Br J Haematol 1992;82:615–619.
104. Ragni MV, Miller BJ, Whalen R, Ptachcinski R: Bleeding tendency, platelet function, and pharmacokinetics of ibuprofen and zidovudine in HIV(+) hemophilic men. Am J Hematol 1992;40:176–182.
105. Ballem PJ, Belzberg A, Devine DV, et al: Kinetic studies of the mechanism of thrombocytopenia in patients with human immunodeficiency virus infection. N Engl J Med 1992;327:1779–1784.
106. Wuk V, Kotze HF, Heyns AP: Kinetics of indium-111-labelled platelets in HIV-infected patients with and without associated thrombocytopaenia. Eur J Haematol 1999;62:332–335.
107. Prasad VK, Kim IK, Farrington K, Bussel JB: TTP following ITP in an HIV-positive boy. J Pediatr Hematol Oncol 1996;18:384–386.
108. Jorda M, Rodriguez MM, Reik RA: Thrombotic thrombocytopenic purpura as the cause of death in an HIV-positive child. Pediatr Pathol 1994;14:919–925.
109. Ellaurie M, Burns ER, Rubinstein A: Platelet-associated IgG in pediatric HIV infection. Pediatr Hematol Oncol 1991;8:179–185.
110. Nardi MA, Liu LX, Karpatkin S: GPIIIa-(49–66) is a major pathophysiologically relevant antigenic determinant for anti-platelet GPIIIa of HIV-1-related immunologic thrombocytopenia. Proc Natl Acad Sci U S A 1997;94:7589–7594.
111. Bettaieb A, Oksenhendler E, Duedari N, Bierling P: Cross-reactive antibodies between HIV-gp120 and platelet gpIIIa (CD61) in HIV-related immune thrombocytopenic purpura. Clin Exp Immunol 1996;103:19–23.
112. Najean Y, Rain JD: The mechanism of thrombocytopenia in patients with HIV infection. J Lab Clin Med 1994;123:415–420.
113. Bel-Ali Z, Dufour V, Najean Y: Platelet kinetics in human immunodeficiency virus induced thrombocytopenia. Am J Hematol 1987;26:299–304.
114. Ellaurie M, Burns ER, Bernstein LJ, et al: Thrombocytopenia and human immunodeficiency virus in children. Pediatrics 1988;82:905–908.
115. Cole JL, Marzec UM, Gunthel CJ, et al: Ineffective platelet production in thrombocytopenic human immunodeficiency virus-infected patients. Blood 1998;91:3239–3246.
116. Espanol I, Muniz-Diaz E, Margall N, et al: Serum thrombopoietin levels in thrombocytopenic and non-thrombocytopenic patients with human immunodeficiency virus (HIV-1) infection. Eur J Haematol 1999;63:245–250.
117. Gatanaga H, Hoshikawa N, Tahara T, et al: Serum thrombopoietin levels correlate with disease progression of AIDS. AIDS 1999;13:1590–1591.
118. Monte D, Groux H, Raharinivo B, et al: Productive human immunodeficiency virus-1 infection of megakaryocytic cells is enhanced by tumor necrosis factor-alpha. Blood 1992;79:2670–2679.
119. Kouri YH, Borkowsky W, Nardi M, et al: Human megakaryocytes have a CD4 molecule capable of binding human immunodeficiency virus-1. Blood 1993;81:2664–2670.
120. Basch RS, Kouri YH, Karpatkin S: Expression of CD4 by human megakaryocytes. Proc Natl Acad Sci U S A 1990;87:8085–8089.
121. Zucker-Franklin D, Termin CS, Cooper MC: Structural changes in the megakaryocytes of patients infected with the human immune deficiency virus (HIV-1). Am J Pathol 1989;134:1295–1303.
122. Zauli G, Capitani S: HIV-1-related mechanisms of suppression of CD34+ hematopoietic progenitors. Pathobiology 1996;64:53–58.
123. Arranz Caso JA, Sanchez MC, Garcia TJ: Effect of highly active antiretroviral therapy on thrombocytopenia in patients with HIV infection. N Engl J Med 1999;341:1239–1240.
124. Glatt AE, Anand A: Thrombocytopenia in patients infected with human immunodeficiency virus: Treatment update. Clin Infect Dis 1995;21:415–423.
125. Maness LJ, Blair DC, Newman N, Coyle TE: Elevation of platelet counts associated with indinavir treatment in human immunodeficiency virus-infected patients. Clin Infect Dis 1998;26:207–208.
126. Andersen JC: Response of resistant idiopathic thrombocytopenic purpura to pulsed high-dose dexamethasone therapy. N Engl J Med 1994;330:1560–1564.
127. Oksenhendler E, Bierling P, Farcet JP, et al: Response to therapy in 37 patients with HIV-related thrombocytopenic purpura. Br J Haematol 1987;66:491–495.
128. Rigaud M, Leibovitz E, Quee CS, et al: Thrombocytopenia in children infected with human immunodeficiency virus: Long-term follow-up and therapeutic considerations. J Acquir Immune Defic Syndr 1992;5:450–455.
129. Landonio G, Galli M, Nosari A, et al: HIV-related severe thrombocytopenia in intravenous drug users: Prevalence, response to therapy in a medium-term follow-up, and pathogenetic evaluation. AIDS 1990;4:29–34.
130. Ragni MV, Bontempo FA, Myers DJ, et al: Hemorrhagic sequelae of immune thrombocytopenic purpura in human immunodeficiency virus-infected hemophiliacs. Blood 1990;75:1267–1272.
131. Pollak AN, Janinis J, Green D: Successful intravenous immune globulin therapy for human immunodeficiency virus-associated thrombocytopenia. Arch Intern Med 1988;148:695–697.
132. Bussel JB, Graziano JN, Kimberly RP, et al: Intravenous anti-D treatment of immune thrombocytopenic purpura: Analysis of efficacy, toxicity, and mechanism of effect. Blood 1991;77:1884–1893.
133. Saulsbury FT, Bringelsen KA, Normansell DE: Effects of prednisone on human immunodeficiency virus infection. South Med J 1991;84:431–435.

134. Tunkel AR, Kelsall B, Rein MF, et al: Case report: Increase in CD4 lymphocyte counts after splenectomy in HIV-infected patients. Am J Med Sci 1993;306:105–110.
135. Needleman SW, Sorace J, Poussin-Rosillo H: Low-dose splenic irradiation in the treatment of autoimmune thrombocytopenia in HIV-infected patients. Ann Intern Med 1992;116:310–311.
136. Caulier MT, Darloy F, Rose C, et al: Splenic irradiation for chronic autoimmune thrombocytopenic purpura in patients with contra-indications to splenectomy. Br J Haematol 1995;91:208–211.
137. Blauth J, Fisher S, Henry D, Nichini F: The role of splenic irradiation in treating HIV-associated immune thrombocytopenia. Int J Radiat Oncol Biol Phys 1999;45:457–460.
138. Soum F, Trille JA, Auvergnat JC, et al: Low-dose splenic irradiation in the treatment of immune thrombocytopenia in HIV-infected patients. Int J Radiat Oncol Biol Phys 1998;41:123–126.
139. Leung JT, Kuan R: Splenic irradiation in HIV-related thrombocytopenia. Australas Radiol 1996;40:324–325.
140. Giraud P, Soum F, Daly-Schweitzer N, et al: Low-dose splenic irradiation in human immunodeficiency virus-related immune thrombocytopenia. Int J Radiat Oncol Biol Phys 1996;35:417–418.
141. Kaushansky K: Thrombopoietin. N Engl J Med 1998;339:746–754.
142. Harker LA, Marzec UM, Novembre F, et al: Treatment of thrombocytopenia in chimpanzees infected with human immunodeficiency virus by pegylated recombinant human megakaryocyte growth and development factor. Blood 1998;91:4427–4433.
143. Denny T, Yogev R, Gelman R, et al: Lymphocyte subsets in healthy children during the first 5 years of life. JAMA 1992;267:1484–1488.
144. The European Collaborative Study: Age-related standards for T lymphocyte subsets based on uninfected children born to human immunodeficiency virus 1-infected women. Pediatr Infect Dis J 1992;11:1018–1026.
145. Moore RD, Keruly JC, Chaisson RE: Neutropenia and bacterial infection in acquired immunodeficiency syndrome. Arch Intern Med 1995;155:1965–1970.
146. Keiser P, Higgs E, Smith J: Neutropenia is associated with bacteremia in patients infected with the human immunodeficiency virus. Am J Med Sci 1996;312:118–122.
147. Eng RHK, Yen K, Tecson-Tumang F, et al: Risk of gram-negative bacteremia during neutropenia in patients with AIDS. Infect Dis Clin Pract 1994;3:373–375.
148. Domingo P, Fontanet A, Sanchez F, et al: Morbidity associated with long-term use of totally implantable ports in patients with AIDS. Clin Infect Dis 1999;29:346–351.
149. Hambleton J, Aragon T, Modin G, et al: Outcome for hospitalized patients with fever and neutropenia who are infected with the human immunodeficiency virus. Clin Infect Dis 1995;20:363–371.
150. McNaghten AD, Hanson DL, Jones JL, et al: Effects of antiretroviral therapy and opportunistic illness primary chemoprophylaxis on survival after AIDS diagnosis. Adult/Adolescent Spectrum of Disease Group. AIDS 1999;13:1687–1695.
151. Kuritzkes DR: Neutropenia, neutrophil dysfunction, and bacterial infection in patients with human immunodeficiency virus disease: The role of granulocyte colony-stimulating factor. Clin Infect Dis 2000;30:256–260.
152. Crowe SM, Vardaxis NJ, Kent SJ, et al: HIV infection of monocyte-derived macrophages in vitro reduces phagocytosis of *Candida albicans*. J Leukoc Biol 1994;56:318–327.
153. Biggs BA, Hewish M, Kent S, et al: HIV-1 infection of human macrophages impairs phagocytosis and killing of *Toxoplasma gondii*. J Immunol 1995;154:6132–6139.
154. Roilides E, Mertins S, Eddy J, et al: Impairment of neutrophil chemotactic and bactericidal function in children infected with human immunodeficiency virus type 1 and partial reversal after in vitro exposure to granulocyte-macrophage colony-stimulating factor. J Pediatr 1990;117:531–540.
155. Elbim C, Prevot MH, Bouscarat F, et al: Polymorphonuclear neutrophils from human immunodeficiency virus-infected patients show enhanced activation, diminished fMLP-induced L-selectin shedding, and an impaired oxidative burst after cytokine priming. Blood 1994;84:2759–2766.
156. McCance-Katz EF, Hoecker JL, Vitale NB: Severe neutropenia associated with anti-neutrophil antibody in a patient with acquired immunodeficiency syndrome-related complex. Pediatr Infect Dis J 1987;6:417–418.
157. Riera NE, Galassi N, de la Barrera S, et al: Anti-leukocyte antibodies as a consequence of HIV infection in HIV+ individuals. Immunol Lett 1992;33:99–104.
158. Rubinstein DB, Farrington GK, O'Donnell C, et al: Autoantibodies to leukocyte alphaMbeta2 integrin glycoproteins in HIV infection. Clin Immunol 1999;90:352–359.
159. Weinberg GA, Gigliotti F, Stroncek DF, et al: Lack of relation of granulocyte antibodies (antineutrophil antibodies) to neutropenia in children with human immunodeficiency virus infection. Pediatr Infect Dis J 1997;16:881–884.
160. Mueller BU, Jacobsen F, Butler KM, et al: Combination treatment with azidothymidine and granulocyte colony-stimulating factor in children with human immunodeficiency virus infection. J Pediatr 1992;121:797–802.

161. Kuritzkes DR: Clinical experience with filgrastim in AIDS. J Hematother Stem Cell Res 1999;8(Suppl 1):S17–S19.
162. Hermans P, Rozenbaum W, Jou A, et al: Filgrastim to treat neutropenia and support myelosuppressive medication dosing in HIV infection. G-CSF 92105 Study Group. AIDS 1996;10:1627–1633.
163. Ambati BK, Perlman DC, Salomon N: Outcomes of granulocyte colony-stimulating factor or granulocyte-macrophage colony-stimulating factor use in neutropenic patients infected with human immunodeficiency virus. Int J Infect Dis 1998;3:70–75.
164. Folks TM, Justement J, Kinter A, et al: Cytokine-induced expression of HIV-1 in a chronically infected promonocyte cell line. Science 1987;238:800–802.
165. Perno CF, Cooney DA, Gao WY, et al: Effects of bone marrow stimulatory cytokines on human immunodeficiency virus replication and the antiviral activity of dideoxynucleosides in cultures of monocyte/macrophages. Blood 1992;80:995–1003.
166. Kitano K, Abboud CN, Ryan DH, et al: Macrophage-active colony-stimulating factors enhance human immunodeficiency virus type 1 infection in bone marrow stem cells. Blood 1991;77:1699–1705.
167. Crowe SM, Lopez A: GM-CSF and its effects on replication of HIV-1 in cells of macrophage lineage. J Leukoc Biol 1997;62:41–48.
168. Scadden DT, Pickus O, Hammer SM, et al: Lack of in vivo effect of granulocyte-macrophage colony-stimulating factor on human immunodeficiency virus type 1. AIDS Res Hum Retroviruses 1996;12:1151–1159.
169. Skowron G, Stein D, Drusano G, et al: The safety and efficacy of granulocyte-macrophage colony-stimulating factor (sargramostim) added to indinavir- or ritonavir-based antiretroviral therapy: A randomized double-blind, placebo-controlled trial. J Infect Dis 1999;180:1064–1071.
170. Hammer SM, Gillis JM: Synergistic activity of granulocyte-macrophage colony-stimulating factor and 3′-azido-3′-deoxythymidine against human immunodeficiency virus in vitro. Antimicrob Agents Chemother 1987;31:1046–1050.
171. Hammer SM, Gillis JM, Pinkston P, Rose RM: Effect of zidovudine and granulocyte-macrophage colony-stimulating factor on human immunodeficiency virus replication in alveolar macrophages. Blood 1990;75:1215–1219.
172. Nielsen SD, Afzelius P, Dam-Larsen S, et al: Effect of granulocyte colony-stimulating factor (G-CSF) in human immunodeficiency virus-infected patients: Increase in numbers of naive CD4 cells and CD34 cells makes G-CSF a candidate for use in gene therapy or to support antiretroviral therapy. J Infect Dis 1998;177:1733–1736.
173. Smith PD, Lamerson CL, Banks SM, et al: Granulocyte-macrophage colony-stimulating factor augments human monocyte fungicidal activity for *Candida albicans*. J Infect Dis 1990;161:999–1005.
174. Wang M, Friedman H, Djeu JY: Enhancement of human monocyte function against *Candida albicans* by the colony-stimulating factors (CSF): IL-3, granulocyte-macrophage-CSF, and macrophage-CSF. J Immunol 1989;143:671–677.
175. Grabstein KH, Urdal DL, Tushinski RJ, et al: Induction of macrophage tumoricidal activity by granulocyte-macrophage colony-stimulating factor. Science 1986;232:506–508.
176. Kedzierska K, Mak J, Mijch A, et al: Granulocyte-macrophage colony-stimulating factor augments phagocytosis of *Mycobacterium avium* complex by human immunodeficiency virus type 1-infected monocytes/macrophages in vitro and in vivo. J Infect Dis 2000;181:390–394.
177. Richardson MD, Brownlie CE, Shankland GS: Enhanced phagocytosis and intracellular killing of *Candida albicans* by GM-CSF-activated human neutrophils. J Med Vet Mycol 1992;30:433–441.
178. Fletcher MP, Gasson JC: Enhancement of neutrophil function by granulocyte-macrophage colony-stimulating factor involves recruitment of a less responsive subpopulation. Blood 1988;71:652–658.
179. Prescribing information for Neupogen for Injection. In Medical Economics editors: Physicians' Desk Reference. Montvale, NJ: Medical Economics Company, 1998.
180. Mueller BU, Burt R, Gulick L, et al: Disseminated intravascular coagulation associated with granulocyte colony-stimulating factor therapy in a child with human immunodeficiency virus infection. J Pediatr 1995;126:749–752.

19

Childhood Malignancies in AIDS

Kenneth L. McClain

Children with HIV infection in the United States are at a substantially higher risk of developing a malignancy than those uninfected. It has been estimated that nearly 2% of HIV-infected children will develop a malignancy, versus approximately 0.013% of non-HIV-infected children, each year.[1,2] However, it is likely that the estimate of malignancies in HIV-infected children is low since another primary AIDS-defining condition may occur first and a cancer, as a second event, may not be registered with the Centers for Disease Control and Prevention (CDC).[1] This thesis has been confirmed for adult AIDS patients in a study by Cote and associates.[3] They found that half of the cases of non-Hodgkin lymphomas (NHLs) that occurred after AIDS were not reported to AIDS registries and that NHLs were part of AIDS-defining conditions in 3.2% of AIDS patients.

The most common cancers of children are NHLs, including small noncleaved cell (Burkitt) lymphoma, large cell lymphomas (immunoblastic), and primary brain lymphomas. These are listed among the AIDS-defining conditions but, in fact, are rarely the first event in children. Leiomyosarcomas are the second most frequent tumors but are not included in the list of AIDS-defining conditions. Other tumors found in children with AIDS are acute leukemias, Kaposi sarcoma, Hodgkin disease, mucosa-associated lymphoid tissue (MALT) lymphomas, and carcinomas of the vagina and trachea.

Granovsky and colleagues[4] surveyed Children's Cancer Group institutions and the National Cancer Institute for cases of AIDS-associated malignancies in children from 1982 to 1997. Of the 64 children identified (39 boys, 25 girls), 37 (58%) acquired HIV vertically and were diagnosed with a cancer at a median of 4.3 years from the time of HIV infection. Patient age at presentation ranged from 1.1 to 9.8 years. Twenty-two (34%) children were infected with HIV from blood or blood product transfusions. The latency for developing a malignancy was much later, with a median of 13.4 years and a range of 0.6 to 13.8 years. The investigators calculated the relative risk of developing NHL as 1203 and that for leiomyosarcomas as 10,000. The latter figure is in agreement with an earlier study.[5]

Initially, adults had a higher incidence of lymphomas with zidovudine treatment.[6] With the advent of highly active antiretroviral therapy, children have had fewer complications involving secondary infections, since their CD4+ counts are higher.[7] Time will tell whether the incidence of malignancies also decreases.

NON-HODGKIN LYMPHOMA

Individuals who are immunosuppressed, whether from HIV infection, from bone marrow or organ transplantation, or as a congenital condition, are well known to have a markedly higher incidence of lymphoproliferative diseases and NHLs (Table 19–1).[8] For HIV-positive hemophilia patients, NHL is 36 times more common than in the HIV-negative patients with factor VIII deficiency.[9] Nearly all the NHLs of these children with AIDS are high-grade B-cell tumors of the Burkitt lymphoma (small noncleaved cell) or immunoblastic (large cell) histologic type. Diffuse, large, noncleaved cell lymphoma has also been reported. The lymphomas often have the t8;14 chromosomal translocation. Since the types of NHL noted above represent approximately 25% to 40% of lymphomas in immunocompetent children, NHL cases may not be recognized as AIDS-associated at first. Thus, it is prudent even now to test all children who develop lymphoma for HIV infection.

Clinical Presentation

Most pediatric AIDS patients with NHL acquired the HIV infection vertically or from transfusion of blood and clotting factor concentrates. The mean age for discovery of malignancy in the vertically infected group is 35 months, with a range of 6 to 62 months.[10] In hemophiliac children, the latency is longer, with cases presenting up to the age of 18 years. The latency from time of HIV seroconversion to onset of the lymphomas was 22 to 88 months. A recent review of the multicenter Hemophilia Malignancy Study data revealed no clinical or lifestyle characteristics, antiviral drug treatment, or blood product usage that had an effect on the development of NHLs in HIV-positive hemophilia patients.[11] In the study of hemophilia patients, all children had CD4+ lymphocyte counts less than 50/mm^3 at diagnosis of the malignancy.[9] Studies of adult AIDS patients with NHL found that a CD4+ count of less than 50/mm^3 correlated very strongly ($P = .0085$) with the higher rate of malignancy.[6] However, other studies have shown that HIV-infected children may develop malignancies even when the CD4+ count is normal.[4] This study showed that of the HIV-positive cancer patients at the Pediatric Branch of the National Cancer Institute, 13% had CD4+ percentages greater than 25%, 6% had moderate suppression (15–24%) and 81% had CD4+ percentages less than 15% (severe depression). Among zidovudine-treated adult AIDS patients, NHL occurred in 29.2% at 36 months after start of treatment with zidovudine, versus 9.5% at that time for the didanosine-treated individuals.[12]

The presenting symptoms of lymphoma in children with AIDS are fever, weight loss, and extranodal manifestations of hepatomegaly, jaundice, or abdominal distention, evidence of bone marrow involvement, or central nervous system (CNS) symptoms. Granovsky and associates reported that gastrointestinal NHLs occurred in 37% and CNS NHLs in 17% of their patients.[4] Occasionally, the AIDS NHL patients will already have had lymphoproliferative diseases such as lymphocytic interstitial pneumonia or pulmonary lymphoid hyperplasia.[13] These children tend to have diffuse (stage III or IV) disease at the time of presentation. As opposed to non-immunosuppressed children whose B cell malignancies are very fast-growing, AIDS patients with NHL or B cell leukemia may have months of vague symptoms before the diagnosis of NHL is made.[14] Although the common symptoms of malaise, weight loss, and fever are index symptoms of many malignancies in children, this is of course confounded by the multiple coincident infections of AIDS patients. Those caring for children with HIV infection must thus have a high index of suspicion for malignancy and pursue biopsies of suspicious lymphadenopathy or imaging studies to define bone, intracranial, intrathoracic, or abdominal tumors. Also, these children may have unusual presenting symptoms when the bone marrow or mandible are involved, including numbness of the chin (a common manifestation of

Table 19–1
Spectrum of Systemic Lymphoproliferations in Children with AIDS

Nonmalignant
  Follicular hyperplasia (lymph node, gastrointestinal tract)
  Lymphoid follicles/nodules (liver, thymus)
  Thymitis and multilocular thymic cyst
  Pulmonary lymphoid hyperplasia/lymphoid interstitial pneumonitis complex, typical and atypical
  Polyclonal polymorphic B cell lymphoproliferative disorder
  Myoepithelial sialadenitis
  Myoepithelial sialadenitis with lymphoma

Malignant
  Non-Hodgkin lymphomas
  B cell acute lymphoblastic leukemia
  Hodgkin disease
  Mucosa-associated lymphoid tissue lymphoma (involving lungs, tonsils, and salivary glands)

peripheral facial nerve compression) without evidence of central nervous system involvement.

Central Nervous System Lymphomas

Among the presenting symptoms of CNS lymphomas in children are developmental delay or regression, dementia, cranial nerve palsies, seizures, and hemiparesis.[15] Since developmental problems and dementia are findings in children with HIV encephalopathy, one must still have a high index of suspicion for a malignancy and pursue appropriate imaging studies.[16] In adults or children with HIV infection, CNS symptoms, and a mass lesion seen on computed tomographic scan, the differential diagnosis must also include infections such as toxoplasmosis or cryptococcosis, although young children are less likely to have one of these infections.[17] Contrast-enhanced computed tomographic studies of the brain show hyperdense mass lesions that are usually multicentric or periventricular. Some centers choose to treat patients empirically for toxoplasmosis before a brain biopsy is done. However, the CNS lymphomas of AIDS patients are very fast growing lesions that often have central necrosis and thus appear to have a rim of enhancement like an infectious lesion. Although a stereotactic biopsy can give a definitive answer to the question of what type of lesion is in the brain, positron emission tomography may provide a helpful noninvasive diagnostic result.[18] In a prospective study of AIDS patients with brain lesions, all of the lymphomas showed *hyper*metabolic lesions and the patients with toxoplasmosis had *hypo*metabolic tissue. A new modality for evaluating CNS lymphomas is the use of thallium-201 single-photon emission computed tomography (SPECT) along with analysis for Epstein-Barr virus (EBV) DNA in the cerebrospinal fluid (CSF).[19] A high level of thallium uptake correlated very closely with the presence of EBV. Together, these two modalities helped to correctly define whether patients had a CNS lymphoma or a non-tumor brain mass lesion. When the mass lesion had low uptake and there was no EBV DNA in the CSF, the investigators recommended treatment for the most likely other lesion: toxoplasmosis infection. If the SPECT scan and EBV data are discordant, these patients would need a brain biopsy to define the nature of the lesion. Granovsky and coworkers[4] reported that all six of the CNS lymphomas from their survey were of large-cell histologic type and supratentorial location. These findings are similar to those of non-HIV–infected patients who have primary CNS NHLs.[20]

Not all CNS lesions of HIV-infected children are NHL or a toxoplasmosis infection. Kingma and associates[21] reported an 8-year-old girl with an EBV-associated monoclonal B cell lymphoproliferative disorder. This child was originally thought to have toxoplasmosis and was given treatment for that infection. When the lesion did not regress, it was biopsied. After steroids and antiretroviral therapy, the lesion decreased in size. The child subsequently died of other HIV-associated complications.

Treatment of AIDS Lymphomas

Children with HIV-associated NHL should be given treatment for their malignancy, since effective chemotherapy plans are available. Higher CD4+ lymphocyte counts (>100/mm^3), lactate dehydrogenase (LDH) levels close to normal, lack of other AIDS-defining illnesses, and good Karnofsky performance score (80–100%) naturally are better prognostic indicators for the patient. The number of pediatric AIDS patients treated for lymphoma is low, and the details of the only two series are reported by Granovsky and associates.[4] These patients were treated with two or more of the following drugs: cyclophosphamide (Cytoxan), vincristine (Oncovin), doxorubicin (Adriamycin), methotrexate (amethopterin), cytarabine (cytosine arabinoside), and prednisone plus intrathecal methotrexate or cytosine arabinoside with some modifications of standard dosages. Patients with AIDS NHL treated at the National Cancer Institute (NCI) had a 60% survival rate at 48 months. However, similar patients older than 5.5 years from the Children's Cancer Group (CCG) institutions had a 20% survival rate, and among those younger than 5.5 years of age, there were no survivors at 48 months. It was noted that many of the CCG patients were not treated on standardized protocols. Other study groups reported durable remissions of 20 months to several years, provided the other complicating factors of HIV infection were controlled.[14,15,22–29] Whatever therapy is chosen, it is critical to maintain optimal hydration and alkalinization during the initial week of therapy because of the danger of the tumor lysis syndrome. It is recommended that, if the child can tolerate the volume, the patient be given 2400 mL/m^2 of D5 1/2NS with no potassium and 40 mEq/L of sodium bicarbonate. If the patient does not have a good urine output consistent with the input or has not achieved an alkaline urine, the use of spironolactone is advised. It is critical to monitor the patient's serum electrolytes, blood urea nitrogen, creatinine, calcium, magnesium, phosphate, and uric acid two to three times daily during the initial days of therapy when tumor breakdown can be rapid. After the tumor masses have begun to resolve and the serum chemistries are stable, it is safe to follow the tests at less frequent intervals.

Central nervous system lymphomas provide the greater challenge because of delay in diagnosis and the greater difficulty in treating these patients.[17] The data from several studies demonstrate that intrathecal therapy is indicated in primary cases and as prophylaxis for NHLs in all other locations.[22,29] Radiation therapy may be a helpful adjunct for CNS involvement.[30] Other groups have reported that radiation therapy can achieve short-term complete responses, but the majority of patients will relapse or succumb to opportunistic infections.[31]

Interferon-α is currently under study by the Pediatric Oncology Group for treatment of AIDS-associated malignancies. This agent was chosen because of no cross-resistance to chemotherapy, known anti-HIV activity, and reported responses of some lymphomas.[32,33]

Etiology

Primary features of HIV infection include lymphadenopathy and atypical lymphoproliferations in many organs.[34] Some of these lymphoproliferative diseases have been associated with EBV infection and include lymphocytic interstitial pneumonitis and CNS lymphoma.[22] Shibata and colleagues[35] showed the frequency of EBV in benign lymph node biopsies of HIV-infected patients. EBV DNA was present in 13 of 35 biopsies of AIDS patients with persistent generalized adenopathy, but in none of the nodes from HIV-negative individuals. Important in this study was the fact that some of these 13 patients had lymphoma concurrent with the hyperplastic node and others developed lymphoma 1 to 22 months later. A study of the molecular characteristics of NHLs and B cell acute lymphoblastic leukemia in 25 children with AIDS revealed EBV in varying frequencies, depending on the histology of the malignancy.[36] EBV was found in the tumor cells of 46% of patients with small noncleaved cell lymphomas, 20% of those with large cell lymphoma, 50% of those with MALT lymphomas, and none of those with the B cell leukemias.

Other studies of AIDS NHL adult and pediatric patients reported EBV DNA in the tumor cells of 35% to 77% of NHLs outside the CNS.[37] CNS lesions are uniformly positive for EBV.[38] In Burkitt-type (small noncleaved cell) lymphomas, only 34% of tumors had EBV in the tumor cells. This confirmed findings by other investigators, who have documented c-myc gene rearrangements rather than evidence of EBV genome in many individuals with AIDS-associated NHL.[39] HIV has been found only rarely in the lymphoma cells, but may be present in surrounding lymphocytes or macrophages.[40,41] It is more likely that any cofactor role of HIV relates to cytokines, which are produced as a result of that virus presence. Interleukins-1, -2, -6, -7, and -10, interferon-γ, tumor necrosis factor, and B cell growth factor have all been identified.[42–44]

Since EBV cannot always be implicated in the etiology of the NHL of AIDS patients, some other factors must play an important role. Leach and associates reported that human herpesvirus-6 (HHV-6) type A was found in four cases of children with AIDS and malignancy but none of the AIDS or malignancy control subjects (C.T. Leach, personal communication). However, the role of HHV-6 and cytomegalovirus in the development of malignancy in these patients was unproven.

New understanding of the chemokine receptors that allow the HIV to infect lymphocytes has provided some important insight into the question of how HIV could affect B or T lymphocytes surrounding infected cells.[45] In this study, 746 HIV-1–infected persons were evaluated for variants of the stromal cell–derived factor 1 (SDF-1), CCR5, and CCR2 chemokines and risk of developing NHL. The SDF-13'A variant is known to occur in a little more than one third of whites and 10% of blacks. Presence of this variant in the heterozygous form doubled the chance of an HIV-infected person developing a B-cell NHL, and in the homozygous form it quadrupled the chance. The presence of the CCR5-triangle up32 chemokine receptor variant was shown to be protective against NHL.

Mutations or rearrangements in the c-myc oncogene are frequent in patients with AIDS NHL. The classic t(8;14), t(2;8), or t(8;22), which position an immunoglobulin gene enhancer near the myc oncogene in Burkitt lymphoma, are well known.[46] The number of HIV-infected patients with NHL and rearrangements in c-*myc* is variable (40–75%) depending on the methodology, type of patients, and locations of the lymphomas.[47,48] In the series of 25 pediatric patients noted above, c-*myc* translocations were identified in 73% of the small noncleaved cell lymphomas, 20% of the large cell lymphomas, in one MALT lymphoma, and 75% of the B cell leukemias. Mutations of c-*myc* were found in 38% of patients with small noncleaved cell lymphoma, 20% of those with large cell lymphoma, 1% of those with MALT lymphoma, and 25% of those with B cell leukemias.[36]

LEIOMYOSARCOMA AND LEIOMYOMAS

Clinical Presentation

The number of children with HIV infection and benign or malignant smooth muscle tumors proved to be the most surprising event in the biology of AIDS-associated malignancies of children.[4,5,9,49] This led to the inclusion of smooth muscle neoplasms (leiomyomas and leiomyosarcomas) as category B symptoms for a revised CDC classification.[50] In non-HIV–infected children, leiomyosarcomas and leiomyomas occur at a rate of fewer than 2 cases per 10 million individuals. As the second most frequent tumor of children with HIV infection, leiomyosarcomas and leiomyomas accounted for 17% of the malignancies in one survey.[4] The most common sites of presentation are the lungs, spleen, and gastrointestinal tract. Patients with endobronchial leiomyomas or leiomyosarcomas may present with cyanosis and fever with pulmonary infections unresponsive to antibiotics. These children often have multiple nodules in their pulmonary parenchyma as visualized by chest CT. Bloody diarrhea, abdominal pain, or signs of obstruction may signal intraluminal bowel lesions that may be numerous. Other sites of presentation include the adrenal glands and brain or dura.[51–53]

Etiology

In situ hybridization studies of the leiomyomas and leiomyosarcomas demonstrated that EBV was present in every tumor cell but not the adjoining normal cells.[5] Quantitative polymerase chain reaction (PCR) studies corroborated the in situ data by demonstrating high copy numbers of EBV in the tumor. Increasing concentrations of EBV DNA were also found in serial studies of patients' plasma before the tumors were diagnosed. In situ hybridization showed no HIV in these tumors, but the sensitive PCR assays found 4 to 45 copies of HIV per 100,000 cells, which would not be seen by in situ hybridization. The EBV receptor (CD21/C3d) was present on tumor tissue at very high concentration, but was lower in normal smooth muscle or control leiomyomas/leiomyosarcomas that had no EBV DNA in them.

In AIDS patients, the EBV receptor may be upregulated, allowing EBV to enter the muscle cells and cause their transformation. This hypothesis is supported by the fact that clonal EBV genome was found in each of the two tumors studied. It is impossible to know whether EBV infected the smooth muscle cells before they were transformed, although finding EBV in both the leiomyoma and leiomyosarcoma of one patient suggests that EBV played an early role in the transformation process from benign to malignant neoplasia. Conceivably, one of the EBV transforming genes such as EBNA2 plays a key role. EBNA2 has been identified in a tumor of liver transplant patients, which is infected with EBV like the leiomyosarcomas.[54] Another transforming product of EBV is the latent membrane protein (LMP).[55] LMP is often elevated in the lymphoproliferative diseases associated with EBV but has not been adequately evaluated in the smooth muscle tumors as yet.

Treatment

Although some patients with AIDS-associated leiomyoma or leiomyosarcoma have been treated with chemotherapy or radiotherapy, there are no convincing data to suggest a benefit to such treatment. Complete surgical resection is the most useful treatment, but recurrences are frequent.

PROLIFERATIVE LESIONS OF MUCOSA-ASSOCIATED LYMPHOID TISSUE

Reactive and proliferative lesions of organized lymphoid tissue associated with mucosa of the gastrointestinal tract (including Waldeyer ring and salivary glands) may also occur in the respiratory tract and other sites (e.g., thyroid, thymus).[56,57]

MALT shows the following features: reactive lymphoid follicles with prominent marginal zones containing centrocyte-like cells, lymphocytic infiltration of the epithelium (lymphoepithelial lesion), and presence of plasma cells immediately underneath the surface epithelium. Proliferative lesions of MALT, including lymphomas, show similar histologic features. The neoplastic lesions are usually of low-grade malignancy, but progression to high-grade MALT lymphomas is also described.[57–59]

Clinicopathologic Features

Six cases of MALT lesions in young people who acquired HIV infection perinatally or during childhood and a pediatric case of pulmonary MALT lymphoma have been reported.[60,61] The lesions involved lung, salivary glands, and tonsils. MALT lymphomas characteristically remain localized but if dissemination occurs, it is usually confined to the regional lymph nodes and other MALT sites.[62,63]

In the series of pediatric patients with MALT lesions, two had low-grade MALT lymphoma and two had high-grade MALT lymphoma.[60] One of the two patients with low-grade MALT lymphoma showed response to interferon-α; in the other patient, no specific therapy was given, since the disease had remained indolent without any sign of progression for several weeks. In one of the patients with histologically high-grade MALT lymphoma, there was response to radiation therapy with no evidence of recurrence with 1 year of follow-up. In the other patient, complete remission occurred after multidrug chemotherapy (vincristine, Adriamycin, prednisone, methotrexate, and cytosine arabinoside).

The MALT lesions represent a new conceptual category of pediatric HIV-associated disease, which may arise from a combination of viral causes.[62–64] The understanding and application of the concept of lymphomas arising in the MALT sites are of practical importance from the point of view of prognosis and therapy. In light of the concept of MALT, the spectrum of lymphoid lesions of lungs (pulmonary lymphoid hyperplasia/lymphoid interstitial pneumonitis complex) and other organs described previously in children should also be considered as MALT lesions.[65] Clinicians should have a high index of suspicion for MALT lesions in children with AIDS, and an adequate biopsy specimen should be obtained. The therapy will be determined by the precise pathologic diagnosis of the lesion.

Of particular interest in the spectrum of MALT lesions in children with AIDS is the polyclonal polymorphic B cell lymphoproliferative disorder (PBLD) involving the lungs, liver, kidneys, lymph nodes, and spleen.[66] In this disorder, lymphoid infiltrates with characteristics of MALT were present in the organs mentioned above. In view of the polyclonal nature of the infiltrate as shown by immunoperoxidase staining for Ig-κ and Ig-λ light chains, multiorgan involvement, and the vascular invasion seen histologically, PBLD may be considered as an intermediate biologic behavior between benign and malignant lymphoproliferation.[67] The lymphoreticular proliferative disorders occurring in adults with AIDS include the diffuse infiltrative CD8 lymphocytosis syndrome characterized by parotid gland enlargement, sicca symptoms, and lymphocytic interstitial pneumonia and have not been reported in children.[68] However, it should be noted that detailed and systematic in situ and flow cytometric immunophenotyping of the lymphocytic infiltrates in various organs in children with lymphoproliferative disorders still needs to be done.

LEUKEMIAS AND HODGKIN DISEASE

Most leukemias of children with AIDS are of B-cell origin, which is consistent with the types of lymphomas.[69,70] They represent the fourth most common malignancy of children with AIDS after NHL, leiomyosarcomas, and various forms of Kaposi sarcoma. The clinical presentation and biologic features are similar to those found in non-HIV infected children. Also, these patients have achieved stable remissions with chemotherapy, which includes intravenous vincristine, prednisone, cyclophosphamide, doxorubicin, and methotrexate and intrathecal cytosine arabinoside.

There is no apparent increase in the incidence of Hodgkin disease in children with AIDS.[71,72] This is surprising, because most of the Hodgkin disease cases reported in adults with HIV have been EBV-positive (78%) and manifest at younger adult ages than in non-HIV-infected individuals. Adult HIV patients with Hodgkin disease have extranodal disease, just like the

NHLs, and present at an earlier age (29 years) than non-HIV-infected individuals (38 years), with systemic symptoms and extensive (stage IV) disease, primarily in males.[73] The survival rate of these patients is markedly worse than that of non-HIV-infected individuals with Hodgkin disease. Despite short responses, the median survival was 13 months in one study[74] and 16 months in another.[75] The latter group had a 90% overall response rate, but more than one third of these relapsed, leaving a survival rate of slightly more than 30% at 3 years of observation.

KAPOSI SARCOMA

Kaposi sarcoma occurs in about 25% of adults with AIDS. The highest prevalence is among white male homosexuals with AIDS. In contrast, Kaposi sarcoma is rare in children. Orlow and coworkers[76] reviewed 30 cases of Kaposi sarcoma in children reported in the literature and added three more cases seen in Romanian children. It is of interest to note that Kaposi sarcoma occurs only in those HIV-infected children who were born to mothers in high-risk groups for Kaposi sarcoma (heterosexual transmission via a bisexual partner) or who acquired HIV infection postnatally via contaminated blood or blood products. Kaposi sarcoma is rare in this country, with less than 1% of children younger than 13 years of age and 3% of those from 13 to 19 years of age have Kaposi sarcoma as an AIDS-defining illness.[50] Because of this rarity, there are no specific recommendations for treatment of Kaposi sarcoma in children, and adult guidelines must be adapted.

There is a potential diagnostic dilemma regarding Kaposi sarcoma in children. From the pathologic point of view, bacillary angiomatosis can mimic some features of Kaposi sarcoma.[77] Bacillary angiomatosis (BA), which is caused by *Bartonella henselae* and *Bartonella quintana*, shows presence of neutrophils, cellular debris, and clumps of bacteria in a vasoproliferative lesion that lacks the spindle cell element and bizarre shapes of the vascular channels seen in Kaposi sarcoma. *B. henselae* is also the etiologic agent of cat scratch disease, and epidemiologic studies have implied a relationship between BA and cat exposure.[78] Therefore, the occurrence of bacillary angiomatosis in children with AIDS may be anticipated.

HUMAN PAPILLOMA VIRUS–RELATED GENITAL LESIONS

Only three cases of human papilloma virus (HPV)–associated condylomatous lesions with or without dysplasia have been reported in children and adolescents with AIDS.[65] In one of these cases (an 18-year-old girl) the uterine cervix was the site of the lesion. However, with increasing incidence of HIV infection in adolescents in recent years and the possibility of HIV transmission via sexual abuse of children, HPV-related uterine cervical epithelial preneoplastic and perhaps even neoplastic lesions are likely to become more prevalent.[79,80] Invasive cervical carcinoma has been reported in a 16-year-old girl infected with HIV.[81]

Features of Genital Lesions and Their Progression

The HPV-associated lesions comprise a spectrum extending from condyloma acuminatum with minimal, mild, moderate, or severe dysplasia to cervical intraepithelial neoplasia (CIN). The progression of dysplastic lesions and CIN eventually to invasive carcinoma occurs over a period of many years. Therefore, HPV-related cervical neoplasia is unlikely to be seen with measurable frequency in pediatric AIDS. However, it is possible that immunodeficiency may cause more rapid and more frequent progression.[82] Cytologic examination and biopsy of the lesion establish the diagnosis. The morphologic hallmark of HPV-related genital lesions is the presence of koilocytotic atypia. The physicians taking care of adolescent girls with HIV infection should look for the HPV-related genital lesions in their patients. If found, these lesions should be treated promptly, so that their progression to malignancy is prevented. Thus pediatricians can play a major role in the prevention of cervical cancer in AIDS.

MISCELLANEOUS TUMORS

Only single cases of the following types of tumors have been reported in children with AIDS: hepatoblastoma, embryonal rhabdomyosarcoma of the gall bladder, fibrosarcoma of liver, and papillary carcinoma of thyroid.[10,65,83] These tumors probably represent coincidental occurrence rather than true association with HIV infection. As the children with HIV infection live longer, we should not be surprised to see some of them developing the more common malignancies of childhood: acute lymphoblastic leukemia and brain tumors.[2]

SUPPORTIVE CARE GUIDELINES

Children with AIDS and a malignancy are more susceptible to the cytopenic effects of chemotherapeutic agents, so dosages of the antineoplastic agents may have to be modified to keep prolonged neutropenia, thrombocytopenia, and anemia to a minimum. Concurrent use of antiretrovirals is probably essential, so the possible additive toxicities are obvious. Some protease inhibitors may increase the possibility of mucositis.[84]

The routine use of prophylaxis against *Pneumocystis carinii* infections with trimethoprim-sulfisoxazole (Bactrim) or pentamidine is the standard of care for AIDS patients and should be continued when they develop a malignancy. The only caveat is that some patients develop neutropenia with the former and thus the prophylaxis may have to be modified. Cytokines to stimulate granulocyte recovery (granulocyte-colony stimulating factor or granulocyte-macrophage colony stimulating factor) after chemotherapy may be useful in preventing secondary bacterial or fungal infections in these highly vulnerable patients. The prophylactic use of oral fluconazole has been shown to reduce the incidence of mouth and esophageal candidal infections.[85]

REFERENCES

1. Centers for Disease Control and Prevention: US HIV and AIDS cases reported through June 1999. HIV/AIDS Surveillance report, midyear edition. Available at: http://www.cdc.gov/hiv/stats/nasr1101.htm.
2. Robison LL: General principles of the epidemiology of childhood cancer. In Pizzo PA, Poplack DG, (eds): Principles and Practice of Pediatric Oncology. p1–10. Philadelphia; Lippincott-Raven Publishers, 1997.
3. Cote TR, Biggar RJ, Rosenberg PS, et al: Non-Hodgkin's lymphoma among people with AIDS: incidence, presentation and public health burden. AIDS/Cancer Study Group. Int J Cancer 1997; 73:645.
4. Granovsky MO, Mueller BU, Nicholson HS, et al: Cancer in human immunodeficiency virus-infected children: a case series from the Children's Cancer Group and the National Cancer Institute. J Clin Oncol 1998;16:1729.
5. McClain KL, Leach CT, Jenson HB, et al: Association of Epstein-Barr virus with leiomyosarcomas in young people with AIDS. N Engl J Med 1995;332:12.
6. Pluda JM, Yarchoan R, Jaffe ES, et al: Development of non-Hodgkin lymphoma in a cohort of patients with severe human immunodeficiency virus (HIV) infection on long-term antiretroviral therapy. Ann Intern Med 1990;113:276.
7. Palella FJ, Delaney KM, Moorman AC, et al: Declining morbidity and mortality among patients with advanced human immunodeficiency virus infection. N Engl J Med 1998;338:853.
8. Filipovich A: Lymphoproliferative disorders associated with immunodeficiency. In Magrath IT (ed): The Non-Hodgkin's Lymphomas. London, Edward Arnold, 1990, p 135.
9. Ragni MV, Belle SH, Jaffe RA, et al: Acquired immunodeficiency syndrome-associated non-Hodgkin's lymphomas and other malignancies in patients with hemophilia. Blood 1989;81:993.
10. Mueller BU, Shad AT, Magrath IT, et al: Malignancies in children with HIV infection. In Pizzo PA, Wilfert CM (eds): Pediatric AIDS: The Challenge of HIV Infection in Infants, Children, and Adolescents. Baltimore, Williams & Wilkins, 1994, p 603.
11. Ragni MV, Belle SH, Bass D, et al: Clinical characteristics and blood product usage in AIDS-associated lymphoma in haemophiliacs: A case-control study. Haemophilia 1998;4:826.
12. Pluda JM, Venzon DJ, Tosato G, et al: Parameters affecting the development of non-Hodgkin's lymphoma in patients with severe human immunodeficiency virus infection receiving antiretroviral therapy. J Clin Oncol 1993;11:1099.
13. Bix DL, Redfield RR, Tosato G: Defective regulation of Epstein-Barr virus infection in patients with acquired immunodeficiency syndrome (AIDS) or AIDS-related disorders. N Engl J Med 1986;314:874.
14. Neumann Y, Toren A, Mandel M, et al: Favorable response of pediatric AIDS-related Burkitt's lymphoma treated by aggressive chemotherapy. Med Pediatr Oncology 1993;21:661.
15. Epstein LG, DiCarlo FJ, Joshi VV, et al: Primary lymphoma of the central nervous system in children with acquired immuodeficiency syndrome. Pediatrics 1988;82:355.
16. Belman AL, Diamond G, Dickson D, et al: Pediatric acquired immunodeficiency syndrome: Neurologic syndromes. Am J Dis Child 1988;142:29.
17. McArthur JC: Neurologic manifestations of AIDS. Medicine 1987;66:407.

18. Pierce MA, Johnson MD, Maciunas RJ, et al: Evaluating contrast-enhancing brain lesions in patients with AIDS by using positron emission tomography. Ann Intern Med 1995;123:594.
19. Antinori A, De Rossi G, Ammassari A, et al: Value of combined approach with thallium-201 single-photon emission computed tomography and Epstein-Barr virus DNA polymerase chain reaction in CSF for the diagnosis of AIDS-related primary CNS lymphoma. J Clin Oncol 1999;17:554.
20. Miller DC, Hochberg FH, Harris NL, et al: Pathology with clinical correlations of primary central nervous system non-Hodgkin's lymphoma. Cancer 1994;74:1383.
21. Kingma DW, Mueller BU, Frekko K, et al: Low-grade monoclonal Epstein-Barr virus-associated lymphoproliferative disorder of the brain presenting as human immunodeficiency virus-associated encephalopathy in a child with acquired immunodeficiency syndrome. Arch Pathol Lab Med 1999;123:83.
22. Andiman WA, Eastman R, Martin K, et al: Opportunistic lymphoproliferations associated with Epstein-Barr viral DNA in infants and children with AIDS. Lancet 1985;2:1390.
23. Arico M, Caslli D, D'Argenio PD, et al: Malignancies in children with human immunodeficiency virus type 1 infection. Cancer 1991;68:2473.
24. Bouquety JC, Siopathis MR, Ravisse PR, et al: Lymphadenopathic Kaposi's sarcoma in an African pediatric AIDS case. Am J Trop Med Hyg 1989;40:323.
25. Chilcote R, Williams T, Siegel S: Therapy of Burkitt's lymphoma in children with HIV infection. Pediatr Res 1989;25:149A.
26. Goldstein J, Dickson DW, Rubenstein A, et al: Primary central nervous system lymphoma in pediatric patient with acquired immune deficiency syndrome. Cancer 1990;66:2503.
27. Kamani N, Kennedy J, Brandsma J: Burkitt lymphoma in a child with human immunodeficiency virus infection. J Pediatr 1988;112:241.
28. Nadal D, Caduff R, Frey E, et al: Non-Hodgkin's lymphoma in four children infected with the human immunodeficiency virus. Cancer 1994;73:224.
29. Patton DF, Sixbey JW, Murphy SB: Epstein-Barr virus in human immunodeficiency virus-related Burkitt lymphoma. J Pediatr 1988;113:951.
30. Del Mistro A, Laverda A, Calabrese F, et al: Primary lymphoma of the central nervous system in two children with acquired immune deficiency syndrome. Am J Clin Pathol 1990;94:722.
31. Formenti SC, Gill PS, Lean E, et al: Primary central nervous system lymphoma in AIDS. Results of radiation therapy. Cancer 1989;63:1101.
32. Lane HC, Feinberg J, Davey V, et al: Anti-retroviral effects of interferon-α in AIDS-associated Kaposi's sarcoma. Lancet 1988;2:1218.
33. Rohatiner AZS: Interferon alpha in lymphoma. Br J Haematol 1991;79(suppl 1):26.
34. Vellatini C, Horschowski N, Philippon V, et al: Development of lymphoid hyperplasia in transgenic mice expressing the HIV tat gene. AIDS Res Hum Retrovirol 1995;11:21.
35. Shibata D, Weiss LM, Nathwani BN: Epstein-Barr virus in benign lymph node biopsies from individuals infected with the human immunodeficiency virus is associated with concurrent or subsequent development of non-Hodgkin's lymphoma. Blood 1991;77:1527.
36. McClain KL, Leach CT, Jenson HB, et al: Molecular and virologic characteristics of lymphoid malignancies in children with acquired immune deficiency syndrome. J AIDS 2000;23:152–159.
37. Hamilton-Dutoit SJ, Raphael M, Audouin J, et al: In situ demonstration of Epstein-Barr virus small RNAs (EBER 1) in acquired immunodeficiency syndrome-related lymphomas: correlation with tumor morphology and primary site. Blood 1993;82:619.
38. MacMahon EME, Glass JD, Hayward SD, et al: Epstein-Barr virus in AIDS-related primary central nervous system lymphoma. Lancet 1991;338:969.
39. Suber M, Neri A, Inghirami G, et al: Frequent c-*myc* oncogene activation and infrequent presence of Epstein-Barr virus genome in AIDS-associated lymphoma. Blood 1988;72:667.
40. Montagnier L, Gruest J, Chamaret S, et al: Adaption of LAV to replication in EBV transformed B lymphoblastomatoid cell lines. Science 1984;225:63.
41. Schittman SM, Lane HC, Higgins SE, et al: Direct polyclonal activation of B lymphocytes by AIDS virus. Science 1986;233:1084.
42. Jelinek DF, Lipsky PE: Enhancement of human B cell proliferation and differentiation by tumor necrosis factor-alpha and interleukin 1. J Immunol 1987;139:2970.
43. Paul WE: Interleukin 4/B cell stimulatory factor 1: One lymphokine, many functions. FASEB J 1987;1:456.
44. Zlotnik A, Morre KW: Interleukin 10. Cytokine 1991;3:366.
45. Rabkin CS, Yang Q, Goedert JJ, et al: Chemokine and chemokine receptor gene variants and risk of non-Hodgkin's lymphoma in human immunodeficiency virus-1-infected individuals. Blood 1999;93:1838.
46. Klein G: Multiple phenotypic consequences of the *Ig/Myc* translocation in B-cell-derived tumors. Genes Chromosomes Cancer 1989;1:3.
47. Ballerini P, Gaidano G, Gong J, et al: Multiple genetic lesions in acquired immunodeficiency syndrome-related non-Hodgkin's lyumphoma. Blood 1993;81:166.
48. Meeker TC, Shiramizu B, Kaplan L, et al: Evidence for molecular subtypes of HIV-associated lymphoma: Division into peripheral monoclonal,

48. polyclonal, and central nervous system lymphoma. AIDS 1991;5:669.
49. Chadwick EG, Connor EJ, Hanson CG, et al: Tumors of smooth-muscle origin in HIV-infected children. JAMA 1990;263:3182.
50. Centers for Disease Control and Prevention: Revised classification system for human immunodeficiency virus infection in children less than 13 years of age. MMWR 1994;43[RR12]:1–17.
51. Rosenfeld DL, Girgis WS, Underberg-Davis SJ: Bilateral smooth-muscle tumors of the adrenals in a child with AIDS. Pediatr Radiol 1999;29:376.
52. Bejjani GK, Stopak B, Schwartz A, et al: Primary dural leiomyosarcoma in a patient infected with human immundeficiency virus: Case report. Neurosurgery 1999;44:199.
53. Brown HG, Burger PC, Olivi A, et al: Intracranial leiomyosarcoma in a patient with AIDS. Neuroradiology 1999;41:35.
54. Lee ES, Locker J, Nalesnik M, et al: The association of Epstein-Barr virus with smooth-muscle tumors occurring after organ transplantation. N Engl J Med 1995;332:19.
55. Wang F, Liebowitz D, Kieff E: An EBV membrane protein expressed in immortalized lymphocytes transforms established rodent cells. Cell 1985;43:831.
56. Hyjek E, Smith W, Isaacson P: Primary B cell lymphoma of salivary gland and its relationship to myoepithelial sialadenitis. Hum Pathol 1988;19:72.
57. Pelstring RJ, Essel JH, Kurtin PJ, et al: Diversity of organ site involvement among malignant lymphomas of mucosa associated lymphoid tissues. Am J Clin Pathol 1991;96:738.
58. Harris NL: Entranodal lymphoid infiltrates and mucosa associated lymphoid tissue (MALT): A unifying concept. Am J Surg Pathol 1991;15:879.
59. Isaacson PG: Gastrointestinal lymphoma. Hum Pathol 1994;25:1020.
60. Joshi V, Gagnon A, Chadwick E, et al: The spectrum of mucosal associated lymphoid tissue (MALT) lesions in pediatric patients infected with human immunodeficiency virus (HIV). Am J Clin Pathol 1997;107:592.
61. Teruya-Feldstein J, Teemeck BL, Sloas MM, et al: Pulmonary malignant lymphoma of mucosa associated lymphoid tissue (MALT) arising in a pediatric HIV-positive patient. Am J Surg Pathol 1995;19:357.
62. Labouyrie E, Merlio JPH, Beylot-Barry M, et al: HIV type I replication within cystic lymphoepithelial lesions. Am J Clin Pathol 1993;100:41.
63. Laimore MD, Poulson JM, Adducci TA, et al: Lentivirus-induced lymphoproliferative disease: Comparative pathogenicity of phenotypically distinct ovine lentivirus strains. Am J Pathol 1988;130:80.
64. Laimore MD, Rosadio RH, DeMartini JC, et al: Ovine lentivirus lymphoid interstitial pneumonia: Rapid induction in neonatal lambs. Am J Pathol 1986;125:173.
65. Joshi VV: Pathology of pediatric AIDS: Overview, update, and future directions. Ann N Y Acad Sci 1993;693:71.
66. Joshi VV, Kauffman S, Oleske JM, et al: Polyclonal polymorphic B-cell lymphoproliferative disorder with prominent pulmonary involvement in children with AIDS. Cancer 1987;59:1455.
67. Joshi VV: Systemic lymphoproliferative lesions in children with AIDS. In Pizzo PA, Wilfert W (eds): Pediatric AIDS: The Challenge of HIV Infection in Infants, Children, and Adolescents. Baltimore, Williams & Wilkins, 1990, p 44.
68. Itescu S, Brancato LJ, Bunbaum J, et al: A diffuse infiltrative CD8 lymphocytosis syndrome in HIV infection: A host immune response associated with HLA-DR5. Ann Intern Med 1990;112:3.
69. Montalvo FW, Casanova R, Clavell LA: Treatment outcome in children with malignancies associated with human immunodeficiency virus infection. J Pediatr 1990;116:735.
70. Rechavi G, Ben-Bassat I, Berkowicz M, et al: Molecular analysis of Burkitt's leukemia in two hemophilic brothers with AIDS. Blood 1987;70:1713.
71. Ames ED, Conjalka MS, Goldberg AF, et al: Hodgkin's disease and AIDS: Twenty-three new cases and a review of the literature. Hematol Oncol Clin North Am 1991;5:343.
72. Newcome SR, Ward M, Napoli VA, et al: Treatment of HIV-associated Hodgkin's disease (HIV-HD): Is there a clue regarding the etiology of Hodgkin's disease [abstract]? Am Soc Clin Oncol 1992;11:44.
73. Tirelli U, Errante D, Dolcetti R, et al: Hodgkin's disease and human immunodeficiency virus infection: Clinicopathologic and virologic features of 114 patients from the Italian Cooperative Group on AIDS and Tumors. J Clin Oncol 1995;13:1758.
74. Serrano M, Bellas C, Campo E, et al: Hodgkin's disease in patients with antibodies to human immunodeficiency virus: A study of 22 patients. Cancer 1990;65:2248.
75. Errante D, Gabarre J, Ridolofo AL, et al: Hodgkin's disease in 35 patients with HIV infection: An experience with epirubicin, bleomycin, vinblastine, and prednisone chemotherapy in combination with antiretroviral therapy and primary use of G-CSF. Ann Oncol 1999;10:189.
76. Orlow SJ, Cooper D, Petrea S, et al: AIDS-associated Kaposi's sarcoma in Romanian children. J Am Acad Dermatol 1992;28:449.
77. LeBoit PE: Bacillary angiomatosis. Mod Pathol 1995;8:218.
78. Tuffero JW, Mohle BJ, Koehler JE, et al: The epidemiology of bacillary angiomatosis and bacillary peliosis. JAMA 1993;269:770.

79. Gutman LT, St. Claire KK, Weedy C, et al: HIV transmission by child sexual abuse. Am J Dis Child 1991;145:137.
80. Adger H: Sexually transmitted diseases. In McMillan JA, DeAngelis CD, Feigin RD, Warshaw JB (eds): Oski's Pediatrics, Principles and Practice, 3rd ed. Philadelphia, Lippincott, Williams & Wilkins, 1999, p 555.
81. Maemain M, Fruchter RG, Serur E, et al: HIV infection and cervical neoplasia. Gynecol Oncol 1992;38: 377.
82. Matoras R, Ariceta JM, Rementeria A, et al: HIV induced immunosuppression: A risk factor for human papilloma virus infection. Am J Obstet Gynecol 1991;164:42.
83. Diamond FB, Price LJ, Nelson RP: Papillary carcinoma of thyroid in a 7 year old HIV positive child. Pediatr AIDS HIV Infect Fetal Adolesc 1994;5:232.
84. Sparano JA, Wiernick PH, Strack M, et al: Infusional cyclophosphamide, doxorubicin, and etoposide in human immunodeficiency virus- and human T-cell leukemia virus type I-related non-Hodgkin's lymphoma: A highly active regimen. Blood 1993; 81:2810.
85. Uzun O, Anaissie EJ: Antifungal prophylaxis in patients with hematologic malignancies: A reappraisal. Blood 1995;86:2063.

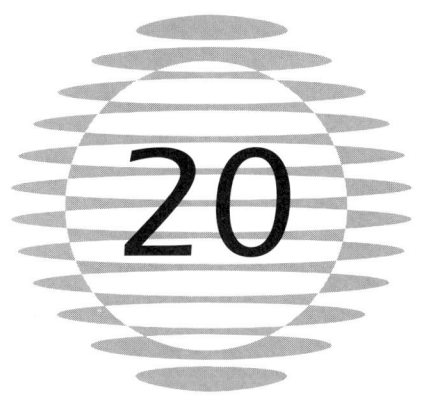

20

Palliative Care for Children Infected with HIV

Samuel Grubman and James M. Oleske

In 1995, the World Health Organization (WHO) reported that, worldwide, there were 12.2 million deaths of children younger than 5 years of age. In 1993, only 1% (<2000) of US hospice patients were children, although it is estimated that 17,000 children die each year in the United States who would benefit from palliative care and hospice services. The lack of attention to palliative care and the lack of access to hospice programs are even more pronounced in less developed countries, which account for 70% of all pediatric deaths worldwide. Many therapies that would prevent disease progression and are part of the continuum of palliative care in more developed countries are not available in these resource-poor areas. The linkage of access to health care (including palliative care), poverty, and human rights has been brought into focus by the epidemic of HIV infection and AIDS. By 2000, 3 million children died from HIV and 10 million children were orphaned as a result of this epidemic. Most children who have died of HIV/AIDS have died in pain. The purpose of this chapter is to begin changing this prospect for children now living with HIV.[1-4]

Palliative care is the combination of active and compassionate therapies intended to comfort and support individuals and families who are living with chronic life-limiting illnesses. It is a continuum of care that addresses the physical, social, psychological, and spiritual needs of the patient and family within the context of standard medical therapies specific for the disease. Problems addressed by palliative care include pain management, suffering, physical and cognitive limitations, and anxiety-provoking signs and symptoms experienced during the course of an illness (Table 20–1).[5-8]

The use of palliative care within the context of other forms of medical treatment should not be reserved for the end of life.[9,10] For children with HIV disease, palliative care is an important aspect of a comprehensive treatment program from the time of diagnosis.[11-13] Antiretroviral therapy and other medical therapies for HIV disease can have a significant adverse effect on quality of life, secondary to medication-related and other side effects, even when patients are otherwise asymptomatic. Essentially, if issues relating to pain management and quality of life are ignored, HIV-specific medical therapy, especially antiretroviral therapy, will

Table 20–1
Problems Addressed by Palliative Care

Pain	Dyspnea
Abdominal	Vomiting
Headache	Anorexia
Extremity	Fever
Oral/skin	Immobility
Neuropathic	Alterations in cognitive
Cough	functioning:
Nausea	Personality change
Diarrhea	Depression
Bleeding	Anxiety
Seizures	Insomnia

ultimately fail because of lack of patient adherence.[14–17]

The principles of palliative care, when applied, improve the quality of life of the child with chronic life-limiting illness. Quality of life, defined in large part by the patient and his or her family, includes the ability of the child to carry out activities of daily living with minimal discomfort while receiving treatment for their illness. The quality of life of patients should be the main concern of any physician and the driving force throughout the course of a chronic illness.[18–23] Hospice care is the continuum of palliative care in end-stage disease. It incorporates the principles of palliative care used in earlier stages of illness but with an enhanced emphasis on easing the burden of end of life care for the patient and family with concern focused on comfort care, while limiting or withdrawing life-sustaining measures. As part of the continuum of palliative care, hospice services maximize patient dignity and allow for a transition to appropriate family and staff bereavement.[24–33]

PAIN AND SUFFERING

Children with HIV infection have acute and chronic pain from the disease, its complications, and the multiple evaluations and treatments required for its management.[34] Acute pain serves a protective function, is symptomatic of a focal site of injury, by definition is self-limited, and usually does not have associated psychological disturbance and its treatment is relatively straightforward. Acute pain can be a manifestation of a treatable medical complication or related to invasive procedures. Chronic pain, however, serves no biologic function, can be diffuse in nature, is unrelenting or recurrent, and has profound psychological implications and its treatment is complex and often difficult.[35–36] With HIV infection, chronic pain is a significant aspect of later stages of disease and can also be secondary to the side effects of medications from early in the course of the illness. In children with chronic disease, repetitive types of acute pain (i.e., those related to diagnostic and therapeutic procedures) can have a similar impact on quality of life as chronic pain.[37] Suffering, like chronic pain, is more difficult to address and may not be associated with acute or chronic physical pain but rather with the psychological effect of altered function experienced by children living with a complex medical condition.

DISEASE-RELATED PAIN

HIV disease-related pain syndromes result from both infectious and noninfectious pathologic conditions in various organ systems and can be acute and chronic. Causes of oropharyngeal pain include candidiasis, dental caries, oral abscesses, gingivitis, aphthous stomatitis, and herpetic stomatitis. Esophageal pain results from several different infectious complications including esophageal candidiasis and cytomegalovirus and herpetic ulcerative esophagitis. Common causes of abdominal pain result from pancreatitis, hepatitis, hepatosplenomegaly, intermittent obstruction secondary to *Mycobacterium avium* complex adenopathy, and inflammatory and infectious colitis. Chronic diarrhea, although not classically considered a pain syndrome, is common in patients with HIV disease and is usually associated with abdominal discomfort, including cramping and spasms.[11,14,15,34,38]

These oropharyngeal and gastrointestinal pain syndromes frequently result in poor oral intake, increased losses, malnutrition, failure to thrive, and progression to wasting syndrome. Even in early stages of illness, chronic and recurrent difficulty with oral intake from various causes has a significant impact on quality of life for HIV-infected children. The joy of eating for many children becomes the job of needing to eat. Wasting syndrome can be associated with cachexia, fatigue, depression, musculoskeletal pain, abdominal pain, and neuropathy secondary to nutritional deficiencies. The chronic pain and suffering experienced by HIV-infected children with wasting syndrome is one of the most challenging to effectively treat and relieve.[39,40]

Neurologic and neuromuscular pain syndromes are common in HIV-infected children. These include hypertonicity, spasticity, peripheral neuropathies, static and progressive encephalopathy, herpes zoster, and myopathy. Skin and soft tissue complications of HIV that are associated with both acute and chronic pain and discomfort include infections (fungal, viral, bacterial) as well as chronic adenopathy, adenitis, and parotitis. HIV-infected children with malignancies have cancer-associated pain syndromes in addition to their HIV-associated symptoms.[11,15,34,38,41–43]

TREATMENT-RELATED PAIN

The procedure-related pain experienced by children with HIV disease is similar to the procedure-related pain experienced by children with cancer.

Published studies indicate that for children with cancer, the pain associated with diagnostic and therapeutic procedures can be more stressful than the disease itself. Common painful procedures, many of which are recurrent, include venipunctures, nasogastric and gastrostomy tube placement, lumbar punctures, and intravenous infusions. The fear, anxiety, and stress associated with medical procedures may be worse than the pain associated with the procedure and needs to be addressed in a comprehensive approach to pain management.[44–48]

A chronic cause of pain experienced by HIV-infected children that significantly affects quality of life is related to the side effects and toxicities of the multiple medications used, especially antiretroviral medications. A detailed description of the specific side effects of each antiretroviral is available in published pediatric treatment guidelines.[49] Many of the antiretroviral medications cause abdominal discomfort, nausea, and diarrhea. This is especially true of the protease inhibitors as a class but is also seen with the nucleoside analogues didanosine and zidovudine. Other painful side effects associated with many antiretrovirals include fatigue, anorexia, headache, pancreatitis, and neuropathy. A unique side effect of efavirenz that affects quality of life is altered mental status, including irritability, amnesia, impaired concentration, hallucinations, and nightmares. Patients often need to continue on the medications causing these symptoms and are asked to "live with" these side effects or risk development of resistance and disease progression. In addition to the pain associated with antiretroviral therapy, the stress of adherence to these complex regimens has an independent adverse impact on quality of life.

PAIN ASSESSMENT AND MANAGEMENT

The goals of pain management in HIV-infected children are multifaceted and include (1) reducing the incidence and severity of acute and chronic pain while providing appropriately aggressive medical therapy; (2) providing adequate pharmacologic pain control with minimal side effects; (3) utilizing nonpharmacologic approaches to pain management; (4) educating children and families to communicate about pain; (5) relieving suffering; and (6) addressing quality of life issues, especially in cases of terminal illness. In children with end-stage disease, pain management often needs to take precedence over other aspects of medical care, including antiretroviral therapy.[50,51]

Unrelieved pain can have physical and psychological consequences that negatively affect the survival and quality of life of children. Anand and associates investigated the impact of the addition of fentanyl to the anesthetic regimen of nitrous oxide and tubocurarine in preterm infants undergoing ligation of a patent ductus arteriosus. Compared with infants who received fentanyl, infants who did not receive fentanyl had evidence of stress responses following surgery with increased catecholamines, growth hormone, glucose, corticosteroids, and insulin suppression. Infants who did not receive fentanyl had evidence of postoperative endogenous protein breakdown with significantly increased urinary 3-methylhistidine/creatinine ratio. None of the infants in the study displayed any outward clinical evidence of pain during the surgery.[52]

The main limitation in preventing children from receiving appropriate palliative care and pain management is the lack of appreciation of pain associated with the disease and its treatment. In general, physicians are not adequately trained in pain assessment and management, and many do not appreciate that newborns and infants experience pain. Specific barriers to management of pain in HIV-infected children include (1) the difficulty of assessing pain in young children; (2) the difficulty of assessing pain in children with neurologic impairment; (3) parental denial of their children's disease; (4) resistance to the use of narcotics by families who have a history of drug use; (5) unfounded fears about the addiction potential and the physical dangers of opioids (including respiratory depression); and (6) resistance by clinicians to treat pain in children because of myths such as the following: children lie about pain to get attention; children who can fall asleep or who can play cannot be in pain; and children who deny pain or do not complain are not in pain.[5,34,53–56]

Even when physicians are aggressive in pain management, family members or caregivers may be resistant. Parental guilt concerning HIV infection can be profound and fosters denial of the severity of the illness and its associated pain. Additionally, the use of pain medications such as opioids may be perceived as heralding disease progression and death, thereby increasing resistance to pain assessment and treatment. Because the treatment of HIV infection is complex, pain management and other supportive care efforts can be overlooked during an acute crisis or hospital admission.[57–59]

The first step in pain assessment is to think and ask about pain regularly. Pain assessment should be part of routine health maintenance in children with chronic life-limiting illnesses. Signs and symptoms that should alert the clinician to the potential that pain is present include listlessness, crying, wincing, change in mood, irritability, change in sleeping pattern, change in appetite, lower activity level, loss of concentration, loss of playfulness, and loss of interest in daily activities. The various characteristics of pain, which should be included in an assessment, are intensity, duration, distribution, and factors that increase or decrease pain. A child's developmental level and parental judgment and insight into pain are important factors to consider in an evaluation. Several pain assessment instruments are available that are age- and developmentally appropriate for children. These include the Poker Chip Tool, Visual Analogue Scales, Oucher Scale, and the Wong-Baker Faces scale (Table 20–2).[60–70] Many clinicians use the Wong-Baker Faces scale, which is shown in Figure 20–1.

PHARMACOLOGIC MANAGEMENT OF PAIN

A simple, validated, and effective stepwise method for treating acute and chronic pain in patients with cancer has been devised by the World Health Organization (WHO) (Fig. 20–2).[71,72] This is based on incremental use of stronger pain medications in conjunction with ongoing pain assessments and treatment of side effects with adjunctive therapies. An adaptation of the WHO pain ladder used for HIV-infected children at the FXB Center for Children in Newark, New Jersey, is presented in Table 20–3 and includes the commonly used analgesics.

Table 20–2
Pain Assessment Instruments

INSTRUMENT	DESCRIPTION
Poker Chip Tool	This instrument rates pain based on "pieces of hurt" from "a little bit of hurt" to "the most hurt you could ever have." The child is asked to choose from a horizontal line of four poker chips, the number of chips that best corresponds to the intensity of his/her pain with the first chip on the left being the least. The number of "pieces of hurt" (1–4) is recorded on a pain assessment flow sheet.
Visual Analogue Scales	This instrument is either a horizontal or a vertical line with verbal, facial, or numerical end points designed to represent the two extremes of pain intensity. Children are asked to indicate the strength of their pain by marking the line from the left (no pain) end point. These scales are best for children over the age of 7 or 8.
Oucher Scale	This scale consists of six photographs of a young child's face indicating various intensities of pain. The photographs are ranked from 0 ("no hurt") to 5 ("biggest hurt you could ever have") with a vertical scale with number 0–100 running next to the pictures. The child is asked to choose the picture that is most similar to the way he/she feels. Older children can use the number scale. Culturally sensitive photographs are available.
Wong-Baker Faces Scale	This scale consists of six drawings of a face indicating various intensities of pain, ranging from face 0, which represents a happy face with no pain, to face 5, which represents the most pain you can imagine. The face number is recorded on a pain assessment flow sheet.
FLACC Behavioral Scale	This is a scale that can be used in young children who may not be able to accurately verbalize pain and discomfort. FLACC is an acronym for Face, Legs, Activity, Cry and Consolability and the scale consists of five behavioral indicators. Each indicator is rated on a 3-point scale (0,1,2) yielding a total score ranging from 0–10. The FLACC scale is used for children 29 days to 4 years old and developmentally impaired children.
CRIES Scale	This is a neonatal pain scale that consists of five physiologic and behavioral indicators. CRIES is an acronym for Crying, Requires 02 for saturation >95%, Increased HR and BP, Expression, and Sleeplessness. Each indicator is rated on a 3-point scale (0,1,2) yielding a total score ranging from 0 to 10.

WONG-BAKER FACES SCALE

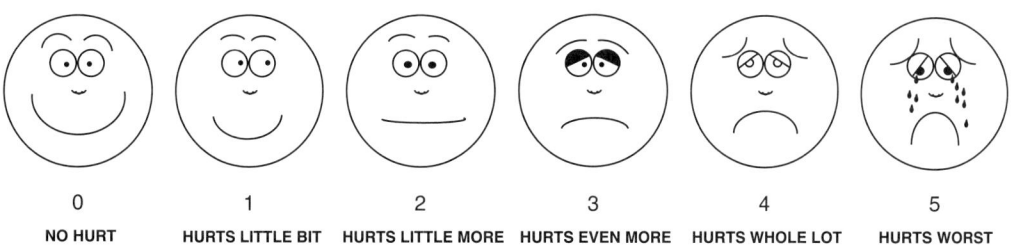

Instruction:
1. Explain to child that each face is for a person who feels happy because there is no pain (hurt) or sad because there some or a lot of pain:
   Face 0 is very happy because there is no hurt.
   Face 1 - hurts just a little bit.
   Face 2 - hurts a little more.
   Face 3 - hurts even more.
   Face 4 - hurts a whole lot.
   Face 5 - hurts as much as you can imagine, although you don't have to cry to feel this bad.
2. Ask child to choose the face that best describes their own pain. Record the number under the chosen face on pain assessment record.

Figure 20–1. Wong-Baker Faces Scale. (From Wong DL, et al: Wong's Essentials of Pediatric Nursing, 6/e. St. Louis, Mosby; 2001:1301; with permission.)

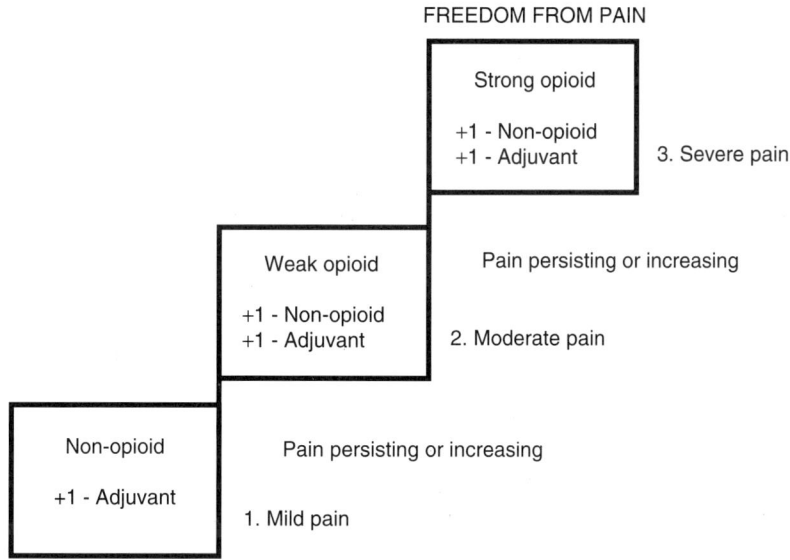

Figure 20–2. WHO analgesic ladder: management of pain in cancer.

The general approach to pediatric pain management should be a preventative one, with the continuous use of medications rather than as-needed dosing. This is especially important in infants, young children, and neurologically impaired children who cannot express a need for pain medication.

Table 20-3
Pain Management for HIV-Infected Infants and Children

MEDICATION	STARTING DOSE*, ROUTE, AND FREQUENCY	MAXIMUM DOSE
Mild pain		
Acetaminophen	10–15 mg/kg PO q4–6h	60 mg/kg/day or 4 gm/day
	15–20 mg/kg rectally q4h	
Aspirin	10–15 mg/kg PO q6h	60 mg/k/gday or 4 gm/day
Ibuprofen	4–10 mg/kg PO q6–8h	40 mg/kg/day
Naproxen	5–7 mg/kg PO q8–12h	15 mg/kg/day
Ketorolac	0.5 mg/kg PO q6h	
	Assess pain relief. If not relieved, go to MODERATE PAIN	
Moderate pain	Continue above and ADD weak opioid	
Codeine	0.5–1 mg/kg PO q4h	60 mg/day
Hydrocodone with acetaminophen	0.2 mg/kg PO	4 g/day or 75 mg/kg/day (acetaminophen component)
	Assess pain relief. If not relieved, go to SEVERE PAIN	
Severe pain	Continue nonopioid medication if tolerated and ADD stronger opioid	
Morphine	0.2–0.4 mg/kg PO q4h	No maximum, titrate to effect
	0.1–0.15 mg/kg IM or SC q3–4h	
	0.08–0.1 mg/kg IV q2h	
	0.05–0.06 mg/kg/hr IV infusion	
Morphine timed release (MS-Contin)	0.3–0.6 mg/kg PO q12h	No maximum, titrate to effect
Methadone	0.1 mg/kg IV or PO q4h initially for two or three doses, then q6–12h	No maximum, titrate to effect
Oxycodone	0.2 mg/kg PO q3–4hr	No maximum, titrate to effect
Fentanyl (transdermal)	25 µg/hr (children over 50 kg)	No maximum, titrate to effect
Assess pain relief. If inadequate, increase dosages of opioids until comfort is achieved or limited by side effects. Consider adding adjunctive medications such as tricyclic antidepressants for neuropathic pain and sleep disorders.		
Monitor for side effects of pain medications. Opioid side effects include nausea and vomiting, constipation, miosis, pruritus, urinary retention, and respiratory depression. Treat opioid-related side effects early and aggressively using antiemetics and laxatives. Nonsteroidal anti-inflammatories inhibit platelet aggregation and may cause gastrointestinal irritation and bleeding with chronic use.		

*All dosages should be modified based on individual circumstances. These represent starting dosages. Opioid doses can be increased steadily dependent on need until pain is relieved or dose limited by side effects. For infants younger than 3 months of age, initial dosages of opioids should be one quarter to one third the doses listed above.

Therapy should be individualized for each patient. Intramuscular and subcutaneous routes of administration should be avoided when possible in favor of oral, transdermal, or intravenous routes. Side effects of analgesics should be monitored for and treated. Although side effects are not indications for discontinuing analgesics, switching from one opioid to another may alleviate side effects. Consultation with a pain management service should be considered when available.[60,73,74]

Opioids are the backbone of the pharmacologic management of pain and can be safely used in infants and children. It is important for practitioners to be aware of the common side effects of opioids, such as constipation, nausea, vomiting, pruritus, and sedation. Constipation should be anticipated with chronic opioid use and treated prophylactically. Nausea should be addressed aggressively with antiemetics such as prochlorperazine (Compazine), trimethobenzamide (Tigan), ondansetron (Zofran), and granisetron (Kytril). Respiratory depression is an uncommon side effect and is dose dependent.[75–80]

Tolerance, which is a state in which an individual is less susceptible to the effects of a drug, is commonly seen with the chronic use of opioids. Upward dose adjustments are frequently necessary.

Physical dependence, which is manifested by a physiologic abstinence syndrome upon withdrawal of opioids, can occur with long-term use. Children can be gradually weaned off of this physiologic state of dependence if pain medication is no longer necessary. Tolerance and physical dependence should not be confused with addiction, which is a psychological disorder characterized by a behavior pattern of compulsive drug use and preoccupation with drug acquisition. Children treated with opioids for chronic pain rarely become addicted.[60,74]

Adjuvants are medications whose primary indication is not for pain but which can be used as supplemental therapy for pain management and the management of opioid-related side effects. Tricyclic antidepressants, such as amitriptyline, and anticonvulsants, such as phenytoin and gabapentin, are often used for neuropathic pain. Other adjuvants include laxatives, antiemetics, steroids, anxiolytics (benzodiazepines), and barbiturates for sedation.[46,79,81–84]

MANAGEMENT OF PROCEDURE-RELATED PAIN

Many techniques are available to minimize pain from medical procedures. Adequate preparation of children and families for the procedure is an important first step. It is helpful to give a simple and age-appropriate explanation to all children and anyone accompanying them about what the child can expect during the procedure. Allow the parents to be with their children during the procedure. If it is anticipated that the child will have repeated procedures, provide appropriate pain management starting with the first time the procedure is performed.

Pharmacologic and nonpharmacologic interventions during painful tests or therapies should be utilized jointly. EMLA (Eutectic Mixture of Local Anesthetic) is a topical anesthetic consisting of a mixture of prilocaine and lidocaine. It is highly effective if applied 60 minutes prior to venipuncture or lumbar puncture. Nonpharmacologic techniques such as relaxation, hypnosis, play therapy, visualization, and particularly distraction should be applied in the control of procedure-related pain.[85]

Pharmacologic management also includes the use of conscious sedation for more invasive procedures. Conscious sedation is a medically controlled state of depressed consciousness obtained through the administration of medications to obtund, dull, and reduce the intensity of pain and awareness. Through conscious sedation, the patient's ability to maintain a patent airway is retained, there is no loss of protective reflexes, and the patient retains the ability to respond appropriately to physical stimulation or simple verbal commands. Guidelines for the monitoring and managing of children receiving conscious sedation have been published and include the need for a dedicated person, not involved in the procedure itself, to provide ongoing cardiopulmonary monitoring.[86]

GUIDING PRINCIPLES OF PALLIATIVE CARE AND HOSPICE SERVICES

HIV infection is an unpredictable disease in infants, children, and adolescents with multisystem involvement resulting in a chronic and very complex illness. It is a multigenerational disease, because other family members, especially parents, are also infected and have varying symptoms and substantial psychosocial problems. At the onset of the HIV epidemic, most perinatally infected infants died before they reached the age of 4 years, but with improvements in antiretroviral therapy, prophylaxis for opportunistic infections, and good supportive care, many are now long-term survivors living well into the teen-aged years and beyond, and many have multiorgan system disease.[42,87]

Palliative care for children with chronic, multisystem, and life-limiting disease, such as HIV, should ensure the child's comfort and maximum function through the course of their illness. Children need to know about their disease, which raises the difficult issue of disclosure of diagnosis. Studies on disclosure of diagnosis have been based on children with cancer and have shown that, in general, disclosure should occur some time after the age of 6 years and that this adds to the quality of life for the child and the family. Age-appropriate disclosure may affect adherence to complex medical regimens and therefore has specific importance in perinatal HIV infection. The unique characteristics of HIV infection make disclosure more difficult than the disclosure of cancer, especially to those outside the family. These unique characteristics include social stigmatization and the multigenerational nature of the infection. Nevertheless, there is a growing consensus among care providers of HIV-infected children that disclosure is as important in this disease as in cancer. In general, children should be told about their illness, its treatment, and its consequences, in accordance with the United

Nations convention on the rights of children. During this time, they need to be supported and loved and should participate in decisions appropriate to their age and understanding.[37,87,88]

At end-stage disease, children should know they are dying and be given the opportunity to discuss their fears with their loved ones. Likewise, families of a dying child also need to be knowledgeable, supported, and active participants in decisions about end-of-life care for their child. Health care providers need to recognize the multiple difficulties and psychosocial issues in end-of-life care, including ambivalence, fear, isolation, anger, loss of control, helplessness, and sadness. The physician needs to maintain a physical presence that is compassionate, recognizing the need to relieve the multiple causes of pain and suffering while balancing the need for restorative care (disease-specific management with aggressive antiretroviral therapies and prophylaxis and treatment of opportunistic infections) and supportive care (nutrition, pain management, and other aspects of palliative care). The guiding ethical principles of palliative care include autonomy, beneficence, non-malfeasance, and justice. Thus, the family and child are full partners with the health-care team in management decisions, the child's best interests are paramount, care is provided in an atmosphere of kindness, and access to appropriate palliative care is maintained.[15,89–94]

The continuum of palliative care for HIV-infected children begins from the time an HIV-infected woman becomes pregnant through the course of disease and eventual death of her child. Ideally, pregnant women should receive comprehensive prenatal care, which is most important for the well-being of the infant and mother. For HIV-infected children, all care should be aggressive, and during the course of illness some types of restorative care are also the best palliative care. For example, the prevention of *Pneumocystis carinii* pneumonia with co-trimoxazole oral prophylaxis is compatible with a continuum of palliative care that provides comfort by avoiding the substantial morbidity of this infection. Other treatments for HIV disease complications that improve quality of life include antiretroviral therapy (except at the end of life), treatment of and continuing prophylaxis for selected opportunistic infections (e.g., *Pneumocystis carinii* pneumonia, cryptococcal meningitis, toxoplasmosis, cytomegalovirus retinitis, herpes simplex virus infection), and the prevention of recurrent bacterial infections. The use of antiretroviral therapy has had a significant impact on quality of life by improving survival, prolonging the time free from opportunistic infection, and improving and maintaining immunologic health. However, at end-stage disease, decisions relating to the continuation of antiretroviral therapy must be made, balancing the ultimate futility of current treatment after a certain point and the side effects of the medications. Nutrition is an important part of supportive care and a critical component in health maintenance while adding to quality of life.[39,95,96]

Although HIV-infected children can show great variability in the clinical course of their disease, end-stage disease is characterized by the progression to CDC class C3 disease (severe clinical disease with substantial immunosuppression). HIV encephalopathy and wasting syndrome, which may be associated with cytomegalovirus infection, cryptosporidiosis, and atypical mycobacterial infection, are commonly part of this progression. End-stage disease is also associated with the development of HIV-specific malignant disease, such as leiomyosarcoma and central nervous system lymphoma. Multiple organ failure is evident in end-stage disease, and despite aggressive antiretroviral therapy, high HIV RNA load persists with progressive loss of CD4+ lymphocytes. At this stage, there is a shift from restorative care to more supportive care; the physician and the family therefore need to recognize when end-stage disease is present and hospice care is an appropriate option.[21,29,34,93,97–100]

CRITICAL COMPONENTS OF END-OF-LIFE CARE

At some point in the care of children with AIDS, the issue of medical futility in continuing restorative care is raised by the child, the family, or a health care worker. A discussion with the family about the medical status and prognosis needs to be initiated at this point, including an age-appropriate discussion of death and dying with the child. The components and meaning of a "do not resuscitate" (DNR) order should be explained and a joint plan developed to recognize the need for control by the patient and family and to ensure a comfortable and pain-free death at home, in the hospital, or in a hospice setting. It is important that this plan is recorded in the medical records. If a conflict or disagreement arises between the patient's family and health care providers, the case should be referred to an ethics committee.

The discussion of the dying process should include signs and symptoms of impending death with assurances to the family about continuous support. Implementation of the end-of-life care plan includes withdrawal of interventions that detract from quality of life (unnecessary medication and procedures), written notification to community ambulance and emergency room services of the child's DNR status, and, if not already done, referral to a hospice program. All DNR orders should be reviewed regularly with the health-care team and family. Despite obvious difficulties and sensitivities, this is an appropriate time to discuss the role of autopsy, including benefits and drawbacks and its importance in adding to the knowledge of this tragic disease.

At the time of death, the health-care and case-management teams need to be available to make funeral arrangements and complete the death certificate. Bereavement support for survivors should be provided, along with an opportunity for the family to discuss the cause of death with supportive professionals. Finally, programs that care for children with chronic terminal illnesses such as HIV infection and AIDS need to arrange appropriate opportunity for staff to grieve.

LIMITATIONS IN PROVIDING PALLIATIVE CARE AND HOSPICE SERVICES

Barriers to the provision of palliative and hospice care to HIV-infected children exist. Perinatal HIV infection is a family disease. Guilt, denial of disease progression, and resistance to the use of opioids and hospice services are often seen. The course of HIV infection is unpredictable, and physicians have difficulty knowing when the child is truly dying. Clinicians who are preoccupied with the management of HIV infection sometimes neglect adverse symptoms and offer pain and symptom management only in the terminal phase of the disease. Few hospice services are designed specifically for children. Methods of delivering pain and symptom management to children throughout the disease, rather than at some arbitrary endpoint, are needed.[11,56]

The research agenda for palliative care and hospice services has been mainly limited to descriptive studies, apart from clinical trials of pain management in patients with end-stage cancer. The research agenda for non-cancer patients, and children in particular, needs to be developed and expanded. The development of research programs in palliative and hospice care will partly stimulate educational and training programs at all levels of medical training. Unfortunately, there is little attention paid in most medical school curricula to palliative care, and even less in residency training programs, mainly because there are few trained specialists in palliative and hospice care who can serve as role models, educators, and research leaders. A tradition of palliative care teaching and research is seen in nursing schools. Collaborative multidiscipline programs will therefore provide the best environment to provide palliative and hospice care while enhancing training, education, and research.[53,54,93]

Table 20–4
Principles for Providing a Continuum of Palliative Care and Improving Quality of Life for Children with HIV

1. Palliative care begins at the time of diagnosis.
2. Pain management is critical and includes:
   a. Thinking about the possibility of pain on an ongoing basis.
   b. Regular assessment and evaluation of pain.
   c. Aggressive pharmacologic and nonpharmacologic interventions.
   d. Reassessment of pain and adjustment of treatment.
3. Assess for and alleviate physical and psychological suffering.
4. Provide supportive care as appropriate, including:
   a. Nutritional support
   b. Psychological/psychiatric services
   c. Social work services
   d. Rehabilitative services
5. Evaluate the need for a shift to end-of-life care on an ongoing intermittent basis as disease progresses.
6. Implement hospice care when appropriate.
7. Respect the spiritual and bereavement needs of child, family, and staff.

There are two essential qualities that physicians and other caregivers must possess to meet the obligation to provide care and relieve suffering. The first quality is *humility*, the willingness to listen to others, including patients and their families and to avoid arrogance, which is the greatest threat to the well-being of patients and biggest deterrent to the professional growth of physicians and other caregivers. The second quality is *perseverance* in the commitment to work each day to be effective caregivers and strong patient advocates, and to meet the trust of families and children.

The continuum of palliative care, when all is said and done, is about quality of life (Table 20–4). Quality of life means having the encouragement and support to dream about tomorrow; to wake up each day with purposes and goals while living, playing, and working as normally as possible in the home, school, or workplace; to be free of pain and other symptoms through the progression of the disease; and to be held and comforted at the time of death by loved ones. The quality of life for most individuals depends on the presence of others and the actions of others. A child with a life-limiting illness, regardless of diagnosis, socioeconomic status, or geographic location, should receive a continuum of palliative care and have access to hospice services that give them the best quality of life and ease the burden of dying.

REFERENCES

1. Martinson IM: An international perspective on palliative care for children. J Palliat Care 1996;12:13–15.
2. Oleske JM, Czarniecki L: Continuum of palliative care: Lessons from caring for children infected with HIV. Lancet 1999;354:1287–1290.
3. World Health Organization: The World Health Report 1995: Bridging the gap. Report of the Director General. Geneva, WHO, 1995.
4. World Health Organization: Report on the global HIV/AIDS epidemic, June 1996. Geneva, UNAIDS/WHO, 1998.
5. Davies B, Steele R: Challenges in identifying children for palliative care. J Palliat Care 1996;12:5–8.
6. Davies B: The development of pediatric palliative care. In Doyle D, Hanks G, MacDonald N (eds): Oxford Textbook of Palliative Medicine, 2nd ed. Oxford, Oxford University Press, 1998, pp 1097–1106.
7. Levetown M: Ethical aspects of pediatric palliative care. J Palliat Care 1996;12:35–39.
8. Storey P: Primer of Palliative Care. Gainesville, FL, American Academy of Hospice & Palliative Medicine, 1996.
9. Frager G: Pediatric palliative care: Building the model, bridging the gaps. J Palliat Care 1996;12: 9–12.
10. Frager G, Shapiro B: Pediatric palliative care and pain management. In Holland JC (ed): Psycho-Oncology. New York, Oxford Press, 1998.
11. Ferris F, Flannery J (eds): A comprehensive guide for the care of persons with HIV disease—Module 4: palliative care. Toronto, Mount Sinai Hospital/Casey House, 1995.
12. Boland M, Burr C, Harvey D: Pediatric AIDS revisited: Family, social and legal issues. Semin Pediatr Infect Dis 1995;6:40–45.
13. Oleske JM, Ruben-Hale A: Enhancing supportive care and promoting quality of life: Clinical practice guidelines. Pediatr AIDS HIV Infect Fetus Adolesc 1995;6:187–203.
14. Foley F, Flannery S: AIDS palliative care: Challenging the palliative paradigm. J Palliat Care 1995;11:34–37.
15. Grothe TM, Brody RV: Palliative care for HIV disease. J Palliat Care 1995;11:48–49.
16. Reiter G, Kudler N: HIV and palliative care: Part I and II. AIDS Clin Care 1996;8:21–34.
17. Von Gunten CF, Martinez J, Neely KJ, von Roenn JH: AIDS and palliative medicine: Medical treatment issues. J Palliat Care 1995;11:5–9.
18. Lewis SY, Haiken HJ, Hoyt LG: Living beyond the odds: A psychosocial perspective of long-term survivors of pediatric human immunodeficiency virus infection. J Dev Behav Pediatr 1994;15:S12–17.
19. Liben S: Pediatric palliative medicine: Obstacles to overcome. J Palliat Care 1996;12:24–28.
20. Fleischman AR, Nolan K, Dubler NN, et al: Caring for gravely ill children. Pediatrics 1994;94:433–439.
21. Attig T: Beyond pain: The existential suffering of children. J Palliat Care 1996;12:20–23.
22. Robinson WM, Ravilly S, Berde, et al: End-of-life care in cystic fibrosis. Pediatrics 1996;100:205–209.
23. Walco GA, Cassidy RC, Schechter NL: The ethics of pain control in infants and children. N Engl J Med 1994;331:541–544.
24. Martinson IM: Hospice care for children: Past, present, and future. J Pediatr Oncol Nurs 1993;10:93–98.
25. American Academy of Pediatrics Committee on Psychosocial Aspects of Child and Family Health: The pediatrician and childhood bereavement. Pediatrics 1992;89:516–518.
26. Davies B, Clarke D, Connaughty S, et al: Caring for dying children: Nurses' experiences. Pediatr Nurs 1996;22:500–507.
27. Faulkner KW, Armstrong-Dailey A: Care of the dying child. In Pizzo P, Poplack D (eds): Principles and Practice of Pediatric Oncology, 3rd ed. Philadelphia, Lippincott-Raven, 1997, pp 1349–1351.
28. Goldman A: Home care of the dying child. J Palliat Care 1996;12:16–19.
29. Institute of Medicine: Approaching death: Improving care at the end of life. Washington, DC, National Academy Press, 1997.

30. Lauer M, Carmitta B: Home care for dying children: A nursing model. J Pediatr 1980;97:1032–1035.
31. Martinson IM, Moldow DG, Armstrong GO, et al: Home care for children dying of cancer. Res Nurs Health 1986;9:11–16.
32. Martinson IM: Pediatric hospice nursing. Ann Rev Nurs Res 1995;13:195–214.
33. Stevens MM, Jones P, O'Riordan E: Family responses when a child with cancer is in palliative care. J Palliat Care 1996;12:51–55.
34. Czarniecki L, Boland M, Oleske JM: Pain in children with HIV disease. PAAC Notes 1993;5:492–495.
35. Anand KJ, Craig KD: New perspectives on the definition of pain. Pain 1996;67:3–6.
36. Carr DB, Jacox AK, Chapman CR, et al: Acute pain management: Operative or medical procedures and trauma, clinical practice guidelines. AHCPR publication No. 92-0032. Rockville, MD, US Public Health Service, Agency for Health Care Policy and Research, 1992.
37. Oleske JM: The many needs of the HIV-infected child. Hosp Pract 1994;29:81–87.
38. Hirschfeld S, Moss H, Dragisic K, et al: Pain in pediatric human immunodeficiency virus infection: Incidence and characteristics in a single-institution pilot study. Pediatrics 1996;98:449–452.
39. Oleske JM, Rothpletz-Puglia PM, Winter H. Historical perspectives on the evolution in understanding the importance of nutritional care in pediatric HIV infection. J Nutr 1996;126:2616S–2619S.
40. Connolly GM, Hawkins D, Harcourt-Webster JN, et al: Oesophageal symptoms, their causes, treatment and prognosis in patients with acquired immunodeficiency syndrome. Gut 1989a;30:1033–1039.
41. Futterman D, Hein K: Medical care of HIV-infected adolescents. AIDS Clin Care 1992;4:95–98.
42. Grubman S, Gross E, Lerner-Weiss N, et al: Older children and adolescents with perinatally acquired HIV infection. Pediatrics 1995;95:657–666.
43. Epstein LG, Sharer LR, Oleske JM, et al: Neurological manifestations of human immunodeficiency virus infection in children. Pediatrics 1986;78:678–687.
44. World Health Organization: Cancer pain relief and palliative care in children. Geneva, WHO, 1998, p 19.
45. Rhiner M, Ferrell BR, Shapiro B, et al: The experience of pediatric cancer pain, part II: Management of pain. J Pediatr Nurs 1994;9:380–387.
46. Portenoy RK, Waldman SD: Adjuvant analgesics in pain management: Part 1. J Pain Symptom Manage 1994;9:390–391.
47. Katz ER, Kellerman J, Siegel SE: Distress behavior in children with cancer undergoing medical procedures: Developmental considerations. J Consult Clin Psychol 1980;48:356–365.
48. Breitbart W, Rosenfeld B, Passik S, et al: The undertreatment of pain ambulatory AIDS patients. Pain 1996;65:239–245.
49. Centers for Disease Control and Prevention: Guidelines for the use of antiretroviral agents in pediatric HIV infection. MMWR Morb Mortal Wkly Rep 1998;47: 1–43.
50. Yaster M, Schechter N: Pain and human immunodeficiency virus infection in children. Pediatrics 1996;98:455–456.
51. Galloway KS, Yaster M: Pain and symptom control in terminally ill children. Pediatr Clin North Am 2000; 47(3):711–746.
52. Anand KJS, Sippell WG, Aynsley-Green A: Randomized trial of fentanyl anaesthesia in preterm babies undergoing surgery: Effects on the stress response. Lancet 1987;1:243–247.
53. Billings JA, Block S: Palliative care in undergraduate medical education. JAMA 1997;278:733–738.
54. Charlton R: Medical education—addressing the needs of the dying child. Palliat Med 1996;10: 240–246.
55. Cook LA, Watchko JF: Decision making for the critically ill neonate near the end of life. J Perinatol 1996;16:133–136.
56. Corner J: Is there a research paradigm for palliative care? Palliat Med 1996;10:201–208.
57. Oleske J, Boland M: When a child with a chronic condition needs hospitalization. Hosp Pract 1997; 32:167–191.
58. Pellegrino ED: Emerging ethical issues in palliative care. JAMA 1998;279:1521–1522.
59. Nelson LJ, Rushton CH, Cranford RE, et al: Forgoing medically provided nutrition and hydration in pediatric patients. J Law Med Ethics 1995;23:33–46.
60. Agency for Health Care Policy and Research: Acute pain management in infants, children, and adolescents: Operative and Medical Procedures Quick Reference Guide for Clinicians. Publ. 92-0020. Rockville, MD, Department of Health and Human Services, 1993.
61. Baker CM, Wong DK: QUEST: A process of pain assessment in children. Orthoped Nurs 1987;6:11–21.
62. Bieri D, Reeve RA, Champion GD, et al: The faces pain scale for the self-assessment of the severity of pain experienced by children: Development, initial validation, and preliminary investigation for ratio scale properties. Pain 1990;41:139–150.
63. Champion GD, Goodenough B, von Baeyer CL, et al: Measurement of pain by self-report. In Finley GA, McGrath JP (eds): Measurement of Pain in Infants and Children. Seattle, IASP Press, 1998, p 141.
64. Craig KD, Grunau RVE: Neonatal pain perception and behavioral measurement. In Anand KSJ, McGrath PJ (eds): Pain in Neonates. New York, Elsevier Science, 1993, pp 67–105.
65. Hain RDW: Pain scales in children: A review. Medicine 1997;11:341–350.
66. Hester NKO, Foster R, Kristensen K: Measurement of pain in children: Generalizability and validity of the pain ladder and the poker chip tool. In Tyler DC, Kane EJ (eds): Advances in Pain Research Therapy. New York, Raven Press, 1990, pp 79–84.
67. McGrath PJ, Johnson G, Goodman JT, et al: CHEOPS: A behavioral scale for rating postoperative

pain in children. In Fields HL (ed): Advances in Pain Research and Therapy. New York, Raven Press, 1985, pp 395–402.
68. Robertson J: Pediatric pain assessment: Validation of a multidimensional tool. Pediatr Nurs 1993;19:209–213.
69. Wong DL: Whaley and Wong's Essentials of Pediatric Nursing, 5th ed. St. Louis, Mosby-Yearbook, 1997.
70. Varni JW, Seid M, Rode CA: The PEDSQL: Measurement model for the Pediatric Quality of Life Inventory. Med Care 1999;37:126–139.
71. Jacox A, Cart DB, Payne R, et al: Management of cancer pain: Clinical practice guideline no. 9. AHCPR publication no. 94-0592. Rockville, MD, US Public Health Service, Agency for Health Care Policy and Research, 1994.
72. WHO Expert Committee: World Health Organization: Cancer pain relief and palliative care. WHO Technical Report Series 804. Geneva, WHO, 1990.
73. deStouz ND, Bruera E, Suarez-Almazor M: Opioid rotation for toxicity reduction in terminal cancer patients. J Pain Symptom Manage 1995;10:378–384.
74. McGarth PJ, Finley GA: Attitudes and beliefs about medication and pain management in children. J Palliat Care 1996;12:46–50.
75. Berde CB, Lehn BM, Yee JD, et al: Patient-controlled analgesia in children and adolescents: A randomized, prospective comparison with intramuscular morphine for postoperative analgesia. J Pediatr 1991;118: 460–466.
76. Collins JJ, Grier HE, Kinney HC, et al: Control of severe pain in children with terminal malignancy. J Pediatr 1995;126:653–657.
77. Collins JJ, Grier HE, Stehna NF, et al: Regional anesthesia for pain associated with terminal pediatric malignancy. Pain 1996;65:63–69.
78. Kenny NP, Frager G: Refractory symptoms and terminal sedation of children: Ethical issues and practical management. J Palliat Care 1996;12:40–45.
79. McGrath PA: Development of the World Health Organization guidelines on cancer pain relief and palliative care in children. J Pain Symptom Manage 1996;12:87–92.
80. McGrath PA: Pharmacological interventions for alleviating children's pain. In McGrath PA (ed): Pain in Children: Nature, Assessment and Treatment, 2nd ed. Amsterdam, Elsevier, 1990.
81. Roila F, Aapro M, Stewart A: Optimal selection of antiemetics in children receiving cancer chemotherapy. Support Care Cancer 1998;6:215–220.
82. Siever BA: Pain management and potentially life-shortening analgesia in the terminally ill child: The ethical implications for pediatric nurses. J Pediatr Nurs 1994;9:307–312.
83. Vargas-Schaffer G, Pichard-Léandri E: Neuropathic pain in young children with cancer. Eur J Palliat Care 1996;3:95–98.
84. Watanabe S, Bruera E: Corticosteroids as adjuvant analgesics. J Pain Manage 1994;9:442–445.
85. Guttormsen AB, Nordahl SH, Olofsson J: Home application of EMLA cream prior to venipuncture. Is it feasible in pediatric ENT day care surgery? Int J Pediatr Otorhinol 1995;31:47–52.
86. Committee on Drugs: Guidelines for monitoring and management of pediatric patients during and after sedation for diagnostic and therapeutic procedures. Pediatrics 1992;89:1110–1114.
87. United Nations: Convention on the rights of children. New York, United Nations, 1991.
88. Tasker M: How can I tell you? Secrecy and disclosure with children when a family member has AIDS. Bethesda, MD, Association for the Care of Children's Health, 1992.
89. Welch K, Kessinger P, Bessinger R, et al: The clinical profile of end stage AIDS. AIDS Patient Care STD 1998;12:125–129.
90. American Academy of Pediatrics Committee on Fetus and Newborn: Perinatal care at the threshold of viability. Pediatrics 1995;96:974–976.
91. American Academy of Pediatrics Committee on Fetus and Newborn: The initiation or withdrawal of treatment for high-risk newborns. Pediatrics 1995;96:362–363.
92. Collins JJ: Intractable pain in children with terminal cancer. J Palliat Care 1996;12:29–34.
93. Committee of Bioethics on the American Academy of Pediatrics: Guidelines for forgoing life-sustaining medical treatment. Pediatrics 1994;93:532–536.
94. DeTrill M, Kovalcik R: The child with cancer: Influence of culture on truth-telling and patient care. Am NY Acad Sci 1997;809:197–210.
95. Oleske JM: Preventing disability and providing rehabilitation for infants, children and youths with HIV/AIDS. NIH publication no. 95-3850. Bethesda, MD, US Department of Health and Human Services/National Institute of Child Health and Human Development, 1995.
96. Paris JJ, Schreiber MD: Physicians' refusal to provide life-prolonging medical interventions. Clin Perinatol 1996;23:563–571.
97. McQuillan R, Finlay I: Facilitating the care of terminally ill children. J Pain Symptom Manage 1996;12: 320–324.
98. Meyers HI: Spiritual care in pediatric hospice. Am J Hospice Care 1989; 6(3):12.
99. Nelson LJ, Nelson RM: Ethics and the provision of futile, harmful or burdensome treatment to children. Crit Care Med 1992;20:427–433.
100. Rothpletz-Puglia PM: Perspectives in practice: Case report of children infected with HIV. Topics Clin Nutr 1997;12:69–77.

21

Primary Care of the HIV-Infected Infant and Child

Maggi Coyne, Kim Evans, and Celine Hanson

The incidence of perinatal transmission of HIV in the United States has dramatically declined in the last decade, with transmission rates currently reported at less than 5%.[1,2] Both the increasing use of antiretroviral therapy and modifications in obstetric practices during pregnancy and labor and delivery have been causally associated with the dramatic reduction in perinatal HIV transmission.[2-4] Perinatal HIV transmission has not, however, been eliminated and is still reported in association with high maternal viral load (related to viral resistance or lack of compliance to prescribed therapy), lack of maternal prenatal care (failed opportunities to provide antiretroviral therapy during labor and delivery or postpartum), and selected cofactors (other infections, e.g., hepatitis C virus infection; genetic predisposition, e.g., chemokine receptor expression; maternal/infant immunologic response).[3,5-8] Suggested guidelines to prevent perinatal transmission of HIV include recommendations for the care of the newly diagnosed perinatally HIV-infected child.[9] This chapter provides standards for well-child care for HIV-infected infants and children. Specific recommendations for the medical management of acute illnesses in the HIV-infected infant or child are also reviewed.

GENERAL EXAMINATION CONSIDERATIONS

During the neonatal period, the physical examination of the HIV-exposed infant does not differ significantly from that of the unexposed newborn.[10] Children born to HIV-infected mothers in this decade are likely to have antiretroviral therapy exposure in utero, at a minimum zidovudine therapy. Hence, attention to common side effects of such drug interventions are important, for example, zidovudine-induced reversible macrocytic anemia.[11] As new drug interventions to interrupt perinatal HIV transmission are more commonly used in the HIV-infected pregnant women, attention to potential adverse outcomes will need to be carefully reviewed.[9] Recent examples include reports of mitochondrial defects following nucleoside reverse transcriptase inhibitor or protease inhibitor use in both infected and HIV-exposed infants.[12,13] Such reports have prompted very careful reviews of US cohorts without identifying similar findings to date.[14-16]

In early infancy (first 6 months of life), the HIV-infected child can often be distinguished from the exposed but uninfected infant by clinical examination. Specifically, systemic signs of chronic HIV infection—lymphadenopathy, hepatomegaly, or splenomegaly—may be present as early as 3 months of age. Independent of gender, growth failure, as manifested by lower weight, height, and head circumference for age, may also distinguish infected children from their exposed but uninfected counterparts.[10,17] Without intervention, progressive growth delay or neurodevelopmental delay, or both, can be detected through 18 months of life.[18-20]

HIV-infected children require regular health care visits with their primary care providers to ensure health maintenance and prevention of disease and should follow the same schedule as their noninfected peers. These visits should follow the American Academy of Pediatrics guidelines for well-child care (6–8 weeks, 4 months, 6 months, 9 months, 1 year, 15 months, 18 months, 2 years, and then yearly). The health status of the individual HIV-infected child will determine when additional visits are needed. In addition, initiation or changes in HIV-specific therapy will determine the frequency of not only general examinations but also relevant laboratory determinations.

HIV-exposed infants should be evaluated on a similar time schedule and with appropriate HIV diagnostic tests at each visit until the diagnosis of HIV is either confirmed or eliminated (Table 21–1).[21] Nonantibody tests, such as the HIV DNA polymerase chain reaction (PCR) test, should be performed to determine whether a child born to an HIV-infected woman has acquired the infection. Two such tests are necessary to confirm the diagnosis. In children older than 6 to 12 months of life, serologic assays such as the enzyme immunoassay and Western blot tests can be used to determine the infection status of the child (see Chapter 6). Laboratory tests that should be performed on a routine basis once HIV infection is confirmed include a complete blood cell count with cell differential and platelet counts, lymphocyte subsets, and HIV RNA PCR. These should be performed at 1- to 3-month intervals but can vary based on the clinical status of the child. Serum immunoglobulin (IgG, IgA, IgM) levels can be obtained at 4 months of age. Cytomegalovirus, toxoplasmosis, and syphilis serology should be done initially and repeated after the child is older than 12 months. Urine cytomegalovirus culture should be done at birth, at 1 month, and at 6 months. A battery of chemistry evaluations (liver function tests, triglyceride levels, and pancreatic enzyme tests) may need to be performed at each visit for the child on HIV-specific therapy. Scheduled evaluations of bone marrow function and solid organ function can be important to identify early complications that relate either to primary HIV infection and its accompanying immunosuppression or to the effects of HIV-specific therapy. These can be coordinated with specialists providing HIV care to minimize duplicate tests and trauma to the child. Initial examinations for a newly diagnosed HIV-infected child include baseline chest radiographs, computed tomography or magnetic resonance imaging of the brain (if neurologic or Denver examination results are abnormal), electrocardiogram, and ophthalmologic and dental examinations.

Therapy for HIV infection is a dynamic field. Highly active antiretroviral therapy (HAART) used to minimize the viral burden in the peripheral blood and other tissues often mandates the use of medication combinations that must be monitored carefully. Guidelines for HIV therapy are discussed in detail in Chapters 9 and 10. Antiretroviral agents often interact with medications used in routine pediatric care. Anticonvulsants, antimycobacterials, antihistamines, antiarrhythmics, sedatives, and anti-reflux medications are examples of common drugs with potential for adverse interactions with HAART. Gathering an accurate drug history at each pediatric visit is very important for the general health of the HIV-infected child. Since an individual child's caregiver may change or have imperfect recollection of the child's medication history, it is important for the primary physician to communicate directly with specialists and their staff to obtain the most current medication information. This team approach to chronic HIV care cannot be understated, as it facilitates an understanding of the potential side effects of HIV-specific medications for each child and allows the primary physician to participate in monitoring for signs and symptoms of drug toxicity at each well-child visit.

Although it is often tempting to relegate the care of children with chronic HIV illness to specialists who manage their antiretroviral treatment, it is the primary care provider who is best suited to provide general care and coordinate the multiple subspecialty care that ensures optimal patient management. Working with appropriate specialists, the primary care provider can and should provide anticipatory individual and family guidance and education in relation to the child's illness. The importance of developing a consistent and strong relationship with the primary care provider cannot be overstated.[22] In the following sections, specific general examination needs of the HIV-infected infant or child are outlined.

Evaluation of Growth Parameters

Traditional measurement of growth parameters, that is, height, weight, head circumference, and weight for height, should be done at every visit and, when possible, in a consistent fashion (e.g., same scale, stadiometer) and charted on standardized growth charts. Children younger than 2 years of age should be weighed in a dry diaper only, and their length should be measured in a supine position. Children older than 2 years of age should be weighed in their underwear only, and their height measured in a standing position in bare feet. A major emphasis for growth evaluation of HIV-infected children should be placed on consistent readings that allow

Table 21–1
Suggested Evaluations for the HIV-Infected Child

VISIT	GENERAL CONSIDERATIONS	LABORATORY TESTS	RADIOGRAPHIC EXAMINATIONS	REFERRALS
First	Complete physical examination	CBC, differential, and platelet counts urinalysis	Chest radiograph	Ophthalmologic
	Growth measures	BUN, creatinine, albumin	Electrocardiogram*	Dental
	Vital signs (including blood pressure)	AST, ALT, bilirubin	Computed tomography, magnetic resonance imaging[†]	Gynecologic[‡]
	Denver Developmental Examination	Amylase, Triglyceride, cholesterol[§]		
	Immunization record review	CMV, Epstein-Barr Virus, toxoplasmosis, syphilis serology		
	Social history	CMV urine culture		
	Nutritional history	Serum immunoglobulin levels		
		CD4+ and CD8+ T cell counts[¶]		
		HIV/DNA RNA PCR[¶] HIV enzyme immunoassay/Western blot**		
Second or subsequent	Complete physical examination	CBC, differential, and platelet counts	As indicated	As indicated
	Growth measures	BUN, creatinine, albumin		
	Vital signs	ALT, AST		
	Denver Development Examination	Amylase triglyceride, cholesterol[§]		
	Immunization record review	CD4+ and CD8+ T cell counts[¶]		
	Social history	HIV RNA PCR[¶]		
	Nutritional history			

*Echocardiogram, if chest radiograph and/or electrocardiogram is abnormal.
[†]If neurologic or Denver examination is abnormal.
[‡]For all sexually active females or adolescents ≥18 years (see text).
[§]Intervals for testing depend on individual child's HIV-specific treatment.
[¶]Every 3 months or as needed: HIV DNA PCR is used in infants; HIV RNA PCR is used in children >6 months of age.
**If not already performed.
ALT, alanine transaminase; AST, aspartate transaminase; BUN, blood urea nitrogen; CBC, complete blood cell count; CMV, cytomegalovirus; PCR, polymerase chain reaction.

changes in growth curves to become quickly noticeable. Infants with rapid progression of their disease may show deviation from previous growth patterns. Growth disturbances can indicate progression of disease but can also be a sign of other complications of HIV infection. Examples include association of weight loss with secondary infections such as oral candidiasis, chronic diarrhea, fat malabsorption, and so on. Head circumference measurements should be done at every visit for the first 2 years and then every 6 months until the child is 6 years of age. Since delayed sexual maturation can often accompany wasting, Tanner staging can be done at regular intervals to evaluate growth and body maturity. Body fat composition measurements may be necessary if a child exhibits poor weight gain or other signs of wasting. Evaluation for evidence of unusual growth patterns such as lipodystrophy (truncal obesity with peripheral wasting) should be conducted at each visit to evaluate potential adverse events related to HIV-specific therapy.

Nutrition

Adequate nutritional intake is necessary for optimal growth and body function, such as proper immune function and maturation of the central nervous system. As part of regular health maintenance visits, a nutritional assessment should be made by the health care provider or, if possible, a registered dietician, to ensure adequate caloric intake with proper amounts of protein and fat. Nutritional assessments should be done every 3 months in the normally growing HIV-infected child. This will allow for early identification of abnormal patterns of nutritional intake, optimally before growth is affected. These nutritional assessments should be coupled with careful evaluation of the aforementioned growth parameter measurements. Nutrition perturbations or growth failure can be an important prognostic indicator of mortality in HIV-infected children. Aggressive measures, including the addition of appetite stimulants or physical interventions with exogenous feeding measures (feeding tubes, central venous catheters), may be needed to ensure adequate nutritional intake. Before high-calorie supplements or appetite stimulants are added to the patient's drug regimen, the HIV-infected child with clinical evidence of malnutrition should be evaluated (routine stool cultures including evaluation for ova and parasites, stool evaluation for protein, fat, and red and white blood cell content, breath hydrogen test if applicable, and radiographic studies) for underlying causes of growth failure.[23]

Neurodevelopment

Children with HIV infection can have a wide range of central nervous system sequelae, ranging from no symptoms to severe encephalopathy. The severity of HIV-related central nervous system disease has been correlated with the stage of HIV disease, age at which first symptoms appeared, rates of disease progression, and response or compliance to prescribed antiretroviral therapy.[24] Routine developmental screening such as with the Denver Developmental Screening Test should be performed as part of the routine pediatric well-child examination. This provides the primary care provider with an objective basis for detecting early evidence of developmental delay that can be coupled with collection of historical information on infant and child acquisition of developmental milestones. When deviations from routine developmental patterns are suspected, either by caregiver history or by direct health care provider observation, referral to a clinical psychologist or neurologist for comprehensive neurodevelopmental testing is indicated. Early cognitive and motor deviations in the HIV-infected child can be identified by comprehensive evaluations and may be the earliest signs of clinical failure of HIV-specific therapy.[19] Neuroimaging studies of the brain, including ultrasonography in infants and computed tomography and magnetic resonance imaging, are indicated for children with new onset or past evidence of neurologic abnormalities or developmental delay. The frequency of such testing should be tailored to the specific needs of the individual child.

Manifestations of central nervous system disease in HIV-infected children may be subtle and include expressive language delay, attention deficit or hyperactivity symptoms, lack of appropriate socialization, changes in academic achievement, and loss of daily living skills. In identifying such changes, it is important to ensure that the child is evaluated by an expert familiar with the individual child's native language and in the context of the child's cultural environment. Motor dysfunction may also manifest in subtle signs that are often overlooked, such as feeding and swallowing difficulties, articulation problems, and fine hand and finger skills. Through regular and careful neurologic and neurodevelopmental evaluation, the primary care provider is in an excellent position to assist the family in obtaining early referrals for treatment and potential prevention of progression of these HIV-related symptoms.

Oral Care and Dental Evaluations

Oral fungal lesions are common in HIV-infected children, with very few escaping infection. Topical therapy is indicated but often fails and systemic therapy is required. A thorough oral examination is indicated at each clinical visit. In addition to medical examinations of the oral cavity by the primary care provider, a dentist should examine the HIV-infected child at regular intervals. The initial referral should be made by 1 year of age, and follow-up visits are recommended every 6 to 12 months. Daily standard hygienic practices are encouraged. Advancing HIV disease and immunosuppression place the HIV-infected child at risk for oral and dental disease, including opportunistic infections, gingivitis, aphthous ulcers, caries, and abscesses. Many oral medications contain sugar, increasing the risk of caries in this population.

Eye Care and Ophthalmologic Referral

As part of routine ocular evaluation, vision screening should be performed. For the HIV-infected child, a more extensive baseline ophthalmologic examination is indicated at the time of diagnosis. Subsequent examinations are recommended annually, at a minimum. More frequent examinations may be indicated for children with severe immunosuppression, because they are at risk for ocular opportunistic infections that affect vision, such as cytomegalovirus retinitis, fungal infections, and viral infections. Early detection of such diseases is imperative to initiation of early treatment, with the goal of preserving vision. Because some HIV therapies have been associated with ocular abnormalities, children receiving such medications may also warrant more frequent eye examinations. Examples of potential ocular adverse effects from HIV-related medications are as follows:

Didanosine: retinal pigment epithelium alterations

Ethambutol: optic neuritis (decreased visual acuity)

Rifabutin: uveitis, hypopyon

Cidofovir: uveitis

Interval ophthalmologic examinations are indicated for children with new symptoms or newly diagnosed cytomegalovirus disease.

Genitourinary Evaluation

This section provides brief guidelines for genitourinary evaluations in HIV-infected children. A pelvic examination is not routinely indicated in HIV-infected girls without a history of sexual intercourse. HIV-infected females with a history of sexual activity should be evaluated. Independent of sexual activity status, a history of severe dysmenorrhea unresponsive to routine treatment, vaginal discharge, unexplained vaginal bleeding, amenorrhea, or sexual assault warrants gynecologic referral for evaluation. The Public Health Service guidelines to prevent opportunistic infection in HIV-infected individuals recommend a pelvic examination with Pap smear twice in the first year after diagnosis of HIV infection and, if the results are normal, annually thereafter.[25] Because the frequency of cervical dysplasia increases with immunosuppression, some experts advise that HIV-infected females with CD4+ counts less than 500 cells/mm^3 be evaluated every 6 months.[26,27] Family planning services should be easily accessed by the sexually active HIV-infected child. In addition to contraception, age-appropriate counseling regarding barrier precautions for safer sex should be an ongoing part of care.

PREVENTION OF INFECTIONS

Infection control for the HIV-infected child includes immunizations, both active and passive, prevention of opportunistic infections, and implementation of general measures to prevent transmission of infectious diseases.

Active Immunization

Guidelines for the protection of HIV-infected children from vaccine-preventable diseases have been revised over the past years.[25,28] Table 21–2 provides a listing of vaccines that should be delivered to HIV-infected children with the following exceptions:

1. The varicella vaccine, an attenuated live virus vaccine, is currently recommended only in asymptomatic HIV-infected children without evidence of immunosuppression. HIV-negative household contacts (HIV exposed but seronegative infants) should be immunized to protect HIV-infected children and adults.[25]

2. The measles-mumps-rubella vaccine is recommended in HIV-infected children without severe

Table 21-2
Vaccinations for the HIV-Infected Child

VACCINE	SYMPTOMATIC	ASYMPTOMATIC
Diphtheria, tetanus, and pertussis	Yes	Yes
Poliovirus, inactivated	Yes	Yes
Haemophilus influenzae type B	Yes	Yes
Hepatitis B Virus	Yes	Yes
Measles, mumps, rubella*	Yes	Yes
Varicella	No	Yes
Pneumococcal	Yes	Yes
Influenza	Yes	Yes
Hepatitis A†	Yes	Yes

*See text for indications for children with severe immunosuppression.
†As indicated for areas with endemic hepatitis A.

immunosuppression. This live virus vaccine is recommended for HIV-infected children with moderate to no immunosuppression because it poses less risk than the occurrence of natural measles.[25]

3. The rotavirus vaccine was withdrawn in July 1999. No child is currently advised to receive the rotavirus vaccine.[28]

4. A conjugate pneumococcal vaccine (PCV7) has been approved by the Food and Drug Administration (FDA) for use in children. Since the incidence of invasive infection due to *Streptococcus pneumoniae* has been reported at rates of 6.1 cases per 100 patient-years among HIV-infected children, PCV7 is recommended using the same guidelines suggested for HIV-uninfected children.[29] Namely, infants younger than 23 months should receive three doses of PCV7 at 2-month intervals up to 6 months of age, followed by a booster vaccine at 12 to 15 months of age. HIV-infected children aged 24 to 59 months are considered at high risk for pneumococcal infection, and two doses of PCV7 are recommended (2 months apart) followed in 2 months by delivery of the 23-valent pneumococcal vaccine (PCV23). For children who have already received PCV23, PCV7 can be used to prime their immunologic response, with two doses of PCV7 recommended at 2 or more months following receipt of PCV23. The use of PCV7 in children older than 5 years of age and in adults is not contraindicated. However, in older individuals, PCV7 provides protection to only 50% to 60% of the pneumococcal isolates that cause invasive disease as compared to PCV23, which provides protection to 80% to 90% of isolates. The efficacy of PCV7 as compared to PCV23 does not appear to be enhanced in older individuals.[30]

5. An annual influenza vaccine is recommended for HIV-infected children and should follow routine vaccine schedules. Current data suggest that increased viral load (RNA PCR) in HIV-infected children following influenza vaccine delivery is a rare event and should not prohibit the use of the vaccine to protect against natural influenza disease.[31]

Passive Immunization

Because unchecked HIV infection results in progressive immunologic dysfunction, antibody responses to infectious agents may be inadequate or with time may wane. Therefore, independent of vaccination status, prophylaxis following select vaccine-preventable disease exposures is indicated, as follows[32]:

Measles: human immunoglobulin within 6 days of exposure (This may be unnecessary in children who have received intravenous immunoglobulin in the 2 to 3 weeks preceding the exposure.)

Management of tetanus-prone wounds: tetanus immunoglobulin

Varicella or zoster: varicella-zoster immunoglobulin as soon as possible (within 96 hours of exposure) for children without a history of clinical varicella (This may be unnecessary in children who have received intravenous immunoglobulin in the 2 to 3 weeks preceding the exposure.)

Prevention of Opportunistic Infections

In 1999, the US Public Health Service and the Infectious Diseases Society of America published revised guidelines for the prevention of opportunistic infections in HIV-infected children and adults.[25] These recommendations contain detailed information about the prevention of infectious disease exposures, prevention of disease following exposures, and prevention of recurrence for many infectious agents. A rating system is provided to score both the strength of each recommendation and the quality of supporting evidence. Highlights of these recommendations are provided below; the reader is referred to the referenced document for more extensive information.

Pneumocystis carinii pneumonia remains the most frequent AIDS-defining condition in children, although its incidence has decreased in recent years.[1] HIV-infected children should receive prophylaxis for the first year of life. Subsequent prophylaxis is based on age-specific CD4+ lymphocyte count thresholds. Children aged 1 to 5 years with CD4+ counts less than 500 cells/mm^3, children aged 6 years and older with CD4+ counts less than 200 cells/mm^3, and children aged 1 to 12 years with CD4+ percentages less than 15% should receive prophylaxis. Prophylaxis is also recommended for children with a history of *Pneumocystis carinii* pneumonia, regardless of CD4+ count and percentage. Trimethoprim-sulfamethoxazole (TMP-SMZ) is the preferred agent for prophylaxis. Alternative agents include dapsone, pentamidine, and atovaquone. These drugs also offer protection against other opportunistic infections, namely bacterial infections and toxoplasmosis.

Prophylaxis for *Mycobacterium avium* complex is recommended for children based on age-specific CD4+ lymphocyte count thresholds. Children younger than 1 year of age with CD4+ counts less than 750 cells/mm^3, children aged 1 to 2 years with CD4+ counts less than 500 cells/mm^3, children aged 2 to 6 years with counts less than 75 cells/mm^3, and children 6 years and older with CD4+ counts less than 50 cells/mm^3 should receive prophylaxis. Azithromycin and clarithromycin are first-choice agents for prophylaxis; rifabutin is offered as an alternative agent for children aged 6 years and older.

Annual tuberculin skin testing should be considered for HIV-infected children who are tuberculin-negative on initial evaluation and who reside in areas in which there is a substantial risk for exposure to *Mycobacterium tuberculosis*. Primary prevention guidelines for *M. tuberculosis* infection suggest that these children be screened using developed screening questionnaires to determine risk and tested if (1) screening is positive or (2) contact with active cases of tuberculosis are reported or documented.

Children with hypogammaglobulinemia or recurrent invasive bacterial infections despite TMP-SMZ prophylaxis may benefit from routine intravenous immunoglobulin administration. Frequent or severe recurrences of herpes simplex virus and *Candida* infection (oropharyngeal and esophageal) may warrant specific prophylaxis.

Highly active antiretroviral therapy has been documented to have an impact on the immunologic dysfunction associated with HIV infection by significantly improving CD4+ counts and percentages. Until the protective value of these new populations of CD4+ cells are better understood in the pediatric population, it is advisable to continue prophylaxis.[33] Currently, Pediatric AIDS Clinical Trials Group studies are evaluating the safety of prophylaxis withdrawal in children younger than 13 years of age with evidence of immunorestoration on HAART therapy.

General Infection Control Measures

Education concerning transmission and control of infectious diseases is an essential component of infection control for the family of an HIV-infected child. The basic tenets of standard precautions for exposures and preventing infectious diseases should be presented in an age-appropriate manner, with careful consideration of the educational level of caretakers.[34] Potential exposures to infections (e.g., varicella, measles, hepatitis A or B) in day care or school settings should be discussed and appropriate plans made for prompt notification of the health care provider. Chapter 12 provides in-depth descriptions of infection control measures appropriate for HIV-infected children and their families.

SCHOOL AND SOCIAL ISSUES

Most HIV-infected children will attend school. Existing laws and policies regarding their education ensure that they are neither excluded from school nor isolated within the school setting. They should be encouraged to participate in all school activities, including competitive sports, for which they have an interest and to the extent their health permits. Childhood activities need not be restricted to the school site alone but can include activities such as camping and other recreational events that are considered part of routine childhood socialization and educational opportunities. Transmission of HIV infection during activities of daily living is rare, and there have been no reported cases of HIV transmission in the school setting.[35] Standard precautions, incorporated into health policies established for schools and child care facilities, ensure that the risk of HIV transmission (and other blood-borne pathogens) is minimal. Exposure of the HIV-infected child to readily communicable diseases, however, is not as easily controlled. Varicella, measles, hepatitis A, and tuberculosis all pose a risk to the immunodeficient child. Proper notification procedures can assist in the timely provision of preventive measures outlined earlier.

Disclosure

Maintaining confidentiality of an individual's HIV status is protected by law. Hence, informing school and child care personnel of a child's HIV status is not mandated. A decision to disclose information regarding HIV status should be made in the best interests of the child and is the responsibility of the parents or caregiver. Benefits and risks associated with disclosure to the day care or school should be carefully weighed at different times in the child's life, for example, in toddler years with entry into day care or during early childhood with entry into school. Benefits may include (1) facilitating prompt parental notification by the faculty of the child's exposure to communicable diseases, (2) facilitating appropriate attention to the individual child's health care needs should he or she become ill at the caring facility, (3) planning for anticipated absences, and (4) relief of secrecy. Possible detrimental effects may include discrimination and social isolation.

Disclosure of HIV status to the infected child is a complex issue that demands attention to the unique circumstances that surround each child and family. This disclosure demands an individualized approach that includes a sensitive evaluation of the educational, cultural, societal sophistication, and language needs for each child and family. The American Academy of Pediatrics strongly encourages disclosure to school-aged children.[36] Knowledgeable health care professionals can assist families with disclosure to ensure that the process is positive. This may include several open discussion sessions with disclosing family members prior to approaching the HIV-infected child. Adolescents deserve full disclosure of their HIV status to enable them to assist with and participate in decision-making about their own care and to reduce the risk of HIV transmission to others through high-risk behaviors (e.g., sex, drug use). Newly infected adolescents may need both encouragement and assistance in disclosing their HIV status to their parents, sexual partners, and peers.

Empowerment and Compliance with Medical Care

Just as adherence to prophylactic medication regimens can prevent unnecessary infections, adherence to antiretroviral regimens can delay progression of HIV disease. Ongoing encouragement and support from family, friends, and health care workers can help the HIV-infected child or adolescent and his or her family become successful in adherence.

Following simple environmental safety guidelines (regarding pets, soil, water, and food handling and preparation) can reduce the risk of infectious exposures and disease. A balanced diet, adequate rest and sleep, regular exercise, and stress reduction techniques all contribute to an increased quality of life and improved immune function.

It is advisable for HIV-infected individuals of any age to reduce or discontinue the use of alcohol, tobacco, and recreational drugs, as these substances can increase immunosuppression, which in turn can lead to HIV disease progression. Sexually active HIV-infected youth should understand and follow safe sex practices, not only to prevent the transmission of HIV infection but also to protect themselves from other sexually transmitted diseases. Additional infections such as sexually transmitted diseases place increased stress on an already compromised immune system, again increasing the risk of HIV disease progression. Sexually active HIV-infected youth should be educated about the risks associated with pregnancy, including additional risks with HIV disease: immunosuppression and risk of HIV transmission to the infant.

Case Management

The needs of the HIV-infected child are complex, often involving multiple specialists and numerous special medical services. The use of case management services can assist in accessing resources, streamlining care, and providing client advocacy. Case management services are often needed to reach beyond the needs of the infected child, assisting other infected or affected family members, and enhancing family-centered care.

SICK-CHILD EVALUATIONS

The HIV-infected child with acute illness poses some diagnostic dilemmas. In perinatally infected infants, HIV infects the important CD4+ lymphocyte, directly impacting a developing immune system. The result is that the normal host response to infection may be significantly altered. In HIV-infected children, immune response to first exposures to infectious agents may be significantly compromised. More widespread use of HAART therapy has significantly reduced morbidity and mortality for all HIV-infected individuals. Of note, however, the HIV-infected child on HAART may, even in the face of immunorestoration, still have unusual clinical manifestations of routine childhood illnesses, such as Kawaski disease.[37]

Fever Management

The HIV-infected infant or child with fever should receive the same medical attention afforded to the uninfected child. This includes a general physical examination to evaluate the cause of the fever and delivery of appropriate dosing of antipyretics (acetaminophen or ibuprofen) to reduce fever magnitude and provide fever control. Evaluation for contraindications to antipyretic use is necessary for children on HIV-specific therapy because of overlapping toxicity. It is important for the clinician to identify during well-child visits which antipyretics are acceptable for use in each individual HIV-infected child. For example, HIV-infected children with thrombocytopenia or renal disease should avoid the use of nonsteroidal anti-inflammatory agents for fever control, if possible.

The source of fever in the HIV-infected child may represent common illnesses that are routinely found in uninfected children, namely upper respiratory infections, systemic viral illnesses (e.g., influenza, coxsackievirus, enteroviruses), otitis media, pharyngitis, sinusitis, and pneumonia. However, fever may also herald the onset of common infections that plague HIV-infected children, namely, invasive bacterial infections or opportunistic infections. Many investigators suggest that the well-appearing HIV-infected child with fever with no clearly defined origin on physical examination should be evaluated with a complete blood cell count. Published studies have not always convincingly linked the results of a complete blood cell count in this setting as predictive of serious infection. However, HIV-infected children are almost uniformly on some degree of HIV-specific therapy, most of which can cause bone marrow suppression. A pragmatic use of the complete blood cell count in this setting may be to evaluate the child for evidence of neutropenia or bandemia to assist with decisions about further outpatient management versus hospitalization. Ill-appearing HIV-infected children should receive both blood and radiographic evaluations. For ill-appearing febrile infants with no identifiable source on physical examination, empiric antimicrobial therapy should not be provided unless blood and urine cultures are obtained before initiation of treatment. Additional analyses should target those organ systems that are uniquely affected in the individual child. For example, the HIV-infected child with fever, wasting, and chronic diarrhea is likely to have many tests performed, including liver functions (including evaluations of nutritional parameters), extensive stool evaluations (cultures for bacterial, fungal, parasitic, and viral agents; enzyme immunoassay for rotavirus; fat/protein losses), and blood cultures, PCR, or serology to identify disseminated disease (atypical mycobacterial disease, cytomegalovirus, Epstein-Barr virus). Of note, interpretation of serologic (specific antibody levels) analyses will be compromised if the individual child is receiving intravenous immunoglobulin. In such a case, IgM antibody responses or antigen detection methodologies should be used.

The HIV-infected child may require individualized therapeutic consideration for the treatment of even simple infections because of significant immunosuppression or HIV-related multiorgan dysfunction. For example, HIV-infected children with severe immunosuppression and oral thrush may require systemic antifungals in place of simple topical therapy. Children with HIV-related chronic diarrhea and routine illnesses will require therapeutic interventions that are easily absorbed and least likely to themselves induce diarrhea. Drug selection for the HIV-infected child must always be evaluated in the context of the child's HIV-specific therapy, since the potential exists for altering HIV-specific drug levels and overlapping toxicity to certain organs (bone marrow suppression, pancreatitis, hepatitis).

CONCLUSION

The general care of the HIV-infected child is challenging for many reasons, including the complex and dynamic nature of therapeutic interventions;

the presence of unique and persistent infections; the occurrence of complicated social issues that often require specific interventions; and the need for ongoing family and individual education about infectious disease prevention, lifestyle choices, and compliance with prescribed medical regimens. Active participation of the primary care physician in partnership with a multispecialty team that delivers medical care is the optimal approach to health care management for the HIV-infected child.

REFERENCES

1. Lindegren ML, Byers RH Jr, Thomas P, et al: Trends in perinatal transmission of HIV/AIDS in the United States. JAMA 1999;282:577.
2. Cooper ER, Charurat M, Burns DN, et al: Trends in antiretroviral therapy and mother-infant transmission of HIV. The Women and Infants Transmission Study Group. J Acquir Immune Defic Syndr 2000;1:24.
3. Sperling RS, Shapiro DE, Coombs RW, et al: Maternal viral load, zidovudine treatment, and the risk of transmission of human immunodeficiency virus type 1 from mother to infant. Pediatric AIDS Clinical Trials Group Protocol 076 Study Group. N Engl J Med 1996;335:1621.
4. Read JS, Tuomala R, Kpamegan E, et al: Mode of delivery and postpartum morbidity among HIV-infected women: The Women and Infants Transmission Study. J Acquir Immune Defic Syndr 2001;1:26.
5. Welles SL, Pitt J, Colgrove R, et al: HIV-1 genotypic zidovudine drug resistance and the risk of maternal-infant transmission in the women and infants study. The Women and Infants Transmission Study Group. AIDS 2000;14:263.
6. Conte D, Fraquelli M, Prati D, et al: Prevalence and clinical course of chronic hepatitis C virus (HCV) infection and rate of HCV vertical transmission in a cohort of 15,250 pregnant women. Hepatology 2000;31:751.
7. Teglas JP, N'Go N, Burgard M, et al: CCR2B-64I chemokine receptor allele and mother-to-child HIV-1 transmission or disease progression in children. French Pediatric HIV Infection Study Group. J Acquir Immune Defic Syndr 1999;1:22.
8. MacDonald KS, Embree JUE, Nagelkerke NJ, et al: The HLA A2/6802 supertype is associated with reduced risk of perinatal human immunodeficiency virus type 1 transmission. J Infect Dis 2001;183:503.
9. Public Health Service Task Force: Recommendations for the use of antiretroviral drugs in pregnant women infected with HIV-1 for maternal health and for reducing perinatal HIV-1 transmission in the United States. MMWR 1998;47;1.
10. Diaz C, Hanson C, Cooper ER, et al: Disease progression in a cohort of infants with vertically acquired HIV infection observed from birth: The women and infants transmission study (WITS). J Acquir Immune Defic Syndr Hum Retrovirol 1998;18:221.
11. Connor EM, Sperling RS, Gelber R, et al: Reduction of maternal-infant transmission of human immunodeficiency virus type 1 with zidovudine treatment. Pediatric AIDS Clinical Trials Group Protocol 076 Study Group. N Engl J Med 1994;331:1173.
12. Vigouroux C, Gharakhanian S, Salhi Y, et al: Adverse metabolic disorders during highly active antiretroviral treatments (HAART) of HIV disease. Diabetes Metab 1999;25:383.
13. Blanche S, Tardieu M, Rustin P, et al: Persistent mitochondrial dysfunction and perinatal exposure to antiretroviral nucleoside analogues. Lancet 1999;354:1054.
14. Culnane M, Fowler M, Lee SS, et al: Lack of long-term effects of in utero exposure to zidovudine among uninfected children born to HIV-infected women. Pediatric AIDS Clinical Trials Group Protocol 219/076 Teams. JAMA 1999;281:151.
15. Hanson IC, Antonelli TA, Sperling RS, et al: Lack of tumors in infants with perinatal HIV-1 exposure and fetal/neonatal exposure to zidovudine. J Acquir Immune Defic Syndr Hum Retrovirol 1999;20:463.
16. The Perinatal Safety Review Working Group: Nucleoside exposure in the children of HIV-infected women receiving antiretroviral drugs: Absence of clear evidence for mitochondrial disease in children who died before 4 years of age in five United States cohorts. J Acquir Immune Defic Syndr 2000;1:261.
17. Moye J Jr, Rich K, Kalish LA, et al: Natural history of somatic growth in infants born to women infected by human immunodeficiency virus. Women and Infants Transmission Study Group. J Pediatr 1996;128:58.
18. Alfaro MP, Siegel RM, Baker RC, et al: Resting energy expenditure and body composition in pediatric HIV infection. Pediatr AIDS HIV Infect 1995;6:276.
19. Chase C, Ware J, Hittelman J, et al: Early cognitive and motor development among infants born to women infected with human immunodeficiency virus. Women and Infants Transmission Study Group. Pediatrics 2000;106:E25.
20. Smith R, Malee K, Charurat M, et al: Timing of perinatal human immunodeficiency virus type 1 infection and rate of neurodevelopment. The Women and Infant Transmission Study Group. Pediatric Infect Dis J 2000;19:862.
21. Hutto C: Routine pediatric care. In Zeichner SL, Read JS (eds): Handbook of Pediatric HIV Care, 1st ed. Philadelphia, Lippincott Williams & Wilkins, 1999, p 122.
22. Hines SE: Primary care for HIV-exposed and infected children: Translating progress into practice. Lippincotts Prim Care Pract 2000;4:43.
23. O'Hara MJ, D'Orlando D: Ambulatory care of the HIV-infected child. Nursing Clin North Am 1996;31:179.

24. Cooper ER, Hanson C, Diaz C, et al: Encephalopathy and progression of human immunodeficiency virus disease in a cohort of children with perinatally acquired human immunodeficiency virus infection. Women and Infants Transmission Study. J Pediatr 1998;132:808.
25. 1999 USPHS/IDSA Guidelines for the Prevention of Opportunistic Infections in Persons Infected with Human Immunodeficiency Virus. MMWR 1999;48:1.
26. Stratton P, Gupta P, Riester K, et al: Cervical dysplasia on cervicovaginal Papanicolaou smear among HIV-1-infected pregnant and nonpregnant women. Women and Infants Transmission Study. J Acquir Immune Defic Syndro Hum Retrovirol 1999;20:300.
27. Maiman M: Management of cervical neoplasia in human immunodeficiency virus-infected women. J Natl Cancer Inst Monogr 1998;23:43.
28. Withdrawal of Rotavirus Vaccine Recommendation. MMWR 1999;48:1007.
29. Mao C, Harper M, McIntosh K, et al: Invasive pneumococcal infections in human immunodeficiency virus-infected children. J Infect Dis 1996;173:870.
30. Preventing Pneumococcal Disease Among Infants and Young Children. Recommendations of the Advisory Committee on Immunizations Practices (ACIP). MMWR 2000;49:1.
31. Keller M, Deveikis A, Cutillar-Garcia M, et al: Pneumococcal and influenza immunization and human immunodeficiency virus load in children. Pediatric Infect Dis J 2000;19:613.
32. Human Immunodeficiency Virus Infection. In Pickering LK, Peter G, Baker CJ, et al (eds): Redbook 2000, Report of the Committee on Infectious Diseases, 25th ed. Elk Grove Village, Ill, American Academy of Pediatrics, 2000, p 341.
33. Ledergerber B, Mocroft A, Reiss P, et al: Discontinuation of secondary prophylaxis against *Pneumocystis carinii* pneumonia in patients with HIV infection who have a response to antiretroviral therapy. Eight European Study Groups. N Engl J Med 2001;18:168.
34. Hospital Infection Control Practices Advisory Committee: Guidelines for isolation precautions in hospitals. Infect Control Hosp Epidemiol 1996;17:53.
35. AAP Committee on Pediatric AIDS and Committee on Infectious Diseases: Issues related to human immunodeficiency virus transmission in schools, child care, medical settings, the home, and community. Pediatrics 1999;104:318.
36. AAP Committee on Pediatric AIDS: Disclosure of illness status to children and adolescents with HIV infection. Pediatrics 1999;103:164.
37. Johnson RM, Little JR, Storch GA: Kawasaki-like syndromes associated with human immunodeficiency virus infection. Clin Infect Dis 2001;32:1628.

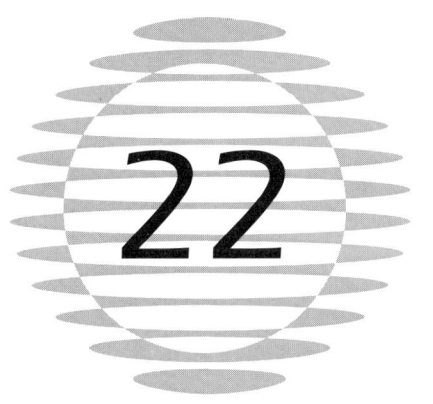

22

Psychosocial Challenges in Pediatric HIV Infection

Lori S. Wiener,
Jennifer F. Havens, and
Yiu Kee W. Ng

Pediatric HIV infection in the United States has always been associated with complex and significant psychosocial issues. During the last decade, HIV infection in women and children has concentrated in socioeconomically deprived, urban populations living in communities affected by endemic substance abuse. Advances in the prevention of vertical transmission and in antiretroviral treatment over the last 5 years have had a dramatic impact on the prevalence and the prognosis of children and adolescents living with HIV. However, the steady increase in the number of women with HIV/AIDS has led to large numbers of children and adolescents losing parents to AIDS or living with parental illness.[1]

As HIV-related mortality has decreased, issues in psychosocial management have evolved from a model largely focused on bereavement and stabilization of families struggling with loss to one of maximizing quality of life in the face of chronic illness. Issues related to HIV illness, such as disclosure, planning, and bereavement, remain important. However, there has been increasing awareness of the psychosocial needs associated with the complex backgrounds of many HIV-infected children and their parents. These include familial substance abuse, histories of trauma and family disruption, mental illness, socioeconomic stressors, and urban violence. In this chapter, issues in psychosocial and psychiatric management of HIV-infected and affected children are described. For the purposes of clarity, these are separated categorically; however, in clinical presentation they will overlap and intertwine.

MENTAL HEALTH ISSUES ASSOCIATED WITH FAMILIAL SUBSTANCE ABUSE

In the United States, AIDS in women and children represents a confluence of two major epidemics plaguing American cities, HIV infection and substance abuse. Injecting drug use is the risk factor for HIV infection in 43% of the AIDS cases in women; heterosexual contact with a drug user accounts for a significant percentage of the remaining cases.[2] Reflecting the risk factors for HIV infection in women, 58% of children with AIDS were born to women whose risk factor for HIV infection is their own or their partner's intravenous drug use.[2] For clinicians working with HIV-infected children and their caregivers, the close link between HIV infection and substance abuse in women calls for an in-depth understanding of the mental health problems common in families affected by substance abuse.

Mental Health Risk Factors Associated with Parental Substance Abuse

For children with drug-abusing parents, risk factors for mental health problems cluster in two areas. These can be broadly conceptualized as

All material in this chapter is in the public domain with the exception of any borrowed figures or tables.

follows: (1) sequelae of parenting deficiencies associated with parental substance abuse (neglect, abuse, discontinuity of attachments, and disruption of placement) and; (2) the biologic risks associated with parental drug addiction (prenatal drug exposure, heritable parental psychiatric disorder).

Neglect, Abuse, and Disrupted Attachment Associated with Parental Drug Addiction

One of the most devastating effects of substance abuse is the erosion of parenting capacities essential to children's development and well-being. Children living with substance-abusing parents are at increased risk for neglect, abuse, exposure to domestic violence, and disruption of attachments,[3–5] all of which have been shown to increase children's risk for mental health problems.[6–8]

Biologic Risks Associated with Parental Drug Addiction

Prenatal Drug Exposure

Several studies have described the developmental and behavioral problems of prenatally drug-exposed children.[9–11] Methodologic problems in much of the research on prenatally drug-exposed children limit definitive conclusions regarding the link between specific drug exposures and behavioral or cognitive outcomes.[12,13] However, it is clear that maternal drug use during pregnancy with its associated problems, such as inadequate prenatal care, premature birth, and low birth weight may act to increase children's risk for developmental, cognitive, and mental health problems.

Heritable Psychiatric Disorders

Adults with substance abuse disorders have high rates of psychiatric comorbidity, in particular affective and anxiety disorders and childhood histories of attention deficit-hyperactivity disorder.[14–16] Children born to adult substance abusers are at increased risk for mental health problems, due to the heritable nature of the psychiatric disorders prevalent in adult substance abusers.[17–19]

Furthermore, for both genetic and environmental reasons, substance abuse in the parental generation frequently clusters in extended families. It is not unusual to find extended families with two or more substance-abusing adult siblings, nor, in fact, is it rare to encounter two or even more adult siblings with HIV infection associated with substance abuse or substance-abusing sexual partners. In these families, material and emotional resources may be too strained to intervene effectively on behalf of grandchildren, nieces, or nephews who are HIV-infected or affected; this lack of extended family capability may place the child at further risk.

In summary, HIV illness commonly strikes families already struggling with substance abuse and its associated problems, including impairment of parenting capacities and psychiatric disorders. When a child's parent is substance abusing and HIV positive, the HIV disease may play a less significant role in the child's mental health problems than do issues related to the substance abuse.

MENTAL HEALTH NEEDS ASSOCIATED WITH HIV INFECTION

Infants and Toddlers

The biological mother often learns of her own infection at the same time she discovers that her child is HIV positive. This is clearly a crisis point and an essential time for psychosocial intervention, education, and family support. Almost immediately, these mothers begin questioning how and when they became infected with the HIV virus and whom they can share this diagnosis with. Understanding the disease and the complex medical regimens associated with treatment of the infection can be quite overwhelming. Learning to administer medication to their young child and finding a way to balance hope with fear of becoming severely ill is one of the first major tasks to be accomplished.

Children younger than 2 years of age are unable to grasp the concept of being diagnosed with a life-threatening disease. As a result, the psychological trauma of the diagnosis falls primarily on the child's caregiver.[20] The caregiver's own level of distress will be largely defined by the support that she can receive from others and her ability to help the child deal with medical procedures and medications.

Generally speaking, children up to age 6 or 7 are not told their HIV diagnosis due to concern about their capacity for discretion in sharing this information. Toddlers and young children do not understand the concept of chronic illness and experience episodes of HIV-related illness as discrete events rather than as part of an ongoing process. However, they do benefit from ongoing and developmentally appropriate explanations of illness and treatment.

School-Aged Children

How a child copes with his or her illness depends on many factors. These include the age and developmental stage of the child, parental adaptation, social skills, and the child's psychological make-up. When considering the psychological make-up of a child, one must examine the child's ability to trust, to use and reach out for help, to tolerate pain, to make and maintain friendships, to cope with change and separation, and whether or not support from family and others is available. One must also assess the child's cognitive abilities, disclosure status, and stage of illness. All of these factors determine the meaning that the illness carries for the child. These factors will also determine the kind of psychological and intellectual resources the child has available to cope with the disease and to meet each challenge.

Clearly, this is a period of developmental inquiry and universal questions that begin with "why," "what," "when," "how," and "what if" need to be anticipated. Trust between the parent and child is imperative. A bond between physician and child will often enhance understanding and compliance. Honesty is essential. Both the parent and the health care team must respect the comfort level of the child and the parent when it comes to disclosing information about the infection to the child.

Disclosure

Despite extensive research with other disease processes that have documented the risks of nondisclosure and benefits of open communication about illness in the family, disclosure poses unique difficulties in families affected by HIV/AIDS. Even as we enter the third decade of this disease, stigma continues to prevent open discussion of the illness in most families. For many parents, behaviors associated with the acquisition of HIV (substance abuse, relationships with substance-abusing partners) are sources of shame and guilt and complicate open communication. Many parents remain reluctant to discuss the diagnosis with their children, their own parents, extended family members, friends, or employers; in essence, those who would traditionally provide support in time of need. Within the immediate family, the diagnosis frequently becomes a guarded family secret, one that is felt to be shameful, embarrassing, and potentially explosive if revealed.

Maintaining this secret places tremendous stress on all members of the family unit, especially the children who are themselves infected. It is primarily for this reason that parents put off sharing information about the virus with their infected children. In a study that examined the factors associated with parents' decision to disclose or not disclose an HIV diagnosis to their child,[21] the reasons listed by nondisclosing caregivers for not telling their child his or her diagnosis and the factors they listed that would need to be in place before disclosing primarily reflected the protective nature of parents. Parents feared that their children would be psychologically harmed or ostracized by others. The fear of ostracization was reflected in the fact that 45% of the children were not allowed to share their diagnosis with *anyone*. They also desperately wanted to protect their children from losing the innocence of childhood or having to burden the children with the need to lie to others. As previously identified in parents who transmitted a deleterious gene or chromosome abnormality resulting in a birth defect, the additional parameter of maternal guilt remains a factor for some HIV-positive parents.[22,23] These parents expressed great pain about not being able to shelter their children from the illness. A primary concern was that once the child understood the source of infection, he or she might harbor tremendous anger toward the parents or outwardly reject them. Since learning about the source of infection often means having to reveal information about other family members who are also infected, and either sexual contact, drug use, or paternity issues not previously known,[24] fear of rejection is a real issue for many parents. Conversely, parents who decided to disclose the diagnosis to their children opposed keeping family secrets, reported a strong belief that the children have a right to know about the illness, feared that their children would learn about the diagnosis elsewhere, were concerned about transmission to others, found lying too stressful, or desired greater intimacy with their children.

Disclosure of the HIV diagnosis to children is an individualized and dynamic process. Patterns of disclosure vary from full disclosure (the name of the virus, ways to treat the disease, and transmission routes are provided) to partial disclosure (a child is given a description of symptoms and treatment but the exact name of the illness is not revealed).[25] Patterns of nondisclosure vary as well, from deception (the illness is hidden behind another condition) to complete nondisclosure (there is no communication about the illness at all).[25]

Timing of disclosure is essential. Research shows that the majority of parents wait approximately 2 years and until they feel their children could both understand and cope with the diagnosis before sharing this information with their children. Their intuition must be respected, especially when 65% of children in the earlier cited study[21] reported that they felt the right person told them and 86% at the right time. In almost all cases, this was the child's parent or parents. Disclosure seems to best take place in a supportive atmosphere of cooperation between health professionals and parents. It should be conceived of as a process rather than as a single episode and may need to occur in sequence.[26] See Table 22–1 for a guide to helping parents through the disclosure process.

Emotional reactions following disclosure of the diagnosis vary. Reactions tend to be consistent with the way the child has responded to earlier crises. A parent might report that the child "had no reaction" while others might describe acute panic or anxiety. Delayed reactions are not uncommon. Most prevalent are the onset of new psychosomatic complaints, nightmares, emotional lability, regressions, and anxiety symptoms (often in the form of tics). Others present with an adult-like acceptance. In spite of what appears to be acceptance of the illness, careful assessments must be made. For many HIV-infected children, the sense of shame and personal defectiveness can be profound and is often exacerbated by the stigma and the need for secrecy associated with their infection.[27] These issues frequently surface in counseling either in play or through artwork where themes about being "bad" or "devilish" appear. Counseling can be enormously helpful for these children. Almost all children demonstrate considerable pride with mastery of

Table 22–1
Guiding a Family Through the Disclosure Process

- Listen carefully to the factors associated with the parent's reasons for wanting to disclose or not disclose the diagnosis to the child. This is a highly emotional topic that patients often do not discuss with many people.
- Talking to children about the HIV diagnosis takes preparation and careful thought.
- Help parents to understand that differences among diseases are not understood by the preschool-aged child.
- The school-aged child often asks a barrage of questions. Role-playing prior to disclosure is always helpful.
- Parents should provide an explanation that is appropriate to the child's cognitive, emotional, and developmental stage and one that they could build on with more specific detail later. Using words the child is familiar with is helpful.
- The preadolescent and adolescent child will ask more sophisticated questions related to how the disease was acquired and their future. One should be prepared to answer these questions honestly before disclosing the diagnosis.
- All children should be informed that they, in no way, caused this illness to occur.
- Disclosure is a process that usually takes place over time—one cannot expect children to understand all aspects of the HIV diagnosis after one discussion. Revisiting the issue to assess understanding and emotional responses is essential.
- The impact of the diagnosis may take the child weeks to years to absorb. If the child has specific questions, answer them. Let the child know that no matter how difficult the subject matter, he or she can always ask questions or share feelings. Be careful, however, not to provide more information than the child wants or is prepared to cope with.
- Having someone outside the immediate family available that the child can talk to has been helpful. Offer the child time alone with his or her physician.
- Offer the child the opportunity to talk to or meet other children with the same illness.
- Following disclosure, parents may seek reassurance that they made the right decision by disclosing the diagnosis to their child. Offer ongoing support to the parent and child.
- Encourage parents to maintain or re-establish routines at home. The child needs to understand that the only thing that has changed is his or her knowledge of their illness.
- Trust between the parent and child should always be the highest priority.

From Wiener L, Battles HB, Heilman NE: Factors associated with parents' decision to disclose their HIV diagnosis to their children. Child Welfare 1999;77:115.

information, increased knowledge about the illness, reduction of guilt, and the ability to tolerate procedures such as blood draws and pill swallowing.

School

Any kind of chronic illness can result in setbacks in school or even avoidance of school. Being out of school due to illness can increase the child's loneliness, isolation, and the feeling of being different from or behind other schoolmates. Although HIV/AIDS is no different in this regard, the stigma associated with this disease results in concerns that parents have about whether they need to inform the school of their child's diagnosis. Many families have had positive outcomes after informing the school of their child's diagnosis. Other situations in which parents have informed the school of their child's diagnosis have resulted in school battles pertaining to inappropriate class placement, discrimination, or a breach of confidentiality. Currently, the number of situations in which legal intervention is needed is being drastically reduced as school districts are beginning to develop their own HIV policies. Many of these policies include "no-disclosure" laws, although each policy varies as to which personnel are still required to be informed of the child's diagnosis. As a result, parents' anxiety associated with informing school personnel about their child's diagnosis and the fear of disclosure remains tremendous. Many parents remain anonymous and keep the diagnosis from the school for as long as possible.

There are many ways that the health care team can assist families with the school process. These include (1) informing parents of a child's right to an education, (2) meeting with school officials and school personnel to educate them about HIV infection and apprise them of the individual needs of a specific child, (3) health care providers accompanying parents to school board meetings when they feel this would be of support, (4) providing consultation to teachers and principals in talking to the other classmates about HIV and AIDS, and (5) providing up-to-date information to the school pertaining to the child's progress if the child has been out ill for a period of time.[24] One publication that has been especially helpful to school districts and teachers is *Someone at School Has AIDS: A Guide to Developing Policies for Student and School Staff Members Who Are Infected with HIV*. This is available from the national association of state boards of education.

For many parents, the threat of their child's death at a young age results in a lack of stress on the importance of school, work ethics, or a sense of independence within the family.[24] Balancing academic expectations for the child and being flexible in terms of what the child can keep up with (due to frequent clinic visits) is a challenge to both parents and teachers. Nevertheless, it is of great importance in terms of preparing the child for the responsibilities of adolescence and young adulthood.

Adolescents

The number of AIDS cases reported each year among adolescents (13 to 19 years of age) in the United States has steadily increased from one case in 1981 to 3564 cases by June 1999.[28] Even more alarming is that many young adults aged 21 to 29 who present with AIDS almost certainly acquired their infection as adolescents. The developmental tasks of adolescence such as risk-taking, struggles for independence, experimenting with adult behavior, impulsivity, and a sense of invulnerability, coupled with awakening sexuality, make adolescents vulnerable to HIV.[29]

Levels of HIV-related stress appear to change over the course of time, increasing with the onset of adolescence, the need for a change in therapy, when dating begins, when decisions about informing the school need to be made, and when future goals are being considered. A key issue for HIV-infected adolescents is how or when to inform sexual partners of their status. The effect of peer pressure cannot be underestimated. It is important that the care provider talk openly to adolescents concerning their peer relationships, sexuality, and sexual practices. Adolescents appreciate acknowledgment concerning the difficulty of disclosing their diagnosis to potential sexual partners. It helps to have them review the pro's and con's out loud and for them to hear about successful disclosures, as well as ones that did not go well and why. It is also important that the care provider avoid attempts to convince the adolescent by moral argument either not to become sexually active or to inform their partners immediately. Most often, this strategy only alienates the teen and has no positive effect on his or her choices. Rather, exploring his or her underlying fears of stigmatization and rejection may better facilitate open discussion and behavior change.[30] Reviewing safer sexual behaviors and making barrier protection available is invaluable.

Regardless of how the teenager acquired his or her infection, the most damaging result is its effect on the formation of relationships outside of the family.[24] These adolescents fear rejection more than they fear dying from the disease. Most have no access to or will not participate in mental health services. When unaddressed, these powerful emotions manifest in either physical symptoms (anxiety reactions, fatigue, aches and pains that are psychosomatic in nature) or psychological and social symptoms (social withdrawal, poor social judgment, depression, substance abuse, or sexual acting out).[24]

Many of the adolescents living with HIV have already experienced significant hardships prior to their diagnosis, including poverty, violence, abandonment, and living environments that consist of constant threats and dangers.[30–32] Several outpatient clinics reported that as many as half of the teenagers they have seen have also suffered from neglect or physical or sexual abuse, necessitating intervention by social service agencies or the courts.[31–35]

AIDS will affect every aspect of an HIV-positive adolescent's life. Establishing a sense of trust from which a therapeutic alliance can be formed is one of the most important interventions and greatest challenges for the health care provider working with adolescents. Such a relationship will allow the provider the opportunity to openly discuss issues related to sexuality, disclosure, family, treatment options, and future planning. It will allow essential ongoing evaluations of how he or she is doing in school and at home, and to assess for any problems with depression, anxiety, substance abuse, or safety. However, for this to happen, clinic and hospital visits may need to be conducted differently. For adolescents, confidentiality and privacy are key issues. Although these adolescents may present as mature and sexually active, they are often modest and anxious about bodily changes and have a poor understanding of their anatomies.[36] Health care providers may routinely need to ask the caregiver to step out of the room so privacy during the physical examination can be ensured. This is also the time when confidential information is mostly likely to be raised.

The related issues of adherence and responsibility are crucial as these children enter adolescence. The provider must have a solid understanding of adolescent development prior to engaging adolescents in treatment.[36] For example, during the early teen years, many parents begin feeling that their child should be responsible for his or her own medications. However, emotionally, many of these adolescents are not ready for this responsibility. Moreover, the triple combination regimens, with their rigid schedule of medications and meals, are very difficult for even adults to adhere to. For adolescents, it is even more challenging. Their impulsivity, shorter attention spans, and desire to fit in with their peers' schedules and eating habits often leads to poor adherence. One must also consider the side effects that many individuals on these therapies develop, such as diarrhea, nausea, skin rashes, and unusual deposits of body fat. Others express great concern that the medications may no longer be effective against the virus. When one adds the fact that the teenager may also be tired of obeying parents' and doctors' orders and of having to take medications all of his or her life, there is a great likelihood that these teens will not be compliant with their medication regimens. Any psychosocial crisis can also lead to a period of nonadherence, such as a death, a break-up with a girlfriend or boyfriend, a family fight, or a problem in school or on the job. Teenagers in crisis or teenagers who are depressed may not only stop taking their medications but also stop taking care of themselves in other ways, such as no longer eating well, not getting enough rest, or having unprotected sex.[37] Those who are the most adherent are usually well informed about their treatment and feel that taking the medications is their own decision. Therefore, it is wiser to wait before starting a teenager on a protease inhibitor until he or she feels strongly that he or she may benefit from treatment and will be able to adhere to it.

Interventions designed to best understand the individual adaptation of these teens are essential. The Montefiore Adolescent AIDS Program has identified four key time points for HIV-positive adolescents in coping with changes in their health status.[36,38] These are (1) receiving an HIV diagnosis, (2) disclosing the HIV status to parents, partner, and others, (3) coping with HIV illness, and (4) preparing for death. At other times, which are not perceived as crisis points, many of these adolescents seem to be doing fine. Their symptoms of maladaption go along unnoticed or are perceived as "normal adolescent behavior" until a major episode such as a suicidal gesture, acute illness resulting from nonadherence with medications, or an episode with the law brings attention to them. Frequent phone calls are helpful.

The health care provider must acknowledge and address difficult areas such as disclosure issues and side effects to medications. Many adolescents respond well to opportunities to talk with other HIV-positive youth, especially those who are also on similar medication regimens. Without early and ongoing psychosocial intervention, the mental health outcome of these teens could be seriously jeopardized, especially as they are transferred to adult clinics, where the change in staff and routines provides one more loss of their past.

The Transition to Young Adulthood/Long-Term Survivors

A decade ago, there was a dismal direction to the illness. Almost all children died before their young adult years. Today, the outcome is much more favorable. A significant number of children are expected to live well into their adolescent years and hopefully beyond. With the dramatic health improvements for many HIV-positive adolescents since the introduction of protease inhibitors and combination therapies, one would expect to see dramatic excitement in now being able to plan an independent future. For some, this is exactly what is happening. A growing number of children transfused with contaminated blood in the early years of their life and those with vertically acquired infection have survived the earlier years of this epidemic. Many are now graduating high school and attending trade schools or colleges, while others are holding down part-time or full-time jobs. But for others, the transition from expecting to die to now planning for their future has been severely anxiety provoking. Most of these young adults have survived life-threatening events. They saw themselves as needy and dependent. Many have no long-term plans or goals. Adherence to complex medication schedules is arduous. With the uncertainty of how long these drug regimens will work and the fear associated with losing the security of their parent's health insurance or SSI benefits, many others do not want to obtain steady employment.

Many of these youngsters have experienced multiple losses in their early years and they find themselves grieving for their parents, siblings, and close friends who did not live long enough to benefit from the drug treatments currently available. Others have been shuffled between households, schools, neighborhoods, and community programs. Often the most consistent part of their lives has been their medical care. Even for the most fortunate of these children, those who have not lost parents, all have known at least one other person well who has died from the same disease they have. It is often not until they reach late adolescent years that the impact of these losses "hits home." Depression, anxiety, trouble making decisions, feeling "lost," guilt surrounding survival, complicated grief reactions, and uncertainty can lead to disabling mental health problems.

Many teens are reluctant to attend traditional support groups, although clearly such an intervention has the potential to offer tremendous benefit. Support groups can offer a sense of belonging to these teens, a place where they can undo the shame and stigmatization that has isolated them from their peers. It is also a place where their pain can be validated, the trauma understood, and a deep connection with others made. Camping programs for teens can also provide this effect, especially those that take place away from their home (Table 22–2). Many of these teens find themselves without the language to define their pain. Through therapeutic activities, such as artwork, challenge courses, campfire chats, and rap sessions, connections with repressed emotions and with others can lead to enormous healing and growth.

Along with social support and a sense of belonging, attitude appears to be most essential. Those who keep themselves mentally active, have a sense of purpose in their lives, have a sense of humor, adapt to loss and change, and create a back-up plan in case they become ill appear to be thriving under the continued uncertainties associated with this disease. Despite the many stresses inherent in living with HIV/AIDS, these young adults need to be given the opportunity to develop and pursue individual aspirations and goals. If recognized and nurtured, they have the potential to significantly contribute to society.[24]

Siblings: Well Children in Affected Households

The majority of children who survive the death of a parent from AIDS or who live with a HIV-infected family member are not themselves HIV-infected. Sandra Thurman, former Director of the Office of National AIDS Policy, declared at a conference on families with AIDS in 1997 that "as a nation, we've only begun to deal with the fact that an estimated 80,000 to 125,000 American children and youth will lose their mothers to AIDS by the end of the century, and worldwide, 40 million

Table 22-2
Summer Camps for Children Infected with or Affected by HIV

CAMP	DESCRIPTION	CONTACT INFORMATION
Camp AmeriKids	Serves children infected and affected with HIV/AIDS.	Contact: Camp Director 161 Cherry St. New Canaan, CT 06840 Phone: (203) 972-5500
Birch Family Camp	Serves children and families living with HIV/AIDS.	Contact: Herbert G. Birch Services Summer Camp Program 145-02 Farmers Blvd. Springfield Gardens, NY 11434 Phone: (718)528-5754
Boggy Creek Gang	Serves children with chronic and life-threatening illnesses, including HIV/AIDS.	Contact: Boggy Creek Gang 30500 Brantley Branch Road Eustis, FL 32736 Phone: (352)483-4200
Camp Chrysalis	Serves children and their families who are affected by HIV/AIDS in the state of Maine.	Contact: Camp Chrysalis Waldo-Knox AIDS Coalition P.O. Box 990 Belfast, Maine 04915 Phone: (207)338-5089
St. Claire's Summer Camp	Serves children with HIV/AIDS and their families. Offers a summer camp program.	Contact: AIDS Resource Foundation for Children 182 Roseville Ave. Newark, N.J. 07107 Phone: (973)483-4250
Imani Village	Serves infected and affected children between the ages of 3 and 14 years in a day camp environment.	Contact: Children's AIDS Program at Boston Medical Center 255 River St. Mattapan, MA 02126 Phone: (617)543-2050. 1844 Commonwealth Ave. Newton, MA 02166 Phone: (617)243-2156
Camp Good Days and Special Times	Serves children between the ages of 8 and 17 years who are living with AIDS. The sister camp, TLC, serves children who have a parent or sibling who has AIDS or who has died from the disease.	Contact: Camp Good Days and Special Times, Inc. 1332 Pittsford-Mendon Road Mendon, NY 14506-9732 Phone: (585)624-5555
Camp Dream Street	Serves children aged 4 to 16 years with cancer, blood disorders, and other life-threatening illnesses.	Contact: Dream Street Foundation 9536 Wilshire Blvd., Suite 310 Beverly Hills, CA 90212 Phone: (310)274-7227
Camp Funshine	Serves children with HIV/AIDS and their families for a weekend camping program.	Contact: Special Love 117 Youth Development Court Winchester, VA 22602 Phone: (540)667-3774
Hakuna Matata	Serves children and their families in Arizona who are infected and affected by HIV/AIDS.	Contact: AIDS Project Arizona 115 East Camelback Road Phoenix, Arizona 85012 Phone: (602)265-3300
Camp Heartland	Serves children infected and affected by HIV/AIDS. Teen/Young adult retreat also provided.	Contact: Camp Heartland Project 3326 East Layton Ave. Cudahy, WI 53110 Phone: (414)272-1118 or 800-724-4673

Table 22–2
Summer Camps for Children Infected with or Affected by HIV *Continued*

Camp	Description	Contact
Camp Pacific Heartland	Summer camp program and other programs for children infected and affected by HIV/AIDS.	Contact: Camp Pacific Heartland 5358 Cartwright Ave N. Hollywood, CA 91601 Phone (818)753-6190
The Hole In The Wall Gang Camp and The Double "H"-Hole in the Woods Ranch	Serves children 7 to 15 years of age with cancer and other serious blood conditions who, because of their disease, its treatment, or its complications, cannot attend an ordinary summer camp. They have a special immunology session. They offer a 1-week session for brothers and sisters.	Contact: The Hole In The Wall Gang Camp 565 Ashford Center Road Ashford, CT 06278 Phone (860)429-3444 *or* Contact: The Double "H"-Hole in the Woods Ranch 97 Hidden Valley Road Lake Luzerne, NY 12846-3318 Phone: (518)696-5676
Camp High Five	Serves children between the ages of 6 and 16 years who are HIV affected.	Contact: Camp High Five 3130 Vista Brook Drive Decatur, Georgia 30033 Phone: (404)616-9809
Camp Knutson	Serves families in which any member is infected with HIV/AIDS, for a 1-week residential camp.	Contact: Lutheran Social Service 11169 Whitefish Ave. Cross Lake MN 56442 Phone: (218)543-4232
Camp Laurel	Serves children aged 6 to 17 years and their families living with HIV/AIDS.	Contact: Camp Laurel P.O. Box 93204 Los Angeles, CA 90093 Phone: (323)653-5005/(323)801-2113
Camp Rise and Shine	Serves children and teens affected by HIV/AIDS.	Contact: Camp Rise and Shine 1305 4th Avenue, 910 Cobb Building Seattle, WA 98101 Phone: (206)628-0461
Safe Haven Project	Serves children infected with and affected by HIV/AIDS. Family events, community-based camps/retreat experiences, and year-long programs are held.	Contact: The Safe Haven Project, Inc. PO Box 24 Vineyard Haven, MA 02568 Phone: (508)693-1767
Stepping Stones	Serves children infected with and affected by HIV/AIDS.	Contact: Camp Stepping Stones Swearer Center for Public Service Brown University Box 1974 Providence, RI 02192 Phone: (401)863-2338
Camp Sunburst	Serves children and adolescents with and affected by HIV/AIDS and their families.	Contact: SunBurst Projects 5350 Commerce Blvd., Suite I Rohnert Park, CA 94928 Phone: (707)588-9477
Tataya Mato	Serves children aged 4 to 17 years who have or live with a family member who has HIV/AIDS.	Contact: Jefferson Camp, Inc. 2001 South Bridgeport Rd. Indianapolis, IN 46231 Phone: (317)241-2661

Information from Wiener L, Septinius A, Grady C: Psychosocial support and ethical issues in pediatric AIDS. In Pizzo PA, Wilfert C (eds): Pediatric AIDS, 3rd ed. Baltimore, Lippincort Williams & Wilkins, 1998, p 703.

children will be orphaned by the year 2010."[39] The social, psychological, and legal implications for the children who survive are immense. Many of their parents are likely to have had a series of preexisting and longstanding stressors such as poverty, substance abuse, and violence, so these children suffer not only from chronic disruption to family life, they also suffer from widespread anxieties about future losses. They wonder who will care for them if all family members die and about their own health. However, it is the pervasive threat of death and fear of being left alone that constitutes chronic trauma for child survivors of HIV infection.[40] Psychotherapeutic interventions for the well children in HIV-affected households must concentrate on the need for permanency planning, building legacies and social support networks, and ongoing mental health services. These children must be allowed to grieve, feel appropriate anger for the tragedies in their life, and find ways of channeling these emotions. Special attention must be given to the envy and rivalry that might be present when the HIV-infected child is receiving special medical care and parental attention. Survivor guilt must not be underestimated.[24]

Similar to the long-term survivors of HIV, some of these children manifest behavioral symptoms, become involved with the law, and do not want to go on living, while others attempt to make sense of their world and keep hope alive in spite of the continual threat of abandonment. Camps geared toward the HIV-affected family members have been enormously helpful for many of these children (see Table 22–2). In such a setting, these children are provided a place where they feel they belong. They are provided the opportunity to be open about their family's plight, can meet others facing similar challenges, and can even assume a sense of responsibility as they have the option of also training to become camp counselors.

MENTAL HEALTH SERVICES FOR HIV-INFECTED AND AFFECTED CHILDREN AND FAMILIES

Mental health treatment for HIV-infected and affected children, adolescents, and caregivers must take into account potentially complicating factors associated with familial substance abuse (where present) as well as the dynamic course of HIV illness, which moves through specific predictable psychosocial stages roughly paralleling the natural history of the disease.[41] These stages begin with the diagnosis of HIV infection and continue through illness progression, late-stage illness, death, and reconfiguration of the family, with many of the children in new care arrangements.

At any stage in this process, children may exhibit a variety of responses to HIV diagnosis, illness, or loss. These responses may be characterized as (1) normative responses requiring supportive counseling or increased access to existing social supports; (2) responses complicated by familial histories of poor or disrupted attachment or trauma, indicating a need for individual or family psychotherapy; and (3) exacerbations of a preexisting psychiatric disorder or precipitations of new-onset disorder, in which syndrome-specific treatment must be among the interventions.

In general, mental health services are best delivered by a multidisciplinary team, which includes child and adolescent psychiatry, psychology, social work, and case management. Given the complex backgrounds of many HIV-affected children, psychosocial and mental health staff must have the sophistication to distinguish problems related to trauma and the sequelae of HIV illness from preexisting or new-onset psychiatric problems.

Several modifications of traditional mental health service models are helpful in increasing the accessibility and acceptability of mental health services to HIV-affected families. First, close coordination of mental health services with medical care increases the identification and engagement of families in need of mental health services. Second, active outreach strategies and flexibility in appointments helps overburdened families frequently juggling HIV infection in multiple family members. Third, integrated case management services to address the significant concrete service needs in these families is essential. Addressing basic issues such as entitlements, housing, or educational placement is one of the most effective ways to engage treatment-resistant families in ongoing mental health work.

Whenever possible, mental health services to HIV-affected families should be delivered with continuity across the stages of HIV illness. Children who are engaged in mental health services prior to parental or sibling death should be maintained in those services following that loss. Unfortunately, many services are organized to primarily serve the HIV-infected individual and are terminated with the death of that individual, leav-

PSYCHIATRIC MANIFESTATIONS

The psychiatric manifestations of HIV infection in children present many diagnostic and treatment challenges. In understanding the child with HIV, the first step is to effectively define the problems and designate different diagnostic categories, such as neurobiologic, psychiatric, and psychosocial. The challenge lies in the fact that these entities are often difficult to differentiate and are often still in evolution, as the research attempts to characterize the clinical entities. Without the research to influence treatment guidelines, clinicians can only rely on current knowledge after doing a careful comprehensive psychiatric evaluation. Using existing paradigms and extrapolating data from pediatric and adult HIV research will help the clinician understand the clinical presentations and assist treatment approaches. Integrating all of the components of a psychiatric evaluation involves paying attention to the medical, psychosocial, psychiatric, and family histories with a developmental perspective.

The majority of the research has focused on the neurodevelopmental effects of HIV and has established the findings of significant neurologic, developmental, cognitive, and language deficits in children.[42–46] The limited research on the psychiatric manifestations of HIV infection has suggested that these children are at high risk for anxiety, depression, guilt, and low self-esteem,[47,48] while Havens and associates[49] found high rates of attention deficit hyperactivity disorder (21%) and oppositional defiant disorder (17%). Treatment needs to be comprehensive, with an emphasis on the particular needs of the child without ignoring the issues of the HIV-infected and affected family members. Psychopharmacology can be a useful adjunct to the treatment armamentarium when thoughtfully practiced with a keen awareness of drug interactions and adverse effects.

Concerns regarding the use of psychotropic medications in pediatric HIV patients tend to be analogous to those in geriatric psychopharmacology. Valuable clinical research is often nonexistent, which necessitates the careful extrapolation and interpretation of adult research. This is clearly problematic, since many differences such as altered pharmacodynamics and pharmacokinetics are not addressed. One shared caveat with the geriatric population is that the medication titration should be slow and initiated at a lower dosage. Anecdotal reports in HIV-infected children has suggested that the overall clinical response to psychotropic medications may be less robust.

Complicating the psychiatric picture further is often multiple medical illnesses requiring concurrent treatment. Meticulous attention needs to be paid to understanding the neuropsychiatric adverse effects of any antimicrobial, antifungal, and antiviral agents used in the management of the HIV infection. It is important to educate the patients and their families about potential side effects. Due to the inevitability of polypharmacy, increased awareness and avoidance of possible drug-drug interactions is critical. Of particular concern with psychotropic medications is the family of cytochrome P-450 isoenzymes in combination with antiviral medications, with special attention to the protease inhibitors.[50,51] The risks and synergies of complicated medication regimens are complex and changing. It is important to have a reference and a medication table or pharmacist to check for any possible contraindications to medications.[52–54] The paucity of research to provide guidance in this arena of child psychopharmacology warrants significant caution, since many aspects of the disease manifestation in children are not known.

Attention Deficit Hyperactivity Disorder

Attention deficit hyperactivity disorder (ADHD) may be the most common presenting complaint to the child psychiatrist. Despite the high prevalence of symptoms compatible with ADHD in HIV-infected children,[55,56] it is imperative that the same diagnostic criteria be used to exclude other disorders manifesting with disruptive behaviors. Mood, anxiety, and adjustment disorders in addition to bereavement reactions in children could easily mimic aspects of ADHD or may represent comorbid diagnoses. In one of the few studies focusing specifically on ADHD, Havens and colleagues[49] reported that 5 of 24 HIV-infected children (21%) met the diagnostic criteria. In the study, the background factors in this population, such as parental substance abuse and the constellation of related risk factors, conferred similar rates of ADHD in a matched control sample.

The scarcity of research in the treatment approaches for ADHD in HIV-infected children require that the clinician evaluate each child's case individually. Extrapolating guidelines generated by the MTA study for the treatment of ADHD can be used to help design a multimodal approach and intervention.[57] Psychosocial and psychotherapeutic interventions build a foundation, which can be enhanced by psychopharmacologic treatments. In a case series, Havens and McCaskill[58] described the psychostimulant treatment of 12 HIV-infected children and adolescents, 8 with ADHD and 4 with dementia related to HIV disease. Two thirds of children tolerated psychostimulants, methylphenidate or dextroamphetamine, with good efficacy as measured by the Efficacy Index of the Clinical Global Impressions. The maintenance dosage of methylphenidate ranged from 0.2 to 1.2 mg/kg, and the one child on dextroamphetamine required 0.6 mg/kg. Four of the 12 (3 out of the ADHD sample) experienced adverse side effects precluding their continuation of the methylphenidate. While the neuropsychiatric adverse effects argue for caution in the psychostimulant treatment of this population, such treatment should not be withheld when clinically indicated. Two of the three children who required termination of their methylphenidate trial were switched to clonidine as their second-line medication. The only study describing the use of clonidine was a case study by Cesena and associates[59] in the treatment of behavioral symptoms in a preschool-aged child with HIV encephalopathy.

Despite the concerns about adverse effects, including sedation or orthostatic hypotension in uninfected children,[60] clonidine can be a possible alternative. Clonidine should be initiated with a bedtime dosage of 0.025 to 0.05 mg and slowly titrated upward weekly. Multiple administrations during the day are often necessary, with close attention to any adverse effects. The transdermal preparation, Catapres-TTS, can be an option for children who have marked sedation effects or who have difficulty taking oral preparations.

Dementia

Dementia in pediatric HIV cases is just one of a range of symptoms in a complex entity, HIV-related encephalopathy. Encephalopathy is a common occurrence, the rate of which was found to be 21% in a cohort of 128 perinatally infected children studied by the Women and Infants Transmission Study Group, a national collaborative study.[61] Other studies, have quoted higher rates, but factors such as zidovudine prophylaxis in pregnancy and the effects of early highly active antiretroviral treatment need to be considered in interpreting data. The current classification of encephalopathy in children encompasses a continuum of presentations; however, two relatively distinct neurodevelopmental patterns emerge: static encephalopathy and progressive encephalopathy.[42,43] In affected children, the recognition of dementia-related behavioral sequelae and accurate differential diagnosis is clinically important for several reasons. First, parents and medical staff can misinterpret a child's increasing fatigue, decreased interest in and resistance to regular activities, and regressive behavior as volitional oppositional behavior or as a pure depressive disorder. This can result in efforts to encourage the child to alter his or her behavior when in actuality the behavior represents sequelae of the disease process and is not within the child's control. Second, early in the presentation of HIV-related dementia in children, stimulants such as methylphenidate can be very helpful to them in raising their energy level and improving their quality of life.[58] Third, progressive organic involvement in children is an important clinical sign, indicating a need for change in the antiretroviral treatment to include agents that may have greater penetrance to the central nervous system (CNS) with greater blood-brain barrier permeability.

Only zidovudine has demonstrated improved neurocognitive functioning in children,[62] but other antiviral agents such as nevirapine, abacavir, and stavudine may also have CNS penetrance. There have been concerns about possible sequestered CNS reservoirs or sanctuaries of HIV infection unresponsive to antiviral regimens, which have inadequate CNS penetration.[43]

Delirium

There is no literature on the treatment of delirium in HIV-infected children with psychotropic medications. In adults with more advanced HIV disease, medical illness, or encephalopathy,[63] there is an increased susceptibility to extrapyramidal side effects[64] and neuroleptic malignant syndrome.[65] Effective management of the agitated delirious patient should be conservative and include acute observation and containment with an urgent identification of the underlying cause. If neuroleptics are used, there are risks and benefits for both high- and low-potency antipsychotics. The latter is often associated with orthostatic hypotension and tachycardia in addition to anticholinergic effects. Careful use of neuroleptics is critical, since they may alter the blood levels of antidepressant, antiviral, and antifungal medications due to their pharmacokinetics and metabolism.[63] Most neuroleptics are either metabolized by the 2D6 isoenzyme of the cytochrome P-450 system, such as risperidone and thioridazine, or by 1A2 such as clozapine, or by both, such as haloperidol. Despite the risks, the use of neuroleptics should be considered when clinically appropriate.

Anxiety

Several studies found children who are living with HIV to have high rates of anxiety disorders.[49,66–68] Likely confounding factors contributing to anxiety include the greater levels of psychosocial stressors related to being HIV infected, including frequent illness and hospitalization, concerns over health status, stigma, secrecy, family illnesses, and level of stability. Alternatively, it is possible that the effects of HIV infection on brain structures, such as the basal ganglia, would be involved in the regulation of anxiety.[69] There is no literature on the psychopharmacologic treatment of anxiety disorders in HIV-infected children. However, the data collected from the use of selective serotonin reuptake inhibitors in uninfected children can be helpful in addressing treatment approaches for the HIV-infected child.[70,71]

Drug-Drug Interactions

Pharmacokinetic and pharmacodynamic principles govern our understanding of effective psychopharmacology, especially with medically ill children who take many medications. *Pharmacokinetic* interactions relate to how the body handles the medication, and *pharmacodynamic* interactions relate to how the medication affects the body. Key concepts in pharmacokinetics include absorption, distribution, metabolism, and excretion of the drug. In HIV-infected children, specific concerns regarding absorption are pertinent because of changes in the gastrointestinal system or the route of administration. Different medications, including antacids and antidiarrheal medications or intestinal infections can alter absorption. Distribution commonly relates to the degree that the medication is freely dissolved in the blood or bound to plasma proteins. Many medications can alter the relative bioavailability and serum concentration of other medications, depending on their level of protein binding and solubility. Different factors affect the permeability that a medication will have on the blood-brain barrier and therefore its effect on the brain. This is particularly relevant for psychotropic medications, since the site of action is the central nervous system. New antiretroviral medications, particularly protease inhibitors, demonstrate poor permeability into the brain, which is an important factor in the treatment of progressive encephalopathy.

Metabolism, or biotransformation, is particularly important in the pharmacology for HIV-infected children, since many of the antiretroviral medications depend on the family of cytochrome P-450 isoenzymes.[72] The protease inhibitors potently inhibit the 3A4 isoenzyme in addition to affecting other isoenzymes. This affects many psychotropic medications in addition to antimicrobial, antifungal, antiseizure, and antiarrhythmia agents.[73] With altered pharmacokinetics, medications can exhibit more adverse effects or even toxicity. Since medications can act as substrates for the isoenzymes or actively induce or inhibit them, a careful review of the metabolic pathway of any medication should be reviewed with the entire pharmacologic regimen.[52,53] This will help prevent adverse drug reactions and medication contraindications.

The genetic heterogeneity of the isoenzymes adds another layer of complexity, since the deficiency of the 2D6 isoenzyme is reported to be 5% to 8% in the white population.[74]

WORKING WITH CAREGIVERS OF HIV-INFECTED CHILDREN AND ADOLESCENTS

The best models for psychosocial and mental health intervention acknowledge AIDS as a family disease with profound effects on both infected and noninfected members of the family. Family-based interventions, which take into account the mental health needs of individual family members (both adults and children) and the needs of the family unit as a whole, are optimal. Frequently, intervention with children without addressing the needs of caregivers is ineffective, particularly when families bring histories of substance abuse and disruption to their struggles to cope with HIV infection.

HIV-Positive Mothers

Parents living with HIV disease reflect considerable diversity in cultural heritage, socioeconomic circumstances, life experiences, and geographic location, and psychosocial interventions must be individualized. However, a significant number of HIV-positive mothers are also struggling with their own substance abuse or that of their partners, as well as living in communities characterized by poverty and violence. For this population, clinicians should be vigilant for mental health problems known to be comorbid with substance abuse in women. These include depressive and anxiety disorders as well as high rates of traumatization and post-traumatic stress disorder.[15,16,75,76] Appropriate identification and intervention in these mental health problems when they present is essential to optimizing a woman's adaptation to her own HIV illness and that in her family members.[41]

Many HIV-infected women are socially isolated and have experienced discrimination due to substance abuse and poverty prior to their HIV diagnosis. This baseline isolation can impede access to social and mental health supports as well as health care. In addition, guilt and shame about behaviors associated with the acquisition of HIV can impede effective communication about their HIV diagnosis, further isolating women from social supports. For women struggling with drug addiction, the stress of an HIV diagnosis can lead to relapse in women in recovery or escalation of use in active users.

Progression of HIV Illness

The necessity of communicating with family members about illness and the need to plan for their children's future increases with the progression of HIV illness in parents. Quite commonly, parents with advancing HIV illness have difficulty communicating effectively with their children about their illness. Andrews and coworkers[77] found that only 33% of HIV seropositive mothers had disclosed to children younger than 16 years of age, whereas 67% had disclosed to those older than 16. Similarly, Mellins and Ehrhardt[46] found, in a study of 40 HIV-infected mothers, that the majority had not told their children of their HIV status, particularly when children were younger than 12 years of age. Although adults often perceive the lack of disclosure to children as protective, it can serve to increase the anxiety of children experiencing the ongoing physical and mental deterioration in their parents.

Clearly, one of the most difficult and painful realizations for parents with HIV to face is that they must plan for the placement of their children and adolescents after their death. Although this is less prevalent with the advances in medical treatment over the last several years, it remains an important issue for those parents with progressing HIV illness. However, approaching a parent about legal permanency issues before establishing a therapeutic alliance will often lead to resistance, as will raising this issue at inappropriate times. Once a relationship is established and the parent has raised the issue or the medical stage indicates the need for such planning, it is important to begin this process.

Legacy projects—activities that help people express their thoughts, experiences, hopes, and dreams and provide lasting, tangible evidence of their love for family members—make it easier for families to cope with the losses associated with the disease. Examples of legacy projects include letters to their children, audiotapes of their child's favorite stories, memory boxes, memory books, and videotapes. Videotapes create a powerful visual legacy. They can provide a vivid and lasting sense of intimacy that is cherished by the family for generations to come.[78]

It is also especially important that providers help family members explore the potential roles of extended family members and friends. Unfortunately, several emotional and legal barriers discourage mothers from making formal custody plans for their children. These include denial or resistance to thinking about their future death, fear of disclosing their illness to others, reluctance to "give up" their children, and unwillingness to involve the biological father.[79] A complex legal system also drives parents who are unfamiliar with legal processes away from permanency planning. Some legal barriers include lack of information or misinformation about planning options and a general fear of the legal system. A range of custody options should be available to parents to meet the short- and long-term care needs of their children. These include the creation of a will and legal proceedings such as standby guardianship, guardianship, coguardianship, subsidized guardianship, and adoption (Table 22–3).

Legal counseling about parent-friendly custody options can help parents understand their legal options and reduce the fear and intimidation many often feel about the legal system.[79] Other activities that encourage mothers to make custody plans include talking with other HIV-positive parents, discussing their concerns about their children with family members, attending permanency planning and legacy workshops, and discussing the plan with the child's father. Parents also find great comfort in having mental health services available for their children. These services should be made available during the time of parental illness and should continue to be available after the parental death to assist with issues associated with loss and grief as well as with the transition to a new home and family.

Late-Stage Illness

In the final phase of HIV illness, loss of parental functioning becomes paramount. Families with minimal social support can find themselves in crisis in this phase of the illness. The care of younger children may be left to older adolescents or young adult family members, who are themselves facing the impending loss of a parent. In those parents who develop AIDS-related dementia, children experience the changes in their parent's mental status, often without a clear understanding of the cause or implications of these changes. In cases in which parents develop AIDS-related organic brain syndromes, their disinhibited or disorganized behavior can be dangerous to children in their care.

Optimally, parents affected by AIDS have begun the communication and permanency planning process prior to the final stage of parental HIV illness, and other adults are available to provide care and support for affected children. However, some parents, particularly those struggling unsuccessfully with mental illness or substance abuse, present to medical care settings in end-stage AIDS without having addressed these issues. These are usually the most disorganized families with the highest burden of psychiatric and substance abuse disorders. In these families, special attention to the mental health needs of the children and adolescents is essential. Both the lack of family preparation and the factors associated with that lack of preparation indicate increased risk for mental health problems in these children.

Fathers

Women are the predominant caregivers of children infected with the virus, and most HIV-infected children live within single-parent, female-headed families. Consequently, the majority of attention, programs, interventions, and research have focused on women and children. There is very limited demographic and psychosocial information available on fathers, despite the fact that these individuals may outlive their partners. As the mother becomes increasingly symptomatic or when she dies, some of these men become the sole caregivers of their infected children. A recent investigation[80] revealed that compared with parents of children with congenital heart disease, fathers of HIV-infected children reported elevated levels of distress in their parenting roles. They also suffered from increased psychological distress and reported a number of service-related needs.[80] Many women do not even mention the availability of the father to health care personnel because of their concern about losing financial benefits if they do. The father's role as a parent and as a resource merits careful attention and consideration.

Extended Family and Foster Caregivers

HIV-infected children whose parents are unable to care for them due to the physical demands of their own HIV/AIDS disease, substance use, emotional dysfunction, or death are often left to extended family members. It has been estimated that 45% of children born to HIV-infected mothers live with primary caregivers other than a biological parent, with the strongest predictor of such placement being maternal drug use. Most of these children reside with another relative, usually aunts, great aunts, older siblings, or, most frequently, grandparents.[24] Grandparents and great-grandmothers are increasingly called on to care for children infected with HIV in addition to the need to care for their own child living with HIV/AIDS. They have the daunting task of dealing with the loss of their own child at the same time they are helping the surviving grandchildren endure the loss of their parent and their own illness.[24]

The percentage of grandmothers raising children is highest among African American children, with estimates as high as 30% to 70% in Detroit and New York City.[81] Many of these women have extensive medical needs of their own but tend to neglect their own health care, since they consider their grandchild's needs more urgent.

Table 22-3
Legal Options in Permanency Planning: Responsibilities and Rights of Guardians, Adoptive Parents and Biological Parents

	LEGAL STATUS	DECISION MAKING	FINANCIAL RESPONSIBILITY	RELATIONSHIP WITH BIRTH PARENTS	CAREGIVER REQUIREMENTS
GUARDIANSHIP: ABUSE AND NEGLECT CASES, CHILD WELFARE INVOLVEMENT	Biological parents retain residual parental rights. Guardian is public child welfare entity or its designee. Guardian has right to custody, educational, medical, and other decisions. Child is a ward of the court.	Most major decisions (including educational and medical) are made by guardian, but parents retain rights that include visitation with the child and the right to consent to adoption.	Guardian is responsible for the care and support of the child. Birth parent(s) may be required to contribute. In most cases, caregivers (licensed foster parents, relatives) receive some financial payment from child welfare system.	Birth parent(s) has (have) the right to visit the child. Guardian can regulate how the visits are structured but cannot prevent visits from occurring. Court may also order visits to be supervised.	Child welfare agency/designee acts as guardian. Substitute caregivers, including foster parents, group homes and institutions, and relatives (or kinship care providers), must meet various licensing requirements as promulgated by child welfare.
GUARDIANSHIP: NON-ABUSE OR NEGLECT, NO CURRENT CHILD WELFARE SYSTEM INVOLVEMENT	Birth parents' rights are not terminated. Guardian has right to day-to-day custody, educational, medical, and other decisions.	Most major decisions (including educational and medical) are made by guardian, but parents retain rights that include visitation with the child and the right to consent to adoption.	The guardian is responsible for the care and custody and ensuring the support of the minor. The guardian may also apply for some types of benefits on behalf of the minor.	Birth parent(s) has (have) right to visit the child. The guardian will have input into how the visits are structured but cannot prevent visits from occurring. If the guardian and the parents cannot work out visitation, the court may determine circumstances under which visitation may take place.	In general, guardian must be at least 18 years of age and a resident of the United States, not adjudged disabled, and have no felony convictions. Court also may want criminal background check and may want child abuse/neglect check. Some courts also require home investigation and report.

STANDBY GUARDIANSHIP*	Birth parents' rights are not terminated. Standby guardian acts only when a future event or condition occurs. Usually the "triggering" event or condition is associated with a parent's "terminal" or "chronic" illness, such as the parent's death or physical or mental incapacity.† Standby status vests only after written designation by parent, or court appointment, or both, depending on state. To become permanent guardian, usually court-approved standby guardian must apply to court for full guardianship.	Until the standby guardian's duties are activated, parent(s) make all decisions. In most states, once duties are activated, most major decisions are made by guardian, but parents retain rights that include visitation with the child and the right to consent to adoption.*	The standby guardian is not responsible for the care, custody, or ensuring the support of the minor until his/her duties are activated. The standby guardian may also apply for some types of benefits on behalf of the minor once duties are activated.	Standby guardian works in cooperation with the birth parent, and assumes duties only when birth parent dies or is unable to make and carry out day-to-day child care decisions.	Most states require that standby guardian must be at least 18 years of age and a resident of the United States, not adjudged disabled, and have no felony convictions. Court also may want criminal background check and may want child abuse/neglect check. Some courts also require home investigation and report.
ADOPTION	Rights of birth parent(s) are terminated. Adoptive parent(s) has all rights and responsibilities formerly attributed to birth parents. Adoption is a permanent legal relationship.	All major decisions are made by the adoptive parent(s)—e.g., school, medical treatment, religion, etc.	Adoptive parents are responsible for the care, custody and support of the minor. If parental rights are terminated due to abuse and neglect and the child has special needs, in many cases adoption assistance is available through child welfare. Adoption assistance can include a cash payment, a medical card, and payments for nonrecurring expenses related to the adoption.	In general, adoptive parents have right to determine the type of relationship that the child will have with birth parent(s). A few states permit open adoption, with court approved postadoption visits.	Usually state requires some period of residency prior to filing petition for adoption. Some exceptions to residency requirement may be made for adoption of a related child or adoption of a child placed by an agency. Adoptive parent must be under no legal disability. Must be of legal age and, if married, state may require spouse to be a party to the adoption.

Table 22-3
Legal Options in Permanency Planning: Responsibilities and Rights of Guardians, Adoptive Parents and Biological Parents *Continued*

	LEGAL STATUS	DECISION MAKING	FINANCIAL RESPONSIBILITY	RELATIONSHIP WITH BIRTH PARENTS	CAREGIVER REQUIREMENTS
STANDBY ADOPTION[‡]	Standby adoption is an adoption in which a terminally ill parent consents to custody and termination of parental rights to become effective upon the occurrence of the parent's death, or the parent's request that the adoption be finalized. Parental rights of terminally ill parent preserved until birth parent dies or wants adoption finalized. Child's other parent may consent to adoption or rights may be otherwise terminated. Standby adoptive parent acts only when birth parent dies or wants adoption finalized.	Until standby adoptive parent's duties are activated, birth parents make all the decisions. Once duties are activated, standby adoptive parents become the legal parents of the child.	The standby adoptive parent is not responsible for care, custody, or support of the minor until his/her duties are activated. Once duties are activated and the adoption is finalized, standby adoptive parent becomes completely financially reponsible for the child.	Standby adoptive parent works in cooperation with the birth parent, and assumes duties only when birth parent dies or requests that the adoption be finalized. Once the adoption is finalized, the standy adoptive parent becomes the legal parent of the child.	Same as adoptive parent.

[*]As of September, 2002, the following had standby guardianship laws: Arkansas, Colorado, District of Columbia, Florida, Georgia, Illinois, Iowa, Maryland, Massachusetts, Minnesota, Nebraska, New Jersey, New York, North Carolina, Ohio, Pennsylvania, Virginia, West Virginia, Wisconsin, and Wyoming. California and Connecticut have "joint guardianship" laws that permit shared decision-making while providing for a future care and custody plan.
[†]Some states (IL, MD, MA, NC, VA, WV) include parental consent alone as sufficient to trigger the standby guardianship. In those states, no disability or illness is required to trigger the guardianship.
[‡]Standby adoption became effective in Illinois on January 1, 2000. As of September, 2002, Illinois was the only state that had enacted a standby adoption statute.
From Coons LS: Legal Options in Permanency Planning Responsibilities and Rights of Guardians, Adoptive Parents, and Biological Parents. Chicago, LS Coons, Esq, copyright 2002.

A number of prevention efforts are available to help these caregivers. These include engaging community resources that can provide practical and emotional services, in-home support, respite care, and financial assistance. It is important to help the caregiver to anticipate, prevent, and cope with excessively stressful events. If the medication regimens are too complex or difficult, drawing up syringes in advance, making charts, or purchasing alarm watches can be helpful in assisting these caregivers. Assessing for depression and symptoms of anxiety and providing early treatment as necessary are crucial. Through a sensitive response, these women can carry on their responsibilities and take care of their own emotional and physical needs while working through the painful consequences of AIDS.

While efforts to place HIV-positive children with relatives should always be made first, in some cases, no appropriate relatives are identified. These children frequently end up in foster care. For the most part, foster parents, who have made a commitment to care for children infected with HIV, have been courageous and excellent care providers. Nevertheless, foster home placement presents many psychosocial challenges. If the child was removed from the biological home due to abuse or neglect, the foster family has the challenge of helping the child cope with the consequences of such treatment as well as the disruption of removal from their parent's care. For children placed in foster care after the death of their parents, there are significant losses, including the loss of relationships within the family and loss of neighborhood friends and teachers.[24]

Loss is a key issue for the foster parent as well, as he or she becomes attached to the child and grieves for the child's potential loss of health or death. Caregiver problems related to raising an HIV-positive child such as disclosure to the child and school, potential isolation, stigmatization, or ostracism, uncertainty, and preparation for the HIV-infected child's future and/or death are not unique to the biological relative. Mental health services for all care providers that address these issues are essential.

CONCLUSION

Psychosocial interventions for children living with or affected by HIV are best delivered by a multidisciplinary team that includes a child and adolescent social worker, a psychologist, and a psychiatrist, who can help the child and family develop psychologically healthy ways of living with the disease and its long-term effects. For many families, HIV/AIDS represents another item on a long list of socioenvironmental problems, such as poverty, substance use, limited access to health care and health information, and discrimination. A multisystem model of care that coordinates numerous social service and health care systems provides a much-needed framework for health care providers that limits duplication of services and clarifies the roles of various providers.[82] Systems of care that have the expertise and capacity to meet the needs of all involved family members in a coordinated manner also are important in reducing family burden and fragmentation of care.[83] Just as recent advances in medical treatment have increased hope and optimism in the face of HIV medical illness, increasing knowledge and systems development in the psychosocial arena has the potential to improve quality of life and adaptation to illness.

REFERENCES

1. Michaels D, Levine C: Estimates of the number of motherless youth orphaned by AIDS in the United States. JAMA 1992;268:3456.
2. Centers for Disease Control and Prevention. HIV/AIDS Surveillance Update 1998;10:2.
3. Singer L, Farkas K, Kliegman R: Childhood medical and behavioral consequences of maternal cocaine use. J Pediatric Psychol 1992;17:389.
4. Kelley S: Parenting stress and child maltreatment in drug-exposed children. Child Abuse Neglect 1992; 16:312.
5. Rodning C, Beckwith L, Howard J: Characteristics of attachment organization and play organization in prenatally drug-exposed toddlers. Dev Psychopathol 1989;1:277.
6. Cicchetti D, Carlson V (eds): Child Maltreatment: Theory and Research on the Causes and Consequences of Child Abuse and Neglect. New York, Cambridge University Press, 1989, p 529.
7. McLeer S, Callaghan M, Delmina HJ, et al: Psychiatric disorders in sexually abused children. J Am Acad Child Adolesc Psychiatry 1994;33:313.
8. Pelcovitz D, Kaplan S, Goldenberg B, et al: Post-traumatic stress disorder in physically abused adolescents. J Am Acad Child Adolesc Psychiatry 1994;33:305.
9. Griffith DR, Azuma S, Chasnoff I: Three-year outcome of children exposed prenatally to drugs. J Am Acad Child Adolesc Psychiatry 1994:33:20.

10. Coles C, Platzman K, Smith IE, et al: Effects of cocaine and alcohol use in pregnancy on neonatal growth and neurobehavioral status. Neurotox Teratol 1993;15:289.
11. Wilens TM, Biederman J, Kiely K, et al: Pilot study of behavioral and emotional disturbance in the high risk children of parents with opioid dependence. J Am Acad Child Adolesc Psychiatry 1995;34:6:779.
12. Hutchings D: The puzzle of cocaine's effects following maternal use during pregnancy. Are there reconcilable differences? Neurotox Teratol 1993;15:281.
13. Gonzalez NM, Campbell M: Cocaine babies: Does prenatal drug exposure to cocaine affect development? J Am Acad Child Adolesc Psychiatry 1994; 33:1.
14. Carroll KM, Rounsaville BJ: History and significance of childhood attention deficit disorder in treatment-seeking cocaine abusers. Compr Psychiatry 1993;34:75.
15. Haller DL, Knisely JS, Dawson KS, et al: Perinatal substance abusers: Psychological and social characteristics. J Nerv Ment Dis 1993;181:509.
16. Regier DA, Farmer Rae DS, et al: Comorbidity of mental disorders with alcohol and other drugs of abuse. JAMA 1990;264:2511.
17. Weissman MM, Gershon ES, Kidd KK, et al: Psychiatric disorders in the relatives of probands with affective disorders. Arch Gen Psychiatry 1984;41:13.
18. Biederman J, Faraone SV, Keenan K, et al: Family-genetic and psychosocial risk factors in DSM-III attention deficit disorder. J Am Acad Child Adolesc Psychiatry 1990;29:526.
19. Goodman R, Stevenson J: A twin study of hyperactivity: II. The aetiological role of genes, family relationships, and perinatal adversity. J Child Psychol Psychiatry 1989;30:691.
20. Lewert G: Children and AIDS. Soc Casework 1988;69:348.
21. Wiener L, Battles H, Heilman N, et al: Factors associated with disclosure of diagnosis to children with HIV/AIDS. Pediatr AIDS HIV Infect 1996;7:310.
22. Cohen FL: Research on families and pediatric human immunodeficiency virus disease: A review and needed directions. J Dev Behav Pediatr 1994;15:S35.
23. Cohen FL: Clinical Genetics in Nursing Practice. Philadelphia, JB Lippincott, 1984.
24. Wiener L, Septimus A, Grady C: Psychosocial support and ethical issues in pediatric AIDS. In Pizzo PA, Wilfert C (eds): Pediatric AIDS, 3rd ed. Baltimore, Lippincott Williams & Wilkins, 1998, p 703.
25. Funck-Bretano I, Costagliola D, Seibel N, et al: Patterns of disclosure and perceptions of the human immunodeficiency virus in infected elementary school-age children. Arch Pediatr Adolesc Med 1997;151:978.
26. Lipson M: Disclosure of diagnosis to children with HIV or AIDS. J Dev Behav Pediatr 1994;15:S61.
27. Pollock SW, Thompson CL: The HIV-infected child in therapy. In Boyd-Franklin N, Steiner G, Boland M (eds): Children, Families and HIV/AIDS. New York, Guilford Press, 1995, p 127.
28. Centers for Disease Control and Prevention: AIDS cases in adolescents and adults under age 25, by sex and exposure category, reported through June 2001, United States. HIV/AIDS Surv Rep 2002; 13(1).
29. Samples CL, Goodman E, Woods E: Epidemiology and medical management of adolescents. In Pizzo PA, Wilfert C (eds): Pediatric AIDS, 3rd ed. Baltimore, Lippincott Williams & Wilkins, 1998, p 615.
30. Lightfoot M, Rotheram-Borus MJ: Negotiating behavior change with HIV-positive adolescent girls. AIDS Patient Care STDs 1998;12:395.
31. Lyon ME, Silber TJ, D'Angelo J: Difficult life circumstances in HIV-infected adolescents: Cause or effect? AIDS Patient Care STDs 1997;11:29.
32. Kissinger P, Clark RA, Abdalian SE: Psychosocial characteristics of HIV-infected adolescents in New Orleans. J Adolesc Health 1997;20:258.
33. Henderson R, et al: A survey of the mental health care needs of HIV+ adolescents and young adults. Paper presented at the 12th World AIDS Conference, Geneva, Switzerland, 1998, abstract 24230.
34. Hein K, Dell R, Futterman D, et al: Comparison of HIV+ and HIV− adolescents: Risk factors and psychosocial determinants. Pediatrics 1995;96.
35. Futterman D, et al: Human immunodeficiency virus-infected adolescents: The first 50 patients in a New York City program. Pediatrics 1993;91:730.
36. Hoffman ND, Futterman D, Myerson A: Treatment issues for HIV-positive adolescents. Mass Med Soc AIDS Clin Care 1999;11(3):17–19, 21, 23–24.
37. Engle L: Growing up positive. Body Positive 1999;XII(8). (Available at http://www.thebody.com/bp/aug99/growing.html.)
38. Kunins H, et al: Guide to adolescent HIV/AIDS program development. J Adolesc Health 1993;14:36S.
39. Casey Family Services: Planning Children's Futures: Meeting the Needs of Children, Adolescents, and Families Affected by HIV/AIDS. Shelton, CT, Casey Family Services, 1999.
40. Mendelsohn A: Pervasive traumatic loss from AIDS in the life of a 4-year-old African boy. J Child Psychother 1997;23:399.
41. Havens J, Mellins CA, Pilowski D: Mental health issues in HIV-affected women and children. Int Rev Psychiatry 1996;8:217.
42. Epstein LG, Sharer LR, Goudsmit J: Neurological and neuropathological features of human immunodeficiency virus infection in children. Ann Neurol 1988;23(suppl):S19.
43. Brouwers P, Wolters P, Civitello L: Central nervous system manifestations and assessment. In Pizzo PA, Wilfert C (eds): Pediatric AIDS, 3rd ed. Baltimore, Lippincott Williams & Wilkins, 1998, p 293.

44. Diamond GW, Kaufman J, Belman AL, et al: Characterization of cognitive functioning in a subgroup of children with congenital HIV infection. Arch Clin Neuropsychol 1987;23:245.
45. Swayles TP, Scorr GB, Cohen DS, et al: Neurocognitive functioning among infants exposed perinatally to HIV. Paper presented at the Fifth International Conference on AIDS, Montreal, June 14, 1989. Vol. 9(5), abstract 317.
46. Mellins CA, Ehrhardt AA: Families affected by pediatric AIDS: Sources of stress and coping. J Dev Behav Pediatr 1994;15;S54.
47. Spiegel L, Mayers A: Psychosocial aspects of AIDS in children and adolescents. Pediatr Clin North Am 1991;38:153.
48. Wiener L, Battles H, Reikert KA: Longitudinal study of psychological distress symptoms in HIV-infected, school-aged children. J HIV/AIDS Prevent Educ Adolesc Child 1999;3:13.
49. Havens JF, Whitaker AH, Feldman JF: Psychiatric morbidity in school-age children with congenital human immunodeficiency virus infection: A pilot study. J Dev Behav Pediatr 1994;15:S18.
50. Gonzalez, A, Everall IP: Lest we forget: Neuropsychiatry and the new generation anti-HIV drugs. AIDS 1998;12:2365.
51. Sahai J: Risks and synergies from drug interactions. AIDS 1996;10:S21.
52. Fauci AD, Bartlett JG, Goosby EP, et al: Guidelines for the use of antiretroviral agents in HIV-infected adults and adolescents. Panel of clinical practices for treatment of HIV infection. Living Doc 1999;24–26.
53. Oleske J, Scott GB, et al: Guidelines for the use of antiretroviral agents in pediatric HIV infection. Working group on antiretroviral therapy and medical management of HIV-infected children. Living Doc 1999;24–26. www.HIVatis.org/trtgdlns.html.
54. Heylen R, Miller R: Adverse effects and drug interactions of medications commonly used in the treatment of adult HIV positive patients. Genitourin Med 1996;72:237.
55. Corsi A, Albizzati A, Cervini R, et al: Hyperactive disturbance in the behavior of children with congenital HIV infection. In Abstracts of the Seventh International AIDS Conference, Volume 2, Florence Italy, 1991.
56. Hittleman J, Nelson N, Shah V, et al: Neurodevelopmental disabilities in infants born to HIV-infected mothers. AIDS Reader 1996;6:126.
57. Arnold LE, Abikoff HB, Cantwell DP, et al: National Institute of Mental Health Collaborative Multimodal Treatment Study of Children with ADHD (MTA). Design challenges and choices. Arch Gen Psychiatr 1997;54:51.
58. Havens JF, McCaskill EO: Psychostimulants in HIV-infected children and adolescents: A case series. In Greenhill LL, Osman BB (eds): Ritalin Theory and Practice, 2nd ed. Larchmont, NY, Mary Ann Liebert, 1999, p 165.
59. Cesena M, Douglas LO, Cebollero AM, et al: Case study: Behavioral symptoms of pediatric HIV-1 encephalopathy successfully treated with clonidine. J Am Acad Child Adolesc Psychiatry 1995;34:302.
60. Hunt RD, Minderaa RB, Cohen DJ: Clonidine benefits children with attention deficit disorder and hyperactivity: Report of a double-blind placebo-crossover therapeutic trial. J Am Acad Child Psychiatr 1985;24:617.
61. Cooper ER, Hanson C, Diaz C, et al: Encephalopathy and progression of human immunodeficiency virus disease in a cohort of children with perinatally acquired human immunodeficiency virus infection. J Pediatrics 1998;132:808.
62. Pizzo PA, Eddy J, Falloon J, et al: Effect of continuous intravenous infusion of zidovudine (AZT) in children with symptomatic HIV infection. N Engl J Med 1988;319:889.
63. Ayuso JL: Use of psychotropic drugs in patients with HIV infection. Drugs 1994;47:599.
64. Hriso E, Kuhn T, Maslev J, et al: Extrapyramidal symptoms due to dopamine-blocking agents in patients with AIDS encephalopathy. Am J Psychiatry 1991;148:1558.
65. Breitbart W, Marotta RF, Call P: AIDS and neuroleptic malignant syndrome. Lancet 1988;2:1488–1489.
66. Bussing R, Burket RC: Anxiety and intrafamilial stress in children with hemophilia after the HIV crisis. J Am Acad Child Adolesc Psychiatry 1993;32:562.
67. Hooper SR, Whitt JK, Tennison M, et al: Behavioral adaptation to human immunodeficiency virus-seropositive status children and adolescents with hemophilia. Behav Adapt 1993;147:541.
68. Riekert KA, Wiener L, Battles H: Prediction of psychological distress in school-age children with HIV. Children's Health Care 1999;28:201.
69. Wise SP, Rapoport JL: Obsessive-compulsive disorders: Is it basal ganglia dysfunction? In Rapoport JL (ed): Obsessive-Compulsive Disorder in Children and Adolescents. Washington, DC, American Psychiatric Press, 1989.
70. Riddle MA, Scahill L, King RA, et al: Double blind cross-over trial of fluoxetine and placebo in children and adolescents with obsessive-compulsive disorder. J Am Acad Child Adolesc Psychiatry 1992;31:1062.
71. Birmaher B, Ryan N, et al: Fluoxetine for childhood anxiety disorders. J Am Acad Child Adolesc Psychiatry 1994;33:993.
72. Molla A, Granneman GR, Sun E, et al: Recent developments in HIV protease inhibitor therapy. Antiviral Res 1998;39:1.
73. Nemeroff CB, DeVane CL, Pollock BG: Newer antidepressants and the cytochrome p450 system. Am J Psychiatry 1996;153:311.
74. Broly F, Gaedigk A, Heim M, et al: Debrisoquin sparteine hydroxylation genotype and phenotype:

Analysis of common mutations and alleles of CYP2D6 in a European population. DNA Cell Biol 1991;10:545.
75. Najavitz LM, Weiss RD, Shaw SR: The link between substance abuse and posttraumatic stress disorder in women: A research review. Am J Addict 1997;6:273.
76. Mellins CA, Ehrhardt AA, Grant WF: Psychiatric symptomatology and psychological functioning in HIV infected women. AIDS Behav 1997;1:233.
77. Andrews S, Williams AB, Neil K: The mother child relationship in the HIV-1 positive family. Image 1993;25:193.
78. Taylor-Brown S, Wiener L: Making videotapes of HIV-infected women for their children. Fam Soc 1993;74:468.
79. Shanker R, Budner N, LaGamma D, et al: Barriers and facilitators: Planning for the future care of HIV/AIDS affected children. In Planning Children's Futures, Conference Report. Baltimore, Annie E. Casey Foundation, 1999, p 119.
80. Battles H: Brief report: Fathering of a child living with HIV/AIDS: Psychosocial adjustment and parenting stress. J Pediatr Psychol 2001;26:333–338.
81. Minkler M, Rose KM: Grandmothers as Caregivers. Raising Children of the Cocaine Epidemic, Newbury Park, Calif, Sage Publications, 1993.
82. Lewis SY, Haiken HJ: Contact with social service agencies. In Zeichner SL, Read JS (eds): Handbook of Pediatric HIV Care. Baltimore, Lippincott Williams & Wilkins, 1999, p 572.
83. Havens J, Mellins C, Ryan S: The mental health treatment of children and families affected by HIV/AIDS. In Wicks L (eds): Psychotherapy and AIDS. Washington, DC, Taylor & Francis, 1997, p 101.

23

Nursing Care in Pediatric HIV Infection

Carol A. Vincent

For the past two decades, HIV and AIDS have devastated the world and the families who live in the wake of the disease day to day. The number of deaths worldwide is staggering. The North American continent has seen the ravages of the disease in small proportions compared with other continents, in particular Africa and Asia. Throughout Sub-Saharan Africa and in areas of Asia and Latin America, HIV has become, after malnutrition, the second greatest threat to the well-being of infants and children.[1] The United States has tempered HIV disease with its ability to garner resources to fight the epidemic. As a result, perinatal transmission in the United States is at an all-time low. Treatment of people infected with HIV has improved with the development of new drugs and the availability of intensive services for those with few or no resources.

The epidemic of pediatric HIV-1 in the United States mirrors that of HIV-1 infection in women of childbearing age.[2] The epidemic has disproportionately affected African American and Hispanic women and their children.[2,3] The needs of children in these minority groups are intensified by the fact that poverty also disproportionately affects racial and ethnic minorities.[4] The number of children living with HIV disease in the United States is estimated by the Centers for Disease Control and Prevention (CDC) to be more than 2000 children.[5] Although HIV is less prevalent in the United States in comparison with other countries, the needs of those infected are no less. The disease is ever present and inevitably fatal.

The focus of this chapter is to discuss the role of nursing care in the provision of health care for HIV-infected infants and children. In addition, it discusses the unique needs of HIV-infected children and their families and identifies ways in which nurses can help to lessen the impact of the disease through the formulation of a dynamic plan of care.

THE ROLE OF NURSING CARE IN PEDIATRIC HIV

Nurses, by virtue of their education, are in a unique position within the multidisciplinary team to deliver care and treatment to children with HIV and their families. Because knowledge regarding the diagnosis, management, and treatment of HIV infection is constantly changing, nursing practice must keep pace in order to serve clients in the best manner possible.[6] In recent years, HIV has emerged as a chronic disease. Like other chronic illnesses, HIV forces families to interact with the health care system on a regular basis.[7] The hope that most children with HIV would survive into adolescence with an improved quality of life has been realized with the use of new antiretroviral medications, the ability to monitor the status of infection through laboratory testing, and, in general, better medical management strategies. Unpredictability and uncertainty are still a mainstay of the disease. Nurses need to be prepared to anticipate, to the best of their ability, the needs of children as technology advances.

Pediatrics encompasses a wide range of groups, including infants, toddlers, preschoolers, early school-aged children, late school-aged children, and adolescents. Each group has a unique set of needs surrounding chronic illness and HIV as well as their developmental age. As more children are surviving to adolescence, the special needs of adolescents should be considered.[8]

Developing a plan of care with the child and family is an essential role of the nurse. Nurses can assist families in understanding the plan of care, which includes, but is not limited to, the treatment regimen, multiple appointments, and nutritional needs. Nurses can serve as advocates for children who are affected by HIV disease and their families.

Nurses as Part of the Multidisciplinary Team

The complexity of HIV disease requires that the child and family have access to multidisciplinary health care services. Care that is coordinated and collaborative is essential for successful outcomes. The multidisciplinary team can help to identify the obstacles that families encounter in accessing care.[9] The multidisciplinary team consists of nurses, social workers, primary and specialty care physicians, registered dieticians, neuropsychology and child development professionals, pharmacists, mental health professionals including drug and alcohol counselors, occupational therapists, physical therapists, speech therapists, home care practitioners, foster care agencies, state and local child-related agencies, educators, child life specialists, legal professionals, and the religious clergy.[10] The needs of families are multidimensional, hence the need for multiple disciplines working to help families cope with the enormous physical, emotional, and psychosocial issues secondary to HIV infection. Working as a team assists families in meeting goals and needs. It is essential for health care professionals to be cognizant of the need for many services and of the importance and challenge of coordinating these services. Without coordination, services can be duplicated or can go unmet.[11,12] Coordinating care in the management of this complex disease can be overwhelming for both the health care professional and the family. The family may have difficulty navigating the health care system. Although the need for multiple services is great, this too can become an obstacle to providing care.

As the HIV epidemic has grown and has affected a diverse population, hospitals and communities need to keep pace with the needs of these patients. Addressing the challenges, such as having little or no insurance, is important. Health care providers must facilitate coordination of services, limit duplication of services, and clarify the roles of various providers, not only for the family but also for the team members.[12]

The Populations We Serve

The original cases of HIV in the United States were identified in men who have sex with other men. Over the years, the demographics of persons with HIV have changed. The disease now affects not only men but also women and children of varied backgrounds. Although the virus does not discriminate on the basis of race, color, or creed, a disproportionate number of HIV cases in adults and children are among minority populations. More and more, we are seeing how this disease disproportionately affects unempowered minorities: women, children, African Americans, Hispanics, homosexuals, and intravenous drug abusers. The number of HIV-infected children have paralleled the reported cases of HIV infection and AIDS in women.[13] Perinatally exposed (i.e., mother-to-child HIV transmission) children often live in compromising situations related to great poverty, parental substance abuse, and loss of parents.[12,14,15] Poverty undermines a family's ability to carry out their functions. Being poor with insufficient resources is the strongest predictor of poor health outcomes for children.[15] This creates special challenges when providing care for clients who are affected by poverty and now are affected by HIV. The undue stress this places on children and their families cannot be overstated.

The stigma of HIV goes beyond that of the fear of the disease as a contagion. The social milieu associations with HIV disease are strong. The mode of transmission may invoke stigma. Often, whether or not it is fact, there is an association that an HIV infected individual is homosexual or a drug user.

Almost all cases of pediatric HIV are acquired through perinatal transmission. Less commonly, HIV is acquired through breastfeeding, sexual abuse, and transfusion with HIV-tainted blood products. HIV weaves itself through the fabric of an entire family where the mother, father, child and siblings may be infected. In addition to the ravages of the disease, families must often endure self-imposed isolation from their communities for fear of being "found out." It is a stigma that is painful.

The Communities We Serve

At one time in the HIV pandemic, infection control recommendations based on regional geographic preference were appropriate. These recommendations are no longer appropriate.[13] HIV knows no geographic boundaries. Urban and rural settings pose different challenges, as beliefs among rural and urban families are often different.[4] Planning nursing care for children and their families affected by HIV can be difficult whether there are many or few resources.

Urban Communities

Nurses working in urban settings see and understand the difficulties facing inner city populations. Hopelessness, poverty, and lack of alternatives to drugs and violence, both in the home and in the neighborhoods, are part of urban living.[6,16]

Within cities, there are ethnic populations who live and congregate together. Identifying the needs of these communities is essential to meeting their needs. Language barriers, cultural beliefs, and varied health practices within urban communities pose special challenges in preventing HIV infection as well as caring for those already infected. Nurses who have not grown up in poverty, who have not been the targets of violence, and who have not been discriminated against must listen carefully to families.[17] Nurses can play a key role in working with communities to identify their needs related to HIV prevention, treatment, and education.

Rural Communities

Rural settings pose different challenges to the provision of health care. Poverty is a constant dimension of life in rural areas. The lack of health care professionals is another dimension of inadequate health care in rural areas. The demands of every day life, survival, lack of discretionary income, and the underinsured status of rural inhabitants contribute to the seeking of health care only after pain and illness occur and not as a part of preventative care.[18] Typical rural influences, such as the attributes of self-reliance and independence, emphasis on religion and church, conservative moral values, adherence to the community norms, and the expectation that others will do the same may constitute threats to the health of these populations.[18]

There are several barriers to health care in rural communities. Some examples are the complexity of care provision, limited experience of regional providers, long travel distance for expert care, financial concerns for hospitals and providers, limited mass transportation, concerns about confidentiality, lack of community support groups, and patient isolation from the community and providers.[18,19]

Nurses, as the largest group of health care providers, can plan a key role in developing HIV-related care and prevention programs in rural, suburban, and urban settings.[18] Nurses must work within community-based settings to effectively monitor, coordinate, and manage the care of HIV-affected children and their families. Not only can nurses provide expert care, they can also provide outreach education to the communities in an effort to decrease fear, stigma, and transmission. Assessing for the needs of the communities we serve may help in planning for and providing geographically and culturally sensitive cost-effective care in all settings.

PEDIATRIC HIV AS A CHRONIC DISEASE

Chronic conditions are characterized by relatively stable periods that may be interrupted by acute episodes that require more intense care, including hospitalization.[20] Chronic illnesses have many characteristics, including the need for ongoing medical care; need for subspecialty care; slow degeneration of health; premature death; pain; discomfort; painful, embarrassing, or disruptive procedures; psychological and emotional impact on the child and family; financial burdens; disruption of the usual activities such as school; and impaired ability to engage in usually expected activities.[21] Over the past 20 years, HIV has evolved as an illness that has the attributes of chronic illness.

Aspects unique to HIV as a chronic disease include perinatal transmission, association with poverty and drug use, its nature as an infectious disease, stigma, secrecy, social isolation, and interaction with previous family problems such as drug addiction, multigenerational impact, multiple losses, the intensity of services needed to maintain family functioning and optimal health, the dramatic potential for prevention, and the disproportionate reliance on public financing and health care institutions for medical care.[10,21] In chronic care, the goal of treatment is not to cure the disease but to enhance coping, adaptation, and day-to-day as well as long-term functioning.[22]

The child's chronic health care problem will eventually affect the entire family.[10] By virtue of their extended duration, chronic illnesses place a significant burden on children and their families.[6,23] HIV becomes a part of every hour of the day with the need for medication and, in general, good health maintenance activities such as nutrition, exercise, and good hygiene. Daily family routines are affected by the many routine outpatient visits to monitor infection as well as those unexpected exacerbations of the disease that may necessitate hospitalization.[10]

The secrecy a family has to maintain may drain their energy on a daily basis. The need to prevent "outsiders" from knowing the diagnosis is sometimes essential, owing to the fear and stigma our society has created. Despite a massive education campaign directed at the general public regarding HIV, the stigma still exists. Fear and stigma create social isolation for families, which in turn may create depression, guilt, anxiety, and grief.[10] Although difficult, the nurse can assist families to confront these feelings and move beyond them so as to function effectively in society.

The effect of chronic illness on the child is equally impactful. Children may suffer the untoward physical effects of the disease as well as altered social experiences.[10] They may also experience isolation from their peers and family. Another dramatic finding specific to HIV is that the child may be expected to cope with the loss of a parent, sibling, or perhaps multiple family members, sometimes before the diagnosis is even disclosed to the child.

Health care services can be organized to meet the following objectives of care during chronic illness: treating the illness and preventing the illness and treatment regimen from disrupting the development of the child as well as the family.[11] This becomes especially important for those families who have few or no resources and view health care as a low priority.

The service delivery team needs to be child focused, family centered, comprehensive, and community based.[24]

MANAGING CHRONIC ILLNESS FROM A NURSING PERSPECTIVE

Managing a chronic illness is not as simple as managing the physical effects of the disease. Children with chronic illnesses require assistance with minimizing the physical effects of the disease as well as the emotional, educational, financial, and health care needs. Nursing, from a holistic perspective, addresses the whole child and family. There are many nursing care models that effectively address the management of a chronic illness such as HIV. One such model is the Neuman Systems Model. Management of the disease from the Neuman Systems Model perspective helps nurses look at the child and family's coping strategies. More specifically, it helps define how they coped prior to diagnosis and how the family's support system will help them cope throughout the illness.

Within chronic illness, there are varying states of health and wellness.[25] Neuman defines innate variables that constitute the client system. These innate variables are defined as physiologic, psychological, sociocultural, developmental, and spiritual.[25,26] In cases of HIV, all innate variables can assist the nurse and family in recognizing those aspects of their life that have been most affected and the care plan can be re-evaluated to meet the family's needs.

One of the central themes about a child with chronic illness is parental anxiety and uncertainty surrounding their child's future.[10] HIV disease is unique in the aspect of guilt felt by the parents, particularly mothers, over the fact that their own infection caused the child's infection. Parents worry about how long the child will live and grieve the loss of a perfect child.

Managing chronic illness from a nursing perspective requires not only input from other nurses but also input from the families we serve. Nurses develop relationships with families over the course of the child's illness. These relationships evolve because of the varying needs that are present throughout this chronic illness.[6] Listening to parents and assessing their needs on a continual basis is critical in providing assistance. Family-centered care must be culturally sensitive. In addition, nurses must serve as advocates for families with chronically ill members. Policy makers must listen to families to decrease barriers to families. Some of the barriers encountered by families are based on financial needs, transportation needs, and service delivery system barriers.[27] By the nurses' assisting families in identifying these barriers and by advocating for families, the families may have a stronger voice in influencing policy makers to formulate more sensitive and realistic health care policies.

Family-Centered Care

Family can be defined in many ways. It can consist of parents, siblings, grandparents, and a host of persons who help in the daily care of the child. The philosophy of family-centered care is based on the premise that the child's family is pivotal in the child's care.[28,29]

Children depend on their families to help them live day to day. The family is the most important social context shaping and influencing the health and development of the child.[30,31] No one knows the child better than the family who cares for the child. Since HIV is a disease of the family, it is important for the nurse to provide family-centered care.[10] The challenge to provide family-centered care is embodied in the fact that nurses must assess the needs of the family while examining their own values. Nurses can adapt their own practices based on what they have learned from the family.[32] Family-centered care is built on the belief that informed individuals are capable of making decisions regarding their health while assisting the family to become self-efficacious.[12,28] The Association for the Care of Children's Health (ACCH) has defined eight elements of family-centered care (Table 24–1).[28,29,32,33]

Nursing strategies to promote the family's role as the primary caregivers for the child include recognizing and accepting diverse styles of coping, helping families recognize their strengths and methods of coping, reassuring parents regarding their essential roles, and facilitating family involvement in caregiving.[32] Despite the presence of chronic illness, nurses can assist families in increasing their resources and in their coping behaviors for managing the daily demands and stressors in life, as well as those brought on by the chronic illness.[30] This becomes especially challenging when there are few resources and multiple problems. Chronic illness may disrupt the routines and rituals of families. Maintaining a balance is essential in coping with the daily stressors that accompany having a child with chronic illness. Nurses can assist families by identifying their needs and helping the family develop a plan by which all family members' needs are met in such a way that the child with chronic illness does not get a disproportionate share of the family's time and energy.[30]

Essentials of family-centered care also include having respect for family strengths and resources and willingness to listen, communicate, and collaborate with families and communities.[22,34] Families deserve recognition of their efforts and sacrifices. Nurses should recognize that as each new crisis arises within the family, the support needs of the family will change. What may have been adequate support before may no longer suffice. The impact of having a child with special needs on a family varies depending on their family's beliefs, coping style, and resilience as well as the availability of community resources.[34] Nurses as part of the multidisciplinary team can assist the family to function optimally by integrating appropriate resources and respecting the family's strengths, weaknesses, values, and routines when formulating a care plan.

OVERVIEW OF THE NURSING PROCESS IN CARING FOR CHILDREN AND FAMILIES AFFECTED BY HIV

From the initial diagnosis of HIV, the child and family need nursing support. Nursing roles in the care of the child and family affected by HIV are varied but ultimately require the nurse to be educated about the disease in order to make an effective plan of care. Denial and anger may surface through a

Table 23–1
Eight Elements of Family Centered Care*

1. Recognizing that the family is the constant in a child's life, whereas service systems and personnel within those systems fluctuate.
2. Facilitating parent/professional collaboration at all levels of health care.
3. Recognizing family strengths and individuality and respecting different methods of coping.
4. Sharing unbiased and complete information with parents about their child's care on an ongoing basis in an appropriate and supportive manner.
5. Encouraging and facilitating parent-to-parent support.
6. Understanding and incorporating the developmental needs of infants, children, adolescents, and their families into health care systems.
7. Implementing appropriate policies and programs that are comprehensive and provide emotional and financial support to meet the needs of families.
8. Assuring that the design of the health care delivery system is flexible, accessible, and responsive to family needs.

*As defined by the Association for the care of Children's Health.

tumultuous time when uncertainty becomes a daily struggle and fear is abundant. Nurses can assist families in coping with these feelings.

Case Management and Individualized Plans of Care

As unique as the disease is, so must be the plan of care for children and families infected with and affected by the disease. Protecting health and promoting growth and development are essential in pediatric nursing practice. Caring for children with HIV as a chronic illness, minimizing disability related to HIV, and maximizing the child's quality of life are essential.[6] Ongoing assessment of the family's interpretation of the test results is necessary to clarify misinformation related to the possibility that the child might "outgrow" the virus or just be a "carrier" of maternal antibodies.[35] By utilizing the nursing process of assessing the needs of the child and family, planning care both for and with the family, implementing the plan of care, and evaluating the plan of care so that it can be revised, nurses can assist families to the goal of a positive outcome in health care.

The need for ongoing services that are comprehensive yet individualized enough to meet the needs of the entire family pose one of the greatest challenges in the care of the HIV-infected patient. The social context of family problems often overwhelms attempts to individualize health care planning and intervention.[35] The range of services available for families affected by HIV may include outpatient ambulatory care, inpatient care, dental care, home care, hospice care, child care, school care, transportation, housing, food and nutrition, and legal and financial assistance. In addition, assistance with activities of daily living and the need for health education are important.[6,36] Quality of life concerns become paramount as persons with HIV live longer.[37]

Nurses are in a key position within the health care team to be case managers. Case management can promote collaboration among all disciplines to provide ongoing care involving family in the process.[36,38] In many cases, better management leads to keeping families engaged in care. Case management is systematic and collaborative. Case managers assist in decreasing fragmentation of care, enhancing a child and family's quality of life, and assist with cost containment for both the family and service agencies.[36]

The daily struggle to meet basic needs often overshadows the need for health care for most families.[11] Nurses are in a key position within the team to assist families in identifying what they need and to coordinate the services in such a manner that both their basic needs and the needs brought on by HIV are met.

By utilizing the basics of the nursing process, assessment, planning, implementation of the plan of care, and evaluation of the plan of care, the nurse can develop a plan of care that not only meets the needs of the family but will help the family recognize and meet their own identified needs. It is important to realize that the nursing process is not static but, rather, dynamic. Planning care is a team process. For the care plan to be successful, the nurse must take into account the needs of the child, of the family, and of the disease. Identification of these needs comes through the first part of the nursing process: Assessment.

Assessment/Triage

Assessment is the initial and essential step in the nursing process and creates a foundation for all interventions.[20] It is dynamic and requires the nurse to continually reassess the child and family in formulating a plan of care that will assist the child and family in living an optimal quality of life.

One very important step in assessment is careful documentation, including an account of each encounter as well as a summary of the child's and the family's needs and problems. Keeping a summary of family contact numbers is important, as the family constellation may change. It is also essential to know which family members know the HIV diagnosis, so that breach of confidentiality does not become an issue. Treating the child as an individual and not as a disease or condition is essential in respecting the child and family. Children have unique health care needs related to their age group and developmental status. These needs must be considered as part of the overall care for the child.

Common Health Care Problems Encountered by Children with HIV: The Constellation of Symptoms

The clinical spectrum of HIV disease is as varied as the children infected with it.[35] Two general patterns of presentation emerge in children with HIV infection. The first pattern of presentation, which affects approximately one third of children with perinatally acquired HIV infection, is one of an early fulminant disease course that will result in rapid disease progression and subsequently a poor prognosis. The second pattern of presentation involves later onset of disease symptoms and is associated with a better prognosis.[2,21,31] As in adults, HIV disease appears in infants and children with a broad spectrum of manifestations, some of which are unique to children.[31]

Children with HIV have complex pathophysiologic, psychological, psychosocial, and economic needs. These needs present a unique cluster of clinical challenges to the promotion of general well being, prevention of problems, treatment of symptoms, and restoration of general well-being.[39] Children with HIV experience a constellation of symptoms, unlike those of many other illnesses. One of the reasons there is so much difficulty managing the illness is that the immune system dysfunction affects virtually every body system. An important clue to and a consistent finding in children with immunodeficiency is the presence of atypical clinical scenarios for illnesses that are otherwise not found in healthy children.[2]

HIV in children is categorized by the presence of symptoms as well as their immunologic status. In 1994, the CDC revised the classification system for HIV infection in children younger than 13 years of age.[40] Children with HIV may range from having no symptoms to being severely symptomatic and immunosuppressed throughout their illness.

On examination, children with HIV may present with one or more of the following findings: lymphadenopathy, hepatomegaly, splenomegaly, oral manifestations (most commonly thrush), weight loss, abnormal distribution of body fat, dermatitis, parotitis, and respiratory abnormalities.[41] Infections, both serious and chronic, including pneumonias and chronic otitis media, hematologic disorders, impaired respiratory function due to chronic respiratory conditions, neurodevelopmental disorders including developmental delay, impaired cardiovascular function, gastrointestinal/nutrition disorders including thrush, chronic diarrhea, generalized fatigue, and energy deficits, hearing loss, and impaired vision are all potential findings in the child with HIV infection.[41–45] Nurses, working as part of the health care team, must work to identify those physical findings that will have an impact on the child's well-being and address ways to lessen their clinical impact when possible.

Nutritional assessments should be conducted routinely so that new problems can be identified and treated. Patients may experience numerous complications that compromise nutritional status.[43,46,47] Many families impacted by HIV are affected socioeconomically as well; they may qualify for nutritional supplement programs such as the Women, Infants and Children (WIC) Program.[48] Local food banks as well as church pantries may be of assistance in providing food beyond what is available through government subsidy. Supportive care, particularly nutrition, continues to play a major role in decreasing morbidity and improving the quality of life for children infected with HIV. Using a proactive approach to nutritional assessment is important.

There are many reasons that children with HIV have poor nutritional status. Nutritional problems can lead to impaired growth, inadequate weight gain, increased susceptibility to opportunistic infections, and, ultimately, death. Ongoing nutritional assessments are essential due to the manifestations of the disease over time, change in caregivers, and developmental preferences.[39] Physical symptoms such as anorexia, oral lesions, decreased energy level, food refusal, and neurologic problems may be compounded by psychosocial issues such as lack of resources to purchase food as well as lack of adequate refrigeration.[39] Cultural influences and side effects of medications or complementary or alternative medicines may have a profound effect on nutritional status as well. Ongoing assessment will help to identify those issues that most affect nutritional status and will allow the nurse and family to find ways to improve the child's quality of life when possible.

Pain can be a chronic issue in patients with HIV disease. The spectrum of HIV-related pain is varied and complex. There are many types of pain associated with HIV, including physical (abdominal, headache, extremity, oral/oropharyngeal, generalized), and treatment-related pain (such as those related to procedures).[43,49] Pain management can be confounded by many variables, including the child being unable to report pain; parental denial of their child's pain because of association with disease progression, either their child's or their own; resistance of caregivers and health care providers to give opioids because of previous experiences with drug abuse and fears of addiction; oversight of pain as a symptom in a child with multiple complex symptoms; and lack of adequate research in the area of pain in children with HIV.[38,49] Identifying pain and helping the child and family manage it is essential for the child to live comfortably.

As children age, it is important to discuss bodily changes, including the possible need for a gastrostomy tube, puberty issues, and issues related to body shape changes associated with antiretroviral medications (particularly protease inhibitors). It is important to recognize that changes in body shape cause changes in body image, which ultimately will affect the child's self-esteem and perhaps ability to participate in peer activities.

In addition to all of the problems the child may have as a result of HIV infection, it is important to remember that normal childhood illnesses are a part of the child's growth and development process. Routine childhood immunizations should be given with few exceptions, including inactivated polio in lieu of oral polio. The measles, mumps, and rubella (MMR) vaccine should be avoided in severely immunocompromised children.[50] Varicella vaccine is not recommended at this time for HIV-infected children. Currently, there are ongoing studies of varicella vaccine in the immunosuppressed HIV-infected child. Working closely with the child's primary care provider in managing all illnesses is important.

Beyond the physical health care needs of the child are the psychosocial needs that threaten his or her full integration into society. Often, the child's needs cannot be separated from the overwhelming difficulties faced by their families.[1] Nurses need to look at the overall picture to identify the holistic needs of the child and family and create a plan of care that is satisfactory.

Family Education

Children with HIV and their caregivers need to know information about the disease and its management. It is important to ascertain what a child and various family members know about HIV as well as general health care. Taking into account that disclosure is an issue for many, if not all, families, education should be tailored to accommodate this information. Assumptions that all HIV-infected persons know about HIV prevention, transmission, and risk-reductive measures should be dismissed. Basic education about HIV disease, its transmission, and its prevention is a must.

Caregivers should be educated regarding the myriad of clinical presentations of HIV infection, including recurrent infections, unusual infections, failure to thrive, hematologic manifestations, renal disease, and neurologic manifestations.[51] Any exposure to infectious diseases, particularly varicella or measles, should be reported to the child's health care provider. Providing information for families regarding who and when to call when the child presents with an illness or problem is an important way to stay connected with families.

All persons responsible for the care of children with HIV need to understand appropriate infection control practices, not only to protect the child but also to prevent the transmission of infections to caregivers, family members, and playmates.[13] General good health habits should be emphasized. Basic hygiene, including handwashing, bathing, and dental care, are essential. Avoiding pets, particularly cats, is important in the prevention of contracting diseases such as toxoplasmosis and salmonella.

Nurses should counsel families of HIV-infected or HIV-exposed children about food safety. Avoidance of raw, undercooked, or improperly stored food can cause serious food-borne illnesses such as salmonella.[51] For families who live in poverty and who may not have access to electricity or refrigeration, this is problematic. Food safety education should be included in the family's education. Avoidance of drinking or swimming in lake or river water is important to prevent *Cryptosporidium* or *Giardia* infections.[51]

The education of children and their caregivers about HIV should include a discussion of the potential risk and modes of transmission of HIV.[13] For children who do not know their diagnosis, the nurse can teach the child general good health habits regarding blood and body fluids. Although household transmissions are rare, standard precautions should be taught to all persons who may have exposure to body fluids, including blood. At each clinical visit, as the child approaches puberty, education regarding puberty and sexuality should be incorporated.

Nurses need to develop a comfort level with discussing sensitive topics such as puberty, disclosure, prevention of HIV transmission, and sexuality with children.

Family Assessment

Assessment of the family is essential in developing a plan of care. Knowing who cares for the child, who lives with the child, who supports the family both financially and emotionally, and the family's coping, problem-solving, and parenting styles is important to planning a comprehensive care plan.[22]

Family support and assigning meaning to the illness are strategies crucial to coping with a chronic illness.[22,52] For many families, HIV and AIDS are part of a long list of socioenvironmental issues that they face, including poverty, homelessness, limited access to health care and health information, and discrimination.[12] Since the family is the central point in the child's life, it is essential that assessment of the family occur so that, in the overall assessment of the child's disease, family issues that may affect the care and health of the child are not missed. Children with HIV inevitably strain a family's emotional, financial, organizational, and adaptive resources.[20] Fragmentation of families is common. The key is for the team to assess those factors that will have the greatest impact on the care and health of the child and ultimately on the well-being of the family.

Pediatric HIV poses a unique circumstance for the entire family. A diagnosis of HIV in a child usually necessitates testing of other family members in an effort to engage them in care. Because more than one family member is usually infected with HIV, it creates a circumstance that debilitates a family. Frequently families are without savings, employment, income, insurance, and medical and social support.[53] HIV can literally change a family's life overnight.

Knowing that some HIV-infected women are already seriously ill and may have partners or other family members who are infected as well calls to attention the fact that family assessment is essential to providing adequate care for children in these families. Poverty, lack of health care coverage or fear of losing existing coverage, substance abuse involving drugs or alcohol, difficulty finding housing, domestic violence, and depression are all factors that may require increased use of social services to enhance proper care of the child affected by HIV.[44]

Assessing the caregiver's education level is critical because some of the activities related to caring for children with HIV require reading, writing, and administering medications. In addition, assessing education level helps the health care provider know whether the caregiver is capable of negotiating the health care system to obtain care.[54]

Foster Care and Kinship Care Issues; Child Protective Issues

Sometimes a parent is unable to care for his or her child. The reason might be parental illness, parental death, and child abuse and/or neglect resulting from issues with substance use, mental health, poverty, or homelessness. In these cases, the child must live with someone else who can care for him or her until the time when the child can be reunited with the parent or until parental rights have been legally terminated by the court system. Frequently, families are already known to social service agencies. HIV can overwhelm a family already weakened by severe socioeconomic vulnerability.[53]

Foster care and kinship care are two manners by which children are cared for when their biological parent cannot. Foster care usually consists of care given by those unrelated to the child. The child is usually in the legal custody of the state's social services and the physical custody of the foster parent. Foster parents care for children day to day, but major decisions involving medical care, including investigational drug trials or stopping aggressive medical treatment, are made by the child welfare agency or the biological parent. Foster parents may experience frustrations that come with caring for someone they have no legal rights to make decisions for, yet whom they care for day to day. Whatever the composition of the family, the nurse can provide support and education in the manner that best serves the interests of the child.

Kinship care is provided by a family member when a parent is unable to care for the child. Kinship caregivers may be grandparents, aunts, uncles, or other family members. There may or may not be a formal custody agreement in place. Grandparents, in particular, may be thrust into the caregiving role when their own children are dealing with issues related to HIV or substance use. The emotional impact of raising children, dealing with feelings of anger and resentment of their own children, financial concerns, and the inability to reclaim parts of their own lives can be problematic for kinship caregivers.[20,32] Assisting the family in learning how to access benefits and entitlements as well as resources at the local, state, and national level is important in decreasing unnecessary financial and health care burdens. Nurses should be cognizant that with these resource referrals, the need for confidentiality is great.

Diagnosis and Disclosure

Comprehensive medical care includes disclosure of the HIV diagnosis to the child (when developmentally appropriate) and to the family. How and when disclosure takes place is an essential issue and a key part of the plan of care. As a child ages, the importance of disclosure comes to the forefront as the child assumes more responsibility for his or her own care.[38] Disclosure may become a pivotal point around such issues as medication adherence, treatment compliance, sexual exploration, fears associated with a premature death, and the child' developing autonomy.[55] Disclosure may mean that parents have to come to terms with their own illness and eventual death. It also means that the child may have questions that the parent is not ready to answer. Ethical issues may arise with disclosure in terms of sexual exploration and conflict between the health care provider's judgment and the parents'. Families choice of when and whether to disclose should be discussed openly. Every family of a child with a catastrophic illness experiences the stress of knowing there is no cure. Families of children with HIV also experience another set of stressors, which act with a domino effect. These stressors are the stigma of the illness, which leads to secrecy, which leads to isolation and ultimately lack of support and services.[56] These challenges in caring for children and their families with HIV disease illustrate the need for nurses to plan care throughout the course of the disease.

Disclosure of HIV status is not as easy as it sounds. With disclosure comes the need to tell someone that HIV is a part of your life. Disclosures to a parent, partner, sibling, or child all have different connotations and require different levels of communication. Parents commonly choose not to tell young infected children for fear that they will be unable to keep a secret as well as to shield them from societal response.

As children with HIV approach school age, the question of when and how to talk to children about their illness surfaces. Caregivers often maintain a veil of secrecy around the child's illness to avoid diagnosis disclosure to the child because the results have ramifications.[57] Parents worry that when their children know the diagnosis, they will ask how they became infected. This opens up the potential for many questions about the parent's past, including sexual history and drug use history.[12,38] Given the social stigma surrounding the disease, it is not surprising that most families do not share disclosure with their children.[57]

Discussing the caregiver's perspective on disclosure is essential in the process. Culture may also play a role in the choice to disclose HIV status. Nurses can assist families in the process of disclosure. The key point is that disclosure is a process. It may take days, months, or years of discussion with families to plan the disclosure process. Planning disclosure is important, so that the caregiver is prepared to handle situations that might arise as the result of disclosure. All variables must be taken into account, so that the family's experience with disclosure is positive.

Cultural Considerations and Health Beliefs

Because of the cultural diversity that exists with HIV disease, assessment must include the family's culture and health beliefs. Simply described, culture is the sum of socially learned beliefs, values, and traditions that influence patterns of behavior, including beliefs about health and illness.[58] Respecting the uniqueness of family culture and viewpoint is essential in family-centered care.[22] Although parents from all ethnic and economic groups share similar child care goals, they may have significantly different world views, communication styles, and perceptions of time.[4] It is important to acknowledge that it is difficult to know all of the subtle nuances of all cultures but rather recognize that each patient has a unique cultural heritage that will influence the illness experience.[4,58]

The concept of mutuality fits well with cultural consideration when planning care. It is essential for both the family and the nurse to respect the worth and dignity of the other person and truly want to seek understanding of and in the other.[59] Culture must be integrated in every aspect of care, including education. Developing culturally sensitive health intervention programs is a continuous process of adapting the program to the cultural characteristics of the ethnic group being targeted.[60]

Nurses should acknowledge that immigrants may have come from a persecuted background and stressful social circumstances. Immigrants of racial and ethnic minority are at increased risk of suffering from political, economic, and social inequalities. Immigrants are more likely to have disjointed health care.[58] Compliance and treatment failure may come from the patient's inability to follow directions. Children may experience difficulty when cultural traditions are to be followed in the home but while at school they are expected to look and act like their peers. Different languages, cultural practices, and beliefs are all parts of culture that may affect HIV care.[60]

PLANNING CARE FOR AND WITH THE CHILD AND FAMILY WITH HIV

When planning care for a child with chronic illness, it is important to consider the impact that chronicity has on the child as well as the family. Chronic illness brings with it the need for repeated clinic visits or the need for inpatient stays; long-term drug regimens; chronic episodes of pain or discomfort due to the disease itself or interventions to manage it; repeated separations from family, friends, and school; changes in caregivers; and, in the case of HIV, the threat of death.[20] Since the illness is lifelong, there are many aspects of care that must be considered.

Confidentiality

There is no other disease affecting children or adults in which the need for confidentiality is so great.[10] After all these years, the stigma attached to the diagnosis of HIV remains strong. One of the greatest fears of families is breach of confidentiality.[20] Fear of being "found out" is one reason that individuals do not seek health care despite the risks HIV poses.

Confidentiality within the hospital or home care setting is important. Recognizing that friends or acquaintances may work in these settings can create problems for the family when accessing health care. Disclosure of HIV in these setting should be done with regard to its importance in the patient's care and within legal guidelines set forth within the state where the patient is being cared for.

School Issues

Children with HIV should be allowed to balance their periods of illness and hospitalizations with the playing, growing, learning, and socializing of normal childhood.[42] School is one place where these normal childhood activities occur. With better medicines, children are now frequently living to school age and beyond with relatively long periods of good health.

Helping children have positive school experiences is essential if they are to "fit in." Knowledge of a child's HIV status is unnecessary for school entry.[13] Disclosure should be on a case-by-case basis. Written consent is essential for disclosure to schools. Limiting the information to the school principal or school nurse can minimize discrimination. Nurses can help families assess whether telling the school the HIV diagnosis is in the best interest of the child.

School nurses can collaborate with the health care team and assist the child with having the least disruption during the school day, giving medications and acting as a buffer to those who do not know the diagnosis. As the illness progresses and the child becomes more medically fragile, the child may require increased medical interventions during the school day.[21] Ongoing assessment of the child's physical, nutritional, neurologic, developmental, and immune status are important and may be key to helping the child have a positive school experience.[42] Because HIV can effect cognition, it is essential that the child have at least yearly developmental testing by a neuropsychologist, to assist with recommendations to place the child in appropriate educational settings. In settings where the school does not know the diagnosis, concerns about the child's school performance can be voiced and requests for formal evaluation can be made independent of the knowledge of HIV infection.

The disease has the potential to disrupt school performance. Absenteeism, physical appearance, cognitive deficits, and grief may all play a part in the child's performance. Children with HIV tend to be smaller than their peers and are subject to wasting, dermatologic conditions, and distended abdomens.[21] Children should be taught to cope with these body changes. Children may have lost one or more key people to death, which has great potential to affect school performance because of the grief the child experiences as well as the changed dynamic at home.

Nurses can play an important part in educating schools, day care facilities, and the community. This education should include basic education about communicable diseases, standard precautions, confidentiality, and health screenings, particularly for school personnel. Policies and procedures should be developed to cover first aid and medication administration.[42] In addition, this education should cover first aid in athletic events, since many children are well enough to take part in physical activities. Education should be ongoing and include information on community resources as well.

Respite Care

Care of children is time consuming. When a child has a chronic illness, the care requires time and energy that a parent suffering from the same illness may not be able to muster. Stress and potential for caregiver burnout are high among caregivers of children with HIV.[54] Children with HIV frequently require multiple medications and tube feedings, or may be technology dependent in other ways, requiring the caregiver to meet not only the child's everyday needs but also the needs of the disease.

Respite care provides a break from the day-to-day care that is so demanding. There are several types of respite care, including center-based respite, where children are cared for in an out-of-home agency such as a day care or school facility; in-home respite, where a trained respite worker comes to the home to give the caregivers a break from caring for the child; and emergency respite, which is provided on short notice when the caregiver is unable to care for the child due to illness or hospitalization.[34]

Respite can also be provided via recreational resources, such as summer camps or local activities.

Death and Dying: Family Perspectives

Planning for children whose parents are dying from the disease is another important step in planning individualized care. With the advent of new medications, HIV has become a chronic illness. Long before death and dying becomes an issue, there are issues of chronic sorrow.[6,11] Having a chronic yet fatal illness puts stress on a family that results in physical fatigue and health problems as well as ongoing social and financial stressors.[6]

Helping families plan realistically for the future is challenging not only because of the unpredictable nature of HIV but because of the lack of available resources.[53]

Supportive and Terminal Care

When a person is diagnosed with HIV, the subject of death becomes very real. Because HIV has no cure, terminal care is a part of the comprehensive plan of care. Quality of life issues come into conflict with treatment decisions. Issues regarding how and where a child should die come to the forefront.[38,49] This disease presents a difficult challenge for nurses because the parent and the child will require end-of-life planning. For parents, there is the painful realization that they may not live to see their child grow, nor will they be able to care for their children or take an active part in planning their futures.[61] For children, there is the realization that the stability of family life is gone with the death of a parent. Children need to know that they are loved and that they will be taken care of when their parents die. Proactive permanency planning will assist in meeting the child's needs when a parent dies.

Preparing a family for a child's death is difficult but necessary. Long before death and dying become a part of the daily care plan, some families will rely on spirituality and, in most cases, organized religion to help them with the daily issues associated with HIV infection. Health care providers can assist families by helping them make the connection with someone who shares their spiritual faith.[53,62] When the time comes for terminal care, spirituality can be of great comfort for families. When the prognosis is bleak for a child, the focus of care changes. Listening to the patient, helping the family cope, acknowledging your own grief, discussing the full implications of a Do Not Resuscitate (DNR) order, and concentrating on palliation are important.[1,38,63]

Pain management becomes the primary goal. Signs of impending death such as changes in breathing patterns, cognition, skin color, and elimination and the possibility of bleeding or seizures must be addressed.[49,64] The child may also be frightened by what is happening and by the reactions of people around him or her. Helping children through the experience in a developmentally appropriate way is just as important as preparing the family. In planning, it should be remembered that honesty on the part of health care providers is expected and ambivalence on the part of the family should be anticipated.[49] Hospice care is one way to offer coordinated multidisciplinary services while not leaving the caregiver alone to make choices regarding the child's life. Additionally, spiritual support should be offered by way of involvement of clergy or pastoral care.

Additionally, it is essential to include social service agencies in the planning for children, to ensure that the child is placed in the custody of those persons the parents have chosen. There are many resources available to assist in these planning stages. Discussing the need for this type of care early on in the disease may allow the family to spend less time worrying about what will happen to the survivors. In this planning, the nurse needs to be sensitive to the fact that even within the family, discussion about the illness and cause of death may be avoided, and extended family members may be kept uninformed.[62]

Terminal care should be viewed as part of the comprehensive services required by HIV-infected children and their families, deserving of careful planning and completion.[1]

Care in the Inpatient Setting

Caring for children in the inpatient setting is challenging because there is usually an acute problem in a child with a chronic illness. Remembering that there is a chronic illness that has routine medications as well as important nutritional needs is essential in the inpatient care plan.[63] Confusion can come when the routine that the family is used to is suddenly changed because of the acute illness. Communication between the primary and specialty care providers, the hospital staff, and the child and family is important. Discharge planning should incorporate and address the needs of the acute illness as well as those of the chronic illness. Including the child, family, health care providers (both for the acute and chronic illness), and the home care health care provider is necessary to be sure that all involved know the care plan. No matter what the outcome of the hospitalization, families need consistent messages, not conflicting information.[63]

Care in the Outpatient Setting

Routine health care is primarily provided in the outpatient health care setting. Whether in a general pediatrician's office, a hospital-based clinic, or a rural clinic setting, the importance of getting the child to the clinic appointment on a routine basis is essential to managing HIV as well as general pediatric care, including growth and development. Transportation assistance to visits may be necessary. Minimizing long clinic waits and respecting a family's time is important in helping with adherence with clinic visits.

Continuity of Care and Long-Term Follow-Up Care

Decreasing the burden of the disease and its management is essential throughout the disease. Helping the child to enroll in school as well as assessing the child's developmental and learning needs will help children succeed in school. Health care providers need to be aware that a family's involvement in the health care system with such frequency and vigor is tiresome.

Financial supports and resources are necessary. Federal, state, and local programs are available, including Supplemental Security Income (SSI) and medical assistance.[34] Helping people through the process of accessing services may help with the continuity of care. Health care providers must be prepared to offer continuity of care despite a changing family constellation that may include not only the extended family but foster and adoptive care settings as well as kinship care settings.[1,29]

Because HIV is still a fatal disease, there will be a time when providing supportive care and not providing "all out" care will be the goal. The child, the family, and the health care team will need care. Every effort should be made to guide the family in making choices that they can live with after the death of the child.[6]

CHOICES IN CARE

With the availability of new medications came the hope of helping children and adults with HIV live longer. At the beginning of the epidemic, there were few antiretroviral medications for use in adults and even fewer for children. Monotherapy was the standard. Today, use of multiple antiretroviral medications is the standard of care. The current antiretroviral drugs cannot limit HIV reproduction indefinitely, nor can they correct the immunodysfunction that accompanies HIV disease.[65]

Managing disease symptoms and treatments related to HIV and its sequelae are part of the nurses work with families.[6]

Standard of Care versus Experimental Therapy

HIV is still a relatively new disease to the world. Great effort has been made to define therapies and to help children and adults live quality lives with minimal disruption in their day-to-day activities. The progressive destruction and dysfunction that HIV causes is especially challenging to the scientist who develops new therapies. This devastation is one of the major reasons that development of drugs to stop or reverse the destruction is so important. The progressive destruction and dysfunction that HIV causes is especially challenging to the scientists who develop drugs to fight HIV. Experimental therapy is especially important because, at this time, there is no single regimen that works to completely destroy HIV. In addition to identifying new regimens, examining the emergence of viral resistance to antiretroviral drugs, examining long-term benefit, and appreciating the complexity that immunopathogenesis of HIV has on the body are important.[65]

Entering a clinical trial can be a frightening prospect for a child and family.[62] Every effort should be made to respect the feeling of the participants and to discuss their fears, possible risks, and possible benefits. The family is choosing an unknown by choosing clinical research for care.[66]

The patient and family must never be made to feel that the only way to obtain medical care is through clinical research. By making comprehensive care available for all children, not just those who are privileged with health care and finances, we ensure that the choice to participate in drug trials is made freely, rather than in response to the "coercion of poverty."[1] Clinical trials should be another choice in care, not a necessity or a way to obtain health care and medications. Families who are informed, not just "talked at," may be able to make better decisions when choosing care.

Nurses must understand all aspects of clinical research to effectively support and meet the needs of children who participate in clinical research.[66] Nurses who understand the process can act as better advocates for the patient.

Complementary or Alternative Therapies

Another choice in care is complementary or alternative therapies. Complementary medicine has been around for centuries and emphasizes the body's ability to heal itself.[67] Alternative therapy means replacing or using another form of medicine.[68] Some examples of complementary therapies are meditation, imagery, visualization, acupuncture, homeopathy, nutrition, vitamins, nutritional supplements, herbal therapy, exercise, and relaxation and massage. There are several fields of alternative medicine, including bioelectromagnetic applications, ayurvedic medicine, homeopathic medicine, traditional Chinese medicine, mind-body medicine including biofeedback, herbal medicine, and diet and nutrition in the treatment and prevention of chronic illnesses.[68,69] Many factors play into the choice to use nonconventional therapies. Culture, religion, and distrust of traditional Western medicine are three of these factors. The motivation to use complementary or alternative therapies may be that there is no recognized cure, or that conventional treatments show promise but the side effects are too much to bear.[68]

Despite the widespread use of complementary or alternative therapies in the United States, knowledge of its theoretical basis and practical application among conventional health care providers remains scant.[69] Potential issues with complementary or alternative therapies are that there may be little or no controlled research to support the claims of these therapies, they may be expensive, and there is poor quality control. Complementary or alternative therapies may require foreign travel, and they may be expensive and not covered by insurance.

Health care providers are encouraged to become familiar with the complementary or alternative therapies used by patients to encourage their safe and rational use.[67] Families should be encouraged to talk about their beliefs in complementary or alternative therapies.

IMPLEMENTING, MANAGING, AND EVALUATING CARE

Implementing care and managing the day-to-day as well as the long-term care plan are some of the most important parts of the plan of care. The needs of families change frequently, causing a change in how the child's care is managed. Evaluation of the plan of care is essential in determining whether it is working.

Mutually Negotiated Goals

When initiating and implementing a plan of care for the child and family, it is essential to include the child, the family, and the health care team in the planning. Only a family can judge whether a plan of care will fit into their daily lifestyle. What is practical and what is possible for the family are often polar opposites. Setting goals in the child's care is essential so that the care can be measured as effective and therapeutic or ineffective. Mutually negotiated goals are more likely to be realistic and more likely to be achieved.[20] Mutuality not only embodies the philosophy of family-centered care, it also acknowledges and supports the evolution of parents and nurses toward greater competency in their roles as caregivers.[59] Mutuality also gives the child and family some control over a situation that often seems out of control.

Adherence to Care Issues

Adherence to care as well as adherence to the medication regimen is one of the most challenging parts of the plan of care. There is no gold standard for assessing medication adherence. To assess adherence to medications, there is a baseline of information that must be collected. Some of the information is reliable, some less than reliable. Self-report, pill counts, biologic measures, drug levels in blood or urine, and other laboratory measures including T cell count and viral load are all ways to assess adherence.[70]

None of these measures, either alone or in combination, will predict to 100% accuracy whether the child and the caregiver are compliant with medication administration.

Adherence to medication, adherence to medical appointments, and in general adherence to the overall plan of care is essential if the goal of keeping the child as healthy as possible is to be met. Common-sense would seem to dictate that if the medicine works, the patient will take it, but it is not quite that simple. Although families may articulate the knowledge that nonadherence will result in the child not faring well, adherence is still a major issue in the care of children and adults with HIV. There are many variables that affect adherence to care. Since children are largely dependent on their caregiver to give medications, if the caregiver is affected with illness or has beliefs inconsistent with giving medication, adherence to therapy will suffer. In addition, as children grow older, they may be given the responsibility of taking medications. Some children, out of necessity of living in a chaotic household, take their own medications. Disclosure may also affect adherence.

A practical step in improving adherence is education. Teaching children and caregivers the importance of therapy and the dangers of stopping and starting medications is necessary.[38] Consideration of literacy, education level, and culture are important if the teaching is to be effective. Culture plays a large part in adherence. Possible language barriers, nonavailability of community resources, and characteristics of the sick role in culture may be problematic.[71,72] Also, it is difficult for individuals who live in poverty, regardless of ethnic or racial identity, to communicate with health care providers about their economic or social situation.[4] There are many strategies to enhance adherence. Table 24–2 gives 10 examples of strategies for establishing and maintaining optimal adherence.

Table 23–2
Ten Examples of Strategies for Establishing and Maintaining Optimal Adherence

1. Clarify the regimen.
2. Tailor the regimen to the family's lifestyle.
3. Show the family how to keep a medication diary.
4. Establish a time to set out pills/liquid medications.
5. Establish set places for pill taking.
6. Plan ahead for changes in routine.
7. Make special plans for weekends and holidays.
8. Invite families to become partners in care—create a therapeutic alliance.
9. Refer patients to social services.
10. Follow-up—a plan of care cannot succeed if it is set forth and never revisited.

From Chesney MA: New antiretroviral therapies: Adherence challenges and strategies. Clin Care Options HIV Treat Issues 1997; (See reference 73).

Using aids such as colored stickers on medicine bottles can assist illiterate caregivers and children. Assisting caregivers in setting up times that coincide with routine activities can be helpful. Assessment of adherence to therapy is as dynamic as adherence itself. Stability of social circumstances contributes to adherence.

Nonadherence to therapy is complicated by many factors. Complexity of the regimen, timing of the regimen, duration of therapy, perceived value of the need for therapy, untoward side effects, and the presence of social support are but a short list of these complicating factors.[70,72–74] Providing clients with permission to tell the truth about their medications is essential in continuing to assist the family in finding a regimen that works for them.[73]

When medication adherence in a child becomes impossible, consideration of placement of a gastrostomy tube is essential, though controversial, for the administration of medication in a child who may otherwise be doing well. It is often difficult for parents as well as children to accept gastrostomy tube placement because of the physical appearance and the perception of pain and discomfort. Gastrostomy tube placement is a viable option to ease the burden of medication administration and behavioral issues surrounding medication taking.[75]

Because nonadherence is common and responsible for most failures to achieve virologic control, maximizing and monitoring adherence must be the major focus of pediatric HIV therapy.[76] The inability to predict which families will be adherent makes the job of the health care team difficult. Some characteristics are consistent but not necessarily predictive.[72]

Adherence should be discussed at every visit. Not penalizing patients for not taking medications but actually discussing the obstacles in taking medications may sometimes be the simplest way to address the needs of the client and caregiver. Referral to appropriate services is essential. Realizing that there are limitations to the clinical visit is important. There may not be enough time to cover all the issues relating to the child's care.

Home Care Issues

Because of the high cost of inpatient hospital care, home care has become an important part of HIV care. The setting for the delivery of care has changed focus as a result and now resides within the community, specifically the home setting.[54]

Identifying caregivers who are willing to be supportive and provide assistance to children with HIV is essential in helping them manage their care. The family also needs assistance in integrating to the community.

Resources available in the community are often limited. No matter how well prepared the family may be for problems of disease exacerbation and progression and the general problems that may arise with daily living, all families will need assistance at some point in the child's illness. The needs of the family fluctuate, and the needs may be greater than normal at the time of each new crisis.[34] Many families do not know how to access community support, may not be aware of community support, or may encounter barriers that prevent access to care.[34,77]

Clinical staff caring for persons with HIV in home care has enormous challenges. A home care nurse is on the patient's turf, and, as such, respect for that person's home is imperative. Assessing the home for safety and those environmental issues that assist with daily living such as refrigeration and adequate cooling and heating systems is important. Providing the highest quality care in a nonmedical setting that provides the best possible quality of life is one of the aims of home care. The home care nurse can help the family assess what their strengths and weaknesses are and encourage them to be a part of their care planning, as well as the implementation and evaluation of their care.[54] An ongoing source of updated education is essential, so that health care providers can have greater knowledge of new and investigational treatments.[16]

The safety of home care workers must be considered, particularly in urban areas where crime and substance abuse exist openly. Violence and abuse, whether actual or perceived, may be a frightening reality for those living in the household or those visiting the household.[16]

ISSUES AFFECTING HIV NURSING CARE

The very same issues that affect children and families with HIV can affect nurses and the care they provide as well. Lack of knowledge, prejudices, the influence of the community, and stress are all problems with the potential to have a negative impact on nursing care. In addition, nursing stress may lead to occupational burnout. The nursing process of assessment, planning, implementation, and evaluation can help the nurse introspectively look at his or her own practice.

KNOWLEDGE BASE: WHAT NURSES NEED TO KNOW TO ADEQUATELY CARE FOR CHILDREN WITH HIV AND THEIR FAMILIES

There are some essential concepts that add to the knowledge base of nurses who care for children with HIV. They should have a basic understanding of HIV infection (including transmission and immunology), etiology and epidemiology of HIV infection, CDC classification of pediatric HIV infection, methods of diagnosis, prognosis and course of illness, as well as nursing implications.[6]

Knowledge of community resources and the ability to access these resources are essential parts of comprehensive nursing care of children with chronic illnesses, including HIV. Many clients will resist using certain services if they are targeted toward particular groups.[20] Being sensitive to confidentiality is paramount in referrals to AIDS service organizations.

There are many formal supports in place for children and families with special health care needs, including children with HIV.[34] Federal and state governments have mandated programs to assist families who are affected by illnesses that change their ability to function. There are educational supports such as Individualized Education Plans (IEPs), financial supports such as SSI and medical assistance, and physical and legal supports such as the Americans with Disabilities Act, which mandates public and private transportation resources as well as freedom from architectural barriers in buildings.[34] In addition, many services are available for families who live at or below the poverty level, such as Women, Infants, and Children (WIC), which provides financial assistance with securing formula and food for mothers and children under 5 years of age. Families may be reluctant to seek out resources for fear that they may have to disclose HIV diagnosis or their financial income. Nurses can assist families in accessing these supports confidentially and proactively.

Examining Fears in Caring for HIV-Positive Children

The fear of contracting HIV through an occupational exposure is legitimate. Although statistically the odds of contracting HIV through occupational exposure via needlestick, for example, are extremely low, the risk exists. Even providers who specialize in HIV care have a fleeting bout of anxiety now and then about occupational exposure.[78] The unknowns about HIV disease, its cure, the exact mechanism of transmission, the triggers of the disease progression, and fear of harming loved ones heighten the perception that the virus is contagious and add to the fear of being out of control and vulnerable.[78,79]

Although attitudes have changed somewhat over the past two decades, the stigma of AIDS affects patients, their caregivers, and, in some instances, the health care providers who care for these patients.[7] It is difficult, if not impossible, to separate professional and personal life.[79]

By learning more about HIV and increasing their own knowledge base, nurses can learn more about what is making them uncomfortable and effectively address their fears so that they can provide optimal and safe care for children with HIV. Discussing of these fears, with those knowledgeable about the virus, may help in dealing with and conquering the fears.[79]

Use of Standard Precautions and Prevention of Occupational Exposure

Personal safety is important for those employed in the health care professions as well as caregivers caring for HIV-infected children within the home setting. Accidental exposure is a real issue. Standard Precautions (once termed Universal Precautions) are designed to reduce transmission of all pathogens, including HIV. Standard precautions apply to all health care settings, as well as schools, child care settings, and the home.[13] Safe disposal of sharp and contaminated equipment is mandatory. Avoidance of potentially dangerous situations when dealing with families where drug use is prevalent and violence is present should be undertaken when possible.[20] All health care providers must be educated in the use of standard precautions and consistently use them.

Education regarding prevention of occupational exposures and the availability of resources and protocols to ensure effective treatment and care when exposures do occur are critically important.[80] The CDC provides guidance related to occupational exposure and prophylaxis for health care providers.

Prejudices and Judgments Affecting Nursing Care

One essential aspect of nursing care is the ability of the nurse to examine his or her own prejudices and judgments in regards to the patient, the disease, and the patient's chosen lifestyle. In an ideal world, the nurse would be able to care for the child and family without regard to his or her own prejudices or judgments. Unfortunately, the world is not ideal and these feelings may consciously or subconsciously be reflected in the quality of patient care delivered. This too is true for all health care providers. Recognizing prejudice and judgmental behavior is an essential part of addressing these behaviors. Clients with HIV may come from culturally diverse backgrounds or have a history of drug use. Nurses should seize the opportunity to learn about these backgrounds. Additionally, it may be necessary to include health care providers who are knowledgeable of the culture and language to facilitate care that both meets the needs of the client and is respectful of the client's culture and health care beliefs. Personal values, religious ideals, and cultural background are challenged in health care providers caring for children with HIV.[6]

Frequently, the caregivers of children with HIV are also HIV infected. When a child has missed more than one appointment, it should be considered that the caregiver may also be chronically tired or experiencing problems with his or her own health. Additionally, those who provide kinship care may be experiencing health care issues of their own. Many kinship caregivers are older and have healthcare issues, requiring their attendance at clinic appointments of their own. Members of the health care team need to provide flexible, realistic services in light of this information. First and foremost, it should be determined that the child is not in danger when health care appointments are missed. In cases in which the child is at risk, state laws regarding child welfare should be adhered to. In providing care for clients from different cultures and lifestyles, health care providers need to be empathetic.[78]

Death and Dying: Assisting Clients with Personal Issues

Children in the final stages of illness must be assured as much as possible that they will be cared for. Families need support to accomplish this and not pull away from the child at a time when the child needs them most. In the final stages of life, care will focus on the prevention of infection, maintenance of adequate fluid balance, prevention of constipation, maintenance of age-appropriate self-care, provision of pain control, and provision of adequate sleep and rest.[6] Any care plan must include input from the child (when age appropriate), the family, and the health care team. If goals of the plan are to change, each person should be included so that clarity is not lost.

The multigenerational nature of HIV raises issues seldom confronted in other chronic childhood issues.[7] Comprehensive care includes the stressful task of raising issues related to death, dying, and permanency planning. This is stressful not only for the client but also for the health care provider.

In the terminal stages of the illness and throughout the illness, nurses need to think through their own values regarding quality of life concerns and guard against imposing their values on clients for whom they are caring.[37]

Professional Development

Nurses must keep current about new information related to HIV, including its treatment, current research, and application of that research to practice. There are several ways to do this. Attending professional conferences, accessing electronic media, reading scientific journals, and consulting with professional colleagues who specialize in HIV are among the ways to keep current.[54] Networking with others is an important way to develop professionally.

IDENTIFYING AND COPING WITH STRESS AND BURNOUT: UTILIZING RESOURCES

One of the great rewards of caring for families affected by HIV is the positive relationship that can develop from knowing a family and providing health care over many years. Of great importance in dealing with the daily care of HIV-infected children and their families is coping with the stress that comes with helping people deal with issues that are stressful not only for them but for the health care professionals who care for them. The daily challenges of case-managing illness and family needs coupled with the intensity of services needed to maintain optimal health and family functioning are daunting tasks requiring immense energy.

The stress of chronic and terminal illness is well defined in the literature; however, the effect of stress on the HIV health care provider is an area needing more study. Nurses working in HIV/AIDS care may experience an array of stressors from multiple sources and are therefore vulnerable to emotional exhaustion and eventually to occupational burnout.[81] Occupational burnout may result in physical and emotional exhaustion, absenteeism, tardiness, loss of work motivation, and conflicts within and outside the working environment.[82-84] Occupational burnout may also result in the perception that the job no longer has positive rewards. Eventual job turnover or career separation may occur.[83] In the worst case scenario, pathologic responses such as alcoholism, drug abuse, and suicide may result.[84] The clients whom nurses serve may experience the anger, apathy, emotional exhaustion, depersonalization, and disorganized care that is provided as a result.[83]

The emergence of HIV infection has added new stress factors for the health care profession. Stigma from working with patients with HIV, fear of contagion, perceived risk of infection, lack of knowledge, and the young age of patients are all stressors that can affect the care provider.[84] Nurses suffer the effects of personal depletion, the stress of maintaining a therapeutic relationship, work overinvolvement, and frustration related to difficult client behaviors such as nonadherence and drug use.[85] Patient advocacy at the hospital, local, national, and global level can illicit stress as well. The disease itself as well as its effect on patients can evoke emotions of sadness, anger, and fear.

Stress is usually multifactorial. Many of the causes of stress for nurses lie not only within the individual but also within the health care system that supports the nurses. Feeling devalued, short staffing, and inability to provide quality care without lowering nursing standards may lead to job dissatisfaction.[85] Institutions can assist nurses by recognizing that nurses who provide care to families affected by HIV may need to have rigid institutional policies changed to accommodate them.[7] Providing time off for mental health is essential. Providing adequate staffing is also essential in ensuring that nurses receive the time off they need to cope with stress and generally take care of their own needs.

The realization that comprehensive care is a balancing of health care services and supportive, community-based services is in itself a stressful proposition.[38,86] Managing the health care system as well as the family system is difficult and consumes time and resources.

Stressors in HIV work arise both from specific issues related to HIV and from more generic concerns that stem from being a helping professional working with clients with a chronic illness in an environment of limited resources.[7] The very same issues that draw nurses to the profession may be those that lead to the more serious occupational burnout.

Stress reduction is essential, especially if the care provided is to be effective. Often, nurses forget that parents of chronically ill children are dependent on the nurse for emotional support and approval.[20] There is continual stress created when the nurse must address difficult issues and the caregiver may not be ready to deal with them.[7] Routinely assessing personal needs, client needs, and environmental needs may help in keeping stress within its boundaries.

The existence of a stress-relieving relationship or activity is essential for the physical, mental, emotional, and spiritual well-being of health care providers specializing in HIV and chronic illness in general.[78] For some, spirituality is an important part of coping with stress. By acknowledging and nurturing their spiritual component, nurses can find another avenue for renewal and respite from the rigors of HIV work.[7] Positive coping with job stress and burnout requires a concerted effort.[85] The very same advice given to patients, such as stress reduction, stress management, prioritizing, looking for support systems both at work and outside of work, taking care of physical needs such as adequate rest, nutrition, and exercise, planning for personal time and work-related tasks, avoiding destructive behaviors (e.g., smoking, alcohol, and drug abuse), and maintaining a realistic outlook may also be helpful.[82,85]

Nurses who specialize in HIV care must identify ways to renew themselves through education, individual support, staff support, and variation in workload so that they can continue to contribute their valuable expertise to families dealing with HIV.[7] Through professional and educational opportunities, nurses can share their care strategies and their frustrations. This sharing may allow them to discover new ideas and incorporate them into the care of their patients as well as themselves. Acknowledging that what nurses do day to day is stressful is an essential step in addressing stress and preventing occupational burnout. Recognizing that nurses are doing their best to battle this virus instead of being in a constant state of frustration will help nurses cope better with a disease that so far has eluded our human understanding. Taking care of ourselves has to be a priority if nurses are to continue to provide effective care.

Educating Colleagues

The education of nursing colleagues can best be accomplished by those health care providers who directly care for HIV-infected children and their families, as well as those who are affected by or infected with HIV themselves. Nurses' fears about contracting HIV, harming loved ones as a result, and doing their best to serve patients is very real.[79] It is essential that there be open dialogue when these fears arise.

The complexity of HIV challenges even the most well informed health care provider. Couple the HIV diagnosis with other comorbidities, and the information becomes overwhelming.

Nurses must understand their own values about sexuality and drug use and how they influence their day-to-day practice as well as their ability to care for children and their families affected by HIV.[7] Education of nursing, medical, and other allied health students is essential if HIV is to be a disease that is recognized, understood, and not feared.

Resources

In a health care climate with dwindling resources due to increased systemic burden, nurses face a difficult situation in providing care for clients whose needs may weigh heavily on the health care system. Patients are discharged from the hospital "sicker and quicker," creating problems for the patient at home. Nursing caseloads are often high, creating the feeling of being rushed and overburdened.[7] This can create a problem in communication between professionals, which ultimately leads to duplication of services or, worse, no services at all. Identifying community resources not only for HIV-affected families but also for nurses and health care professionals who care for HIV-infected individuals may be one way of supporting each other.

Nursing Research

If the science involved with HIV and the services provided to those with HIV are to move forward, research must take it there. Important areas for nursing research can be grouped into three areas: psychosocial issues of infected children, psychosocial issues of families of infected children, and studies providing data for policy formation.[86]

Future directions of nursing research related to children with HIV should include, but are not limited to, family coping styles and their effect on chronic illness, family composition, other psychosocial issues such as diagnosis disclosure, assent and consent, self-image and self-esteem in children, quality of life, and adherence to care.[86] In addition, it is essential that assessment tools be developed that address the needs of minority and disadvantaged populations that are most affected by HIV.[87]

Although the opportunities for research are limitless, research projects must be done in a sensitive, nonintrusive manner to avoid the feeling among families with HIV that they are the subject of endless, nonessential analysis.[20] Confidentiality and patient safety should always come first.

Nurses as Advocates

The HIV epidemic has thrown into somber prominence the aspects of the health care system that have functioned poorly in providing access to health care.[17] Nurses can act as advocates on multiple levels. Whatever the nurse's practice setting, opportunities for advocacy exist. The more nurses know about the issues facing children and their families, and the more they are involved in their patient's care, the greater their effect on the outcome will be.[88] First and foremost, acting as a patient advocate is an important role. Helping patients access the services they need in their health care settings and their communities will enhance the care of the family. Being an advocate on the legislative level is important as well. Bringing to the forefront those issues that are barriers to care on a local, state, and federal level may help policy makers revise laws or create new ones that make services more available and consumer friendly.

Prevention Efforts

Prevention of HIV is the only cure. However, in a world where 100% prevention is impractical because of how HIV is transmitted, education is essential.

Nurses can assist in efforts to prevent HIV transmission. Since heterosexual transmission surpassed all other modes of transmission combined, it is essential to target prevention efforts to those who participate in heterosexual activity. For pediatric nurses and nurses who care for families, it is essential to discuss HIV transmission prevention with men and women who are of childbearing potential. Making an informed choice to have a child is one of the goals of family planning.

Factors that may influence maternal viral burden, and consequently the likelihood of transmission, include immunologic status, general health, nutritional status, repeated HIV exposure, other intercurrent sexually transmitted infections, and response to antiretroviral drug therapy or other treatments of AIDS-associated conditions.[1] Should a woman with HIV become pregnant, prevention can still be a goal. Supporting a mother to have a healthy pregnancy in which both the child and the mother have a positive outcome is important.

CONCLUSION

Since the main mode of acquisition of HIV infection in children is through vertical transmission from mother to child,[89] nurses need to play a key role in the education of health care providers and the general public concerning prevention, particularly women of child-bearing age. The United States has been seriously affected by HIV, but developing countries are under siege by the virus. International efforts have fallen short in curbing the disease. HIV has created a worldwide crisis that demands a full-scale response. It cannot and will not wait.

Every day must be treated as a new opportunity for growth and learning. Building on what we have learned is important if science and successful day-to-day care is to move forward. Searching for new ways to help children and adults live with HIV is essential. Frustration abounds for families and health care providers. Each health care discipline, including nursing, must strive to come together to make meaningful advances that will help not only in prevention of the disease but also in the treatment of those already infected.

Health care providers are faced daily with the daunting challenges of assessing families and their needs. Nurses, as well as other health care providers, need to find a level of comfort within their own practice to address some of the most challenging topics as well as the mundane topics that present themselves.

Children and families who are infected with or affected by HIV must be the focus of care. Listening to what works and what does not work is essential to moving forward to the development of new therapies. Those who care for children and families with HIV will continue to do so, tirelessly and with great effort, until there is a cure.

REFERENCES

1. Oleske JM: The many needs of the HIV-infected child. Hosp Pract 1994;29:81–87.
2. Wiznia AA, Lambert G, Pavlakis S: Pediatric HIV infection. Med Clin North Am 1996;80:1309–1336.
3. Centers for Disease Control: Update: AIDS among women—United States. MMWR 1994;44:81–86.
4. MacKune-Karrer B, Taylor EH: Toward multiculturality: Implications for the pediatrician. Pediatr Clin North Am 1995;42:21–30.
5. Centers for Disease Control: US HIV and AIDS cases reported through December 1999: Year-end edition. HIV/AIDS Surveill Rep 1999;11:45.
6. Boland MG, Santacroce SJ: Nursing roles in care of child and family. In Pizzo PA, Wilfert CM (eds): Pediatric AIDS: The Challenge of HIV Infection in Infants, Children and Adolescents, 2nd ed. Baltimore, Williams & Wilkins, 1994, pp 785–808.
7. Burr CK: Supporting the helpers. Nurs Clin of North Am 1996;31:243–251.
8. Riddel J, Moon MW: Children with HIV becoming adolescents: Caring for long-term survivors. Pediatric Nursing 1996;22:220–227.
9. Burns-Tisdale S, Duprat L, Wells C: Caring for people with human immunodeficiency virus: Incorporating the patient's perspective. JONA 1994;24:52–60.
10. Meyers A, Weitzman M: Pediatric HIV disease. Pediatr Clin North Am 1991;38:169–194.
11. Boland MG, Czarniecki L, Haiken HJ: Coordinated care for children with HIV infection. In Stuber ML (ed): Children and AIDS: Clinical Practice, No 19. Washington, DC, American Psychiatric Press, 1992, pp 165–181.
12. Lewis SY, Wesley Y, Haiken H: Pediatric and family HIV-psychosocial concerns across the continuum of disease. Nurs Clin North Am 1996;31:221–229.
13. American Academy of Pediatrics: Issues related to human immunodeficiency virus transmission in schools, child care, medical settings, the home and community. Pediatrics 1999;104:318–324.
14. Sherwen LN, Boland M: Overview of psychosocial research concerning pediatric human immunodeficiency virus infection. Dev Behav Pediatr 1994;15:S5–S11.
15. Schor E: The influence of families on child health: Family behaviors and child outcomes. Pediatr Clin North Am 1995;42:89–102.
16. Ungavarski PJ: Challenges for the urban home health care provider: The New York City experience. Nurs Clin North Am 1996;31:81–95.
17. Krener PKG: Clinical care of pediatric HIV infection: Caregiver and institutional issues. In Stuber ML (ed): Children and AIDS: Clinical Practice, No 19. Washington, DC, American Psychiatric Press, 1992, pp 197–212.
18. Sowell RL, Christensen P: HIV infection in rural communities. Nurs Clin North Am 1996;31:107–123.
19. Grace CJ, Soons KR, Kutzko D, et al: Service delivery for patients with HIV in a rural state: The Vermont model. AIDS Patients Care 1999;13:659–666.
20. Duggan C, Mitchell F: The role of the nurse. In Mok JYQ, Newell ML (eds): HIV Infection in Children: A Guide to Practical Management. Cambridge, Cambridge University Press, 1995, pp 235–250.
21. Lewis SY, Haiken H, Hoyt LG: Living beyond the odds: A psychosocial perspective on long-term survivors of pediatric human immunodeficiency virus infection. J Dev Behav Pediatr 1994;15:S12–S17.
22. Hamel SC, Feldman HM: Focus on families: Caring for children with special needs. Contemp Pediatr 1998;15:141–155.
23. Burroughs MH, Edelson PJ: Medical care of the HIV-infected child. Pediatr Clin North Am 1991;38:45–67.
24. Stuber ML: Psychotherapy issues in pediatric HIV and AIDS. In Stuber ML (ed): Children and AIDS: Clinical Practice, No 19. Washington, DC, American Psychiatric Press, 1992, pp 213–226.
25. Capers CF: The Neuman systems model: A culturally relevant perspective. ABNF J 1996;7:113–117.
26. Neuman B: The Neuman Systems Model, 2nd ed. Norwalk, CT, Appleton & Lange, 1989.

27. Garwick AW, Kohrman C, Wolman C, et al: Families' recommendations for improving services for children with chronic conditions. Arch Pediatr Adolesc Med 1998;152:440–448.
28. Bruce B, Ritchie J: Nurses' practices and perceptions of family-centered care. J Pediatr Nurs 1997;12:214–222.
29. Ahmann E, Shepard-Vernon B: Kinship care: An emerging issue. Pediatr Nurs 1997;23:598–600.
30. Patterson JM: Promoting resilience in families experiencing stress. Pediatr Clin North Am 1995;42:47–63.
31. Boland M, Rothpletz-Puglia P, Oleske J: Infants and children: HIV disease care management. In Ungvarski PJ, Flaskerud JH (eds): HIV/AIDS: A Guide to Primary Care Management, 4th ed. Philadelphia, WB Saunders, 1999; pp 65–97.
32. Ahmann E: Family-centered care: Shifting orientation. Pediatr Nurs 1994;20:113–117.
33. Shelton TL, Jeppson ES, Johnson BH, et al: Family centered care for children with special health care needs. Washington, DC, Association for the Care of Children's Health, 1987.
34. Johnson CP, Blasco PA: Community resources for children with special healthcare needs. Pediatr Ann 1997;26:679–686.
35. O'Hara MJ: Care of children with HIV infection. In Kelly P, Holman S, Rothenberg R, Holzemer SP (eds): Primary Care of Women and Children with HIV Infection: A Multidisciplinary Approach. Boston, Jones and Bartlett, 1995, pp 103–131.
36. Merrill EB: HIV/AIDS case management: A learning experience for undergraduate nursing students. ABNF J 1996;7:47–53.
37. Durham JD: The changing HIV/AIDS epidemic: Emerging psychosocial challenges for nurses. Nurs Clin North Am 1994;29:9–18.
38. Boland MG: Caring for the child and family with HIV disease. Pediatr Clin North Am 2000;47:189–202.
39. Deatrick JA, Lipman TH, Thurber F: Nutritional assessment for children who are HIV-infected. Pediatr Nurs 1998;24:137–141.
40. Centers for Disease Control and Prevention: 1994 Revised classification system for human immunodeficiency virus infection in children less than 13 years of age. MMWR 43:1–19, 1994.
41. Abrams E: Opportunistic infections and other clinical manifestations of HIV disease in children. Pediatr Clin North Am 2000;47:79–108.
42. Gross EJ, Larkin MH: The child with HIV in day care and school. Nurs Clin North Am 1996;31:231–241.
43. O'Hara MJ, D'Orlando D: Ambulatory care of the HIV-infected child. Nurs Clin North Am 1996;31:179–205.
44. Lane-McAuliffe EM, Lipshultz SE: Cardiovascular manifestations of pediatric HIV infection. Nurs Clin North Am 1995;30:291–316.
45. Mintz M: Neurological and developmental problems in pediatric HIV infection. Am Inst Nutr 1996;126:2663S–2673S.
46. Bentler M, Stanish M: Nutrition support of the pediatric patient with AIDS. Perspect Pract 1987;87:488–491.
47. Nicholas SW, Leung J, Fennoy I: Guidelines for nutritional support of HIV-infected children. J Pediatr 1991;119:S59–S62.
48. Oleske JM, Rothpletz-Puglia PM, Winter H: Historical perspectives of the evolution in understanding the importance of nutritional care in pediatric HIV infection. Am Inst Nutr 1996;126:2616S–2619S.
49. Czarniecki L: Advanced HIV disease in children. Nurs Clin North Am 1996;31:207–219.
50. Rutstein RM, Starr SE: Immunizing the HIV infected child. AIDS Patient Care STDs 1997;11:149–160.
51. American Academy of Pediatrics: Evaluation and medical treatment of the HIV exposed infant. Pediatrics 1997;99:909–917.
52. Holaday B: Challenges of rearing a chronically ill child: Caring and coping. Nurs Clin North Am 1984;19:361–368.
53. Wiener L, Septimus A: Psychosocial support for child and family. In Pizzo PA, Wilfert CM (eds): Pediatric AIDS: The Challenge of HIV Infection in Infants, Children and Adolescents, 2nd ed. Baltimore, Williams & Wilkins, 1994, pp 809–828.
54. Baker S: Home care: Addressing the needs of people living with AIDS and their caregivers. Nurs Clin North Am 1999;34:201–211.
55. Lee C, Johann-Liang R: Disclosure of the diagnosis of HIV/AIDS to children born of HIV-infected mothers. AIDS Patient Care 1999;13:41–45.
56. Baker L: The perspectives of families. In Stuber ML (ed): Children and AIDS: Clinical Practice, No 19. Washington, DC, American Psychiatric Press, 1992, pp 147–161.
57. Ledlie SW: Diagnosis disclosure by family caregivers to children who have perinatally acquired HIV disease: When the time comes. Nurs Res 1999;48:141–149.
58. Kinsman SB, Sally M, Fox K: Multicultural issues in pediatric practice. Pediatr Rev 1996;17:349–355.
59. Curley MA: Mutuality: An expression of nursing presence. J Pediatr Nurs 1997;12:208–213.
60. Airhihenbuwa CO, DiClemente RJ, Wingood GM, et al: HIV/AIDS education and prevention among African-Americans: A focus on culture. AIDS Educ Prev 1992;4:267–276.
61. American Academy of Pediatrics: Planning for children whose parents are dying of HIV/AIDS. Pediatrics 1999;103:509–511.
62. Siegel K, Gorey E: Childhood bereavement due to parental death from acquired immunodeficiency syndrome. Dev Behav Pediatr 1994;15:S66–S70.

63. Oleske J, Boland M: When a child with a chronic condition needs hospitalization. Hosp Pract 1997;32:167–181.
64. Rushton CH, Hogue EE, Billett CA, et al: End of life care for infants with AIDS: Ethical and legal issues. Pediatr Nurs 1993;19:79–83.
65. Engle J: Immune-based therapy for HIV. Nurs Clin North Am 1996;31:15–23.
66. Hutchins SA, Eckes R: Clinical research: Considerations for prospective participants. Nurse Clin North Am 1996;31:125–135.
67. Oliveira AL, Crowe RL: Complementary therapies. In Kelly P, Holman S, Rothenberg R, Holzemer SP (eds): Primary care of women and children with HIV infection: A multidisciplinary approach. Boston, Jones & Bartlett, 1995, pp 207–215.
68. Anastasi JK: Alternative and complementary therapies. In Ungvarski PJ, Flaskerud JH (eds): HIV/AIDS: A guide to primary care management, 4th ed. Philadelphia, WB Saunders, 1999, pp 394–409.
69. Freeman EM, MacIntyre RC: Evaluating alternative treatments for HIV infection. Nurs Clin North Am 1999;34:147–162.
70. Levine A: Antiretroviral therapy: Adherence. Clinical Care Options for HIV: 8th Clinical Care Options for HIV Symposium 1998, pp 1–9; http://healthcg.com/hiv/journal/scottsdale98/04.html.
71. Narayan MC: Cultural assessment in home healthcare. Home Healthcare Nurse 1997;15:663–670.
72. Williams AB: Adherence to highly active antiretroviral therapy. Nurs Clin North Am 1999;34;113–129.
73. Chesney MA: New antiretroviral therapies: Adherence challenges and strategies. Clin Care Options HIV Treat Issues; http://healthcg.com/hiv/treatment/ICAAC1997/adherence/chesney.html.
74. Mehta S, Moore RD, Graham MNH: Potential factors affecting adherence with HIV therapy. AIDS 1997;11:1665–1670.
75. Shingadia D, Viani R, Dankner W, et al: Gastrostomy tube insertion for improvement of adherence with highly active antiretroviral therapy in pediatric HIV patients. Pediatrics 2000;105:E80.
76. Watson DC, Collins-Jones TL, Lovelace S: Antiretroviral therapy of pediatric HIV infection: Making hope a reality. 1999;13:587–599.
77. Roizen NJ, Shalowita MU, Kowie KA, et al: Acquisition of services recommended by a multidisciplinary medical diagnostic team for children under three years of age evaluated for developmental delays. Devel Behav Pediatr 1996;17:399–404.
78. Meisenhelder JB: Caring for the caregiver. In Kelly P, Holman S, Rothenberg R, Holzemer SP (eds): Primary Care of Women and Children with HIV Infection: A Multidisciplinary Approach. Boston, Jones & Bartlett Publishers, 1995, pp 291–299.
79. Fry-Revere S: A bioethics consultant's thoughts on caring for pediatric patients with HIV. Pediatr Nurs 1994;20:177–180.
80. McClinsey SC: Occupational exposure to HIV: Considerations for postexposure prophylaxis and prevention. Nurs Clin North Am 1999;34:213–225.
81. Kalichman SC, Gueritault-Chalvin V, Demi A: Sources of occupational stress and coping strategies among nurses working in AIDS care. J Assoc Nurses AIDS Care 2000;11:31–37.
82. Walker ME: Stress and adaptation. In Potter PA, Perry AG (eds): Fundamentals of Nursing: Concepts, Process and Practice. St. Louis, Mosby, 1997, pp 370–387.
83. Robinson SE, Roth SL, Keim J, et al: Nurse burnout: Work-related and demographic factors as culprits. Res Nurs Health 1991;14:223–228.
84. Visintini R, Campanini E, Fossati A, et al: Psychological stress in nurses' relationships with HIV-infected patients: The risk of burnout syndrome. AIDS Care 1996;8:183–194.
85. Johnson BS: Introduction to psychiatric-mental health nursing. In Johnson BS: Adaptation and Growth: Psychiatric-Mental Health Nursing, 4th ed. Philadelphia, Lippincott, 1997, pp 3–19.
86. Sherwen LN, Storm DS: Looking toward the twenty-first century: The role of nursing research in care of children and families affected by HIV. Nurs Clin North Am 1996;31:165–178.
87. Cohen FL: Research of families and pediatric human immunodeficiency virus disease: A review and needed directions. Devel Behav Pediatr 1994;15:S34–S42.
88. Ungvarski PJ: Update on HIV infection. AJN 1997;97:44–51.
89. Newell ML: Children and HIV infection. In Mok JYQ, Newell ML (eds): HIV Infection in Children: A Guide to Practical Management. Cambridge, Cambridge University Press, 1995, pp 1–20.

Managed Care for Children with HIV Infection

Sindy M. Paul,
Paul Langevin,
Dawn M. D'Orlando,
Victor S.B. Jorden, and
Jill Simone

The practice of medicine entails many challenges for the modern practitioner, but the most dominant of these may be the emergence and continued growth of managed care. For both primary care physician and specialist alike, managed care has made severe demands on pediatricians attempting to balance competent, compassionate patient care with viable levels of reimbursement. This balance may be especially precarious for physicians caring for a child with HIV disease. These patients and their families, even when not critically ill, often require more time and effort than the more predictable four to six patients per hour. Children with HIV disease usually have at least one infected parent. Familial and social milieus may be such that case management is an integral part of the overall care plan. Finally, these children frequently come from economically disenfranchised backgrounds with commensurately marginal insurance coverage; in many cases, coverage is simply absent.

This combination of factors makes the care of pediatric patients with HIV disease tremendously challenging, not only medically but also economically, as doctors involved in HIV care find themselves struggling to maintain a fiscally sound practice while offering the opportunity for participation in clinical trials. Considering the dominance of managed care within the medical indemnification market, the pediatric HIV provider has little choice but to make a priority of understanding modern medical economics and managed care. Only by combining this understanding with a reasonable appraisal of resources and strong negotiating skills can physicians continue to not only provide a high standard of care but also survive financially so that these high standards can be sustained. This chapter is designed to help pediatricians better understand managed care, what to look for in the contracts, how to actively participate in contract development, and how to work with managed care to help themselves and their patients navigate the system.

BASICS AND ORIGINS OF MANAGED CARE

The American Medical Association defines managed care as "systems or techniques generally used by third party payers or their agents to affect access to and control payment of health care services."[1] It remains controversial whether the term "managed care" refers to the management of the patient's medical care or management of the composition and reimbursement of the provider delivery system.[2]

Managed care and traditional medical insurance have two major similarities. First, both indemnify their policyholders to varying degrees against medical expenses. Second, both types of products are designed to make money for the insuring entity, a goal frequently forgotten by the public. This drive to generate profit for the insurer is what characterizes managed care, because the *means* through which managed care organizations (MCOs) attain and sustain their profits differ greatly from the means used by traditional third-party payers. These differences are discussed briefly here, and then in greater detail in following sections of this chapter.

Older, more traditional insurance plans basically maintained their profit margins by stratifying their clients' risk based on medical, demographic, and actuarial data. This analysis facilitated a statistical prediction of clients' medical costs; premiums were adjusted to provide for these costs, with additional adjustments for administrative costs and a comfortable margin of profit. Traditional health care insurance made no or little attempt to reduce the amount of money that was actually spent on its clients by providers. Physicians and hospitals performed services, submitted a bill to the insurer, and the bill was paid. The outcome was a carte blanche approach to medical testing and patient procedures, with the resulting spiraling medical costs that outpaced the rate of inflation: by 1970, the growth of medical expenses exceeded the growth of the consumer price index.[3]

The MCOs also maintain revenue through premium adjustments, but what differentiates this industry from traditional insurance are the two additional means used to ensure fiscal stability. Firstly, managed care attempts to control provider expenditures and thus the cost of health care for its clients. Secondly, managed care distributes the risk of indemnification among its contractors, including its physician providers. These methods have obviously led to monumental changes in the arena of reimbursement. As importantly, managed care has infringed on what has previously been considered sacrosanct and untouchable: the physician's autonomous authority to make medical decisions for his or her patients. Concern with autonomy has been an issue facing physicians for more than a century. In the early 1900s, physicians employed by companies to provide employee medical care were concerned with retaining relationships with their patients without corporate intervention.[4] This may sound disturbingly familiar to pediatricians in practice today.

MANAGED CARE TODAY AND THE PRACTITIONER MANAGING PEDIATRIC AIDS

Today, managed care is an accepted model for the financing and delivery of health care services. It is becoming increasingly important in the private sector and for public programs such as Medicaid. Until recently, states focussed primarily on enrolling their Aid to Families with Dependent Children populations in managed care. Now there is increased interest in moving other vulnerable populations covered by Medicaid, including persons with HIV disease, into managed care arrangements. Many of these children previously received their health care through a combination of fee-for-service plans and public programs, including Medicaid and state and federal maternal and child health programs.[5]

Many managed care plans for pediatrics focus on providing efficient care for healthy children. They are not routinely designed to respond to the special needs of children with HIV disease.[5] The transition to managed care as health insurance for HIV-infected and perinatally exposed children is fraught with challenges. The providers and patients are concerned with access to providers with experience and expertise in treating children with HIV disease, continuity of care, quality of care, and appropriate reimbursement for the level of care provided. The managed care organizations are gaining expertise in serving HIV-infected children but are doing so at a time when our knowledge of the disease and the methods to provide cost-effective, high-quality care are constantly changing.

The American Academy of Pediatrics has identified three major differences between adults with disabilities and children with disabilities entering managed care. These include (1) the potential impact of HIV disease on a child's normal development; (2) the low and decreasing incidence of perinatal HIV transmission; and (3) the child's dependence on the families' health and socioeconomic status to have adequate adult protection for the child's health and development. When looking into managed care plans, providers and families need to find a plan that can optimize the health outcome for the child and minimize the potential for developmental delay.[5] For HIV disease, this includes access to providers with experience and expertise treating HIV disease. The Health Care Financing Administration (HCFA) sent a letter to all State Medicaid Directors in 1999 defining experience and expertise in treating HIV disease as a licensed physician, nurse practitioner, or physician assistant who has an active, ongoing caseload of at least 25 individuals with HIV/AIDS over the preceding 24 months, either in regular practice or as part of a supervised postgraduate training program. In urban areas with a high incidence of HIV disease, HCFA defines experience and expertise as a minimum of 50 patients over the preceding 24 months.[6]

Medicaid is the single largest payer of direct medical services for people with HIV disease in the United States. Medicaid pays for more than 50% of the care for adults and 90% of the care for children.[7,8] Combined state and federal Medicaid expenditures for fiscal year 2000 are estimated to be $4.1 billion.[8]

It is important for the pediatrician to know that within Medicaid, special income limits exist for pregnant women and their babies. These income limits are higher than the state's regular income limits for families. They are designed to ensure that pregnant women receive prenatal care. The income limits in each state for pregnant women can be found on the Internet at http://www.hcfa.gov/hiv/subpg4.htm.[8]

TYPES OF HEALTH COVERAGE (INSURANCE)

One of the first questions one must ask when considering the question of accessing health care services for any population is "What kind of coverage does the patient have and how does that affect the resources available to him or her?" In the broadest sense, health care coverage falls into three categories: commercial insurance, self-insured plans, and government programs such as Medicare and Medicaid. While at first blush the coverage plans may all look very similar, and in many ways they are, the major differences can be found in a few significant areas that are worth discussing.

Commercial insurance is what most people think of when they talk about health insurance. A private sector company, usually licensed and regulated by the state government, is responsible for assuming the health insurance risk for a given population. That population pays premiums in exchange for the commercial insurer agreeing to pay for the medical expenses, covered by the contract for benefits. Since state governments regulate these types of plans, whenever a new state law is passed mandating some type of coverage, payment scheme, or benefit, the law usually applies to the commercial insurer.

The second type of coverage is available through self-insured health plans. This coverage may look to the consumer and the health care provider to be the same as commercial insurance. However, these plans are generally exempt through the federal Employee Retirement and Income Security Act (ERISA) from regulations by state agencies. Therefore, state mandates such as length of stay laws for maternity and mandatory diagnostic testing laws enacted by state government cannot be applied to these plans.

The third type of coverage is available through government programs such as Medicare and Medicaid. These programs have generally rich benefits packages and, in the case of Medicaid, little out-of-pocket expense for the beneficiary. Historically, government programs were primarily fee-for-service arrangements with some case management. However, there has been an increasing trend of government programs to move toward managed care for delivering coverage to their beneficiaries.

TYPES OF MANAGED CARE PLANS

Health Maintenance Organizations (HMOs). HMOs are organizations that are responsible for financing and delivering a comprehensive range of health services to a defined population within a specific geographic area. The HMO is both an insurer and an organizer of a health delivery network, which it must maintain and for which it must provide some form of quality assurance. An HMO must ensure that its members have access to the full array of physical and mental health services likely to be required by its members. Government regulators of HMOs usually require a demonstration by the HMO that there are sufficient finances and an adequate network of providers (e.g., physicians, hospitals, home health agencies, mental health professionals) to provide reasonable access to services on a timely basis. Such assurances are usually required in advance of the start up of business.[2]

Point–of–Service (POS) Plans. POS plans have frequently been described as "leaky" HMOs. Under a POS plan, members may seek health care outside of the contracted network of providers in exchange for a higher co-pay or other out-of-pocket expense. These plans were originally developed to enhance enrollment and to address the concern of limited access to physicians (notably specialists) by members of HMOs and have become one of the fastest growing types of managed care.[2]

Preferred Provider Organizations (PPOs). PPO plans represent another form of managed care that is gaining rapid acceptance by consumers and purchasers of health care (usually employers or the government). PPOs are best described as discount provider networks that contract with health benefit plans and insurers to provide care for the beneficiaries of the plan. The providers in the PPO agree to participate in utilization management, quality improvement, and certain administrative conventions of the health plan in exchange for a contracted payment structure (prompt payment of fees negotiated in advance, with no balance billing of the member). A significant advantage for the provider is that in exchange for a minimum of administrative effort they receive a steady and predictable case load of patients from the contracting health plan.[2]

Exclusive Provider Organizations (EPO). EPOs are plans that are very similar in design to PPOs, with one significant exception. In an EPO plan, beneficiaries may seek care only from participating providers; there is no out-of-network benefit. EPOs may employ a gatekeeper model or be of an open access design in which beneficiaries can obtain services from any provider with full benefit coverage so long as that provider participates in the network.[2]

Physician Hospital Organizations (PHOs). PHOs are legal entities composed of at least one hospital and one or more physician groups that are empowered to negotiate on behalf of the hospital and physicians with insurers. When licensed to assume insurance risk by the state or federal government, the PHO may negotiate directly with a purchaser of coverage (such as employers).[2]

Disease State Management Programs (DSMPs). DSMPs are increasingly forming to address concerns associated with the treatment of specific types of patients with chronic or complex illnesses. Renal patients, oncology patients, and HIV patients are examples of these populations. Based on the concept of intense case management, DSMPs generally are made up of physicians and other health care specialists with a depth of knowledge and experience in caring for patients with a particular illness who promise higher quality and lower costs to a purchaser of services. The DSMP does not generally provide comprehensive benefits to the population that they manage, but it may. Unlike other forms of managed care, the DSMP does not offer the full array of health care services but relies on the primary insurer to cover the cost of care in areas unrelated to the disease that it is managing.[2]

REGULATION AND ACCREDITATION OF MANAGED CARE PLANS

Regulation of MCOs is accomplished through a variety of entities, both state and federal. The responsibility for regulating the MCO is generally based on the product—that is, HMO, PPO, POS, and so on—and the source of payment for the product such as private insurance, Medicare, or Medicaid.

Medicare is a benefit program run solely by the federal government and is administered by the Center for Medicare and Medicaid Services. The Medicare Plus Choice program created by the Balanced Budget Act of 1997 dictates the benefit design, reimbursement methodology, and regulatory scheme for the plans. For those beneficiaries who wish to choose a managed care option under Medicare, the three general types of MCOs to choose from are (1) coordinated care organizations, which include HMOs, Provider-Sponsored Organizations (PSOs, which could include PHOs mentioned previously) and PPOs; (2) Medicare Plus Choice medical savings account plans; and (3) Medicare Plus Choice private fee-for-service organizations.

Medicaid is a joint state-federal program for low-income and disabled persons with Medicaid MCOs experiencing rapidly increasing membership. Each individual state operates the program within broad guidelines authorized by the federal government (HCFA). Medicaid managed care beneficiaries have a very generous benefits package when compared with the typical commercial package offered through employers; it may include such benefits as transportation, dental services, and prescription drugs and, depending on the need for it, intensive case management services. To participate in Medicaid, the individual entity must have a state authorization to operate an HMO, PPO, POS, or whatever other type of MCO certificate or license is required in the commercial market. In addition, the MCO must meet the contract requirements of the state agency responsible for administering the Medicaid plan approved by HCFA in the particular state and have an in-force contract with the state agency.

Accreditation of MCOs is done primarily by two organizations nationally, the National Committee on Quality Assurance (NCQA) and the Utilization Review and Accreditation Commission (URAC). The Joint Commission on Accreditation of Healthcare Organizations also offers an accreditation program for MCOs but does not have nearly the same level of participation as the NCQA or URAC.

Both NCQA and URAC accreditation are recognized by federal and state authorities as indicators of high-quality programs. In many states, accreditation may substitute in whole or in part for state regulatory activity and is frequently formally recognized in the state licensing and certification regulations.[9]

REIMBURSEMENT OF PHYSICIANS IN MANAGED CARE ORGANIZATIONS

Among the most significant differences between managed care and the more traditional health care delivery system is the method of compensation for physicians. Ideally, the successful MCO will employ a compensation system that is fair, ties increased reimbursement to the delivery of high-quality care, and encourages neither under- nor overutilization of health care resources.

Designing a compensation system is essentially about striking a balance between providing an incentive for physicians to examine the way they practice and providing the care their patients need. It should reward high-quality care and provide no incentive for withholding medically necessary care from patients. The traditional means of reimbursement for physicians is fee for service (FFS). Providers are paid for each encounter or service provided.[10] There is little financial risk to the physician with respect to caring for sicker patients because if the patient's medical condition requires more services, the physician will be paid each time a service is provided. The disadvantage of FFS reimbursement is that it is very difficult to affect the quality or quantity of care being provided without a well-developed encounter data collection system accompanied by a rigorous utilization review plan.

Discounted FFS is the next step along the continuum of reimbursement. Under this system, the event triggering payment is still the provision of a service. The difference is that there is usually a contract between the provider and the payer, which provides a discounted fee in exchange for some benefit to the provider such as prompt payment or directed patient volume. This method is frequently employed in PPOs because it accommodates frequent migration in and out of the network and does not bind patients to a particular physician.

Capitation is the form of reimbursement that most persons associate with managed care, although its use in the managed care environment is by no means the rule. Simply defined, capitation is the prepayment of services on a per member, per month basis. In other words, a fixed amount of money is paid to the provider (e.g., physician, group practice) each month no matter how much or how little health care services are rendered to that individual patient or member.[11]

Incentive compensation is a broad term that can be used to describe a variety of reimbursement methods but essentially ties some portion of the physician's income to performance, either the quality of care provided, the quantity of resources consumed, or both. Incentive compensation can be used in conjunction with other forms of reimbursement, such as salary, FFS, or capitation. Under incentive arrangements, a portion of the physician's reimbursement is dependent upon meeting certain performance objectives in one or a variety of areas. A portion of the physician payment can be withheld and then distributed based on the physician's or group of physicians' achieving predetermined objectives. Many reimbursement methods attempt to incorporate quality, utilization, and patient satisfaction criteria into the reimbursement distribution formula for physicians. Under such plans, those physicians with the best patient outcomes (highest quality care), utilization closest to the target, and highest patient satisfaction ratings receive maximum reimbursement.[12]

At first glance, the incentive compensation method seems best suited for today's health care delivery system; however, the degree of "at-risk" compensation is critical to a successful system, and missing the mark can have detrimental effects on physicians, patients, and the health plan. If the amount of reimbursement at risk is too small, there will be little incentive to achieve target performance in a variety of areas. Boland has cited 20% to 30% as the minimum range for at-risk compensation to be effective.[12]

As the sophistication of reimbursement incentive plans increases, there has been a tendency to divide the utilization pool into better defined units. Creation of these more specific pools can also create adverse reimbursement scenarios for physicians who see a highly complex mix of critically ill patients. Because of this problem, many incentive plans contain special allowances for the unique needs of special populations, such as HIV-positive patients or patients requiring mental health services.[12] Services to these individuals are "carved out" of the general reimbursement arrangement. These patients may be identified for intense case management, using specialists as primary care providers as well as providers of specialty care. Patients may be assigned case managers who are frequently specialty nurses or other health care professionals with a depth of experience with the target population. These individuals will not only have expertise in the particular disease and its management but also will be intimately familiar with both the medical and social support systems necessary for achieving the best outcome for the patient.[12]

ENROLLMENT AND CREDENTIALING OF PROVIDERS

In nearly all MCOs, developing and maintaining the network of providers is an essential part of operations. Once the providers are under contract (a process that must be completed prior to receiving government approval to operate), the process of credentialing physicians must be conducted. New physicians begin by completing an application form, usually specific to the MCO, which contains the information necessary to determine whether the appropriate education, licenses, and certification, among other criteria, are met by the physician.[13]

Once the information necessary for credentialing has been submitted, the process of verification must occur. Health plan consultation with the National Practitioners Data Bank is required by the Health Care Quality Improvement Act of 1986. In addition, the plan will check references with the state board of medical examiners or other state regulatory body to ascertain whether the physician's license is valid and to ensure that there are no limitations or sanctions placed on the license.[13]

If the physician will be seeing members in his or her own office (such as in the case of an IPA model HMO or a PPO), the health plan will also conduct a site visit of the physician's office and determine whether it meets the minimal criteria for participation. Elements such as the size, design, diagnostic services, medical and surgical capabilities, staffing, and administrative support services available will be reviewed during the site visit. Additional items such as compliance with the Americans with Disabilities Act, the extent of office hours, and the provisions for maintaining medical records and their confidentiality may also be reviewed and may be contract requirements of the plan if it participates with government programs such as Medicare or Medicaid. During the site visit, a determination of the physician's ability to accept new patients will also be made, as it is essential to ensuring adequate network capacity of the plan.[13]

With an application verified, a site visit conducted, and a contract in place, the physician is ready to become a participating provider. An abbreviated review of the above-mentioned elements is usually conducted on a biennial basis.[13]

WHAT THE HMO EXPECTS: MONITORING AND EVALUATION

Continuous quality assurance is central to the successful operation of MCOs. Regulatory agencies require quality assurance as part of the licensure process for MCOs. The data are used to monitor and evaluate the delivery of services and are important to ensuring ongoing access to services and delivery of quality care. Although quality improvement should be part of every medical practice, the data collection requirements of managed care may exceed what physicians have traditionally done in their own practices. However, the importance of these data cannot be overestimated: future decisions within the MCO regarding patient care protocols will be predicated on this information, not to mention various incentives and rewards for the practitioner.

The MCOs have an internal system for managing and monitoring quality of care. The medical director of each MCO decides the quality assurance priorities and requests data from practitioners based on their practice.[10] These data may be obtained administratively from data provided to the managed care plan (e.g., billing information) or may be obtained through a retrospective medical record review. The information can be used to look at the average performance for the entire plan, reports that focus on individual physicians, hospital utilization, outpatient utilization, and plan-wide.

Of most concern to physicians are the individual provider profiles. Profiling focuses on the patterns of an individual physician's care, not specific clinical decisions. The provider profile incorporates performance indicators, which are activities or outcomes that can be used to compare providers. It is usually expressed as a rate or a measure of the amount of resources used during a defined period of time for a defined population—for example, the number of children with AIDS admitted to the hospital in the calendar year 2001. The resulting profile can then be compared with a peer group or a standard. MCOs use the provider profile to measure physician performance, to guide quality improvement projects, and to select physicians for deletion from the MCO network.[14]

Regulatory agencies include reporting requirements as a condition of MCO licensure, and these requirements go beyond individual physician profiles. MCOs expect providers to participate in a variety of monitoring methods used by states to evaluate quality of care and health outcomes. These include focus studies, individual medical record reviews, review of utilization data, member satisfaction surveys, review of complaint and grievance processes and statistics, quality improvement studies, and performance outcomes.

Based on provider profiles and plan-wide information, the MCO may expect physicians to participate in quality improvement projects (QIPs). This may be a regulatory requirement for the MCO. QIPs may be defined by the state with input from the MCOs. These projects are intended to define measurable improvement goals and specific measures, which serve as the focus for each QIP. Each MCO may have the discretion to design and implement its own strategies for achieving each of the objectives within the QIP. Each measure includes a baseline performance rate, the target standard, and the minimum required compliance standard. The MCO's performance rate is periodically measured against the compliance standard. The MCO's performance is expected to improve over time, going from the baseline rate toward the targeted satisfactory outcome. Each year, or review period, the compliance rate is raised until the targeted outcome is achieved.

APPEALS PROCESS

Each managed care organization has an internal appeals process. Many states specify how the grievances should be handled.[15] Some states also require both an internal and an external appeals process. The HMO Model Act, which authorized the establishment of HMOs in all 50 states, requires establishment of a grievance procedure to help resolve enrollee complaints. Typically, state regulators require HMOs to inform enrollees of their right to a hearing when they join the HMO. This notification is usually written. Each HMO is also required to form a grievance committee to hear enrollee complaints. Committee decisions may be appealed within the HMO, and, if necessary, the state may step in to hear the complaint. The HMO must report the number of grievances filed and processed to its regulatory authority on a regular basis.[15]

The MCO internal appeals process can be administered by the plan or by a contracted utilization review organization acting on behalf of the plan. The internal appeals process allows patients who are denied treatment or services ordered by a physician to appeal the decision to the health plan. The exact internal appeals procedure varies from plan to plan. However, most have the same basic components. In stage 1 of the appeals process, the patient typically contacts the medical director of the plan or another physician designated by the plan to discuss why the treatment or service was denied. The appeals need to be completed within a specified time frame (e.g., within 5 business days and within 3 days for emergencies or urgent care). If the patient is dissatisfied with the decision rendered in the stage 1 appeal, the health plan must provide a written explanation of the member's right to appeal to the next level, stage 2. The second stage is more formal. The patient can pursue the claim in front of a panel of physicians and other health care professionals. Stage 2 is completed in a specified time frame (e.g., 20 business days or 72 hours for urgent or emergency care). If the stage 2 appeal is denied, the patient will receive a written explanation for the denial. In states that require the opportunity for an external appeal, the patient will also receive instructions on how to arrange an external appeal.[16]

State regulations may have a list of requirements that must be met for the patient or physician to file for an external appeal. These requirements vary from state to state. Information on the appeals process for individual plans should be available from the plan or from the agency within your state that regulates health insurance plans and managed care organizations.

Regulatory agencies as well as state Medicaid programs monitor the MCO appeals process. The regulatory requirements or the appeals process may vary from state to state. Also, the Medicaid appeals process differs from that of other managed care plans. By federal regulation, Medicaid beneficiaries enrolled in a managed care program have the right to a Medicaid Fair Hearing process in addition to the MCO's internal grievance process. In a Fair Hearing process, the complaint is heard before an administrative law judge. Medicaid beneficiaries also have the ability to access any other external appeal process as may be allowed by state law. The Medicaid Fair Hearing process is available to Medicaid enrollees at any time they have a complaint about the services rendered, denied, or reduced. Medicaid enrollees do not have to access the MCO grievance process first before requesting a Fair Hearing.

MALPRACTICE LIABILITY

Physicians are pulled in opposite directions between their responsibility to the patient and their obligation to the MCO. Working under managed care restrictions does not eliminate the physicians' liability[17]; however, managed care liability for malpractice is a controversial and legally complicated issue. For many years, MCOs had relative immunity from malpractice lawsuits. Patients were unable to sue HMOs for medical malpractice by a federal law, ERISA, enacted in 1974. The courts are currently divided on whether patients who belong to employee group health plans are subject to ERISA.[18]

Recently, malpractice plaintiffs have had some success in suing MCOs by using two legal theories. The first legal theory claims that the HMOs are "vicariously liable" for substandard care provided by physicians in their provider networks. The premise is that the MCOs control to some degree the performance of physicians in their networks who act as their agents. Vicarious liability may include both staff model HMOs and physicians in private practice who independently contract with the MCO on an individual basis, through group practice, or through an independent practice association.[18]

The second theory of corporate liability is that managed care companies are directly liable for their negligent acts and omissions (e.g., delaying hospitalization) when delays harm a patient. Plaintiffs argue that the MCOs are practicing medicine because they actively manage patient care and influence treatment by physicians. The traditional defense for managed care companies is that they do not make medical decisions and should not be liable for malpractice. The companies contend that they determine which treatments are covered as benefits, arrange coverage, and administer employee health plans.[18]

A patient typically files a malpractice claim against both the physician and the MCO. The MCO tries to move the case to federal court. This move, which is advantageous to the MCO, argues that the claim should be dismissed because the plan is governed by ERISA, which supersedes state malpractice law. Even if the case is not dismissed, ERISA has more limited legal remedies than state malpractice laws. Under ERISA, the plaintiff cannot receive a settlement for pain and suffering, lost earnings, or the loss of life. The federal judge can side with the MCO and dismiss the claim. This decision occurs more frequently than the court's siding with the patient and sending the case back to state court for trial.[18] Either way, the physician is embroiled in a malpractice suit.

IDEAL LANGUAGE FOR MANAGED CARE PLANS FOR PATIENTS WITH HIV INFECTION

When reviewing a managed care plan to decide on participation, there is some ideal language related to HIV disease that the physician can look for. Not all of the ideal language may be found in any one specific plan or contract.

Most traditional primary care providers do not treat many children with HIV/AIDS. Consequently, they do not have the experience to treat such a complex disease. The managed care plan should include experienced pediatricians and adolescent providers in its network. The current consensus is that a provider with experience and expertise treating these patients should treat children with HIV disease. As mentioned earlier in this chapter, HCFA established criteria for experience and expertise in treating persons with HIV disease. To reiterate, the criteria are an active ongoing caseload of at least 25 individuals with HIV/AIDS over the preceding 24 months, either in regular practice or as part of a supervised postgraduate training program. In urban areas with a high incidence of HIV disease,

HCFA defines experience and expertise as a minimum of 50 patients in the preceding 24 months.[6] Traditional primary care providers should not be prohibited from being able to be the primary treating physician. However, the MCO must have clear guidelines and protocols delineating when primary care providers can function as the primary caregiver for these patients.

In MCOs, the HIV specialist may not be designated as the primary care provider. Consequently, enrollees are required to contact their primary care provider first to obtain a referral or authorization to see a specialist. Frequently, immediate access is critical and the usual or normal managed care referral process may create a barrier for these patients. Therefore, an alternative process must be in place to ensure appropriate, timely care. Several possible alternatives are allowing (1) specialists to be designated as the primary care providers; (2) long-term standing referrals; and (3) self-referral by the patient. These are discussed in more detail below. Allowing patients to enroll at their care sites could facilitate continuity of care. This may be particularly important for pediatricians practicing in areas where Medicaid managed care is soon scheduled to begin.

Not only is access to specialists expert in treating HIV/AIDS patients important, so too is access to diagnostic testing. Viral load and resistance testing, previously reserved for patients in clinical trials, are now part of the routine clinical management of HIV-infected persons. The specialist must have immediate or standing authorization to determine what tests are needed and when they are needed. Equally important is the ability to collect test specimens immediately to ensure that the test will be performed. The opportunity to do the test may be lost if the patient is sent from the physician's office to another site for testing, which may not be convenient or accessible to the patient. MCOs must maintain policies and procedures for specimen collection by the treating physician or specialty center where the patient is being treated at the time testing is required.

The availability of new classes of antiretroviral agents and recommendations for combination therapy starting in the mid-1990s has markedly improved the life span and quality of life for HIV-infected persons. For example, survival of perinatally infected children was longer in the 1996 through 1998 birth cohorts than in children born in the period from 1980 through 1995. This increased survival was attributed to combination antiretroviral therapy.[19] Access to these medications is essential.

There are two concepts involved with access to these medications. First, patients must be able to receive prescribed medications on a timely basis. HIV/AIDS patients must be directed to pharmacies that are conveniently located and stock or are able to obtain all of the medications the patient will need. Secondly, HIV/AIDS patients must have immediate access to any new drug approved by the Food and Drug Administration (FDA). Since the treatment of HIV/AIDS is rapidly changing and improving the quality of life as well as longevity, immediate access to new drugs can be essential to patient care. MCOs must allow for coverage of all new FDA-approved drugs. To contend with the unpredictable and high costs of antiretroviral agents, some Medicaid plans carve out antiretroviral agents. By carving out the antiretroviral agents, neither the MCO nor the physician is at financial risk for prescribing them because they are not included in the capitated payment system.

The MCOs should address prevention for infected and uninfected enrollees. Prevention programs developed by the MCOs could include the following.

1. Methods for promoting HIV prevention to all enrollees. Information on preventive measures must be disseminated to enrollees, including facts about the disease and how to prevent contact, encourage screening, and incorporate preventive measures in their daily lives.
2. HIV prevention information must be consistent with the various ages, sex, and risk factors and be culturally and linguistically appropriate.
3. The establishment of linkages with HIV/AIDS clinical educational programs and clinical trials to keep current on up-to-date treatment guidelines and standards.
4. Mechanisms to encourage providers to cooperate with community prevention programs.
5. In the case of pregnant women with HIV/AIDS, MCOs must have a program in place to educate, counsel, test, and treat the pregnant women with HIV/AIDS to reduce perinatal transmission of HIV from the mother to infant. Education, counseling, and testing (with the mother's consent) should be part of regular prenatal care. The earlier the mother's serostatus is known, the sooner information on the role of antiretroviral agents and elective cesarean section to decrease the risk of transmission can be discussed. The

patient should also be referred to social services. Appropriate treatment options for the mother throughout the pregnancy and to both the mother and child after birth should be discussed, as both will need continuing care by an HIV specialist.

Comprehensive care of HIV/AIDS patients often involves the need for coordination with social service agencies to assist in managing the nonmedical problems of the patient that affect overall quality of life. Some examples of nonmedical problems may include lack of or inadequate housing, lack of access to a telephone, difficulties with transportation, and no access to day care for young children, all of which may prevent a patient from being able to keep a doctor's appointment.

The MCOs must establish linkages with various social service agencies as part of their case management functions to ensure that all of the needs of the patient are being met. Ultimately, the physical health of the patient may deteriorate if other life issues are severely compromised.

Linkages with Ryan White Comprehensive AIDS Resources Emergency (CARE) Act grantees should be established. Ryan White agencies not only provide medical treatment but also have case management experience. Case management services are essential for this population to ensure there is no breakdown in other life functions that impact considerably on the disease status of individuals. Many pediatric HIV patients and their families would benefit from improved coordination between the managed care plan and Ryan White CARE Act grantees. These programs could develop a comprehensive continuum of care for children with HIV disease that includes outreach, primary care services, prescription drugs, laboratory services, home and community-based health care, and related support services, inpatient services, palliative care, respite care, and end-of-life care. This collaboration could include a contractual relationship for services. CARE Act funds may be used to pay for services to Medicaid beneficiaries if the state's Medicaid program does not cover a particular service benefit. However, the CARE Act is the payor of last resort and may not be used to pay for Medicaid-covered services for Medicaid beneficiaries. Representatives from the managed care plan should meet at least every 6 months with either the Ryan White Eligible Metropolitan Area (EMA) involved in enrollee care or the local consortia to develop service coordination protocols and discuss issues of unmet needs and ways to improve service coordination.

Quality of care has also been a concern with managed care plans. Quality of care monitoring should be performed as described later in this chapter. In addition, plans may require providers to attend (or present at) a minimum of 12 hours of continuing medical education on the medical management of HIV disease in pediatrics annually.

EXAMPLES OF MANAGED CARE AND PEDIATRIC HIV CARE

Early in the HIV/AIDS epidemic, care was provided in a variety of settings such as infectious disease clinics, pulmonary clinics, oncology clinics, primary care centers, and private practices. The site of care was determined by the presenting symptoms. Coverage was provided through a variety of public and private payers, including managed care plans. This was effective at the time because care was based on the symptoms and the number of patients seeking care was low. As the number of persons with HIV disease increased in the late 1980s, especially on the East and West coasts, this care model was no longer feasible. New models to address this growing need began to emerge. One example, the Harvard Community Health Plan (HCHP), a major HMO in Boston, developed an "AIDS Team" to focus on meeting the unique needs of this population. This AIDS Team provided support and consultation for the more than 100 primary care physicians in its staff model HMO. HCHP served several hundred HIV-infected persons at the time. The majority were homosexual men, and pediatric care was not yet a major issue. More than 90% of these patients were paying members of HCHP. The team approach provided both access to state-of-the-art care and cost containment.[20]

In the 1990s, the HIV epidemic shifted to Medicaid and Medicare recipients, especially in the North and Southeast United States. As the HIV epidemic in children began to take shape, many children covered by traditional Medicaid plans were able to obtain direct access to HIV specialty care under this fee-for-service arrangement. Primary care providers who had little experience or expertise in HIV care were eager to have specialists handle the lion's share of the care for children with HIV infection. Due to the severity of the symptoms experienced by pediatric HIV patients during the early part of the epidemic, visits to specialists were frequent, necessitating HIV care specialists to additionally function as primary care providers for these children.

Advances in the treatment of HIV infection throughout the 1990s have resulted in increased life expectancy for children with perinatally acquired infection. As most programs have transitioned to a chronic illness model for the treatment of pediatric HIV infection, many families have grown accustomed to and comfortable with the long-term relationship they have established with their child's HIV care provider.

The relative health that many of these children experience today has left them ineligible for disability benefits. This situation, coupled with the rising cost and complexity of HIV management and monitoring, makes them targets for enrollment into managed care plans. As the costs for care of persons with HIV disease rise dramatically, it is clear that states are eager to transition this population into managed care. The only remaining questions in each state are when this transition will occur and what form it will take.[21] Because each state sets its own reimbursement rate, rates and mechanisms for reimbursement vary nationwide. Additionally, not all managed care organizations in each state participate in Medicaid managed care.

Government officials, health care providers, and consumers have concerns about the impact of children with HIV receiving coverage through managed care plans. In New York, evaluation of the potential role of "Special Needs Plans" in providing services to women and children with HIV infection is being studied. The goal is for these managed care companies to provide comprehensive, coordinated services to people living with HIV. Focus groups of adults with HIV and women with HIV who have infected children revealed that the physician was viewed as the most important aspect of care for patients with HIV infection. In fact, many cited the loss of access to their preferred physician provider as their primary concern in a managed care system. Additionally, it was learned that most of the focus group participants had an overall negative opinion of managed care.[22,23]

As might be expected, studies have shown that costs for patients with undetectable viral load are less than those for patients with higher viral loads.[24] Within a Medicaid managed care system, these patients may consume fewer traditional resources, such as hospital or emergency care. However, programs with alternate funding through resources like the Ryan White CARE Act may bear the brunt of the cost of keeping viral loads low through extensive work with patient adherence issues and intensive nursing and social service intervention. Although skepticism toward the managed care approach remains, the full impact of a transition to Medicaid managed care has yet to be realized. There is, however, some evidence suggesting a favorable effect for adults and children with HIV infection.

A successful Kaiser Permanente initiative illustrates the possible benefit of an integrated service model. At the Kaiser Permanente Medical Center in Santa Rosa, a multidisciplinary team for managing HIV according to a clinical path was established within a staff model HMO. In comparison to other Kaiser sites where no such program was in place, team-managed patients received more nursing, nutritional, and social service intervention than the comparison group. The team-managed group also utilized fewer emergency services and experienced a significant decrease in both number of hospital admissions and length of stay. Overall, this team approach was found to have a significant impact on resource use and patient status.[25]

It is clear those children with HIV infection and their families will continue to utilize services and health care resources at relatively high levels. With that in mind, primary care pediatricians and HIV specialty providers must find new ways to partner in-service delivery to facilitate care for this population. The form that this partnership takes must consider the unique demographics and geographic circumstances of the population being served.

Because of the unique characteristics of its state, Wisconsin developed the HIV Primary Care Support Network, a decentralized program for the care of children and families with HIV infection. This system took into account not only the relatively low prevalence of HIV in children and the size of the state but also the need to collect data to determine the effectiveness of the model. The goal of this program of centralized specialists working with primary care providers throughout the state is to ensure uniform quality of care regardless of geographic location. Children are able to obtain services with a managed care system through their primary care providers. These providers receive support via direct referral to specialists and through education and support from specialists who may not be as geographically accessible. Standards of care are supplied to practitioners via state-published materials, and centralized data collection allows for quality assurance, ongoing feedback, and education.[26]

The input of client groups, physicians, public health officials, and insurers is critical to the formulation of an integrated managed program of HIV services.[27] Traditional walls of resistance between these stakeholders must be removed so that, working collaboratively, these groups can formulate a comprehensive plan for addressing the ongoing needs of children and families living with HIV infection who may receive services within a managed care system that may include same-site care for multiple family members.

KEY COMPONENTS OF A MANAGED CARE DELIVERY SYSTEM OF HIV-INFECTED CHILDREN

Providing timely, medically necessary services that meet the health care needs of children living with HIV/AIDS is dependent on a comprehensive, integrated managed care delivery system. Some of the key components of an integrated managed care delivery system include a comprehensive provider network, case management services, member services tailored to address the specific needs of the population, and a well-defined benefits package.

Traditionally, MCOs include primary care providers, typically pediatricians, internists, general and family practitioners, and physician specialists as well as nonphysician practitioners, and ancillary providers and services. In a regular managed care system, patients are enrolled with a primary care provider who, acting as a gatekeeper, provides primary medical care and coordinates all other health care needs of the enrollees. Such coordination includes making referrals to specialists when needed. That requires the patient to contact the primary care provider for authorization before accessing specialty care. Primary care providers are usually not the primary caregiver for treating HIV/AIDS.

As previously discussed, it is essential that providers who treat children with HIV disease have experience and expertise in treating the disease. Most primary care providers are not able or willing to take on this responsibility. The number of patients with HIV disease in a typical community practice may be too few to provide the primary care provider with the degree of hands-on experience to treat and manage these patients. Access to expert specialists becomes essential. Patients with HIV disease frequently need to see these specialists on an ongoing basis, often on an urgent basis due to changes of health status, such as mitigating factors that have an impact on their overall health status. There are various ways to achieve the desired access in a managed care system: (1) allow specialists to function as primary care providers, and (2) have procedures for patient self-referral or direct access to specialty care.

Specialists may take on the role of primary care provider, including all of the gatekeeper/health care coordination functions. This is usually determined through the contracting and credentialing process with the managed care entity. Specialists must be able and willing to provide not only their specialty services for the disease but also their primary care services in addition to coordinating all other services the patient may need. Few specialists may be willing to do so.

Direct access to specialty care is implemented more frequently in a managed care system. MCOs have been developing a variety of methods to recognize the need for direct access. These are summarized below.

1. The patient chooses a primary care provider who will continue to provide primary care services but may authorize long-term referrals for treatment and medical management. For example, a referral, which usually is time limited, may be extended for long periods of time for 6 or 12 months before the patient has to return to the primary care provider's office for additional referral authorization. In essence, the patient can go to the specialist as frequently as needed during that time period without the need for separate authorizations.
2. The MCO may authorize direct access to an HIV/AIDS specialist without the need to obtain any referrals from the primary care provider. The specialist and primary care provider will need to communicate with each other on updates of the patient's medical status and health care needs.

Case management is frequently used for persons with HIV disease because MCOs consider these patients to be high-risk and high-cost from the time that they are diagnosed. Case management is not interchangeable with managed care. Rather, case management is a process that is one component of the managed care strategy. The Commission for Case

Manager Certification defines case management as a collaborative process that assesses, plans, implements, coordinates, monitors, and evaluates the options and services required to meet the health needs of individual patients. Case management occurs across a continuum of care to address the ongoing needs of children infected with HIV and their families.[28] The MCO generally takes the lead in developing a case management plan with the patient, primary care provider, specialists where appropriate, and family or guardians. Many states have agencies that provide protective services for children. These state agencies need to collaborate closely with the MCO case management system.

The case manager has four major areas of activity: medical, financial, behavioral/motivational, and vocational. The physician has most contact with the case manager in the medical context. The case manager may contact the physician to confirm the diagnosis, learn about the treatment plan, and follow the child's progress. The case manager can coordinate with social services or Ryan White CARE Act agencies to procure social services for the child and the family. He or she can also help with adherence by asking if the child is taking the medication as prescribed and, if not, reinforcing the need for adherence.[28]

Practitioners should ensure that adequate MCO services are available to patients. MCO members must have access to a member services unit available to respond to questions, concerns, and complaints, to explain health services, to discuss their rights and responsibilities under the managed care program they are enrolled in, and to perform certain administrative functions such as assisting members with primary care provider selection or changes. The individuals staffing this unit are not the same individuals providing case management services. They must be culturally sensitive and diverse and must be able to assist members with language barriers or communication-affecting conditions. Staff must include, at a minimum, individuals who speak English and Spanish and must be able to accommodate quickly other languages spoken by the MCO's membership. Critical to this function is a member services unit consisting of individuals who are very knowledgeable in the benefits available to each member who contacts them as well as MCO procedures so that correct information is provided to ensure that members receive proper and timely services.

The benefits package must be clearly delineated and communicated to all enrollees and providers by MCO staff. MCOs must (1) clearly understand what medical services are included in the benefits package and available to the enrollee; (2) clearly communicate how the services can be delivered, including the referral processes to be followed; and (3) clearly communicate any other policies and procedures that can help (or hinder access if not followed) the enrollee in obtaining services and assist the provider in delivering services. Since all MCO plans differ, it is important for the physician to know what each plan provides and how to guide his or her patients to the care that they need.

Issues related to experimental treatment may come up in discussions with patients. It is not unusual for patients with HIV disease or their families to inquire about clinical trials. MCOs allow participation in clinical trials. However, MCO payment for experimental treatment is another matter. From the MCO medical director's perspective, denying access to a treatment or therapy because it is considered experimental or investigational is complicated. In general, the medical director will most likely look at it from several aspects. The medical director will review the proposed plan of treatment to determine whether the treatment protocol states implicitly or explicitly that it is experimental. The consent form will be reviewed to determine whether the procedure is considered to be experimental or investigational. The number of academic or tertiary care centers affiliated with a medical school in the United States performing the procedure will be considered. Published papers may also be reviewed. The medical director will need to consider that what appears to be "cutting edge" in a community hospital or practice may already be the standard of care in academic or specialty centers or practices. Finally, the medical director will consider the patient's chances of surviving the procedure or treatment and the potential for a reasonably good quality of life or a positive impact on the patient's life, lifestyle, or career. The MCOs are aware of multimillion-dollar lawsuits that have been filed, won by the plaintiff, and the legal appeals process regarding access to experimental treatments or procedures.[29]

A MODEL FOR PHYSICIAN INPUT INTO MEDICAID MANAGED CARE OF HIV INFECTION

Pediatricians and other HIV providers can be actively involved in the development, implementation, evaluation, and modification of Medicaid managed care in their state. In New Jersey, a model was established in which state agencies are working with HIV providers as Medicaid managed care is starting to enroll persons with HIV disease. In New Jersey, the Medicaid program is administered by the Department of Human Services (DHS). MCOs in New Jersey are regulated by both the Department of Health and Senior Services (DHSS) and the Department of Insurance and Banking. Both DHS and DHSS have been working closely together and working closely with the providers and the MCOs to ensure continuity of care for patients, provider access to the MCO panels, and quality of care. The working group includes both a pediatric HIV specialist and a pediatric adolescent specialist in addition to adult providers.

Collaboration between the physicians, state agencies, and the MCOs is particularly important for Medicaid patients. The Medicaid population is very diverse, with a broad range of medical and social needs as well as diverse cultural differences. These children range from low-income, relatively healthy to those who are very ill with multiple, complex health care and social service needs. Consequently, a managed care program must be able to incorporate the needs of all of the various populations covered under the Medicaid program. Input from the stakeholders, that is, consumers, consumer advocates, providers of service, the managed care industry, legislators, and state agency representatives, is important to understanding the needs of the individuals who will be enrolled in managed care and the kinds of program components that need to be included in the overall program design.

Listening to these groups individually is the first step in the process. Each of the groups must have an opportunity to speak freely about their specific issues and concerns. Separate meetings were held with providers, state agencies, and the MCOs to identify the concerns of each of these entities with the Medicaid managed care contract for persons with HIV disease. This allowed stakeholders to express and discuss their concerns. Their input into the process of designing a comprehensive managed care program was invaluable.

The second step in the process is bringing the stakeholders together to communicate with each other, to hear and understand each other's perspectives. A round table meeting was held with providers, representatives from DHS, representatives from DHSS, and all six Medicaid managed care organizations. Medicaid program staff facilitated the meeting. There were no set agenda and no formal presentations. It was a discussion among the stakeholders of issues related to continuity of care, provider enrollment in the MCOs, quality of care, communication, access to diagnostic testing, and access to antiretroviral agents. This conversation answered a lot of questions that all the stakeholders had. For example, providers could learn from the MCOs about the enrollment process. Many good ideas were discussed regarding implementation of the initial Medicaid managed care contract and suggestions for the next contract. The desired outcome is to obtain at least a consensus of the managed care requirements that best meet the needs of the various Medicaid populations.

To minimize potential unforeseen difficulties as HIV infected children are transitioned into Medicaid managed care, implementation should be phased in over a period of time. Simultaneous conversion of thousands of people from fee-for-service Medicaid to the managed care program is very difficult to coordinate and manage properly. Phasing in a new program allows for an orderly process, evaluation of the transition, changes to the transition process if difficulties are identified, and the ability to reach as many people on an individual basis as possible to allow them enough time to choose an MCO that best meets their needs.

Continuous input from the physicians and other stakeholders is essential. Each group can provide feedback on the progress of the program and problems encountered and make recommendations for improvement. This includes making recommendations for future modification of the Medicaid managed care program. State agencies can bring these groups together periodically for discussions of the implementation, impact, and ways to improve the program. The groups can also be encouraged to communicate with each other for ongoing discussions of how to best achieve desired goals and outcomes for the enrollees. In all cases, it is essential that the various stakeholders remember that they are working together to serve the Medicaid beneficiaries.

CONCLUSION

Managed care has indelibly altered the landscape of medical insurance and the practice of medicine. Although much of the popular media emphasizes the evils of managed care, the potential benefits may be just as significant. Managed care stresses efficiency and cost accountability. As a result, the industry has already stemmed the explosive growth in health care costs that were seen as a threat to the national economy in the 1970s and beyond. MCOs encourage preventive care and a comprehensive approach to the patient through primary care. Finally, managed care has made monitoring and continuous quality improvement not just an accessory but rather a central component of both office-based and hospital practice. As the industry and quality measurement techniques mature, we as physicians may expect MCOs to make strong contributions to health care access, delivery, and practice standards, all of which promote improved care for our patients.

Managed care is clearly here to stay. While practically all practitioners have little choice but to deal with MCOs, astute practitioners will learn what managed care expects from them and their practice, as well as what managed care has to offer. The pediatric HIV physician contemplating association with an MCO has many decisions to make: whether the HIV practitioner should serve as both primary care provider and specialist, the monthly per-patient fees for capitation, FFS discounts, accessibility to expensive medications, reimbursement for experimental protocols, and dozens of other issues that affect both the patient and a financially sound practice. A realistic understanding of resources, costs, and expectations, coupled with forthright communication, are the keys to a successful negotiation. Furthermore, an understanding of the regulations guiding MCOs, on both federal and state levels, may prove helpful in comprehending the demands placed on managed care and how those demands translate into burdens the MCO places on providers.

What is the future of managed care? The answer is not available without clairvoyance, but the success of any prediction will be contingent on the future of American medicine itself. Issues such as universal health care insurance, increasing enrollee copayments into federal medical programs, the growing concept of health care as a right, and the physician oversupply and maldistribution will all affect where our system is going. Considering the revolution that has occurred in health financing, one may develop the impression that MCOs are driving forces in changes that have occurred in reimbursements and health care delivery. In reality, managed care and its growth is a *reaction* to changing health care priorities, most importantly including, but not limited to, costs.

Hopefully, managed care will continue to respond to the needs and desires of not only the health care consumer population but of providers as well. The model of managed care for Medicaid recipients in New Jersey is a good example of the ability of providers to work with and influence managed care. It is important to learn how to work with MCOs and how to work within the system to guide patients to the care and treatment that they need.

REFERENCES

1. American Medical Association, Department of Medical Review: Principles of Managed Care: A Summary of American Medical Association Policy. Chicago, American Medical Association, 1994, p 1.
2. Wagner ER: Types of managed care organizations. In Kongstevdt P (ed): The Managed Health Care Handbook, 3rd ed. Gaithersburg, MD, Aspen Publishers, 1996, pp 33–45.
3. The Health Insurance Association of America: The fundamentals of managed care: Its history, current status, and future. Washington, DC, HIAA, 1991;4:3.
4. Starr P: Escape from the corporation, 1900–1930. In The Social Transformation of American Medicine. New York, Basic Books, 1982, pp 198–234.
5. American Academy of Pediatrics Committee on Children with Disabilities: Managed care and children with special health care needs: A subject review (RE9814). Pediatrics 1998;102:657–660.
6. Health Care Financing Administration Letter to State Medicaid Directors. October 6, 1999.
7. Kaiser Commission on the Future of Medicaid: Medicaid's Role for Persons with HIV/AIDS. Washington, DC, Henry J Kaiser Foundation, 1996.
8. Department of Health and Human Services: Fact Sheet: Medicaid and Acquired Immune Deficiency Syndrome (AIDS) and Human Immunodeficiency Virus (HIV). Washington, DC, DHHS, 2000.
9. O'Kane ME: External accreditation of managed care plans. In Kongstevdt P (ed): The Managed Health Care Handbook, 3rd ed. Gaithersburg, MD, Aspen Publishers, 1996, pp 593–607.
10. Siren PB, Laffel GL: Quality management in managed care. In Kongstevdt P (ed): The Managed Health Care Handbook, 3rd ed. Gaithersburg, MD, Aspen Publishers, 1996, pp 402–425.
11. Kongstevdt PR: Compensation of primary care physicians in open panel plans. In Kongstevdt P (ed): The Managed Health Care Handbook, 3rd ed. Gaithersburg, MD, Aspen Publishers, 1996, pp 120–146.

12. Boland P: Making Managed Health Care Work: A Practical Guide to Strategies and Solutions. Gaithersburg, MD, Aspen Publishers, 1993.
13. Kongstvedt PR: Primary care in open panel plans. In Kongstevdt P (ed): The Managed Health Care Handbook, 3rd ed. Gaithersburg, MD, Aspen Publishers, 1996, pp 104–119.
14. Kongstevdt PR: Using data in medical management. In Kongstevdt P (ed): The Managed Health Care Handbook, 3rd ed. Gaithersburg, MD, Aspen Publishers, 1996, pp 440–454.
15. Green J, Whitfield N: Report cards on cardiac surgeons: Assessing New York State's approach. N Engl J Med 1995;332:1229–1232.
16. New Jersey Administrative Code 8:38–8.4–8.5 Health Maintenance Organizations.
17. Appleby C: How managed care affects the malpractice liability problem. Managed Care Mag 1996;5:1–5.
18. Coleman DL: Will health plans keep their ERISA shield? Managed Care Mag 1997;186:25–31.
19. Martino MD, Tovo P, Balducci M, et al: Reduction in mortality with availability of antiretroviral therapy for children with perinatal HIV-1 infection. JAMA 2000;284:190–197.
20. Gallagher DM: The era of managed care, the struggle of cost containment, and compassionate, effective care of persons with HIV/AIDS. Nurs Clin North Am 1999;34:227–235.
21. Master RM: Managed HIV care. State Health Watch 1995;2:8.
22. Feldman I, Cruz H, DeLorenzo J, et al: Developing a managed care delivery system in New York State for Medicaid recipients with HIV. Am J Managed Care 1999;5:1457–1465.
23. Abramowitz S, Obten N: Attitudes toward managed care by people with HIV/AIDS. Abstract Book/Assoc Health Services Res 1998;1915:8–9.
24. New study showed average costs of care for HIV in managed care were lower for patients with undetectable viral loads [news article]. J Assoc Nurses AIDS Care 1999;10:87–88.
25. Le CT, Winter TD, Boyd KJ, et al: Experience with a managed care approach to HIV infection effectiveness of an interdisciplinary team. Am J Managed Care 1998;4:647–657.
26. Havens PL, Cuene BE, Waters D, et al: Structure of a primary care support system to coordinate comprehensive care for children and families infected/affected by human immunodeficiency virus in a managed care environment. Pediatr Infect Dis J 1997;16:211–216.
27. Singer B, Gamliel S, Conviser R: Developing a managed care delivery system for people with HIV/AIDS. Am J Managed Care 1999;5:1443–1447.
28. Mullahy CM: Case management and managed care. In Kongstevdt P (ed): The Managed Health Care Handbook, 3rd ed. Gaithersburg, MD, Aspen Publishers, 1996, pp 274–300.
29. Quinn C: Avoiding "bad faith" denials of medical claims. Managed Care Mag 1997;6:79–83.

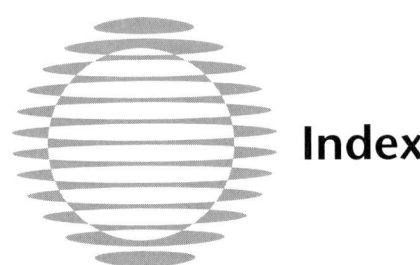

Index

Note: Page numbers followed by f refer to figures; page numbers followed by t refer to tables.

A

Abacavir
 for initiation of antiretroviral therapy, 131t
 in pregnancy, 79
 prophylactic, dosage of, 123, 124t
Abdomen, pain in, 293–294, 293t
Abuse
 legal guardianship in, 388t
 physical, parental substance abuse and, 374
 substance. *See* Substance abuse.
Academic achievement, HIV infection and, 233
Acanthamoeba infection, cutaneous manifestations of, 279, 279f
ACCH (Association for the Care of Children's Health), and elements of family-centered nursing care, 399t
Acidosis, lactic, antiretroviral therapy and, 94
Acquired immunodeficiency syndrome (AIDS)
 clinical case definition of, 18, 18t
 diagnosis of, trends in, 16t
 mortality from, trends in, 16t
 progression to
  epidemiology of, 12t–13t
  plasma HIV-1 RNA and, 130–131, 132t–133t
  pregnancy and, 73–74
  timing of HIV infection and, 34–36, 35f–36f
 wasting in, 297–298
 with cardiovascular disease, 296
Acrodermatitis enteropathica, 285, 285f
ACTG 076. *See* AIDS Clinical Trials Group (ACTG) 076.
Acyclovir
 for herpes virus infection, oral, 253
 for varicella zoster virus infection, 177
 in pregnancy, 95
Adaptive function, HIV infection and, 233–234
ADC(s). *See* AIDS-defining condition(s).
ADCC (antibody-dependent cellular cytotoxicity), 59–61
Adenovirus vector, for HIV vaccine, 145, 145t

ADHD (attention deficit hyperactivity disorder), 383–384
Adherence
 to antiretroviral therapy, 133–134, 368
  in adolescents, 378
 to plan of care, 409–410, 409t
Adolescent(s), psychosocial issues in, 377–379
Adoption, 389t–390t
Adulthood, transition to, psychosocial issues during, 379, 380t–381t
Advocacy, by nurses, 414
Age, and assessment of neurocognitive function, 237
AIDS. *See* Acquired immunodeficiency syndrome (AIDS).
AIDS Clinical Trials Group (ACTG) 076
 study of prophylactic zidovudine by, 120
 study of viral load as risk factor for HIV transmission by, 42
AIDS-defining condition(s)
 in children *vs.* adults, 157t, 158
 percentage of HIV-infected children with, 159t
AIDS Team, in Harvard Community Health Plan, 428
Airway, upper, obstruction of, 201
Albendazole, for microsporidiosis, 171t
Allergic reaction(s), to drugs, cutaneous manifestations of, 284
Alopecia areata, 282
Alternative therapy, 408
Alveoli, diffuse damage to, 200–201
Amniocentesis, HIV infection and, 82, 96–97
AMP. *See* Amprenavir.
Amphotericin B
 for cryptococcosis, 170t
 for *Penicillium marneffei* infection, 172
Amplicor test, 174
Amprenavir
 for initiation of antiretroviral therapy, 131t
 in pregnancy, 81
 prophylactic, dosage of, 123, 124t
Analgesic(s), 354t

Anemia, 323–325, 324t
 etiology of, 324–325, 324t
 incidence of, 323
 significance of, 323–324
 treatment of, 325
Aneurysm(s), incidence of, 311
Angiomatosis, bacillary, 276
 vs. Kaposi sarcoma, 343
Angular cheilitis, in oral candidiasis, 251, 252f
Anorexia, 291–292
Antibodies
 anti-HIV
  intravenous immunoglobulin containing, 147
  monoclonal, for immune-based therapy, 147–148
 HIV-specific, production of, 60–61
Antibody-dependent cellular cytotoxicity (ADCC), 59–61
Antifungal drug(s), for oropharyngeal candidiasis, 251–252
Antipyretic(s), use of, 369
Antiretroviral therapy
 access to, 427
 adherence to, 133–134
  in adolescents, 378
 administration of, via gastrostomy tube, 300
 and anemia, 324, 324t
 and gastrointestinal disorders, 293t
 and immune system reconstitution, 53, 62–64
 and lipodystrophy, 298–299
 and outcome of pregnancy, 89–90
 and plasma HIV-1 RNA levels, 132–134
 and pregnancy outcome, 9
 and psychotropic medications, 383, 385
 and quality of life, 356
 and transmission of HIV infection
  in nonbreastfeeding subjects, 36, 37t–38t, 39
  in pregnancy, 88
 animal models of, 118–119
 central nervous system effects of, 239–240
 choice of drugs for
  during pregnancy, 75

435

Antiretroviral therapy (Continued)
  in postexposure prophylaxis, 212–214, 215t, 218t
  compliance with, 368
  during pregnancy, 92–96
    and fetal toxicity, 93
    and maternal toxicity, 93
    goals of, 93
    initiation of, 92–93
  early use of, and preservation of immune function, 62
  highly active. See Highly active antiretroviral therapy.
  in children, toxicity of, 94–95
  initiation of, 127–129, 128t–129t
    choice of drug for, 130, 131t
    in infants, 127, 128t
    viral load and, 74–75
  limitations of, 139
  monitoring of viral load during, 130–135, 132t–133t
    plasma HIV-1 RNA levels for, 130–131, 132t–133t
  peripartum, 99
  prophylactic
    clinical experience with, 119–122, 122t
    dosage of, 123, 124t
    efficacy of, 13, 16
    for *Pneumocystis carinii* pneumonia, 13
    principles of, 117–118, 118f
    resistance to, 123
    unresolved issues in, 122–123
  resistance to
    assays for, 135t
    testing for, 111–112
  side effects of, 351
  toxicity of, 16
  with interleukin-2, and CD4+ cell count, 141, 142t, 143
Anxiety disorder(s), 385
Aortic root, dilation of, 311
Aphthous stomatitis, 253–254, 254f, 292t
Apoptosis, of lymphocytes, 56
Appeals, in managed care organizations, 425–426
Arrhythmia(s), 312, 312t–313t
Aspergillosis, 172
  cutaneous manifestations of, 278, 278f
  pulmonary, 197
Association for the Care of Children's Health (ACCH), and elements of family-centered nursing care, 399t
Atherosclerosis, incidence of, 311
Athletic program(s), infection control in, 209–210
Atopic dermatitis, 281
Attention, tests of, 239t
Attention deficit hyperactivity disorder (ADHD), 383–384
Attention deficits, 232–233
Autoantibodies, production of, hyperimmunoglobulinemia and, 60–61
Autoimmune hemolytic anemia, 324–325
Autonomic dysfunction, 311

Azithromycin
  for bacterial infection prophylaxis, 164
  for *Mycobacterium avium* complex, 173–174, 196
AZT. See Zidovudine.

B

B cells, pulmonary, HIV infection and, 193
B cell lymphoma, and cardiovascular disease, 314
Bacillary angiomatosis, 276
  vs. Kaposi sarcoma, 343
Bacillus Calmette-Guérin vaccine, for tuberculosis, 175
Bacterial infection(s), 162–165
  CD4+ cell count and, 161t
  cutaneous, 274–276, 276f
  epidemiology of, 162–163
  in children vs. adults, 157t
  neutrophil function and, 61
  percentage of HIV-infected children with, 159t
  prevention of, 163–165
  treatment of, 163–165
Bacterial pneumonia, 194–195
Barrier precaution(s), in delivery room, 211
Behavior, assessment of, 239t
Bile duct, obstruction of, 295
Biologic response modifier(s), for Kaposi sarcoma, 283
Birth weight, and perinatal HIV transmission, 45–46
Bites, transmission of HIV from, 207
Bleeding disorder(s), and dental procedures, 260
Blood
  peripheral, lymphocytes in, HIV infection and, 54, 56
  transmission of HIV infection by, in schools/sports, 208–210, 209t
Blood cells
  production of, factors affecting, 321, 322f
  suppression of, mechanism of, 321–323
Blood product(s), transmission of HIV infection by, epidemiology of, 6, 8
Blood transfusion(s), for anemia, 325
Body composition, assessment of, 297
Body fluids, transmission of HIV infection in, 205–206, 209–210
Bone marrow
  invasive disease of, 323
  suppression of
    drugs causing, 323
    mechanism of, 321–323
Brain
  imaging of
    functional, 235
    in neurocognitive dysfunction, 234–235
  non-Hodgkin's lymphoma in, 339
Breastfeeding, and HIV transmission, 7–8, 99
  intervention trials on, 39–41, 41f
  prevention of, 123
  timing of, 32–34, 34f

Bronchiectasis, 200
Bronchoalveolar lavage
  for tuberculosis, 196
  in *Pneumocystis carinii* pneumonia, 198
Burnout, in health care workers, prevention of, 412–414

C

Calcific vasculopathy, of central nervous system, 228–229
Calcification, cerebral, imaging of, 234
Calories, recommended daily allowance of, 296, 296t
Camp(s), for children with HIV infection, 379, 380t–381t
Canary pox vector, for HIV vaccine, 145, 145t
Cancer, 337–344. See also under specific type, e.g., Lymphoma.
Candidiasis, 167
  CD4+ cell count and, 161t
  cutaneous manifestations of, 276
  esophageal, 292
    in children vs. adults, 157t
    percentage of HIV-infected children with, 159t
    treatment of, 170t
  genital, management of, in pregnancy, 95
  oral, gingival erythema in, 255f
  oropharyngeal, 249–252, 251f–252f
    clinical features of, 250, 251f–252f
    diagnosis of, 250, 292t
    management of, 250–252
  pulmonary, 197
    percentage of HIV-infected children with, 159t
Capitation, 423
Cardiomyopathy
  dilated, incidence of, 308t
  zidovudine and, 316
Cardiovascular disease
  and abnormal cardiac growth, 307
  and autonomic dysfunction, 311
  and left ventricular dysfunction, 307–310, 307t–308t, 309f–310f
    diastolic, 310
    management of, 316
    systolic, 307–309, 307t–308t, 309f–310f
  and myocarditis, 310
  and pericardial effusion, 312, 314–315
  and pulmonary hypertension, 314–315
  congenital, 306
  cross-sectional studies of, 305t
  diagnosis of, 315
  highly active antiretroviral therapy and, 316–317
  management of, 316
  monitoring of, 315–316
  rapid progression of HIV infection and, 303, 306, 306f
  retrospective studies of, 304t
  risk factors for, 303
  with wasting, 308
Cardiovascular tumor(s), 314
Care plan(s), formulation of, 400

Caregiver(s)
  education of, about infection control, 402
  extended family as, 387, 391, 403
  foster, 387, 391, 403
  psychosocial issues of, 385–387, 388t–390t, 391
    and HIV-positive mothers, 386
    in late stage of illness, 387
    progression of illness and, 386–387, 388t–390t
  respite care for, 405–406
Caries, dental, 264, 265t, 266
  plaque and, 263, 263f
Case management, 382, 400
  role of primary care provider in, 368, 430–431
CCR5
  and non-Hodgkin lymphoma, 340–341
  as coreceptor for HIV entry, 144, 230
CD4+ cell count
  after highly active antiretroviral therapy, 62–64
  and bacterial infections, 161t
  and cytomegalovirus infection, 176
  and development of non-Hodgkin lymphoma, 338
  and initiation of antiretroviral therapy, 128–129, 128t–129t
  and opportunistic infections, 155, 160, 161t–162t
    in pregnancy, 82
  and plasma HIV-1 RNA levels, 133t
  and *Pneumocystis carinii* pneumonia, 198
    prevention of, 367
  and risk of pneumonia, 193, 193t
  and skin disorders, 271
  and use of varicella-zoster virus vaccine, 177
  and withdrawal of prophylaxis for opportunistic infections, 181
  during pregnancy, 88
  HIV infection and, 54, 55t, 56
  in long-term nonprogressors, 64
  interleukin-2 and, 141, 142t, 143
  maternal, and HIV transmission, 42–43, 43f
  neurocognitive dysfunction and, 235–236
  pregnancy and, 72–73
CD4+ cells
  HIV replication in, suppression of, CD8+ cells and, 59–60
  loss of, 56
  production of cytokines by, 58
  proliferation of, 58
  with restricted T cell receptor genes, expansion of, 60
CD4-IgG2, for immune-based therapy, 148, 148f
CD4+ molecule, soluble recombinant, research on, 140
CD8+ cell count, HIV infection and, 54, 55t, 56
CD8+ cells
  and replication of HIV, in CD4+ cells, 59–60
  cloning of, 57

CD8+ cells (*Continued*)
  with restricted T cell receptor genes, expansion of, 60
Cellulitis, staphylococcal, 275
Centers for Disease Control and Prevention
  classification of HIV infection by, 10, 14t–15t
  database on opportunistic infections of, 156, 157t
Central nervous system
  antiretroviral therapy and, 239–240
  calcific vasculopathy of, 228–229
  human immunodeficiency virus infection in, 227–230
    pathogenesis of, 229–230
    pathology of, 228–229
  non-Hodgkin lymphoma of, 339
  opportunistic infections and, 227–228
  tumors of, 228
Cerebral calcification, imaging of, 234
Cerebral toxoplasmosis, 179
Cerebrospinal fluid
  Epstein-Barr virus in, and non-Hodgkin lymphoma, 339
  HIV-1 RNA levels in, 134
  quinolinic acid levels in, and disease prognosis, 236–237
Cesarean delivery, 97–99
  and perinatal HIV transmission, 44–45
Cheilitis, angular, in oral candidiasis, 251, 252f
Chemokine(s), for immune-based therapy, 144
Chemokine receptors, in central nervous system toxicity, 229–230
Chemotherapy
  for Kaposi sarcoma, 283
  for non-Hodgkin lymphoma, 339
  supportive care during, 344
Child abuse
  legal guardianship in, 388t
  parental substance abuse and, 374
Child welfare agency(ies), guardianship by, 388t
Chlamydia infection(s), screening for, during pregnancy, 92
Cigarette smoking, and perinatal HIV transmission, 43
CKR5 mutation, and resistance to HIV infection, 206
Clade(s), 111
Clarithromycin, for *Mycobacterium avium* complex, 170t, 173–174, 196
Cleaning, for infection control, 219
Clindamycin, for toxoplasmosis, 171t
Clinical trial(s), 407–408
Clonidine, for attention deficit hyperactivity disorder, 384
c-myc oncogene, and non-Hodgkin lymphoma, 340–341
CNS. *See* Central nervous system.
Coccidioidomycosis, 169, 172
Cognitive dysfunction. *See* Neurocognitive dysfunction.
Colitis, gastrointestinal bleeding in, 295
Community resource(s), access to, 410–411
Compensation program(s), for physician reimbursement, 423–424

Complementary therapy, 408
Compliance. *See* Adherence.
Computed tomography, in neurocognitive dysfunction, 234–235
Condylomata acuminata, 274
Confidentiality, and nursing care, 405
Congenital disorder(s), zidovudine and, 76
Conscious sedation, 355
Continuing education, for nurses, 412
Continuity of care, 407
Corticosteroid(s)
  for *Pneumocystis carinii* pneumonia, 166, 198–199
  for thrombocytopenia, 327
Counseling
  posttest, 71
  pretest, components of, 70–71
Credentialing, in managed care organizations, 424
CRIES Scale, 352t
Crixivan. *See* Indinavir.
Cryotherapy
  for human papillomavirus infection, 274
  for molluscum contagiosum, 273
Cryptococcosis, 167, 169, 169t
  cutaneous manifestations of, 277–278
  prevention of, 169, 169t
  pulmonary, 197
  treatment of, 169, 170t
Cryptosporidiosis, 179–180
  CD4+ cell count and, 161t
  percentage of HIV-infected children with, 159t
  treatment of, 171t
CSF. *See* Cerebrospinal fluid.
CT. *See* Computed tomography.
Culture, and nursing care, 404, 411–412
Custody, of children, after death of HIV-positive parents, 386–387, 388t–390t, 406
CXCR4, as coreceptor for HIV entry, 144
Cyclosporine, for immune-based therapy, 149
Cytokines
  and suppression of hematopoiesis, 323
  for immune-based therapy, 140–144, 142t. *See also specific type, e.g.,* Interleukin-2.
  production of, 58–59
Cytomegalovirus infection
  and myocarditis, 310
  and pneumonia, 197
  CD4+ cell count and, 161t
  clinical features of, 175–176
  cutaneous manifestations of, 274
  epidemiology of, 175–176
  in children *vs.* adults, 157t
  management of, in pregnancy, 95
  oral ulcers in, 254
  percentage of HIV-infected children with, 159t
  prevention of, 168t, 176–177
  transmission of, perinatal, 176
  treatment of, 171t, 176–177
Cytomegalovirus retinitis, CD4+ cell count and, 161t

D

d4T. *See* Stavudine.
Dapsone, for *Pneumocystis carinii* pneumonia, 199
Day care center(s), infection control in, 218–220, 220t
ddC. *See* Zalcitabine.
ddI. *See* Didanosine.
Death/dying
  discussion of, 356, 406
  nursing care before, 412
Delavirdine, in pregnancy, 81
Delirium, 384–385
Delivery
  cesarean, 97–99
  mode of, and perinatal HIV transmission, 44–45
Delivery room, barrier precautions in, 211
Dementia, 384
  and glucose metabolism, 235
Demodicidosis, 279, 279f–280f
Dental care, 266, 365
Dental caries, 264, 265t, 266
  plaque and, 263, 263f
Dental procedure(s), thrombocytopenia and, 260
Dermatitis
  atopic, 281
  seborrheic, 280
Dermatophytosis, 277, 277f
Dextroamphetamine, dosage of, 384
Diabetes, protease inhibitors and, 94
Diarrhea, 293t, 294
  cryptosporidiosis and, 179
  epidemiology of, in developing countries, 22
  transmission of, prevention of, 221
Didanosine
  and transmission of HIV infection, in nonbreastfeeding subjects, 37t, 39
  for initiation of antiretroviral therapy, 131t
  in pregnancy, 77
  prophylactic, dosage of, 123, 124t
Dimorphic fungal infection(s), 169, 172
Disclosure, 209, 222, 355–356, 368
  and primary care, 368
  in school-age children, 375–377, 376t
  nurse's role in, 403–404
  to school personnel, 377
  to sexual partners, by adolescents, 377
Discounted fee for service reimbursement, 423
Disease state management program(s) (DSMPs), 422
Disinfectant(s), 219
Disseminated *Mycobacterium avium* complex
  CD4+ cell count and, 161t
  clinical features of, 173
  epidemiology of, 173
  percentage of HIV-infected children with, 159t
  prevention of, 173–174
  treatment of, 173–174
DNA polymerase chain reaction, 107t, 108–109
DNA vaccine(s), 145t, 146
Do Not Resuscitate (DNR) orders, 356

Drug abuse. *See* Substance abuse.
Drug reaction(s), cutaneous manifestations of, 284
Drug resistance assay(s), recommendations for, 135t
DSMP(s) (disease state management programs), 422
Dying. *See* Death/dying.
Dysphagia, 292–293
Dysrhythmia(s), 312–313

E

EBV infection. *See* Epstein-Barr virus infection.
Echocardiography, diagnostic uses of, 315
Education
  continuing, for nurses, 412
  of colleagues, 413
Efavirenz
  in pregnancy, 81, 93
  prophylactic, dosage of, 123, 124t
Electrocardiogram, abnormal, 312, 312t–313t
Electrocardiography, diagnostic uses of, 315
Emergency room, infection control in, 211
Encephalopathy
  and dementia, 384
  and neurocognitive dysfunction, 230–231
  percentage of HIV-infected children with, 159t
  with wasting, in children *vs.* adults, 157t
End-of-life care, 356–357. *See also* Palliative care.
Energy, expenditure of, wasting and, 297
Enteral nutrition, 299–300
Enzyme innumoassay(s), 107–108, 107t
Eosinophilic folliculitis, 280–281
Epivir. *See* Lamivudine.
EPO(s) (exclusive provider organizations), 422
Epstein-Barr virus infection
  and hairy leukoplakia, 257–258, 258f, 274, 275f
  and leiomyoma, 341
  and non-Hodgkin lymphoma, 339, 341
  cutaneous manifestations of, 274, 275f
  oral manifestations of, 259–260
Eruptive dysplastic nevi, 282–283
Erythropoietin, for anemia, 325
Esophageal candidiasis, 167
  in children *vs.* adults, 157t
  percentage of HIV-infected children with, 159t
  treatment of, 170t
Esophagitis, treatment of, 292–293
Ethambutol, for disseminated *Mycobacterium avium* complex, 170t
European Mode of Delivery Collaborative Study, 45
Exclusive provider organization(s) (EPOs), 422
Experimental therapy, *vs.* standard of care, 407–408

Expressive language, HIV infection and, 232
Extended family, as caregivers, 387, 391, 403
Eye(s), examination of, by primary care provider, 365
Eye protection, use of, 219

F

Fair Hearing Process, of Medicaid, 426
Family(ies)
  assessment of, role of nurse in, 402–403
  education of, role of nurse in, 402
  extended, as caregivers, 387, 391, 403
  impact of chronic illness on, 398
  psychosocial issues of, 385–387, 388t–390t, 391. *See also* Psychosocial issue(s).
Family-centered nursing care, 398–399, 399t
Fat, malabsorption of, and diarrhea, 294
Father(s), psychosocial issues of, 387
Fee for service reimbursement, 423
Fetus
  assessment of, 97
  toxicity to, from antiretroviral therapy, 93
Fever, management of, 369
FLACC Behavioral Scale, 352t
Fluconazole
  for candidiasis, 167
  for cryptococcosis, 169, 170t
Folliculitis
  eosinophilic, 280–281
  staphylococcal, 275
Foscarnet, for cytomegalovirus retinitis, 171t
Foster caregiver(s), 387, 391, 403
Functional brain imaging, 235
Fungal infection(s), 165–172, 168t–171t. *See also specific type, e.g., Pneumocystis carinii* pneumonia.
  CD4+ cell count and, 162t
  diagnosis of, using saliva, 262
  dimorphic, 169, 172
  of skin, 276–278, 277f–278f
  prevention of, 168t
  pulmonary, 197–199

G

Ganciclovir
  for cytomegalovirus infections, 176
  for cytomegalovirus retinitis, 171t
Gastritis, infectious, 294
Gastrointestinal disorder(s), 291–295, 292t–293t
  abdominal pain in, 293–294, 293t
  and nutrition, 295–300, 296t–297t. *See also* Nutrition.
  anorexia in, 291–292
  antiretroviral therapy and, 293t
  bleeding in, 294–295
  diarrhea in, 293t, 294

Gastrointestinal disorder(s)
  dysphagia in, 292–293
  hepatitis in, 295
  jaundice in, 295
  nausea/vomiting in, 293t, 294
  odynophagia in, 292–293
Gastrointestinal infection(s), prevention of, 221
Gastrostomy tube(s)
  for feeding, 299–300
  for medication administration, 409
GCSF (granulocyte colony-stimulating factor), for immune-based therapy, 144
Gen-Probe test, 174
Genital lesion(s)
  from human papillomavirus, 274, 343
  in candidiasis, management of, in pregnancy, 95
Genitourinary function, evaluation of, 365
Gingivitis, 262–263
  thrombocytopenia and, 260f
  ulcerative, necrotizing, 256–257
Gingivitis index, 263
Gingivostomatitis, herpetic, 252
Glossitis, herpetic, 253
Gloves, proper use of, 219
Glucose, metabolism of, dementia and, 235
Glucose-6-phosphate dehydrogenase, deficiency of, and anemia, 325
GM-CSF (granulocyte-macrophage colony-stimulating factor)
  for immune-based therapy, 144
  for neutropenia, 328–329
Gonorrhea, screening for, during pregnancy, 92
Government resource(s), access to, 410–411
Gown(s), use of, 219
Granulocyte colony-stimulating factor (GCSF), for immune-based therapy, 144
Granulocyte-macrophage colony-stimulating factor (GM-CSF)
  for immune-based therapy, 144
  for leukopenia, 328–329
Granuloma annulare, 282
Grievance procedure(s), in managed care organizations, 425–426
Growth, assessment of, 362, 364
  in children/adolescents, 297, 297t
  in infants, 296–297, 296t
Growth factor(s), for immune-based therapy, 144
Growth failure, progression of HIV infection and, 296
Growth retardation, HIV infection and, in developing countries, 19–20
Guardianship, 388t–389t
Guthrie card(s), 111

H

HAART. See Highly active antiretroviral therapy.
Hairy leukoplakia, 257–258, 258f, 274, 275f

Handwashing, 218–219
Harvard Community Health Plan, AIDS Team in, 428
Health care, continuity of, 407
Health Care Financing Administration (HCFA), criteria of, for expertise in care of HIV patients, 426–427
Health care worker(s)
  as liaisons to schools, 377, 405
  burnout in, prevention of, 412–414
  education of colleagues by, 413
  fears of, 411
  postexposure prophylaxis for, 211–216, 213f–214f, 215t. See also Postexposure prophylaxis, occupational.
  transmission of HIV infection by, 208
Health insurance
  indemnification, vs. managed care, 419–420
  types of, 421
Health maintenance organization(s) (HMOs), 421. See also Managed care.
Heart. See also entries under Cardiovascular.
  growth of, abnormal, 307
Heck's disease, 258
Height, serial measurement of, 297, 297t, 362, 364
Hematopoiesis, suppression of
  cytokines and, 323
  mechanism of, 321–323
Hematopoietic precursor cells, direct infection of, 322–323
Hemolytic anemia, autoimmune, 324–325
Hepatitis, 295
  management of, in pregnancy, 96
  screening for, in pregnancy, 92
  transmission of, prevention of, 221
Hepatitis B, prevention of, 168t
Hepatitis C, 178
Herpes simplex virus infection
  chronic, in children vs. adults, 157t
  cutaneous, 272, 272f
  oral, 252–253, 253f
Herpes virus infection
  management of, during pregnancy, 95–96
  screening for, during pregnancy, 91
Herpes zoster virus infection
  CD4+ cell count and, 161t
  oral ulcers in, 255
Highly active antiretroviral therapy
  and cardiovascular disease, 316–317
  and incidence of opportunistic infections, 156, 158, 160t
  and interactions with other drugs, 362
  and neurocognitive function, 66
  and reconstitution of immune function, 62–64
  duration of, before discontinuation of opportunistic infection prophylaxis, 181–182
Histoplasmosis
  cutaneous manifestations of, 277
  disseminated, 172
  oral ulcers in, 255
  prevention of, 169t
  treatment of, 170t

HIV. See Human immunodeficiency virus.
HIV envelope protein, for vaccines, 145t, 146–147
HIV gp 160, for vaccines, 145t, 146
HIV infection. See Human immunodeficiency virus infection.
HIV intravenous immunoglobulin (HIVIg), prophylactic, 121
HIV Primary Care Support Network, 429–430
HIV-related symptom(s), progression to, epidemiology of, 12t–13t
Hivid. See Zalcitabine.
HIVIg (HIV intravenous immunoglobulin), prophylactic, 121
HIVNEt trial, 40
HMO(s) (health maintenance organizations), 421. See also Managed care.
Hodgkin disease, 342–343
Home care, as treatment setting, 410
Hospice care, 349–358. See also Palliative care.
Hospital(s), infection control in, 210–211, 220t
HPV infection. See Human papillomavirus infection.
Human herpesvirus B infection, 177
Human immunodeficiency virus
  and central nervous system, 227–230
  antibodies specific to, production of, 60–61
  culture of, 107t, 109–110
  entry of, coreceptors for, 144
  genetic diversity of, 110–111
  life cycle of, antiretroviral therapy and, 117–118, 118f
  occupational exposure to, 211–216, 213f–214f, 215t. See also Postexposure prophylaxis, occupational.
  replication of, suppression of, in CD4+ cells, 59–60
Human immunodeficiency virus-1, transmission of
  in utero, 30–31, 31t, 32f
  intrapartum, 31–32, 31t, 33f
  rates of, 29–30
  timing of, 30–36, 31t, 32f–36f
    and disease progression in infants, 34–36, 35f–36f
    breastfeeding and, 32–34, 34f
Human immunodeficiency virus-1 DNA, intracellular, monitoring of, 134
Human immunodeficiency virus-1 RNA
  in cerebrospinal fluid, 134
  in plasma
    and initiation of antiretroviral therapy, 129, 129t
    kinetics of, 132–134
    monitoring of, during antiretroviral therapy, 130–131, 132t–133t
  intracellular, 134
  levels of
    and neurocognitive function, 236
    timing of transmission and, 35–36
Human immunodeficiency virus antigens, lymphoproliferative response to, 58

INDEX **439**

Human immunodeficiency virus infection
  age characteristics of, 158, 160t
  and immune function, pathogenesis of, 57–59
  and lymphocyte subpopulations, 54, 55t, 56
    loss/expansion of, 56–57
  and pregnancy outcome, 71–74, 89–90
    in developed countries, 9
    in developing countries, 17
  and psychiatric disorders, 383–385
  as chronic disease, 397–398
  classification of, 10, 14t–15t
  diagnosis of, 107t
    DNA polymerase chain reaction in, 107t, 108–109
    HIV culture in, 107t, 109–110
    in HIV-exposed infants, 362
    Institute of Medicine recommendations for, 71
    p24 antigen assay in, 107t, 110
    prenatal care and, 7
    pretest counseling in, 70–71
    rapid tests for, 69–70, 111
    RNA polymerase chain reaction in, 107t, 110
    serologic tests in, 107–108, 107t
    during pregnancy, 69–82. *See also* Pregnancy, HIV infection during.
  epidemiology of, 1–8, 2f, 3t, 5t
    changes in, 29
    nursing care and, 396
    in children, 6–8
      breastfeeding and, 7–8
      in developed countries, 6–7
      in developing countries, 7–8
      in minority populations, 3
    in women, 2–6, 3t, 5t
      childbearing, 3–4
      in Europe, 4, 5t
      in Latin America/Caribbean, 4, 5t
      in sub-Saharan Africa/Asia, 4, 5t, 6
      in United States, 2–4, 5t
    global distribution of, 2, 2f, 3t
    host susceptibility to, 112
    immaturity of immune system and, 53–54, 55t
    in central nervous system, 227–230
      pathogenesis of, 229–230
      pathology of, 228–229
    morbidity from
      in developed countries, 10, 12t–16t, 13, 16–17
      in developing countries, 18–20, 18t–19t
    mortality from
      in developed countries, 9–10, 11t
      in developing countries, 11t, 17–18
    natural history of, 8–22, 11t–16t, 18t–19t
      in developed countries, 9–10, 11t–16t, 13, 17
      in developing countries, 17–22, 18t–19t
    oral manifestations of, 250t. *See also* specific disease, e.g., Oropharyngeal candidiasis.

Human immunodeficiency virus infection (*Continued*)
  patterns of presentation in, 400–402
  prevention of, 208–211
    educational programs for, 427
    in schools, 208–209, 209t
  prognosis in, neurocognitive dysfunction and, 236–237
  progression of
    after failure of zidovudine prophylaxis, 16–17
    and growth failure, 296
    pregnancy and, 88–89
    rapid, and cardiovascular disease, 303, 306, 306f
    timing of transmission and, 34–36, 35f–36f
    vitamin A deficiency and, 299
  psychosocial issues in, 373–391. *See also* Psychosocial issue(s).
  pulmonary effects of, 193–194
  resistance to
    CKR5 mutation and, 206
    saliva and, 260–262, 261t
  screening for, peripartum, 99
  staging of, during pregnancy, 90–91
  stigma of, 396, 398
  transmission of, 205–208
    breastfeeding and, 99
      intervention trials on, 39–41, 41f
      prevention of, 123
      timing of, 32–34, 34f
    by blood products, epidemiology of, 6
    by health care workers, 208
    from needle sticks, 207
    from sexual activity, 206
    from transfusions, 207
    in body fluids, 205–206
    intervention trials on, 36–41, 37t–38t, 41f
      in breastfeeding subjects, 39–41, 41f
      in nonbreastfeeding subjects, 36, 37t–38t, 39
    perinatal
      antiretroviral therapy and, 88
      cell-mediated immune response and, 46
      hypothetical model of, 36
      maternal viral load and, 42–43, 43f, 87–88
      mode of delivery and, 44–45
      premature rupture of membranes and, 43–44
      public health issues in, 46
      risk factors for, 41–46, 43f
      risk of, minimization of, 87–88
      zidovudine and, 1, 71
    prevention of, nurse's role in, 414
    risk of, 206–207
  treatment of
    alternative therapy in, 408
    immune-based therapy for, 139–150, 139t. *See also* Immune-based therapy.
    standard of care *vs.* experimental, 407–408
  vaccines for, 145–147, 145t
  wasting in, 297–298
  with cardiovascular disease, 308

Human papillomavirus infection
  and oral warts, 258–259, 259f
  cutaneous manifestations of, 273–274, 274f
  genital lesions from, 274, 343
  screening for, during pregnancy, 91
Hyperactive behavior, with attention deficit, 232–233
Hyperbilirubinemia, indinavir and, 81
Hyperimmunoglobulinemia, and production of autoantibodies, 60–61
Hyperpigmentation, 282–283
Hypersensitivity syndrome, cutaneous manifestations of, 284–285
Hypertension, pulmonary, 314–315

I
Iatrogenic/hypersensitivity syndrome, cutaneous manifestations of, 284–285
IDV. *See* Indinavir.
IgA (immunoglobulin A), HIV-specific assays for, 108
Immune function
  HIV infection and, pathogenesis of, 57–59
  preservation of, early therapy and, 61–62
  reconstitution of, after antiretroviral therapy, 62–64
Immune response, cell-mediated, and perinatal HIV transmission, 46
Immune system
  immature, and HIV infection, 53–54, 55t
  reconstitution of
    adoptive lymphocyte transfer for, 148–149
    antiretroviral drugs and, 53, 62–64
Immune-based therapy, 139–150, 139t
  adoptive lymphocyte transfer for, 148–149
  chemokines for, 144
  cytokines for, 140–144, 142t
    action of, 140–141
    interleukin-2 and, 141, 142t, 143
  future of, 150
  immunoglobulins for, 147–148, 148f
  immunosuppressive drugs for, 149
  principles of, 140f
  vaccines for, 145–147, 145t
Immunization. *See also* Vaccination.
  active, 365–366, 366t
  altered response to, 61
  passive, 366
Immunoglobulin(s), for immune-based therapy, 147–148, 148f
Immunoglobulin A (IgA), HIV-specific assays for, 108
Immunosuppressive drug(s), for immune-based therapy, 149
Impetigo, staphylococcal, 275
Incentive compensation, 423
Indemnification insurance, *vs.* managed care, 419–420

Indinavir
  for initiation of antiretroviral therapy, 131t
  in pregnancy, 80–81
  prophylactic, dosage of, 123, 124t
Infection control
  family education about, 402
  for non-HIV diseases, 219–222, 220t
  for sports/recreational activities, 209–210
  handwashing for, 218–219
  in community, 222
  in day care centers, 218–220, 220t
  in delivery room, 211
  in emergency room, 211
  in hospitals, 210–211, 220t
  in schools, 208–209, 209t, 219–220, 220t, 367–368
  procedures for, 218–219, 219t
  role of primary care provider in, 367
  transmission-based precautions for, 218, 219t
Influenza, prevention of, 168t, 366, 366t
Institute of Medicine, recommendations for HIV testing, 71
Insurance
  indemnification, vs. managed care, 419–420
  types of, 421
Intelligence, tests of, 239t
Interdisciplinary collaboration. See Multidisciplinary collaboration.
Interferon-α, for immune-based therapy, 143–144
Interferon-γ, for immune-based therapy, 143
Interleukin(s), production of, 58–59
Interleukin-2, for immune-based therapy, 141, 142t, 143
Interleukin-12, for immune-based therapy, 143–144
Interleukin-16, for immune-based therapy, 143–144
Intrakine(s), for immune-based therapy, 144
Intravenous immunoglobulin
  for bacterial infection prophylaxis, 163–164
  for immune-based therapy, 147
  for pneumonia, bacterial, 195
Intravitreal therapy, for cytomegalovirus retinitis, 176
Invirase. See Saquinavir.
Iron deficiency anemia, 324
Isolation, in HIV-positive mothers, 386
Isoniazid
  for tuberculosis, 170t, 196
  in pregnancy, 95
Isosporosis, 179–180
  treatment of, 171t
Itraconazole, for candidiasis, 167
IVIG. See Intravenous immunoglobulin.

J
Jaundice, 295

K
Kaiser Permanente Medical Center, multidisciplinary team care at, 429
Kaposi sarcoma, 259, 259f, 282–283, 343
  cardiovascular manifestations of, 314
  pulmonary, 201
  vs. bacillary angiomatosis, 343
Kinship care, 387, 391, 403
Knowledge base, for nursing care, 410–412

L
Labor
  antiretroviral therapy during, 99
  management of, 97–99
Lactic acidosis, antiretroviral therapy and, 94
Lactose, malabsorption of, and diarrhea, 294
Lamivudine
  and transmission of HIV infection
    in breastfeeding subjects, 40
    in nonbreastfeeding subjects, 38t
  for initiation of antiretroviral therapy, 131t
  in pregnancy, 78–79
  prophylactic, dosage of, 123, 124t
  with zidovudine
    clinical studies of, 121–122, 122t
    for postexposure prophylaxis, 213–214
Language
  HIV infection and, 231–232
  tests of, 239t
Learning, tests of, 239t
Left ventricular dysfunction, 307–310, 307t–308t, 309f–310f
  diastolic, 310
  management of, 316
  systolic, 307–309, 307t–308t, 309f–310f
Legacy project(s), 386
Legal issue(s), in placement of children of HIV-infected parents, 386–387, 388t–390t
Leiomyoma, 341
Leiomyosarcoma, 314, 341
Leishmaniasis, 180–181
Leucovorin, for toxoplasmosis, 171t
Leukemia, 342–343
Leukocytoclastic vasculitis, 284
Leukoencephalopathy, progressive multifocal. See Progressive multifocal leukoencephalopathy.
Leukopenia, 327–329, 328t
  etiology of, 328, 328t
  incidence of, 327–328
  significance of, 328
  treatment of, 328–329
Leukoplakia, hairy, 257–258, 258f, 274, 275f
Liability, vicarious, 426
Lindane, for scabies, 279
Linear gingival erythema, 255f, 256
LIP. See Lymphoid interstitial pneumonia.
LIP/PLH (lymphocytic interstitial pneumonia/pulmonary lymphoid hyperplasia) complex, 199–200

Lipodystrophy, 298–299
Liver disease, differential diagnosis of, 295
Lopinavir, for initiation of antiretroviral therapy, 131t
Low birth weight, and perinatal HIV transmission, 45–46
Lung(s). See also entries under Pulmonary.
  candidiasis of, 197
    percentage of HIV-infected children with, 159t
  fungal infection of, 197–199
  human immunodeficiency virus and, 193–194
  tumors of, 201
Lymph nodes, pathologic changes in, 55t, 56t
Lymphocytes
  adoptive, transfer of, for immune-based therapy, 148–149
  apoptosis of, 56
  B. See B cell(s).
  HIV antigens and, 58
  subpopulations of, HIV infection and, 54, 55t, 56
  T. See T cell(s).
Lymphocytic interstitial pneumonia/pulmonary lymphoid hyperplasia (LIP/PLH) complex, 199–200
Lymphoid interstitial pneumonia
  in children vs. adults, 157t
  percentage of HIV-infected children with, 159t
Lymphoid tissue, mucosa-associated, 341–342
Lymphoma
  B cell, and cardiovascular disease, 314
  cutaneous manifestations of, 283–284
  non-Hodgkin, 337–341, 338t
    clinical features of, 338–339
    etiology of, 340–341
    latency period in, 338
    of central nervous system, 339
    treatment of, 339–340
  of central nervous system, 228
  oral manifestations of, 260
Lymphoproliferative disorder(s)
  B cell, polyclonal polymorphic, 342
  types of, 338t

M
MAC. See Mycobacterium avium complex.
Macrolide(s), for disseminated Mycobacterium avium complex, 173–174
Magnetic resonance imaging, in neurocognitive dysfunction, 234–235
Magnetic resonance spectroscopy, 235
Malaria, 180
  epidemiology of, in developing countries, 21
Malignancy, 337–344. See also under specific type, e.g., Lymphoma.

Malnutrition
   and anemia, 324
   and lipodystrophy, 298–299
   pain and, 350
Malpractice liability, managed care and, 426
MALT (mucosa-associated lymphoid tissue), 341–342
Managed care
   and malpractice liability, 426
   and special needs of children with HIV infection, 420
   appeals process in, 425–426
   benefits of, 432–433
   challenges from, 419
   contracts for, ideal language in, 426–428
   for Medicaid patients, 420–422, 429
      physician input into, 431–432
   future of, 433
   principles of, 419–420
   quality assurance in, 424–425
   vs. traditional indemnification insurance, 419–420
Managed care organization(s)
   accreditation of, 422–423
   credentialing in, 424
   enrollment of providers in, 424
   regulation of, 422–423
   reimbursement of physicians in, 423–424
   types of, 421–422
Managed care program(s), key components of, 430–431
Mask(s), use of, 219
Measles
   epidemiology of, in developing countries, 21–22
   exposure to, prophylaxis after, 366
   transmission of, prevention of, 221
   vaccination for, 365–366, 366t
Medicaid
   Fair Hearing Process of, 426
   managed care programs for, 420–421, 422, 429
      physician input into, 431–432
Medicare, managed care programs for, 422
Megakaryocytes, direct infection of, 327
Megestrol acetate, for anorexia, 291–292
Memory
   HIV infection and, 233
   tests of, 239t
Mental health, parental substance abuse and, 373–374
Mental health service(s), 382–383
Methylphenidate, dosage of, 384
Microsporidiosis, 179–180
Mineral(s), deficiencies of, 299
Minority population(s)
   HIV infection in, epidemiology of, 3
   nursing care and, 396
Mitochondrial dysfunction
   nucleoside analogues and, 78–79, 94–95
   reverse transcriptase inhibitors and, 94–95, 122–123
Molluscum contagiosum, 273, 273f

Monoclonal antibodies, anti-HIV, for immune-based therapy, 147–148
Montefiore Adolescent AIDS Program, 378
Mother(s), HIV-positive, psychosocial issues of, 386
Motor function
   HIV infection and, 233
   tests of, 239t
Mouth
   HIV infection and, 250t, 292t. See also specific disease, e.g., Oropharyngeal candidiasis.
   tumors of, 259–260, 259f
   ulcers in, 254–255
      and anorexia, 291
   warts in, 258–259, 259f
MRI. See Magnetic resonance imaging.
Mucosa-associated lymphoid tissue (MALT), 341–342
Multidisciplinary collaboration
   for management of HIV infection at Kaiser Permanente Medical Center, 90
   during pregnancy, 90
   nursing care and, 396
Mumps, vaccination for, 365–366, 366t
Mycobacterial infection, cutaneous manifestations of, 275, 276f
Mycobacterium avium complex
   clinical features of, 196
   in children vs. adults, 157t
   prevention of, 168t, 367
   treatment of, 196
Mycobacterium tuberculosis infection. See Tuberculosis.
Myelosuppression
   drugs causing, 323
   mechanism of, 321–323
Myocarditis, 310

N
N-acetyl aspartate/creatine (NAA/creatine) ratio, 235
Natural killer cells, activity of, 59
Nausea/vomiting, 293t, 294
Necrotizing ulcerative periodontitis, 255f, 256–257
Needle stick(s)
   postexposure prophylaxis after, 217, 217t
   transmission of HIV from, 207, 209–210
Neglect
   guardianship in, 388t
   parental substance abuse and, 374
Nelfinavir
   in pregnancy, 81
   prophylactic, dosage of, 123, 124t
Neuman Systems Model, 398
Neurocognitive dysfunction
   and academic achievement, 233
   and disease prognosis, 236–237
   and language, 231–232
   and memory, 233
   and motor function, 233

Neurocognitive dysfunction (Continued)
   brain imaging in, 234–235
   CD4+ cell count and, 235–236
   clinical features of, 230–231
   domains of, 231–232
   HIV-1 RNA levels and, 134, 236
Neurocognitive function
   antiretroviral therapy and, 239–240
   assessment of, 237–239, 239t
      by primary care provider, 364–365
   domains of, 237–238, 239t
   methodologic issues in, 237
   practice and, 238–239
   schedule for, 238–239
Neuroleptic(s), for delirium, 384–385
Neurologic function, HIV infection and, in developing countries, 20
Neutropenia, 327–329, 328t
   etiology of, 328, 328t
   incidence of, 327–328
   significance of, 328
   treatment of, 328–329
      granulocyte colony-stimulating factor in, 144
Neutrophils, function of, 61
Nevirapine
   and transmission of HIV infection, in breastfeeding subjects, 40, 41f
   for initiation of antiretroviral therapy, 131t
   in pregnancy, 81
   prophylactic
      clinical trials of, 122
      dosage of, 123, 124t
      in breastfeeding subjects, 123
   toxicity of, 94
NK cells. See Natural killer cells.
NLV. See Nelfinavir.
N-methyl-D-aspartate (NMDA) receptors, deregulation of, in central nervous system toxicity, 229
Non-Hodgkin lymphoma. See Lymphoma, non-Hodgkin.
Non-nucleoside analogue(s), in pregnancy, 81
Nonprogressor(s), long-term, CD4+ cell count in, 64
Norvir. See Ritonavir.
Nucleoside reverse transcriptase inhibitor(s)
   in pregnancy, 75–79
   toxicity of, 94
Nursing care, 395–415
   advocacy and, 414
   allocation of resources and, 413–414
   and adherence, 409–410, 409t
   and fears of care provider, 411
   and prevention of HIV transmission, 414
   case management in, 400
   changing demographics of HIV infection and, 396
   confidentiality and, 405
   continuity of, 407
   cultural factors in, 404, 411–412
   death/dying and, 412
   disclosure and, 403–404
   family assessment in, 402–403
   family education in, 402
   family-centered, 398–399, 399t

Nursing care (Continued)
  goals of, mutually negotiated, 408
  in inpatient setting, 407
  in outpatient setting, 407
  in urban vs. rural communities, 397
  issues affecting, 410
  knowledge base for, 410–412
  multidisciplinary collaboration and, 396
  palliative, 406–407. See also Palliative care.
  prejudices affecting, 411–412
  professional development and, 412
  research and, 414
  role of, 395–397
Nursing process, application of, 399–404
  for assessment, 400
Nutrition, 295–300, 296t–297t
  and anemia, 324
  and lipodystrophy, 298–299
  and skin disorders, 285, 285f
  assessment of, 296–297, 296t–297t, 364, 401
  enteral, 299–300
  pain and, 350
  vitamin/mineral deficiencies and, 299
  wasting and, 297–298
Nutritional support, 299–300
NVP. See Nevirapine.

O

Occupational exposure, to human immunodeficiency virus, 211–216, 213f–214f, 215t, 411. See also Postexposure prophylaxis, occupational.
Odynophagia, 292–293
Oncogene(s), c-myc, and non-Hodgkin lymphoma, 340–341
Onychomycosis, 277
Opioid(s), 354–355, 354t
Opportunistic infection(s)
  and anemia, 324, 324t
  and leukopenia, 328, 328t
  and myocarditis, 310
  and pericardial effusion, 314–315
  CD4+ cell count and, 155, 160, 161t–162t
  in pregnancy, 82
  central nervous system effects of, 227–228
  databases on, 156, 157t
  in developing countries, 20, 182
  incidence of, highly active antiretroviral therapy and, 156, 158, 160t
  interferon-γ and, 143
  management of, during pregnancy, 91–92, 95–96
  prevention of, 366–367
  treatment of, withdrawal of, 181–182
  trends in, 156–162, 159t–162t
Oral cavity. See also Mouth.
  HIV infection and, 250t. See also specific disease, e.g., Oropharyngeal candidiasis.
Oral health, 266
  assessment of, 365

Oropharyngeal candidiasis, 249–252, 251f–252f
  clinical features of, 250, 251f–252f
  diagnosis of, 250, 292t
  management of, 250–252
Oucher Scale, 352t

P

p24 antigen assay, 107t, 110
PACTG. See Pediatric AIDS Clinical Trials Group.
Pain
  acute vs. chronic, 350
  and nutritional status, 350
  assessment of, 351–352, 352t, 401
  disease-related, 350
  in infants, 351
  management of
    adjuvant drugs in, 355
    goals of, 351
    obstacles to, 351
    pharmacologic, 352–355, 353f, 354t
      pain ladder for, 352, 353f
  treatment-related, 350–351
    management of, 355
Palliative care, 349–358
  access to, 349
  and quality of life, 350, 358
  components of, 349, 349t
  definition of, 349
  end-of-life, 356–357
  nurse's role in, 406–407
  obstacles to, 357–358
  pain management in, 351–355, 352t, 353f. See also Pain, management of.
  principles of, 355–356, 357t
  psychosocial issues in, 356
  spirituality and, 406
Paramomycin, for cryptosporidiosis, 171t
Parasitic infection(s), 179–181. See also specific type, e.g., Toxoplasmosis.
  of skin, 278–279, 278f–280f
  treatment of, 171t
Parent(s)
  death of, and surviving children, 379, 382
  disclosure of HIV diagnosis by, 375–377, 376t
  rights of, in guardianship issues, 388t–390t
Parenteral nutrition, 300
Parenting, substance abuse and, 374
PBLD (polyclonal polymorphic B cell lymphoproliferative disorder), 342
PCP pneumonia. See Pneumocystis carinii pneumonia.
PCR. See Polymerase chain reaction.
PCV7/PCV23, schedule for, 366
Pediatric AIDS Clinical Trials Group, database on opportunistic infections, 156, 158
Pediatric Spectrum of Disease database, 10, 15t, 156, 158, 159t
Pellagra, 285
Penicilliosis, treatment of, 170t
Penicillium marneffei infection, 172

Pentamidine
  cardiotoxicity of, 316, 317f
  for Pneumocystis carinii pneumonia, 166, 199
Pericardial effusion, 312, 314–315
Pericardiocentesis, 315
Periodontal disease, 255–257, 255f
Periodontitis, ulcerative, necrotizing, 255f, 256–257
Permanency planning, legal issues in, 388t–390t
Permethrin, for scabies, 279
PET (positron emission tomography), 235
PETRA study, 38t, 40, 121–123, 122t
Photosensitivity, cutaneous manifestations of, 285
Physician(s), reimbursement of, compensation programs for, 423–424
Physician hospital organization(s), 422
Placement, for children of HIV-infected parents, planning for, 386–387, 388t–390t, 406
Plans of care, formulation of, 400
Plaque, and dental caries, 263, 263f
Plaque index, 263
Platelets, production of, decreased. See Thrombocytopenia.
Pneumococcal infection(s), vaccines against, 164–165, 366, 366t
  indications for, 195
Pneumocystis carinii pneumonia, 165–167, 168t–169t
  age distribution of, 165
  CD4+ cell count and, 161t, 198
  clinical features of, 165–166
  diagnosis of, 166, 198
  epidemiology of, 165, 198
    in developed countries, 10, 13
    in developing countries, 20
  in children vs. adults, 157t
  mortality from, 198
  pathogenesis of, 197–198
  percentage of HIV-infected children with, 159t
  prevention of, 166–167, 168t, 199, 427
    in pregnancy, 82
    withdrawal of drugs for, 181
  transmission of, 165
  treatment of, 166–167, 170t, 198–199
Pneumonia
  bacterial, 194–195
  cytomegalovirus and, 197
Pneumonia
  incidence of, 193
  lymphoid interstitial. See Lymphoid interstitial pneumonia.
  Pneumocystis carinii. See Pneumocystis carinii pneumonia.
  risk factors for, 193, 193t
  viral, 197
Point of service insurance plan(s), 452
Poker Chip Tool, for pain assessment, 352t
Poliovirus vector, for HIV vaccine, 145, 145t
Polyclonal polymorphic B cell lymphoproliferative disorder (PBLD), 342

Polymerase chain reaction
  DNA, 107t, 108–109
  for timing of HIV-1 infection,
    intrapartum, 32
  RNA, 107t, 110
Polyomavirus infection. *See* Progressive
    multifocal leukoencephalopathy.
Porphyria cutanea tarda, 285
Positron emission tomography (PET),
    235
Postexposure prophylaxis
  animal studies of, 211–212
  estimation of risk and, 213f–214f
  nonoccupational, 216–218, 217t–218t
    after sexual assault, 217, 217t
    choice of drugs for, 218t
    in pregnancy, 217
    recommendations for, 216–217
    timing of, 217
  occupational, 7–12, 213f–214f, 215t,
    411
    choice of drugs for, 212–214, 215t
    institutional policies for, 214–216
Postpartum period, HIV infection
  management during, 99–100
Posttest counseling, 71
PPOs (preferred provider organizations),
    422
Practice effect, in neurocognitive
    assessment, 238–239
Preferred provider organizations (PPOs),
    422
Pregnancy
  and progression of maternal HIV
    infection, 88–89
  antiretroviral therapy during. *See*
    Antiretroviral therapy, during
    pregnancy.
  CD4+ cell count during, 72–73, 88
  HIV infection during
    identification of, 69–71
    management of, 74–82
      choice of drugs in, 75, 81–82. *See
        also specific drug, e.g.,
        Zidovudine.*
      maternal monitoring in, 74–75
      multidisciplinary approach to, 90
      obstetric issues in, 82
      postpartum, 99–100
      staging of, 90–91
      standards of care for, 69
    invasive procedures in, 96–97
Pregnancy
  opportunistic infections during,
    management of, 91–92, 95–96
  outcome of
    antiretroviral therapy and, 9
    HIV infection and, 71–74, 89–90
      in developed countries, 9
      in developing countries, 17
  postexposure prophylaxis in, 217
  screening for sexually transmitted
    diseases during, 91
  tuberculosis screening during, 91
  vaccination during, 82
Prejudice, and nursing care, 411–412
Premature birth
  and perinatal HIV transmission,
    45–46
  HIV infection and, 89

Premature rupture of membranes, and
    perinatal HIV transmission, 43–44,
    98–99
Prenatal care, and diagnosis of HIV
    infection, 7
Pretest counseling, components of, 70–71
Primary care, 361–370
  and disclosure of HIV status, 368
  case management in, 368, 430–431
  for prevention of opportunistic
    infections, 366–367
  genitourinary evaluation in, 365
  growth evaluation in, 362, 364
  infection control education in, 367
  infection prevention in, 365–367, 366t
  neurocognitive assessment in, 364–365
  nutritional assessment in, 364
  ophthalmologic evaluation in, 365
  oral health assessment in, 365
  physical examination in, 361–362, 363t
  sick-child evaluation in, 369
  studies performed in, schedule of, 363t
Primary care provider(s), as HIV experts,
    426–427, 429–431
Professional development, for nurses, 412
Progressive multifocal
    leukoencephalopathy
  CD4+ cell count and, 162t
  treatment of, 171t
Protease inhibitor(s)
  and diabetes, 94
  and lipodystrophy, 298–299
  for initiation of antiretroviral therapy,
    131t
  in pregnancy, 79–81
  in saliva, 261, 261t
  interaction with rifampin, 174–175
  toxicity of, 16
Protein, recommended daily allowance
    of, 296, 296t
Proton magnetic resonance spectroscopy,
    235
Provider profile(s), in managed care
    organizations, 425
Pseudomonas aeruginosa infection,
    cutaneous manifestations of,
    275–276
Psoriasis, 281–282, 281f
Psychiatric disorder(s), 383–385
  heritable, parental substance abuse
    and, 374
Psychometric testing, 237–239, 239t. *See
  also* Neurocognitive function,
    assessment of.
Psychosocial issue(s), 373–391
  in adolescents, 377–379
  in infants/toddlers, 374–375
  in palliative care, 356
  in school-age children, 375–377, 376t
  in young adults, 379, 380t–381t
  mental health services for, 382–383
  of caregivers, 385–387, 388t–390t,
    391
    and HIV-positive mothers, 386
    extended family and, 387, 391, 403
    in late stage of illness, 387
    progression of illness and, 386–387,
      388t–390t
  of fathers, 387
  substance abuse and, 373–374

Psychotropic medication(s)
  dosage of, 383
  drug interactions with, 385
Public health issues, and perinatal HIV
    transmission, 46
Pulmonary disease
  chronic, 199–201
  mortality from, 201
Pulmonary hypertension, 314–315
Pyrazinamide, for tuberculosis, 196
Pyrimethamine, for toxoplasmosis, 171t,
    179

Q
Quality assurance, in managed care
    organizations, 424–425
Quality of life
  antiretroviral therapy and, 356
  palliative care and, 350, 358
Quinolinic acid, cerebrospinal fluid
    levels of, and disease prognosis,
    236–237

R
Radiation therapy, for non-Hodgkin
    lymphoma, 340
Receptive language, HIV infection and,
    232
Recreational activity(ies), infection
    control for, 209–210
Recurrent aphthous stomatitis, 253–254,
    254f, 292t
Research, in nursing, 414
Resources, allocation of, 413–414
Respiratory infection(s), transmission of,
    prevention of, 221
Respite care, 405–406
Retinitis, cytomegalovirus
  CD4+ cell count and, 161t
  treatment of, 171t
  intravitreal, 176
Retrovir. *See* Zidovudine.
Reverse transcriptase inhibitor(s)
  interaction with rifampin, 174–175
  mechanism of action in, 118, 118f
  nucleotide analogues of
    and mitochondrial dysfunction,
      122–123
    animal models of, 119
  for initiation of antiretroviral
    therapy, 131t
  prophylactic, history of, 119–120
Rifabutin, for disseminated
    Mycobacterium avium complex,
    173–174
Rifampin
  for tuberculosis, 170t, 196
  interaction with protease inhibitors,
    174–175
  interaction with reverse transcriptase
    inhibitors, 174–175
Ritonavir
  for initiation of antiretroviral therapy,
    131t
  in pregnancy, 79–80
  prophylactic, dosage of, 123, 124t

RNA polymerase chain reaction, 107t, 110
Rubella, vaccination for, 365–366, 366t
Rural community(ies), nursing care in, 397
Ryan White Comprehensive AIDS Resources Emergency (CARE) Act grantees, 428

S
SAINT (South African Intrapartum Nevirapine Trial), 40
Saliva
　and resistance to HIV infection, 260–262, 261f
　isolation of HIV in, 206
Salivary gland(s), dysfunction of, 257, 257f
Saquinavir
　for initiation of antiretroviral therapy, 131t
　in pregnancy, 79
　prophylactic, dosage of, 123, 124t
Sarcoma, Kaposi. See Kaposi sarcoma.
Scabies, 278–279, 278f
School(s)
　infection control in, 208–209, 209t, 219–220, 220t, 367–368
　liaisons to, health care workers as, 377, 405
School-age children, psychosocial issues in, 375–377, 376t
School personnel, disclosure of HIV status to, 377
Scurvy, 285
Seborrheic dermatitis, 280
Secretory leukocyte protease inhibitor (SLPI), in saliva, 261, 261t
Sedation, conscious, 355
Serologic test(s), 107–108, 107t
Sexual activity, transmission of HIV from, 206
Sexual assault, postexposure prophylaxis after, 217, 217t
Sexual partner(s), informing of HIV status, in adolescence, 377
Sexually transmitted disease(s), screening for, during pregnancy, 91
Sibling(s), of HIV-infected children, 379, 382
Sick-child evaluation, 369
Simian immunodeficiency virus infection, transmission of, 118–119
Simian immunodeficiency virus, vaccine research using, 146
Single-photon emission computed tomography (SPECT), in non-Hodgkin lymphoma, 339
Single-Use Diagnostic System (SUDS) HIV-1 test, 111
SIV. See Simian immunodeficiency virus.
Skin disorder(s)
　CD4+ cell count and, 271
　from nutritional deficiencies, 285, 285f
　infectious, 272–279, 272f–280f
　　bacterial, 274–276, 276f
　　fungal, 276–278, 277f–278f

Skin disorder(s) (Continued)
　　parasitic, 278–279, 278f–280f
　　viral, 272–274, 272f–275f
　inflammatory, 280–282, 281f
　neoplastic, 282–284
　prevalence of, 271
　vascular, 284
SLPI (secretory leukocyte protease inhibitor), in saliva, 261, 261t
Smoking, and perinatal HIV transmission, 43
Social service(s)
　access to, 410–411
　types of, 428
Soluble recombinant CD4+ molecule (srCD4), research on, 140
South African Intrapartum Nevirapine Trial (SAINT), 40
SPECT (single-photon emission computed tomography), in non-Hodgkin lymphoma, 339
Spectroscopy, magnetic resonance, 235
Spirituality, and palliative care, 406
Splenectomy, for thrombocytopenia, 327
Sports, infection control issues in, 209–210
Sputum culture, for tuberculosis, 196
srCD4 (soluble recombinant CD4 molecule), research on, 140
Standard precautions, 411
　in hospitals, 210–211
　in schools, 208–209, 209t
Standby adoption, 390t
Standby guardianship, 389t
Staphylococcus aureus infection, cutaneous manifestations of, 275
Stavudine
　and transmission of HIV infection, in nonbreastfeeding subjects, 37t, 39
　for initiation of antiretroviral therapy, 131t
　in pregnancy, 78
　prophylactic, dosage of, 123, 124t
STDs. See Sexually transmitted disease(s).
Stomatitis, aphthous, 253–254, 254f, 292t
Streptococcus pneumoniae infection, prevention of, 168t
Stress, in health care workers, 412–414
Stroke, 228
Substance abuse
　and comorbid psychiatric disorders, 374
　and prenatal drug exposure, 374
　in HIV-positive mothers, 386
　psychosocial issues in, 373–374
SUDS (Single-Use Diagnostic System) HIV-1 test, 111
Sulfadiazine, for toxoplasmosis, 171t
Support group(s), camps as, 379, 380t–381t
Supportive care. See Palliative care.
Syphilis, screening for, during pregnancy, 91

T
T cell receptor genes, restricted, in CD4+ and CD8+ cells, 60

T cell(s)
　activity of, 59
　adoptive, transfer of, for immune-based therapy, 148–149
　fetal, immaturity of, 53–54
　generation of, decreased, 56–57
　production of, by thymus, after highly active antiretroviral therapy, 63
　pulmonary, HIV infection and, 193
　turnover of, 57
Tachycardia, 313t
3TC. See Lamivudine.
Tears, isolation of HIV in, 206
Teeth
　care of, 266
　delayed eruption of, 263–264
　primary, over-retention of, 263–264, 264f
Terminal care, 412. See also Palliative care.
Thalidomide, for immune-based therapy, 149
Thrombocytopenia, 325–327, 326t
　etiology of, 296–297, 326t
　incidence of, 325–326
　oral manifestations of, 260, 260f
　significance of, 326
　treatment of, 327
Thrombocytopenic purpura, 284
Thrush, clinical features of, 250, 250f
Thymus
　pathologic changes in, 55t, 56–57
　production of T cells by, after highly active antiretroviral therapy, 63
Tinea capitis, 277, 277f
Total parenteral nutrition (TPN), 300
Toxoplasmosis, 179
　CD4+ cell count and, 162t
　management of, in pregnancy, 95
　prevention of, 168t
　treatment of, 171t
TPN (total parenteral nutrition), 300
Tracheobronchial candidiasis, 167
Transfusion(s)
　for anemia, 325
　transmission of HIV from, 206
Trichophyton rubrum, 277
Trimethoprim-sulfamethoxazole
　allergic reactions to, cutaneous, 284
　for bacterial infection prophylaxis, 163–164
　for isosporosis, 171t
　for *Pneumocystis carinii* pneumonia, 166, 198
　for toxoplasmosis, 179
Tube feeding, 299–300
Tuberculosis
　CD4+ cell count and, 161t
　clinical features of, 174
　diagnosis of, 195
　epidemiology of, 174, 195
　in developing countries, 20–21
　management of, 170t, 174–175, 196
　in pregnancy, 95
　mortality from, 196
　prevention of, 168t, 174–175, 367
　screening for, during pregnancy, 74, 91
　transmission of, prevention of, 221
Twins, birth order of, and perinatal HIV transmission, 45

U

Ulcer(s), oral, 254–255
Upper airway, obstruction of, 201
Urban community(ies), nursing care in, 397
Urinary tract, evaluation of, 365

V

Vaccination
  altered response to, 61
  during pregnancy, 82
  importance of, 402
  schedule for, 365–366, 366t
Vaccine(s)
  against pneumococcal infections, 164–165, 195, 366, 366t
  anti-HIV, 145–147, 145t
  for tuberculosis, 175
  for varicella-zoster virus infection, 177
Vaccinia vector, for HIV vaccine, 145, 145t
Vaginal delivery, 98
  and perinatal HIV transmission, 44–45
Valacyclovir, for varicella-zoster virus infection, 177
Varicella
  exposure to, prophylaxis after, 366
  vaccination for, 365, 366t
Varicella-zoster virus infection, 177, 221
  cutaneous manifestations of, 272, 273f
  prevention of, 168t
  vaccines for, 177
Vascular disorder(s), 310–311
  cutaneous manifestations of, 284
Vasculopathy, calcific, of central nervous system, 228–229
Venezuelan equine encephalitis (VEE) vector, for HIV vaccine, 145, 145t
Ventricular dysfunction, left. See Left ventricular dysfunction.
Ventricular hypertrophy, 312t–313t
Verruca vulgaris, 258–259
Verrucae, 273–274, 274f
Vicarious liability, 426
Videx. See Didanosine.
Vinblastine, for Kaposi sarcoma, 283
Viral infection(s), 175–178. See also specific type, e.g., Cytomegalovirus infection.
  and myocarditis, 310

Viral infection(s) (*Continued*)
  cutaneous manifestations of, 272–274, 272f–275f
  epidemiology of, 175
Viral load
  and initiation of antiretroviral therapy, 74–75
  maternal
    and HIV transmission, 42–43, 43f, 87–88
    prophylactic zidovudine and, 120
  monitoring of, importance of, 130–135, 132t–133t
Viral pneumonia, 197
Vision screening, 365
Visual Analogue Scale, 352t
Vitamin A, deficiency of, and progression of HIV infection, 299
Vitamin B_{12}, deficiency of, and anemia, 324
Vitiligo, 282
Vomiting, 293t, 294

W

Wart(s), 273–274, 274f
  genital, management of, in pregnancy, 96
  oral, 258–259, 259f
Wasting, 297–298
  pain and, 350
  percentage of HIV-infected children with, 159t
  with cardiovascular disease, 308
  with encephalopathy, in children *vs.* adults, 157t
Weight, serial measurement of, 297, 297t, 362, 364
Western blot assay, 107–108, 107t
WHO. See World Health Organization (WHO).
Women and Infant Transmission Study (WITS), 43
Wong-Baker Faces Scale, 352t, 353f
World Health Organization (WHO)
  clinical case definition of AIDS from, 18, 18t
  pain ladder of, 352, 353f

X

Xerostomia, 257

Y

Yeast infection(s), invasive, 167, 168t–171t

Z

Zalcitabine
  for initiation of antiretroviral therapy, 131t
  in pregnancy, 77–78
  prophylactic, dosage of, 123, 124t
Zerit. See Stavudine.
Ziagen. See Abacavir.
Zidovudine
  and anemia, 324, 324t
  and cardiomyopathy, 316
  and neurocognitive function, 239–240
  and transmission of HIV infection
    during breastfeeding, 8
    in nonbreastfeeding subjects, 36, 37t–38t, 39
    perinatal, 1, 71
      epidemiology of, 7
  for initiation of antiretroviral therapy, 130
  for postexposure prophylaxis, 212–214
  in pregnancy, 75–77, 81
  pharmacokinetics of, animal models of, 119
  prophylactic
    clinical trials of, 121–122, 122t
    dosage of, 123, 124t
    failure of, and rate of disease progression, 16–17
    history of, 119–120
    resistance to, 123
    timing of, 30
  resistance to, in pregnancy, 77
Zinc deficiency, cutaneous manifestations of, 285, 285f